AF807243

Paraproteinemia and Related Disorders

Gaafar Ragab • Luca Quartuccio • Hadi Goubran
Editors

Paraproteinemia and Related Disorders

Springer

Editors
Gaafar Ragab
Rheumatology and Clinical
Immunology Unit
Internal Medicine Department
Faculty of Medicine
Cairo University
Cairo, Egypt

School of Medicine
Newgiza University (NGU)
Giza, Egypt

Hadi Goubran
College of Medicine
University of Saskatchewan
Saskatoon, SK, Canada

Luca Quartuccio
Department of Medicine
University of Udine
Udine, Udine, Italy

ISBN 978-3-031-10130-4 ISBN 978-3-031-10131-1 (eBook)
https://doi.org/10.1007/978-3-031-10131-1

© The Editor(s) (if applicable) and The Author(s), under exclusive license to Springer Nature Switzerland AG 2022, corrected publication 2022
This work is subject to copyright. All rights are solely and exclusively licensed by the Publisher, whether the whole or part of the material is concerned, specifically the rights of translation, reprinting, reuse of illustrations, recitation, broadcasting, reproduction on microfilms or in any other physical way, and transmission or information storage and retrieval, electronic adaptation, computer software, or by similar or dissimilar methodology now known or hereafter developed.
The use of general descriptive names, registered names, trademarks, service marks, etc. in this publication does not imply, even in the absence of a specific statement, that such names are exempt from the relevant protective laws and regulations and therefore free for general use.
The publisher, the authors, and the editors are safe to assume that the advice and information in this book are believed to be true and accurate at the date of publication. Neither the publisher nor the authors or the editors give a warranty, expressed or implied, with respect to the material contained herein or for any errors or omissions that may have been made. The publisher remains neutral with regard to jurisdictional claims in published maps and institutional affiliations.

This Springer imprint is published by the registered company Springer Nature Switzerland AG
The registered company address is: Gewerbestrasse 11, 6330 Cham, Switzerland

This book is dedicated to our beloved families,

Samia, Ahmed, and Sherif

Antonia Vernoni, Diego, and Rita

Hanaa, Mariam and Quinn, Farah and Chance

Foreword

This book is devoted to paraproteinemia, i.e., the appearance of high concentrations of normal or abnormal plasma proteins resulting from an underlying pathologic condition, and its ensuing clinical effects. For the first time, in one book, the reader will find comprehensive analyses of the pathophysiological mechanisms responsible for paraproteinemias and exhaustive descriptions of their consequences.

The first chapters are devoted to the basic aspects of the diseases, focusing on the mechanisms involved in normal and abnormal B-cell activation.

Because B cells are a critical component of the adaptive immune system and mediate the production of immunoglobulins that target pathogens, they have been considered the major actors of humoral immunity. Since the initial description of B-cell functions, 60 years ago, we have learned that the roles of B cells are much more complicated and cannot be simply summarized as the production of antibodies: B-cell subpopulations have been identified and their actions described, and the interactions between B and T cells have progressively become better understood. Over the last decades, drugs targeting B-cell subpopulations have also become available; they have notable clinical impact and help treat diseases arising from B-cell involvement.

Paraproteinemia is characterized by the overproduction of a monoclonal immunoglobulin by plasma cells. That excessive paraprotein synthesis results in paraproteinemia. An excellent chapter on animal models describes the production of paraproteins and the deposition of light chains or whole immunoglobulins in different organs, mainly the kidneys. The clinician will find information on how to diagnose paraproteinemia and analyze monoclonal gammopathy patterns, which could indicate possible outcomes.

Chapters in the second part of the book describe the diseases caused by monoclonal gammopathy. The exhaustive list of those diseases highlights the different clinical manifestations and evolutions of the various paraproteinemias. For some chapters, like those on amyloidosis, the pathogenic mechanisms, classification, and diagnosis are addressed separately from clinical description and management. The most recent drugs, like transthyretin-interfering agents to treat amyloidosis, are given and, in the future, such treatments could revolutionize patients' outcomes.

Multiple myeloma is certainly one of the key entities treated in this book. Monoclonal gammopathy of unknown significance is a premalignant disease, characterized by a low-level plasma monoclonal protein; it has no clinical manifestations during periods which can last for years. Because protein electrophoresis is widely requested by many clinicians in developed countries, peaks of monoclonal gammopathy are quite frequently discovered fortuitously, mainly in elderly patients. For most patients, the outcome is favorable, with no clinical manifestations of malignant disease. For a minority of patients, around 1%/year, these lymphoproliferative diseases can have visceral manifestations, like peripheral neuropathy.

For decades, cytotoxic drugs have been the standard treatment of monoclonal gammopathies. They are still prescribed extensively and are effective, at least transiently.

New drugs are now available and several chapters focus on clone-directed therapies and non-pharmacological interventions, like plasmapheresis for hyperviscosity syndrome. The clone-targeting approach is probably not yet the optimal treatment to cure diseases that are still considered incurable. However, they are a real positive therapeutic advancement, which has improved patients' outcomes and prolonged survival. Treatment of these diseases usually combines new drugs, for example, the 26S-proteasome inhibitor, bortezomib, or/and the anti-CD38 monoclonal antibody, isatuximab, and autologous stem-cell transplantation. Many other monoclonal antibodies, new chemotherapies, and perhaps chimeric antigen-receptor (CAR) T cells might find a place among the future therapeutic strategies for multiple myeloma or malignant lymphoproliferative diseases with paraproteinemia.

This book will be of major interest for many specialists—hematologists, nephrologists, internists, rheumatologists, neurologists, cardiologists—and all other physicians caring for patients with paraproteinemia, its consequences and underlying pathologies.

Académie Nationale de Médecine
University of Paris
Paris, France

Loïc Guillevin

Preface

Dear readers

We invite you to join our expedition to explore the amazing universe of the paraproteinemias. Our team of editors and authors gathered from around the globe. Representing four continents and nine countries: Canada, Egypt, France, Greece, Italy, Lebanon, Taiwan, the United Kingdom, and the United States, in alphabetical order, they volunteered and cooperated to bring this book to light. It is the first of its kind to deal with paraproteinemias as one group and in one tome.

Our team consists of world class experts and practitioners, both clinicians and researchers belonging to many disciplines. You are welcome to this exciting and hopefully fruitful journey throughout the chapters. Whether your discipline is Immunology, Rheumatology, Hematology, Oncology, Nephrology, Neurology, Cardiology, Internal Medicine or you are specialized in the field of Pathology, Radiology, Laboratory investigations, etc., we are confident that you will find interest in the content. It has been our objective to present our readers with the most comprehensive and updated knowledge on the topic.

Louis Pasteur (1822–1895) was quoted to have said "Science proceeds by successive answers to questions more and more subtle, coming nearer and nearer to the very essence of phenomenon." Our measure of success will be the degree to which we managed to incite more questions and to inspire more enthusiasm.

Cairo, Egypt — Gaafar Ragab
Udine, Italy — Luca Quartuccio
Saskatoon, SK, Canada — Hadi Goubran

Contents

Contributors

Mona R. E. Abdel-Halim Dermatology Department, Faculty of Medicine, Cairo University, Cairo, Egypt

Ahmed Abdulhameed Abdulgawad Manchester Royal Infirmary, Manchester, UK

Faculty of Medicine, Cairo University, Cairo, Egypt

Hamdy M. A. Ahmed Division of Rheumatology, Department of Medicine, University of South Alabama, Mobile, AL, USA

Marco Allinovi Nephrology, Dialysis and Transplantation Unit, Careggi University Hospital, Florence, Italy

T. Prescott Atkinson Department of Pediatrics, University of Alabama at Birmingham, Birmingham, AL, USA

Hend Attia School of Medicine, Newgiza University (NGU), Giza, Egypt

James Barton Division of Nephrology, College of Medicine, University of Saskatchewan, Saskatoon, SK, Canada

Ali Bazerbachi Department of Internal Medicine, American University of Beirut Medical Center, Beirut, Lebanon

Mark Bosch Saskatoon Cancer Centre and College of Medicine, University of Saskatchewan, Saskatoon, SK, Canada

Paola Del Bravo Infectious Diseases Division, Verona University Hospital, Verona, Italy

Thierry Burnouf Graduate Institute of Biomedical Materials and Tissue Engineering, College of Biomedical Engineering, Taipei Medical University, Taipei, Taiwan

International Ph.D. Program in Biomedical Engineering, College of Biomedical Engineering, Taipei Medical University, Taipei, Taiwan

Patrice Cacoub Department of Internal Medicine and Clinical Immunology, AP-HP, Groupe Hospitalier Pitié-Salpêtrière, Centre national de références Maladies Autoimmunes et systémiques rares, Centre national de références Maladies Autoinflammatoires rares et Amylose inflammatoire, Paris, France

Sorbonne Université, Paris, France

INSERM, UMR S 959, Immunology-Immunopathology- Immunotherapy (I3), Paris, France

Luca Cantarini Research Center of Systemic Autoinflammatory Diseases, Behçet's Disease and Rheumatology-Ophthalmology Collaborative Uveitis Center, Department of Medical Sciences Surgery and Neurosciences, University of Siena, Siena, Italy

Suchit K. Chatterji Institute of Cancer Therapeutics, University of Bradford, Bradford, West Yorkshire, UK

Stefania Colantuono Department of Translational and Precision Medicine, Sapienza University of Rome, Rome, Italy

Emanuel Della-Torre Unit of Immunology, Rheumatology, Allergy, and Rare Diseases (UnIRAR), San Raffaele Hospital, Milan, Italy

Amr Edrees Department of Internal Medicine, University of Missouri-Kansas City, Kansas, MO, USA

Mohamed Elemary Saskatoon Cancer Centre and College of Medicine, University of Saskatchewan, Saskatoon, SK, Canada

Sherif El-Khamisy Institute of Cancer Therapeutics, University of Bradford, Bradford, West Yorkshire, UK

Shereef Elmoamly Internal Medicine and Haematology Department, Kasr Alainy Faculty of Medicine, Cairo University, Cairo, Egypt

Stavroula Giannouli 2nd Department of Internal Medicine, School of Medicine, National and Kapodistrian University of Athens, Athens, Greece

Hadi Goubran Saskatoon Cancer Centre and College of Medicine, University of Saskatchewan, Saskatoon, SK, Canada

Caroline Hart Saskatoon Cancer Centre and College of Medicine, University of Saskatchewan, Saskatoon, SK, Canada

Mohamed Tharwat Hegazy Rheumatology, and Clinical Immunology Unit, Internal Medicine Department, Faculty of Medicine, Cairo University, Cairo, Egypt

School of Medicine, Newgiza University (NGU), Giza, Egypt

Rami Kotb Department of Medical Oncology and Hematology, CancerCare Manitoba and College of Medicine, University of Manitoba, Winnipeg, MB, Canada

Ahmed Laymouna Department of Medicine, Rheumatology and Clinical Immunology Unit, Faculty of Medicine, Cairo University, Cairo, Egypt

Gianmarco Lugli Department of Biomedical, Experimental and Clinical Sciences, University of Firenze, Florence, Italy

Ayman Abdel-Monem Ahmed Mahmoud Internal Medicine Department, Rheumatology, and Clinical Immunology Unit, Faculty of Medicine, Cairo University, Cairo, Egypt

Mervat Mattar Clinical Hematology Unit, Kasr Alaini Faculty of Medicine, Cairo University, Cairo, Egypt

Adrien Mirouse Department of Internal Medicine and Clinical Immunology, AP-HP, Groupe Hospitalier Pitié-Salpêtrière, Centre national de références Maladies Autoimmunes et systémiques rares, Centre national de références Maladies Autoinflammatoires rares et Amylose inflammatoire, Paris, France

Sorbonne Université, Paris, France

INSERM, UMR S 959, Immunology-Immunopathology- Immunotherapy (I3), Paris, France

Matthew Nicholson Saskatoon Cancer Centre and College of Medicine, University of Saskatchewan, Saskatoon, SK, Canada

Laura Obici Amyloidosis Research and Treatment Centre, IRCCS Fondazione Policlinico San Matteo, Pavia, Italy

Ibraheem Othman Alain Blair Cancer Centre and College of Medicine, University of Saskatchewan, Saskatoon, SK, Canada

Francesco Pegoraro Department of Health Science, University of Firenze, Florence, Italy

Pietro Enrico Pioltelli Haematology Unit, Milano-Bicocca University, San Gerardo Hospital, Monza, Italy

Aikaterini Poulaki Department of Pathophysiology, School of Medicine, National and Kapodistrian University of Athens, Athens, Greece

Luca Quartuccio Rheumatology Clinic, Department of Medicine, University of Udine, Udine, Italy

Gaafar Ragab Rheumatology and Clinical Immunology Unit, Internal Medicine Department, Faculty of Medicine, Cairo University, Cairo, Egypt

School of Medicine, Newgiza University (NGU), Giza, Egypt

Fiammetta Ravaglia Nephrology and Dialysis Unit, Santo Stefano Hospital, Prato, Italy

Elda Righi Infectious Diseases Division, Verona University Hospital, Verona, Italy

Matilde Rocchi Infectious Diseases Division, Verona University Hospital, Verona, Italy

David Saadoun Department of Internal Medicine and Clinical Immunology, AP-HP, Groupe Hospitalier Pitié-Salpêtrière, Centre national de références Maladies Autoimmunes et systémiques rares, Centre national de références Maladies Autoinflammatoires rares et Amylose inflammatoire, Paris, France

Sorbonne Université, Paris, France

INSERM, UMR S 959, Immunology-Immunopathology- Immunotherapy (I3), Paris, France

Waleed Sabry Saskatoon Cancer Centre and College of Medicine, University of Saskatchewan, Saskatoon, SK, Canada

Anna Giulia Salvadori Infectious Diseases Division, Verona University Hospital, Verona, Italy

Steven D. Shnyder Institute of Cancer Therapeutics, University of Bradford, Bradford, West Yorkshire, UK

Julie Stakiw Saskatoon Cancer Centre and the College of Medicine, University of Saskatchewan, Saskatoon, SK, Canada

John H. Stone Division of Rheumatology, Allergy, and Immunology, Massachusetts General Hospital, Boston, MA, USA

Vinita Sundaram Saskatoon Cancer Centre, Saskatoon, SK, Canada

Elena Treppo Rheumatology Clinic, Department of Medicine, University of Udine, Udine, Italy

Augusto Vaglio Department of Biomedical, Experimental and Clinical Sciences, University of Firenze, Florence, Italy

Nephrology and Dialysis Unit, Meyer Children's Hospital, Florence, Italy

Alessandro Visentin Infectious Diseases Division, Verona University Hospital, Verona, Italy

Marcella Visentini Department of Translational and Precision Medicine, Sapienza University of Rome, Rome, Italy

Antonio Vitale Research Center of Systemic Autoinflammatory Diseases, Behçet's Disease and Rheumatology-Ophthalmology Collaborative Uveitis Center, Department of Medical Sciences Surgery and Neurosciences, University of Siena, Siena, Italy

Salvatore De Vita Rheumatology Clinic, Department of Medicine, University of Udine, Udine, Italy

Michael Voulgarelis Department of Pathophysiology, School of Medicine, National and Kapodistrian University of Athens, Athens, Greece

Ashutosh D. Wechalekar National Amyloidosis Centre, University College London, Royal Free Campus, London, UK

Yoh Zen Institute of Liver Studies, King's College Hospital and King's College London, London, UK

Part I
Introductory Chapters

Chapter 1
The Phenomenon of Paraproteinemia

Gaafar Ragab

Introduction

Paraproteinemia or dysproteinemia is characterized by the overproduction of an immunoglobulin by clonal expansion of cells from the B cells lineage which includes the plasma cells. The resultant monoclonal protein can be composed of the entire immunoglobulin or of its components [1]. The identification and categorization of the different representatives of this group of disorders have traveled a long distance. Amyloidosis, for example, which refers to a group of disorders in which protein fibrils accumulate in certain organs disrupting their tissue architecture and impairing the function of the affected organ [2] has for long been identified both clinically and pathologically. Other disease entities have a different history, for instance, the link of autoimmune pancreatitis with immunoglobulin G4 was only revealed in 2001 after a long series of observations [3]. We do not, however, understand the significance of their presence in other disease entities such as infections and autoimmune diseases [4, 5]. It is interesting that paleopathologists described cases of multiple myelomatosis (MM) in their excavations in the Old World, which they dated back to the Middle Ages, whereas in the New World, skeletons showing MM could be traced back to the pre-Columbian era [6].

MM is the second most common blood cancer [7], and the neuropathies associated with plasma cell dyscrasias are a major cause of morbidity for patients managed by medical oncologists [8].

G. Ragab (✉)
Rheumatology and Clinical Immunology Unit, Internal Medicine Department, Faculty of Medicine, Cairo University, Cairo, Egypt

School of Medicine, Newgiza University (NGU), Giza, Egypt
e-mail: gragab@kasralainy.edu.eg

© The Author(s), under exclusive license to Springer Nature Switzerland AG 2022

G. Ragab et al. (eds.), *Paraproteinemia and Related Disorders*,
https://doi.org/10.1007/978-3-031-10131-1_1

A population-based study from Minnesota showed that in individuals aged >50 years, the overall incidence of paraproteins is 3.2% and could be as high as 5.3% for those >70 years [9]. Paraproteins are therefore a common laboratory finding in an elderly population [10].

Recent advances have been introduced in the diagnosis, risk stratifications, and management of many members of this group of illnesses. The diagnostic list of investigations now includes serum protein electrophoresis, immunofixation, immunoglobulin quantification, serum-free light and heavy-light chain arrays, MALDI-TOF mass spectrometric methods, molecular technologies such as fluorescence in situ hybridization and next-generation sequencing, liquid biopsies, and novel immune biomarkers [11–13]. Novel agents (proteasome inhibitors, immunomodulatory drugs, monoclonal antibodies, etc.) and autologous stem cell transplantation have improved the outcome for many patients [1, 2]. These new scientific departures are paving the way to progress in two directions, the first is the expansion of personalized treatment that provides maximum benefit to a specific patient [12]; and the second is the growing tendency towards standardization and networking [14, 15].

To better understand the nature, significance, and characteristics of paraproteinemia, we need to group, classify, and describe its representatives.

Approaching Paraproteinemia

Paraproteinemia is a phenomenon encountered in many diseases and disorders, and it may be detected in apparently healthy individuals, particularly the elderly [9, 10].

Why to group all this in one book and how to introduce them to the reader was our main concern? Exact and precise use of words is needed to describe clear and distinct ideas, and we need our ideas to be conceived very clearly and very distinctly. That is the lesson we learnt from Décartes [1596–1650], the father of modern philosophy [16, 17]. This entails resorting to semantics, the study of the meaning of words, phrases, or systems [18].

Let us now start with a proper description of the words used in this context.

Definitions

In science, we use definitions for a clear and distinct description. Definition is derived from Latin; it is the act of defining an exact description of a thing by its qualities and circumstances or an expression which explains a term so as to distinguish it from everything else [19].

Phenomenon

The Austrian-born German philosopher Edmund Husserl [1859–1938] stated that nothing is known to us except as a condition or a state of consciousness, as a phenomenon [20]. Philosophers and scientists used the term "phenomena" to refer to what appears from nature since some natural events may be unobservable. Following his lead, phenomenologists advised taking a fresh approach, as free as possible from previous presuppositions. They also advised describing a phenomenon as faithfully, or precisely, as possible to attain. They held that we could obtain insights into the essential structures and relationships of these phenomena on the basis of a careful study of concrete examples [21].

Proteins, Paraproteins, and Paraproteinemias

Protein form the functional pattern of animal organisms and all the properties which mark animal organisms as organized units result from their protein constitution [22].

Stedman's Medical Dictionary in 1973, "defines" a paraprotein as an abnormal plasma protein, such as macroglobulin, cryoglobulin and myeloma protein, and paraproteinemia as the presence of abnormal protein in the blood [23]. The word begins with the prefix "para" denoting a departure from normal [23]. It also means "by" or "at the side of" [24].

The expanding knowledge in the field of immunology in general and of the B-lymphocyte line in particular directed the listing of a number of conditions including MM, Waldenstrom macroglobulinemia, primary amyloidosis, and the heavy chain disease in one group. They were given nomenclatures that are used synonymously: monoclonal gammopathy, paraproteinemia, plasma cell dyscrasias, and dysproteinemias [25]. Analysis of these nomenclatures reveals that they point to an abnormality or a disturbance in the proteins or their cell of origin.

Disease and Disorder

The Oxford Advanced Learner's Dictionary defines disease as a medical problem or an illness affecting humans, animals, or plants, often caused by infection. Among the synonyms used for a medical problem, a disorder, which is rather formal and used to describe an illness that causes a part of the body to stop functioning correctly and is generally not an infection. When used to relate to physical problems, it is most often used with blood, bowel, and kidney which are commonly serious, severe, or rare. Normality and abnormality, however, cannot be fully explained by statistical considerations. According to the statistical approach, normality is defined as that which is common, ignoring the fact that sometimes disease is common, and health is rare. Remember how malnutrition can be common for children in many parts of the world. Keeping all this in mind we need to appreciate that paraproteinemia or monoclonal gammopathy may be a common finding [4].

One school of thought considers illness as a deviation from normal biological functioning. Normal functioning does not refer to the common but to what a biological organism needs to thrive, reproduce, and sustain life [26].

We must have noticed that these terms are used broadly in different contexts.

The Nature of the Problem

Earlier on, we discussed the importance of a precise choice of words. As we proceed to address the problem of how to present the phenomenon and its representatives, we have to answer some questions as follows:

- How should we group all the conditions associated with the presence of paraproteins?
  There were attempts by other investigators and experts to group these disorders on a smaller scale.
  Kanzaki and his group [27] recommended that the group of renal diseases attributed to deposition of monoclonal immunoglobulins or their components are arranged as one disease category in order to simplify the understanding of these complicated diseases in plasma cell dysplasia. The group led by Merlini introduced the concept of monoclonal gammopathies of clinical significance (MGCS). They identified their spectrum and classified them based on the mechanisms by which they cause tissue injury [4]. In emulation of this practical approach, we attempt to encompass the whole spectrum of the paraproteinemias in our textbook. This will have the dual benefit of offering the reader a panoramic view of this group of disorders and simultaneously keeping him/her focused on its individual representatives.
  Let us address some possible questions that are likely to arise in this context.
- How do paraproteins evolve and persist in the body and how can we imitate or reproduce this experimentally?
  This entails a review of the B lymphocyte line, as the cell of origin, the immunoglobulins as the protein molecules in question and the bone marrow, as the hotbed for their production. The Principle of the Uniformity of Nature tells us that similar phenomena occur when structurally similar systems are placed in similar situations. It is noteworthy that we are talking of similar and not identical systems [28]. Experimental animal models will also deserve an account as indispensable tools for research.
- When should the medical practitioner or the investigator suspect the presence of paraproteins when dealing with patients, samples, or images? How to detect them and report their findings?

- Since the phenomenon of paraproteinemia is not rare and may pass undetected with unfavorable consequences [4], physicians should be given clues for its early detection and once identified, the available diagnostic modalities should be employed meticulously.
- How to deal with the disorders in terms of understanding, diagnosis, and management?
  Medical science organizes all the knowledge and experience assembled by the careful study of individual patients and transmits it in a concise form through the publication of textbooks. Each disease or disorder is usually given an individual chapter the title of which is the disease name [26]. The conditions which are taking the established shape are better discussed as usual. Other conditions and associations still in the process of acquiring shape should be covered with our up-to-date knowledge based on observations and reports.
- What are the future prospects for therapy?
  As the field is experiencing an expanding horizon, there will be a need for a glimpse of the ongoing research for improving the therapeutic outcome of this group.
  Indeed, answering the above four queries mandates the structure and organization of this text.

The Structure of this Book

We preferred to use the term paraproteinemias for the book title as it describes a specific phenomenon which is the presence of certain proteins in the blood beside the normal proteins. It may be present in normal healthy people, especially the elderly [9, 10]. In certain other well-studied conditions, paraproteinemia is the focal point of attention as in MM since here they account for the pathophysiology, explain the manifestations, and stand as therapeutic targets. We can identify a third group in which the existence of paraproteins is not the center of attention. In the last group, they may represent an epiphenomenon, a transient finding, or a process in evolution. We also preferred disorders as it is more inclusive. Furthermore, blood is the "central stage" of this phenomenon.

This book is divided into three main parts:

Part I:

The introductory part which begins with this chapter deals with the origins of the paraproteins, their structure, and methods of diagnosis.

Chapter 2 describes the B cell lineage, being the cells that produce the paraprotein. Chapter 3 describes the structure and characteristics of immunoglobulins of which the paraproteins, or their fragments are constituted.

Chapter 4 discusses the bone marrow, the hotbed where plasma cells are actively producing paraproteins and also the importance of the matrix, the player that has recently attracted the attention of many researchers.

Chapter 5 deals with the experimental animal models of paraproteinemia with their central importance for understanding its pathophysiology and their significance as an indispensable tool for therapeutic innovations.

Chapter 6 is meant to raise the attention of medical practitioners and direct them to suspect the presence of that phenomenon and to guide their investigative procedures.

Part II:

This part includes Chaps. 7 through 21. It deals with the medical disorders associated with paraproteinemias. It starts with the conditions that have been studied and given the classical account. The list includes several conditions that have been given syndrome entities.

Usually, a chapter is structured as such: definition, causes (etiology and pathogenesis), clinical picture, prognosis, diagnosis, and treatment [26]. We followed this structure whenever possible, but to ensure the balance, the topic of AA amyloidosis is discussed in two successive Chaps. 7 and 8.

Chapters 17 through 20 discuss groups of diseases or disorders that are marked or associated with the existence of paraproteins. We tried to grasp the common features of the phenomenon in each group or class and simultaneously describe the distinctive features or characteristics of its representatives in each entity.

Chapter 18 which deals with infections as potentially causing paraproteinemias also serves as a practical guide to manage infections in the setting of paraproteinemias.

Chapter 21 is dedicated to reporting on a number of miscellaneous conditions and illnesses. We anticipate that some entities in this group will be further studied and elucidated in the future. We also expect the list to be continuously expanding with the discovery and reporting of new members that are likely to be added to our database.

Part III:

Finally, the last two Chaps. 22 and 23 are intended to offer a futuristic outlook on the new departures in the management of some representative diseases and disorders. We present a snapshot of experimental therapies (pharmacological and non-pharmacological) to highlight the current efforts of researchers in their endeavor to find new solutions and fill in many gaps.

Conclusion

Paraproteinemia is a phenomenon that medical practitioners, investigators, and researchers encounter in their practice. Recent advances have been introduced in the diagnostic investigations, risk stratifications, and management of many members of this group with significantly improved outcomes for patients.

For a better understanding of the nature, significance, and characteristics of paraproteinemias, we need to group, classify, and describe its representatives.

This chapter describes the ethos and design of our textbook while adhering to a precise and exact use of terms and definitions.

References

1. Leung N, Drosou ME, Nasr SH. Dysproteinemias and glomerular disease. Clin J Am Soc Nephrol. 2018;13(1):128–39.
2. Vaxman I, Gertz M. Recent advances in the diagnosis, risk stratification, and management of systemic light-chain amyloidosis. Acta Haematol. 2019;141(2):93–106.
3. Hamano H, Kawa S, Horiuchi A, et al. High serum IgG4 concentrations in patients with sclerosing pancreatitis. N Engl J Med. 2001;344(10):732–8.
4. Fermand JP, Bridoux F, Dispenzieri A, et al. Monoclonal gammopathy of clinical significance: a novel concept with therapeutic implications. Blood. 2018;132(14):1478–85.
5. Yang Y, Chen L, Jia Y, et al. Monoclonal gammopathy in rheumatic diseases. Clin Rheumatol. 2018;37(7):1751–62.
6. Riccomi G, Fornaciari G, Giuffra V. Multiple myeloma in paleopathology: a critical review. Int J Paleopathol. 2019;24:201–12.
7. Ledergor G, Weiner A, Zada M, et al. Single cell dissection of plasma cell heterogeneity in symptomatic and asymptomatic myeloma. Nat Med. 2018;24(12):1867–76.
8. Rosenbaum E, Marks D, Raza S. Diagnosis and management of neuropathies associated with plasma cell dyscrasias. Hematol Oncol. 2018;36(1):3–14.
9. Kyle RA, Therneau TM, Rajkumar SV, et al. Prevalence of monoclonal gammopathy of undetermined significance. N Engl J Med. 2006;354(13):1362–9.
10. Cook L, Macdonald DHC. Management of paraproteinaemia. Postgrad Med J. 2007;83 (978):217–23.
11. Pawlyn C, Davies FE. Toward personalized treatment in multiple myeloma based on molecular characteristics. Blood. 2019;133(7):660–75.
12. Levin A, Hari P, Dhakal B. Novel biomarkers in multiple myeloma. Transl Res. 2018;201: 49–59.
13. Willrich MAV, Murray DL, Kyle RA. Laboratory testing for monoclonal gammopathies: focus on monoclonal gammopathy of undetermined significance and smoldering multiple myeloma. Clin Biochem. 2018;51:38–47.
14. Hillengass J, Usmani S, Rajkumar SV, et al. International myeloma working group consensus recommendations on imaging in monoclonal plasma cell disorders. Lancet Oncol. 2019;20(6):e302–12.
15. Gavriatopoulou M, Musto P, Caers J, et al. European myeloma network recommendations on diagnosis and management of patients with rare plasma cell dyscrasias. Leukemia. 2018;32(9):1883–98.
16. Russell B. History of Western philosophy: and its connection with political and social circumstances from the earliest times to the present day. London: Unwin Brothers Limited; 1979. p. 842.
17. Honderich T. The Oxford companion to philosophy. 2nd ed. London: Oxford University Press; 1995. p. 1009.
18. Hornby AS. Oxford advanced learner's dictionary of current English. 8th ed. London: Oxford University Press; 2010.
19. Hayward AL, Sparkes JJ. Cassell's English dictionary: including words & phrases current among the English-speaking peoples of the world, together with many technical & scientific terms in common use. Cassell: The University of Michigan; 1962. p. 1347.
20. Durant W, Durant A. Interpretations of life: a survey of contemporary literature: the lives and opinions of some major authors of our time. New York: Simon and Schuster; 1970.
21. Phenomenology. In: The new Encyclopaedia Britannica, vol. 15. Encyclopaedia Britannica; 1984. p. 210.
22. Whyte LL. The unitary principle in physics and biology. London: Cresset Press; 1949.
23. Stedman TL. Stedman's medical dictionary. 22nd ed. Williams & Wilkins Company: Baltimore; 1973.
24. Godman A. Longman dictionary of scientific usage. Harlow: Longman Group Ltd; 1979.

25. Munshi NC, et al. Plasma cell disorders. In: Kasper DL, et al., editors. Harrison's principles of internal medicine, vol. 2. 20th ed. New York: McGraw-Hill Education; 2018.
26. Gøtzsche P. Rational diagnosis and treatment: evidence-based clinical decision-making. London: Wiley; 2007.
27. Kanzaki G, Okabayashi Y, Nagahama K, et al. Monoclonal immunoglobulin deposition disease and related diseases. J Nippon Med Sch. 2019;86(1):2–9.
28. Toulmin S. The philosophy of science: an introduction. New York: Harper Torchbooks, Harper & Brothers.; 1960.

Chapter 2
B Cell in Health and Disease

Marcella Visentini and Stefania Colantuono

Abbreviations

BCR	B-cell receptor
BM	Bone marrow
BNHL	B-cell non-Hodgkin lymphomas
BTK	Bruton's tyrosine kinase
CD21	Complemenr receptor 2
CSR	Class switch recombination
CVID	Common variable immune deficiency
DLBCL	Diffuse large B-cell lymphoma
FO	Follicular
GC	Germinal center
HC	Heavy chain
HSC	Hematopoietic stem cells
Ig	Immunoglobulin
LC	Light chain
MS	Multiple sclerosis
MZ	Marginal zone
PC	Plasma cells

M. Visentini (✉) · S. Colantuono
Department of Translational and Precision Medicine, Sapienza University of Rome, Rome, Italy
e-mail: marcella.visentini@uniroma1.it; stefania.colantuono@uniroma1.it

© The Author(s), under exclusive license to Springer Nature Switzerland AG 2022
G. Ragab et al. (eds.), *Paraproteinemia and Related Disorders*,
https://doi.org/10.1007/978-3-031-10131-1_2

RA	Rheumatoid arthritis
SHM	Somatic hypermutation
SLE	Systemic lupus erythematosus
TLR	Toll-like receptor
XLA	X-linked agammaglobulinemia

Introduction

B cells are at the center of the adaptive humoral immune system and are responsible for mediating the production of antigen-specific immunoglobulin (Ig) directed against invasive pathogens. For a long time, humoral immunity has been considered pretty simple but in the last decades great effort in the field of B-cell biology revealed the complicated cellular and molecular pathways regulating the many B-cell functions, opening the way to still numerous major challenges that remain to be elucidated. Since the identification of B cells by Cooper in 1965, there has been tremendous progress in our understanding of B-cell development, maturation, and function and today different B cell subsets with specific functions have been identified [1]. B cells are not only responsible for antibody production but are also efficient antigen-presenting cells for CD4+ T cells stimulation and produce cytokines, notably interleukin (IL) 4, IL-6, IL-10, and tumor necrosis factor α, which have regulatory effects. Furthermore, B cells, pivotal actors of the adaptive immune response, also show innate-like features through the production of polyreactive IgM natural antibodies that bridge the innate and adaptive immune responses. These many B-cell activities are appropriately coordinated and tightly regulated and guarantee an efficient immune response. However, these same mechanisms underlying the complexity and integrity of B-cell immune response are tremendously error-prone and subject to repeated controls explaining the possible development of diseases characterized by B-cell dysfunction: (a) loss of B-cell tolerance results in autoimmunity with self-reacting B-cell clones able to produce autoantibodies; (b) loss of B cells, reduction or absence of serum Ig and/or loss of antibody function results in B-cell immunodeficiencies; (c) genetic lesion during B-cell development and activation results in malignant transformation of the B cell at a particular stage of differentiation raising the concept of "cell of origin" of a lymphoma (Fig. 2.1).

In this chapter, physiological B-cell development is described and a focus on the pathogenic mechanisms underlying the development of autoimmune diseases, immunodeficiencies, and B-cell lymphoproliferative disorders is provided.

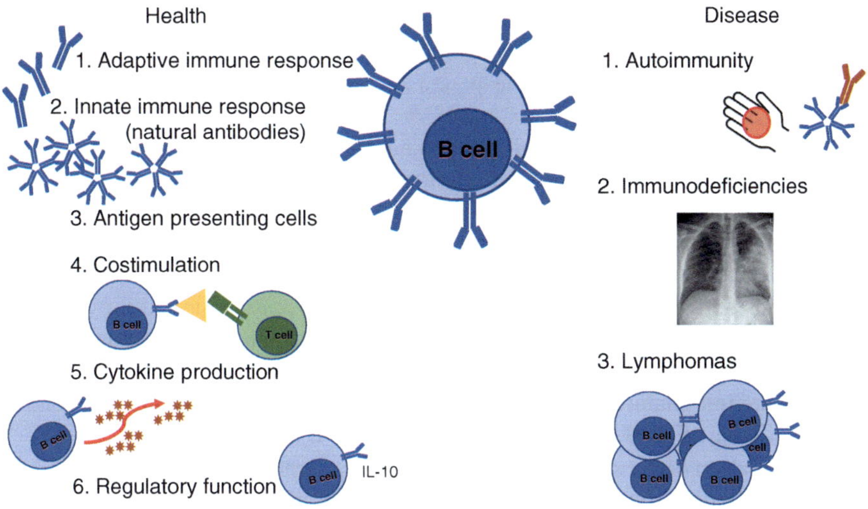

Fig. 2.1 B cells in health and disease. B cells *in health* have different multifaceted roles that allow an efficient immune response. They are part of the adaptive immune system and responsible for its humoral arm through the production of a broad repertoire of antigen-specific antibodies. Marginal zone B cells are able to produce poly-reactive IgM natural antibodies that rapidly respond to blood-borne pathogens, bridging the innate and adaptive immune responses. Beside the well-known role in humoral immunity, B cells are efficient antigen-presenting cells for CD4+ T cells co-stimulation and produce different cytokines. The secretion of IL-10 and transforming growth factor β(TGFβ), that dampen T-cell-driven immune responses, gave rise to the concept of regulatory B cells that have an important role in maintaining peripheral tolerance. In *disease* defects in the mechanisms regulating these many physiological functions of B cells may be at the basis for its development. Loss of B-cell tolerance results in autoimmunity with self-reacting B cell clones able to produce autoantibodies. Loss of B cells, reduction or absence of serum Ig, and/or loss of antibody function results in B-cell immunodeficiencies, and a genetic lesion during B-cell development and activation results in malignant transformation giving rise to B-cell lymphoma development

B-Cell Development

B-cell development proceeds in an orderly fashion and is regulated by intrinsic genetic programs and by external cues such as cytokines, present in the specialized microenvironments of fetal liver, bone marrow (BM), and secondary lymphoid organs. In general, B-cell development can be subdivided into antigen independent, occurring in the BM, and antigen-dependent developing in the secondary lymphoid organs [2]. Each differentiation step is characterized by a specific structure of the B-cell receptor (BCR) and defects in each stage of the B-cell development and maturation pathways can lead to primary immunodeficiencies, autoimmune diseases, and even B-cell malignancies.

The major stages of B–cell development in the BM include the hematopoietic stem cells (HSC), the multipotent progenitor, the common lymphoid progenitor, the progenitor B cell (pro-B cell), the precursor B cell (pre-B cell), and finally the immature B cell [3].

One intriguing feature of B-cell development is that it is accompanied by Ig gene rearrangements [4]. Progenitor B cells rearrange their Ig heavy chain (HC) genes to differentiate into precursor B (pre-B) cells that express μ HCs. Pre-B cells then rearrange their Ig light chain (LC) genes to differentiate into immature IgM^+ B lymphocytes. Lack of a functional surrogate light chain acts as one of the first tolerance checkpoints and those cells carrying receptors with excessive high affinity for self-antigens undergo receptor editing to change the light chains. B cells that express a functional (and non-autoreactive) BCR exit the BM as transitional B cells [5] and differentiate into mature IgM^+IgD^+, naive B cells that will later further differentiate into a follicular (FO) B cell or marginal zone (MZ) B cell [6].

The initiation of the second phase, antigen-dependent development of B cells for an efficient humoral immune response, requires that mature, naive B cells get activated by antigen binding to the BCR. In T-cell-dependent immune responses, antigen-activated B cells undergo clonal expansion in structures called "germinal centers" (GCs) and their affinity to antigens is increased. These encounters predominantly occur in secondary (or peripheral) lymphoid tissues, including the spleen, lymph nodes, and Peyer's patches [7–9].

Upon binding antigen, signaling via the BCR initiates B-cell activation. The actual mechanism by which antigen binding activates the BCR remains an area of active investigation. One model proposes that antigen binding leads to clustering of BCRs on the membrane to initiate signaling [10]. Conversely, an alternative model is that BCR clusters preexist before antigen encounter, and antigen binding dissociates these clusters enabling signaling to occur [11]. A third variant of these models suggests that the mobility of the BCR, relative to co-receptor molecules, may be altered by antigen binding.

Complex antigens engage other receptors on the B cell in addition to the BCR. The ligation of some co-receptors, such as toll-like receptors (TLRs) or complement receptors 2 (CR2), leads to amplification and possibly qualitative modification in the BCR signaling [12, 13].

Upon encounter with an antigen, naive B cells become activated by the interaction with CD4+ T cells in the T-cell-rich area of the lymphoid tissues and aggregate into primary follicles to form GCs. In the GC, B cells are targeted by Ig gene remodeling processes, namely somatic hypermutation (SHM) and class switch recombination (CSR), in order to generate cells with the ability to produce high-affinity antibodies of different isotype classes. The GC structure consists of a dark zone, which almost exclusively contains highly proliferating B cells and a light zone in which B cells are intermingled with follicular dendritic cells, T cells, and macrophages. The dark zone is the site of B-cell division and SHM, whereas the light zone is where B cells undergo activation and selection on the basis of the affinity of their B-cell receptors [14]. Ongoing B-T interactions are critical for the maintenance of GCs. As B cells terminally differentiate into plasma cells, they initially continue proliferating and are referred to as plasmablasts [15]. Once these cells cease dividing and fully mature, they become plasma cells (PCs). The factors that determine whether a B cell undergoes PC differentiation, becomes a GC B cell, or a memory B cell are being actively investigated. These differentiation states are influenced by a variety of signals, such as those from the BCR, co-receptors, and cytokines. PC development is tightly regulated by a panoply of transcription factors, most notably Bcl-6 and BLIMP-1. B cells with higher affinity for antigens give rise to a stronger PC response than B cells responding with lower affinity, and this reflects the strength of the plasmablast proliferative response [16].

Another factor that might influence the propensity to become a PC versus a GC cell is the chronic exposure to low avidity autoantigens. B cells exposed to such antigens show a downregulated expression of IgM and are in an "anergic" state, poorly responsive in vitro to antigen stimulation. However, when exposed to a cross-reactive multivalent antigen and T cell help, such anergic B cells preferentially enter the GC response where they undergo somatic hypermutation to mutate away from self-reactivity and develop increased ability to bind the foreign antigen in a process referred to as clonal redemption [17, 18]. The PCs arising in the early phases of B-cell responses, independently of GCs, typically remain within the peripheral lymphoid tissue and are short-lived PCs (SLPCs). In contrast, GCs give rise to long-lived plasma cells, many of which have a BM tropism and can live for months (Chap. 4).

In B-cell responses, memory may be maintained in two forms, first through the long-term production of antibody by long-lived plasma cells, and second by the generation of a pool of relatively quiescent memory B cells expressing mutated BCRs with enhanced affinities, persisting after antigen challenge and that can be reactivated by subsequent antigen exposures.

Upon re-exposure to antigen, memory B cells can differentiate into GC B cells or PCs, and specific subsets of IgM versus IgG memory B cells, defined by surface markers such as CD73, CD80, and PDL2, show different propensities to undergo particular differentiation programs. GC B cells are thought to give rise to a large fraction of the B-cell memory pool, yet GC-independent memory B cells have also been described to appear very early in the immune response [19, 20].

B Cells and Autoimmunity

B cells play a key role in regulating the immune system by producing antibodies, acting as antigen-presenting cells, providing support to other mononuclear cells, and contributing directly to inflammatory pathways. Accumulating evidence points to disruption of these tightly regulated processes in the pathogenesis of autoimmune disorders. Although the exact mechanisms involved remain to be elucidated, a fundamental feature of many autoimmune disorders is the loss of B-cell tolerance and the inappropriate production of autoantibodies. Furthermore, B cells may contribute to autoimmune pathogenesis by presentation of autoantigen to T cells, or through production of proinflammatory cytokines.

These findings provide the rationale for B-cell depletion as a potential therapeutic strategy in autoimmune disorders and other disease states characterized by inappropriate immune responses [21, 22]. B-cell-targeted therapy focused on restoring normal B-cell function and eliminating pathogenic autoantibodies have been successful in treating rheumatoid arthritis (RA), systemic lupus erythematosus (SLE), and multiple sclerosis (MS).

A major pathway for immune activation and tissue damage for systemic autoantibodies is through formation of immune complexes that induce complement activation by both classical and alternative pathways and can lead to direct cell lysis and damage as well as recruitment of leukocytes to further enhance inflammatory responses. Immune complexes can activate Fc receptors that are expressed by a variety of cells, particularly by immune cells of the myeloid lineage. Autoantibodies have been shown to activate these immune cells through FcγR-dependent pathways or through direct modulation of signaling receptors on target cells [23].

Multiple self-tolerance checkpoints exist to remove autoreactive specificities from the B-cell repertoire or to limit the ability of such cells to secrete autoantigen-binding antibodies. These include receptor editing and deletion of immature B cells developing in the BM, competitive elimination of chronically autoantigen-binding B cells in the periphery, and a state of anergy that disfavors PC differentiation [24, 25]. Autoantibody production can occur due to failures in these checkpoints or in T-cell self-tolerance mechanisms.

However, despite this undisputed involvement of B cells, little is known about B-cell subpopulations with distinct immune functions that may play a role in the spectrum of autoimmunity. One distinct subset that is implicated in the autoreactive B-cell response are the innate-like MZ B cells.

In contrast to FO B cells, which primarily express mono-reactive BCRs and give rise to highly specific, high-affinity antibodies, the innate-like MZ B cells express poly-reactive BCRs and rapidly produce low affinity antibodies with self-reactivity to clear pathogens and apoptotic cell debris [26]. MZ B cells are strategically located at the interface between the circulation and the white pulp of the spleen, where they provide a first line of defense by rapidly producing IgM and class-switched IgG antibodies in response to infections by blood-borne viruses and encapsulated bacteria. MZ B cells have a lower activation threshold than follicular B cells, which permits the rapid initiation of IgM production and of IgG- and IgA-inducing (CSR) in the absence of CD40-dependent help from T follicular helper cells. This T-cell-independent pathway requires dual BCR and TLR engagement by conserved microbial antigens together with co-stimulatory signals from dendritic cells, macrophages, and neutrophils via various cytokines, including BAFF, a proliferation-inducing ligand (APRIL), interleukin-6 (IL-6), IL-10, IL-21, interferon-α (IFNα), IFNβ, and CXC-chemokine ligand 10 (CXCL10).

MZ B cells share the feature of being "innate-like," meaning they exist in a "pre-activated" state and differentiate into antibody-secreting cells very rapidly (within 1–2 days) following antigen encounter. They have a B-cell repertoire enriched with specificities that recognize carbohydrate and lipid moieties present on various life-threatening microbes [27].

Unlike their murine counterpart, human MZ B cells carry mutated BCRs [28]. It was recently suggested that they complete their maturation not in the spleen, but rather in gut-associated lymphoid tissue [29]. Here they can interact with gut bacteria, mutate, and then be selected for (self-/) poly-reactive-binding abilities before circulating back to the spleen. Thus, the microbiota may play a crucial role in shaping the MZ B-cell compartment in humans. This may be one of the mechanisms whereby the microbiome, influenced both by genetics and diet, can play a significant role in the pathogenesis of several autoimmune conditions, for example, SLE, systemic sclerosis, and RA [30].

Another important feature of MZ B cells and other innate-like B cells is the production of natural antibodies [31, 32]. Natural antibodies can be produced in germ-free contexts although their composition is shaped by the microbiota. Natural antibody provides a first line of defense against a range of pathogens and, through opsonization, augments the follicular B-cell response. In general, natural antibodies are characterized by their low affinity, high avidity, and broad/multi-reactivity against self-antigens, but some have the ability to recognize evolutionarily conserved epitopes occurring in foreign antigens. A subset of B cells in mice, named B-1 cells, was recognized as the main source of natural antibodies. B-1 cells are found in various tissues of adult mice, including the peritoneal cavity, pleural cavity, spleen, bone marrow, lymph nodes, and blood and are considered an innate like B-cell population. In humans B1 B cells have not been identified and the main producers of natural antibodies are MZ B cells. Natural antibodies have a key role in the first defense against bloodborne pathogens but also in maintaining the immune homeostasis through the clearance of apoptotic cells and regulation of inflammatory, autoimmune, and allergic responses. Interestingly, natural antibodies seem to have potential functions in the pathogenesis and progression of other chronic inflammatory condition, such as atherosclerosis. It was demonstrated that oxidation-derived epitopes on apoptotic cells and oxidized low-density lipoproteins are recognized by the phosphorylcholine-specific natural antibody that seem to play a protective role in atherosclerosis [33].

Another recently identified B-cell population with a possible role in autoimmune and chronic infectious diseases is a subset of B cells characterized by low expression of the complement receptor 2 (CD21), the so-called $CD21^{low}$ B cells. These B cells have been found expanded also in aged female mice, have an increased expression of the transcription factor T-bet and of CD11c, and were named ABCs (aged B cells) or $T\text{-}bet^{+}CD11^{+}$ B cells. Their formation and expansion rely on TLR7 or TLR9 signals in the context of Th1 cytokines [34]. $CD21^{low}$ B cells are enriched in the peripheral blood of patients with pathogenic infections (malaria, tuberculosis, HIV) as well as in several autoimmune conditions including SLE, RA, common variable immunodeficiency, primary Sjögren's syndrome, hepatitis C virus-associated mixed cryoglobulinemia [35, 36], and MS, but their role in disease development or progression remains elusive. Functionally, this memory subset demonstrated altered responsiveness to stimuli compared to conventional memory B cells, express low or no CD27, and are therefore atypical memory B cells with features of innate-like B cells. It is possible that chronic BCR stimulation due to exposure to self-antigens desensitizes BCR signaling, rendering these cells hyporesponsive and exhausted. Moreover, there is an enrichment of poly-reactive and auto-reactive clones within the CD21^{low} compartment and in chronic infection, such as HIV, these cells produce high titers of virus-specific antibodies. These features suggest that CD21^{low} B cells might not only be an epiphenomenon but may participate in the pathogenic mechanisms of many diseases characterized by B-cell dysfunction. It is curious that TLR7, whose gene is located on chromosome X, is crucial for CD21^{low} B-cell generation is found expanded in aged female mice, raising the question on the strong female bias seen in many autoimmune diseases. In this view, it is widely known that estrogens are immune system modulators, which may influence the induction of autoimmunity [37]. In murine disease models of autoimmunity, it has been established that estrogen potently exacerbates B-cell autoimmunity by promoting the expansion and activation of autoreactive MZ B cells, which are consequently induced to secrete antibodies and undergo class-switch recombination.

Another interesting B-cell population with relevant functions in autoimmunity, allergy, and cancer are the B regulatory cells (Bregs). In addition to the well-established contribution of Tregs in the maintenance of immune homeostasis, immunosuppressive Bregs cells producing IL-10 have been shown to contribute to the maintenance of tolerance and of homeostasis in the immune system. The importance of Bregs is emphasized by the different immune-related pathologies that are associated with abnormalities in the number and function of Bregs, such as SLE, RA, and MS. For these reasons, Breg-based immunotherapies might be an interesting promise and could provide a more improved and targeted approach to treat various immune-related pathologies [38].

B Cell and Immunodeficiency

Among primary immune defects, B-cell immunodeficiencies are clinically predominant. The study of the impairment in B-cell development or function that characterize these conditions represents the most illuminating lesson about B-cell biology. The end product of the multiple steps that include continuous reconfiguration of genes for the B-cell antigen receptors along with the elimination of perhaps 90% of poly-reactive and autoreactive B cells is the generation of functional antibodies. Thus, a variable loss of B cells, reduction or absence of serum immunoglobulins, and/or loss of antibody function are features of most immunodeficiencies [39]. The clinical spectrum of B-cell immunodeficiencies is heterogeneous and reflects the stage of B-cell development impairment, the entity and quality of antibodies defect, and eventually the interactions with other immune cells.

Agammaglobulinemia is characterized by the absence of circulating B cells with severe reduction in all serum immunoglobulin levels. X-linked agammaglobulinemia (XLA) is due to mutations of Bruton's tyrosine kinase (BTK) gene [40]. Member of a family of cytoplasmic tyrosine kinases, it is expressed at all stages of B-cell differentiation except for plasma cells. Mutations in BTK account for approximately

85% of patients presenting with congenital agammaglobulinemia, whereas mutations in components of the pre-BCR, including μ heavy chain, Ig-α, Ig-β, or λ5 are found in 5-7% of patients with isolated defects in B cell development [41]. All the reported mutations of the μ heavy chain are associated with the complete absence of B cells in the peripheral circulation, so patients with μ heavy chain defects tend to have a more severe phenotype and are diagnosed earlier. B-cell linker (BLNK) defects [42] PIK3R1 [43] and E47 Transcription Factor/TCF3 mutations [44] are responsible for rare forms of agammaglobulinemia. The clinical features of homozygous PIK3R1 mutation include almost total loss of B cells (1%) and agammaglobulinemia without abnormalities in the T-cell compartment. Bone marrow findings were consistent with an early block in B-cell development with minimal VDJ rearrangement.

In common variable immune deficiency (CVID), B cells either do not become fully activated, proliferate normally, and/ or terminally differentiate into plasma cells and/or memory B cells, reflecting the various blocks in B-cell development [45]. Although most CVID patients have low to normal numbers of circulating B cells, the main characteristic is the failure in differentiation of B cells into immunoglobulin-secreting plasma cells, resulting in antibody deficiency. Reduced numbers of isotype switched $CD27^+$ memory B cells with increases in $CD21^{low}$ or increased transitional B cells has become a useful basis for subclassification of CVID patients [46].

The clinical spectrum of a/hypogammaglobulinemia predominantly consists of recurrent infection susceptibility, over-represented for encapsulated or atypical bacteria. Autoimmune and/or inflammatory features also coexist [47]. Moreover, individuals with CVID are susceptible to malignancy, particularly non-Hodgkin lymphoma, but also solid cancers [48].

Genetic defects account for only a few patients with CVID and nearly 75% of patients have no known defect. Mutations of transmembrane activator and CAML interactor (TACI), expressed on mature B cells, especially marginal zone B cells, $CD27^+$ memory B cells and plasma cells, are found in 8–10% of CVID patients [49]. More rare gene defects may affect B-cell activating factor of the tumor necrosis family receptor (BAFF-R) [50], TNF-like weak inducer of apoptosis (TWEAK) [51], inducible T-cell co-stimulator (ICOS) [52] and B-cell costimulatory molecule (CD19, CD20, CD21, CD27, CD81) [53–56].

As mentioned above, CSR and SHM result in high-affinity antibody production and the differentiation of B cells into long-lived memory B cells and plasma cells. Immunoglobulin class switch recombination deficiencies, previously termed "hyper-IgM syndromes (HIGM)" are rare primary immunodeficiencies characterized by impaired production of switched immunoglobulin isotypes and normal or elevated IgM levels. Some of the CSR deficiencies are caused by defects in CSR machinery and are predominately intrinsic B-cell defects, which include mutations in activation-induced cytidine deaminase (AID) [57] and uracil-DNA glycosylase (UNG) [58]. In contrast, CD40 ligand (CD40L) and CD40 deficiencies are combined immune defects with impaired interaction between activated CD4+ T cells expressing CD40L and cell types expressing CD40 which include B cells, dendritic cells, monocytes/macrophages, platelets, and activated endothelial/epithelial cells [59].

Selective IgA deficiency (SIGAD), IgG subclass deficiency, selective IgM Deficiency, and the rare Kappa (κ) chain deficiency are antibody deficiencies characterized by generally normal numbers of B cells. In transient hypogammaglobulinemia of infancy (THI), usually, also the low antibodies levels spontaneously return to normal within 2–3 years of age.

B Cell and Malignancies

About 95% of the lymphomas are of B-cell origin, the rest are T-cell malignancies. This high percentage is understandable considering the specific factors that influence the pathogenesis of B-cell lymphomas that are linked to B-cell development. Studies of the status of the Ig genetic regions within lymphoma cells can align their origin in either pre- or post-GC B cells. Malignant B cells seem to be "frozen" at a particular differentiation stage, which reflects their origin. With the exception of the relatively rare lymphoblastic and mantle-cell lymphoma subtypes, all B-cell non-Hodgkin lymphomas (B-NHL) display somatically mutated IgV genes, indicating that they are derived from B cells that are blocked within or have passed through the GC [60–62].

A diverse group of B-cell lymphomas, including follicular lymphoma, Burkitt lymphoma, and diffuse large B-cell lymphoma (DLBCL) are thought to have a GC origin and comprehensive gene expression studies have provided evidence that these malignancies derive from different stages of the reaction.

Burkitt lymphoma seems to derive from dark zone B cells, whereas follicular lymphoma and DLBCLs correspond to B cells arrested by transformation events that occur at various stages of the GC transit.

Follicular lymphoma and the GC B-cell (GCB)-like subtype of DLBCL resemble light zone B cells, whereas activated B-cell (ABC)-like DLBCLs seem to derive from GC cells arrested during the early stages of post-GC plasma cell differentiation (plasmablasts). Primary mediastinal B-cell lymphoma represents a distinct subtype that originates from post-GC thymic B cells in the mediastinum.

Interestingly, the same genetic mechanisms that enable the development of high-affinity immunoglobulin receptors of different isotype classes are involved in the malignant transformation of B cells. It is generally accepted that the GC microenvironment is the main source of memory B cells and plasma cells that produce high-affinity antibodies, which are necessary to protect against invading microorganisms. However, the beneficial role of GC B cells in immunity is somewhat counterbalanced by their detrimental role in lymphomagenesis, as the majority of B-cell lymphomas originate from GC B cells. The GC B cell is at a particularly high risk for undergoing malignant transformation, due to attenuation of certain DNA damage and cell proliferation checkpoints, which is essential for immunoglobulin affinity maturation. Although the GC reaction is tightly regulated, SHM can disrupt this delicate equilibrium by generating off-target mutations that enable B cells to gain selective advantages.

B-NHLs carry numerous genetic aberrations including amplifications, deletions, and non- synonymous point mutations that are associated with gain- or loss-of-function consequences [63]. Two additional types of genetic alterations characterize B-cell NHLs: (a) chromosomal translocations and aberrant SHMs (ASHMs), both of which are dependent on immunoglobulin remodeling mechanisms including V(D)J recombination, SHM, and CSR that occur during the GC reaction. The transit from the dark zone to the light zone, the recycling between the two zones and the post-GC differentiation of B cells are controlled by a complex network of cellular and soluble signals that affect GC B-cell responses by activating and repressing specific transcriptional programs. The pathways driving these programs are commonly hijacked through genetic alterations during malignant transformation. The dissection of these pathways provides insights into the process of lymphomagenesis and contributes to the understanding of the GC physiology. The common denominator of chromosomal translocations associated with B-NHL is the transcriptional dysregulation of genes that regulate GC B-cell development, or the ectopic expression of genes not normally expressed in a particular developmental stage of mature B cells.

Chromosomal translocations associated with GC-derived non-Hodgkin lymphomas frequently involve the immunoglobulin locus, with the breakpoints either in the switch region or in the target region for SHM. Notable exceptions to the SHM- and CSR-associated translocations are represented by the t(14;18) chromosomal translocation involving the immunoglobulin and *BCL2* loci in follicular lymphoma, and a subset of the t(8;14) chromosomal translocation involving the immunoglobulin and *MYC* loci in endemic-type Burkitt lymphoma, which probably represent by-products of an error which could have occurred during V(D)J recombination, presumably in immature pre-GC B cells.

In contrast to BCL-2, BCL-6 is normally expressed in GC B cells, but its expression needs to be switched off for the post-GC differentiation of B cells. Chromosomal translocations involving *BCL6*, commonly associated with DLBCL and less frequently with follicular lymphomas, dysregulate BCL-6 expression by preventing its silencing at the conclusion of the GC response.

A block in post-GC differentiation might also be the functional consequence of the chromosomal translocations affecting *PAX5* and the IgH locus in lymphoplasmacytoid lymphoma. In fact, the constitutive expression of PAX5, which maintains the B-cell phenotype, might prevent the silencing of its program and therefore block the terminal differentiation of B cells into plasma cells.

Translocations of MYC into the immunoglobulin heavy chain or light chain loci are associated with 100% of Burkitt lymphoma cases and up to 10% of DLBCL cases. These tumors are derived from the oncogenic transformation of a GC B cell, as a fraction of tumors shows ongoing IgV SHM and the tumor cells are strongly related in their gene expression profile to GC B cells.

The study of B-cell lymphomas and their associated genetic derangements continues to be illuminating for the understanding of the physiologic B-cell differentiation process, leading to the development of targeted therapies [64, 65]. For example, the finding that CLL cells depend on BCR signaling for survival has led to the development of BTK and PI3Kd inhibitors as treatments for this cancer [66].

Conclusions

B cells are essential for efficient immune responses and the maintenance of health. B cells not only participate in the immune response by producing antibodies but show multifaceted roles that range from antigen presentation to regulatory functions. Emerging data shows that different B-cell subpopulations exist and have specific functions that also include innate-like features through the production of natural IgM antibodies. Thus, it is not surprising that defects in many processes regulating B-cell development, differentiation, and activation result in the development of autoimmune diseases, immunodeficiencies, and lymphoproliferative disorders. Untangling these molecular and cellular pathways may improve the therapeutic strategies of diseases characterized by B-cell dysfunction, not through a generalized B-cell depletion approach but through a more specific and targeted strategy.

References

1. Cooper MD, Peterson RD, Good RA. Delineation of the thymic and bursal lymphoid systems in the chicken. Nature. 1965;205:143–6.
2. LeBien TW, Tedder TF. B lymphocytes: how they develop and function. Blood. 2008;112(5):1570–80.
3. Wang Y, Liu J, Burrows PD, Wang JY. B cell development and maturation. Adv Exp Med Biol. 2020;1254:1–22.
4. Early P, Huang H, Davis M, Calame K, Hood L. An immunoglobulin heavy chain variable region gene is generated from three segments of DNA: VH, D and JH. Cell. 1980;19:981–92.
5. Sims GP, Ettinger R, Shirota Y, Yarboro CH, Illei GG, Lipsky PE. Identification and characterization of circulating human transitional B cells. Blood. 2005;105(11):4390–8.
6. Pillai S, Cariappa A. The follicular versus marginal zone B lymphocyte cell fate decision. Nat Rev Immunol. 2009;9(11):767–77.
7. De Silva NS, Klein U. Dynamics of B cells in germinal centres. Nat Rev Immunol. 2015;15(3):137–48.
8. Victora GD, Nussenzweig MC. Germinal centers. Annu Rev Immunol. 2012;30:429–57.
9. Cyster JG, Allen CDC. B cell responses: cell interaction dynamics and decisions. Cell. 2019;177(3):524–40.
10. Harwood NE, Batista FD. Early events in B cell activation. Annu Rev Immunol. 2010;28:185–210.
11. Yang J, Reth M. Receptor dissociation and B-cell activation. Curr Top Microbiol Immunol. 2016;393:27–43.
12. Suthers AN, Sarantopoulos S. TLR7/TLR9- and B cell receptor-signaling crosstalk: promotion of potentially dangerous B cells. Front Immunol. 2017;8:775.
13. Carroll MC, Isenman DE. Regulation of humoral immunity by complement. Immunity. 2012;37(2):199–207.
14. Klein U, Dalla-Favera R. Germinal centres: role in B-cell physiology and malignancy. Nat Rev Immunol. 2008;8(1):22–33.
15. Nutt SL, Hodgkin PD, Tarlinton DM, Corcoran LM. The generation of antibody-secreting plasma cells. Nat Rev Immunol. 2015;15(3):160–71.

16. Kräutler NJ, Suan D, Butt D, Bourne K, Hermes JR, Chan TD, et al. Differentiation of germinal center B cells into plasma cells is initiated by high-affinity antigen and completed by Tfh cells. J Exp Med. 2017;214(5):1259–67.
17. Burnett DL, Reed JH, Christ D, Goodnow CC. Clonal redemption and clonal anergy as mechanisms to balance B cell tolerance and immunity. Immunol Rev. 2019;292(1):61–75.
18. Reed JH, Jackson J, Christ D, Goodnow CC. Clonal redemption of autoantibodies by somatic hypermutation away from self-reactivity during human immunization. J Exp Med. 2016;213(7):1255–65.
19. Kurosaki T, Kometani K, Ise W. Memory B cells. Nat Rev Immunol. 2015;15(3):149–59.
20. Weisel F, Shlomchik M. Memory B cells of mice and humans. Annu Rev Immunol. 2017;35:255–84.
21. Edwards JC, Cambridge G. B-cell targeting in rheumatoid arthritis and other autoimmune diseases. Nat Rev Immunol. 2006;6(5):394–403.
22. Looney RJ. Treating human autoimmune disease by depleting B cells. Ann Rheum Dis. 2002;61(10):863–6.
23. Takai T. Roles of Fc receptors in autoimmunity. Nat Rev Immunol. 2002;2(8):580–92.
24. Goodnow CC, Crosbie J, Jorgensen H, Brink RA, Basten A. Induction of self-tolerance in mature peripheral B lymphocytes. Nature. 1989;342:385–91.
25. Nemazee D. Mechanisms of central tolerance for B cells. Nat Rev Immunol. 2017;17:281–94.
26. Palm AE, Kleinau S. Marginal zone B cells: from housekeeping function to autoimmunity? J Autoimmun. 2021;119:102627.
27. Lopes-Carvalho T, Kearney JF. Development and selection of marginal zone B cells. Immunol Rev. 2004;197:192–205.
28. Weill JC, Weller S, Reynaud CA. Human marginal zone B cells. Annu Rev Immunol. 2009;27:267–85.
29. Zhao Y, Uduman M, Siu JHY, Tull TJ, Sanderson JD, Wu YB, et al. Spatiotemporal segregation of human marginal zone and memory B cell populations in lymphoid tissue. Nat Commun. 2018;9(1):3857.
30. De Luca F, Shoenfeld Y. The microbiome in autoimmune diseases. Clin Exp Immunol. 2019;195(1):74–85.
31. Ehrenstein M, Notley C. The importance of natural IgM: scavenger, protector and regulator. Nat Rev Immunol. 2010;10:778–86.
32. Panda S, Ding JL. Natural antibodies bridge innate and adaptive immunity. J Immunol. 2015;194(1):13–20.
33. Shaw PX, Hörkkö S, Chang MK, Curtiss LK, Palinski W, Silverman GJ, et al. Natural antibodies with the T15 idiotype may act in atherosclerosis, apoptotic clearance, and protective immunity. J Clin Invest. 2000;105(12):1731–40.
34. Cancro MP. Age-associated B cells. Annu Rev Immunol. 2020;38:315–40.
35. Rakhmanov M, Keller B, Gutenberger S, Foerster C, Hoenig M, Driessen G, et al. Circulating CD21low B cells in common variable immunodeficiency resemble tissue homing, innate-like B cells. Proc Natl Acad Sci U S A. 2009;106(32):13451–6.
36. Visentini M, Conti V, Cristofoletti C, Lazzeri C, Marrapodi R, Russo G, et al. Clonal expansion and functional exhaustion of monoclonal marginal zone B cells in mixed cryoglobulinemia: the yin and yang of HCV-driven lymphoproliferation and autoimmunity. Autoimmun Rev. 2013;12(3):430–5.
37. Grimaldi CM, Cleary J, Dagtas AS, Moussai D, Diamond B. Estrogen alters thresholds for B cell apoptosis and activation. J Clin Invest. 2002;109(12):1625–33.
38. Mauri C, Menon M. Human regulatory B cells in health and disease: therapeutic potential. J Clin Invest. 2017;127(3):772–9.
39. Smith T, Cunningham-Rundles C. Primary B-cell immunodeficiencies. Hum Immunol. 2019;80(6):351–62.

40. Tsukada S, Saffran DC, Rawlings DJ, Parolini O, Allen RC, Klisak I, et al. Deficient expression of a B cell cytoplasmic tyrosine kinase in human X-linked agammaglobulinemia. Cell. 1993;72(2):279–90.
41. Yel L, Minegishi Y, Coustan-Smith E, Buckley RH, Trübel H, Pachman LM, et al. Mutations in the mu heavy-chain gene in patients with agammaglobulinemia. N Engl J Med. 1996;335(20):1486–93.
42. Minegishi Y, Rohrer J, Coustan-Smith E, Lederman HM, Pappu R, Campana D, et al. An essential role for BLNK in human B cell development. Science. 1999;286(5446):1954–7.
43. Conley ME, Dobbs AK, Quintana AM, Bosompem A, Wang YD, Coustan-Smith E, et al. Agammaglobulinemia and absent B lineage cells in a patient lacking the p85α subunit of PI3K. J Exp Med. 2012;209(3):463–70.
44. Boisson B, Wang YD, Bosompem A, Ma CS, Lim A, Kochetkov T, et al. A recurrent dominant negative E47 mutation causes agammaglobulinemia and BCR(−) B cells. J Clin Invest. 2013;123(11):4781–5.
45. Ahn S, Cunningham-Rundles C. Role of B cells in common variable immune deficiency. Expert Rev Clin Immunol. 2009;5(5):557–64.
46. Wehr C, Kivioja T, Schmitt C, Ferry B, Witte T, Eren E, et al. The EUROclass trial: defining subgroups in common variable immunodeficiency. Blood. 2008;111(1):77–85.
47. Quartuccio L, De Marchi G, Longhino S, Manfrè V, Rizzo MT, Gandolfo S, et al. Shared pathogenetic features between common variable immunodeficiency and Sjögren's syndrome: clues for a personalized medicine. Front Immunol. 2021;12:703780.
48. Mayor PC, Eng KH, Singel KL, Abrams SI, Odunsi K, Moysich KB, et al. Cancer in primary immunodeficiency diseases: cancer incidence in the United States immune deficiency network registry. J Allergy Clin Immunol. 2018;141(3):1028–35.
49. Castigli E, Wilson SA, Garibyan L, Rachid R, Bonilla F, Schneider L, Geha RS. TACI is mutant in common variable immunodeficiency and IgA deficiency. Nat Genet. 2005;37(8):829–34.
50. Losi CG, Silini A, Fiorini C, Soresina A, Meini A, Ferrari S, et al. Mutational analysis of human BAFF receptor TNFRSF13C (BAFF-R) in patients with common variable immunodeficiency. J Clin Immunol. 2005;25(5):496–502.
51. Wang HY, Ma CA, Zhao Y, Fan X, Zhou Q, Edmonds P, et al. Antibody deficiency associated with an inherited autosomal dominant mutation in TWEAK. Proc Natl Acad Sci U S A. 2013;110(13):5127–32.
52. Grimbacher B, Hutloff A, Schlesier M, Glocker E, Warnatz K, Dräger R, et al. Homozygous loss of ICOS is associated with adult-onset common variable immunodeficiency. Nat Immunol. 2003;4(3):261–8.
53. van Zelm MC, Smet J, Adams B, Mascart F, Schandené L, Janssen F, et al. CD81 gene defect in humans disrupts CD19 complex formation and leads to antibody deficiency. J Clin Invest. 2010;120(4):1265–74.
54. Kuijpers TW, Bende RJ, Baars PA, Grummels A, Derks IA, Dolman KM, et al. CD20 deficiency in humans results in impaired T cell-independent antibody responses. J Clin Invest. 2010;120(1):214–22.
55. van Montfrans JM, Hoepelman AI, Otto S, van Gijn M, van de Corput L, de Weger RA, et al. CD27 deficiency is associated with combined immunodeficiency and persistent symptomatic EBV viremia. J Allergy Clin Immunol. 2012;129(3):787–93.e6.
56. Thiel J, Kimmig L, Salzer U, Grudzien M, Lebrecht D, Hagena T, et al. CD21 deficiency is associated with hypogammaglobulinemia. J Allergy Clin Immunol. 2012;129:801–10.
57. Minegishi Y, Lavoie A, Cunningham-Rundles C, Bédard PM, Hébert J, Côté L, et al. Mutations in activation-induced cytidine deaminase in patients with hyper IgM syndrome. Clin Immunol. 2000;97(3):203–10.
58. Imai K, Catalan N, Plebani A, Maródi L, Sanal O, Kumaki S, et al. Hyper-IgM syndrome type 4 with a B lymphocyte-intrinsic selective deficiency in Ig class-switch recombination. J Clin Invest. 2003;112(1):136–42.

59. Lougaris V, Badolato R, Ferrari S, Plebani A. Hyper immunoglobulin M syndrome due to CD40 deficiency: clinical, molecular, and immunological features. Immunol Rev. 2005;203:48–66.
60. Shaffer AL 3rd, Young RM, Staudt LM. Pathogenesis of human B cell lymphomas. Annu Rev Immunol. 2012;30:565–610.
61. Basso K, Dalla-Favera R. Germinal centres and B cell lymphomagenesis. Nat Rev Immunol. 2015;15:172–84.
62. Küppers R, Klein U, Hansmann ML, Rajewsky K. Cellular origin of human B-cell lymphomas. N Engl J Med. 1999;341(20):1520–9.
63. Nussenzweig A, Nussenzweig MC. Origin of chromosomal translocations in lymphoid cancer. Cell. 2010;141(1):27–38.
64. Pasqualucci L, Dalla-Favera R. The genetic landscape of diffuse large B-cell lymphoma. Semin Hematol. 2015;52(2):67–76.
65. Jerkeman M, Hallek M, Dreyling M, Thieblemont C, Kimby E, Staudt L. Targeting of B-cell receptor signalling in B-cell malignancies. J Intern Med. 2017;282(5):415–28.
66. Fabbri G, Dalla-Favera R. The molecular pathogenesis of chronic lymphocytic leukaemia. Nat Rev Cancer. 2016;16(3):145–62.

Chapter 3
Immunoglobulins, Structure, and Function

T. Prescott Atkinson

History

The history of immunology and the development of knowledge about the function and structure of immunoglobulins are intimately tied to that of infectious diseases as researchers struggled to find ways to prevent and treat the often-devastating types of infections plaguing humanity [1, 2]. The first evidence that immune serum contains specific activities that can protect from disease was developed in the 1890s by von Behring and Kitasato, who showed that serum from animals that had been rendered resistant to diphtheria through the use of toxoids could protect naive animals [3]. This discovery, for which von Behring received the Nobel Prize in 1901, led directly to the use of immune sera in the treatment of infectious diseases such as diphtheria. In 1897, Paul Ehrlich published his side chain theory, a remarkably prescient concept in which he postulated the existence of certain cells of the immune system with "side chain" molecules on their surfaces which exhibited specificity for toxins such as diphtheria toxin. This proposed mechanism for antibody activity was thus analogous to the "lock-and-key" hypothesis put forward earlier by Emil Fisher for enzyme activity. Ehrlich further postulated that soluble side chains released in large amounts could circulate in the body and protect the host [4]. By the 1930s, the term "*antibodies*" began to be used to describe this specific antigen binding activity in serum, a translation of the term *Antikörper*, which was first employed in 1900 by Karl Landsteiner [2]. A completely different type of highly specific activity was described in 1902 by Paul Portier and Charles Richet, a dramatic and lethal response to antigen which, because it was the opposite of protection of the host, they named "anaphylaxis" [4]. This activity Richet later showed in animal experiments resided

T. P. Atkinson (✉)
Department of Pediatrics, University of Alabama at Birmingham, Birmingham, AL, USA
e-mail: patkinson@peds.uab.edu

© The Author(s), under exclusive license to Springer Nature Switzerland AG 2022
G. Ragab et al. (eds.), *Paraproteinemia and Related Disorders*,
https://doi.org/10.1007/978-3-031-10131-1_3

in and was transferrable by serum, a finding replicated in humans in 1921 by Carl Prausnitz and Heinz Küstner [5].

Physical properties of antibodies also began to be identified in the late 1800s with the observation by Rudolf Kraus in 1897 that toxin/antitoxin reactions could generate a precipitate in solution [2]. John Marrack proposed the lattice theory in 1934, which required both antigens and antibodies to have more than one binding site, in order to explain how the combination of antigen and antibody could combine to form a precipitate [6]. Characterization of the antibodies advanced further with the development of electrophoresis by Arne Tiselius in 1937, which permitted the separation of molecules by their net surface charge in buffer [1]. Tiselius and his post-doctoral student Elvin Kabat used the new technique to prove that the bulk of antibodies were gamma globulins, [7] later named IgG. Using the technique of ultracentrifugation developed a decade earlier by Theodor Svedberg [8], a second high molecular weight antibody that sedimented at 19 Svedberg units (19S) was simultaneously described by Waldenstrom and Pedersen and Kunkel [9, 10]. This, the second of the immunoglobulin isotypes to be defined, was later named IgM for the macroglobulinemia patients described by Waldenstrom. After further improvement of the technique to include precipitation in gel (immuno-electrophoresis), first published by Grabar and Williams in 1953 [11], J.F. Heremans in 1959 proposed the term "immunoglobulins" for all these related proteins after his discovery of IgA [12, 13]. In 1966, the fourth isotype of immunoglobulin, IgD, was described from a myeloma protein by Rowe and Fahey [14] and the last isotype, IgE, was identified from patient sera by the Ishizakas and colleagues in the United States and Johansson and Bennich in Sweden in 1966–1967 [15–17].

Ehrlich's side chain hypothesis proposed that antibody molecules were able to bind with high specificity to antigens, but as the work of immunologists proceeded, it became more and more baffling as to how such a vast number of molecular shapes could be produced. In 1940, the American chemist Linus Pauling proposed a physicochemical mechanism called the instructive theory of antibody formation to explain what was beginning to seem a near infinite variety in chemical compounds to which antibodies could bind [18]. According to this theory, antigen forms a template around which antibody forms a specific configuration. It took over 40 years for the elegant recombinatorial mechanism of immunoglobulin diversity to be revealed with the demonstration of DNA recombination in the immunoglobulin kappa locus by Hozumi and Tonegawa, a stunning achievement for which Susumu Tonegawa received the Nobel Prize in 1987 [19, 20]. In 2004, Zeev Pancer and Max Cooper discovered that lampreys, primitive jawless chordates that lack immunoglobulin genes, instead have their own combinatorial immune system that is markedly similar in organization to that of higher vertebrates but is composed of gene segments coding for leucine-rich repeats instead of the characteristic immunoglobulin-like domains [21]. The astounding parallel evolutionary development of this genetic system for antibody diversity suggests that there must be few if any other solutions to serve this important function.

ImmunoglobulIns Structure

The immunoglobulins are heterodimeric glycoproteins composed of two disulfide-linked heavy chains, each associated through disulfide linkages with a light chain forming a Y-shaped molecular configuration (Fig. 3.1). They are composed of repeating globular immunoglobulin-like domains, a motif that forms a large super-family found in many other proteins [23]. The basic structure of the immunoglobulin domain is a disulfide-linked sandwich of two beta sheets made up of antiparallel strands (Fig. 3.2). Digestion of immunoglobulin with the enzyme papain, a protease derived from the fruit of the papaya tree, results in the release of the light chain-bound arms, termed Fab fragments, which contain the antigen binding activity, and the remainder of the dimeric heavy chains, termed the Fc fragment, which encompasses the Fc receptor and complement-activating effector functions. The molecular weights, glycosylation, Fc binding properties and the ability to activate complement vary with immunoglobulin isotype and subclass (Table 3.1). Differences in the amino acid sequences give rise to other properties such as the number and location of N-linked glycosylation sites, which affect Fc effector functions and can provide protection from bacterial proteases in the lumen of the respiratory and gastrointestinal tracts, and disulfide bridges joining the heavy chains at the hinge region, the region joining the constant and variable domains of the heavy chains. IgM and (variably) IgA are polymeric, composed of (usually) five and two complete immunoglobulin molecules, respectively, that are joined in the final stage of intracellular assembly by the addition by disulfide bridges of a single 15 kD molecule called the J chain that also serves as the ligand for the polymeric Ig receptor (pIgR) at the basal surface of epithelial cells (Fig. 3.2). This receptor mediates the intracellular passage of bound polymeric IgM and IgA across the mucosal epithelium into the lumen [31].

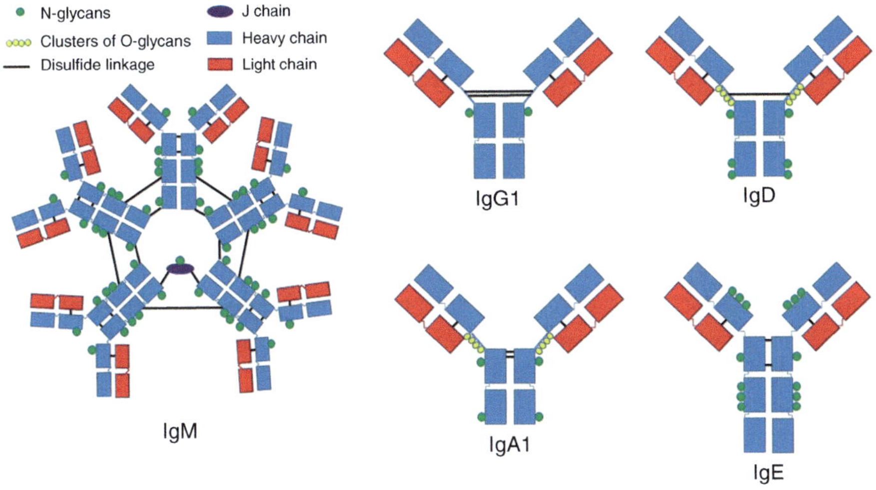

Fig. 3.1 General structure of the five immunoglobulin isotypes (modified from Arnold, 2007 [22])

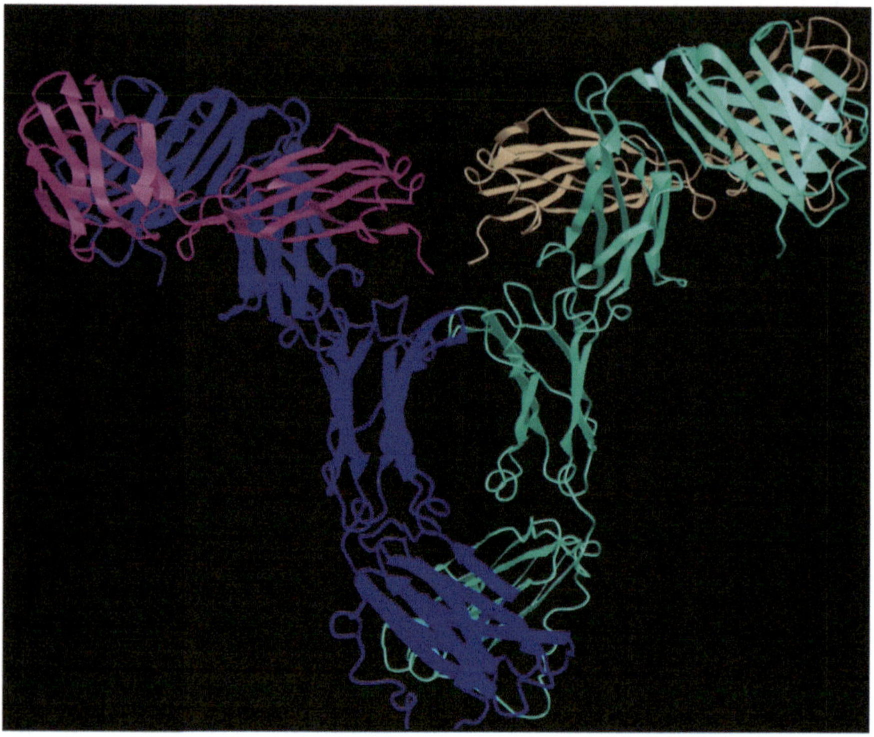

Fig. 3.2 Ribbon diagram of the crystal structure of IgA2 [24, 25]. The heavy chains are shown in blue and green and the light chains in pink and brown. The structural similarities of the 4–5 immunoglobulin domains in each heavy chain and the two in each light chain are evident

The extracellular portion of the pIgR is cleaved and remains associated with the secretory IgA and IgM as the secretory component when they enter the secretions.

Immunoglobulins Function

IgG, the isotype of immunoglobulin that makes up the bulk of serum immunoglobulins was the first to be identified because of its dominance of the gamma region of the serum electrophoretic profile, hence its original designation as gamma globulin. There are four IgG subclasses, two of which activate complement well (IgG1 and IgG3), one of which activates complement poorly (IgG2), and one of which not at all (IgG4) (Table 3.1). IgG subclass-specific production of antibodies is regulated by cytokines, particularly Interferon γ and IL-4, a process better understood in mice than humans at present [32, 33]. IgG4, in particular, has interesting properties that are worthy of comment. In 1974, three different groups published the observation that there was an association between a late rise in IgG4 and the development of

Table 3.1 Immunoglobulin properties [22, 26–30]

Isotype	Subclass	Mol. wt. (kD)	Serum concentration (mg/mL)	Serum half-life (days)	Complement activation	Carbohydrate content	Polymer
IgM		970	0.5–1.5	5	+++	12%	5
IgD		170	0–0.4	3	–	11%	
IgG						3%	
	IgG1	146	5–12	21	++		
	IgG2	146	2–6	21	+		
	IgG3	165	0.5–1.0	7	++		
	IgG4	146	0.2–1.0	21	–		
IgA				6		10%	
	IgA1	160	0.5–2.0	5–9	–		1–2
	IgA2	160	0–0.2	4–5	–		1–2
IgE		190	0–0.002	2	–	12%	

Refs: Middleton Ch 5, Metabolic properties of human IgA subclasses Morell 1973; Metabolic properties of IgG subclasses in man Morell 1970
Carbohydrate content: Muller-Eberhard HJ, Kunkel HG.1959 PMID: 13639270; Cohen S, Porter RB. 1964. PMID: 14333020. Arnold JN 2007. PMID:17029568.

tolerance in patients receiving allergen-specific immunotherapy [34]. It is now known that like IgE, IgG4 is dependent upon IL-4/IL-13 for production and as a consequence tends to be produced in response to nonbacterial antigens [35]. Uniquely, IgG4 undergoes a dynamic process of half-antibody formation, reforming to produce heterodimers with different Fab antigen binding specificities [36]. This process, termed "Fab arm exchange," has also been observed to occur in therapeutic monoclonal antibodies, potentially impairing the desired therapeutic effect or even inducing unwanted effects [27]. The functional consequence of a monovalent antibody is that it can no longer crosslink antigens forming a lattice/immune complex, and it can even potentially break up existing complexes. Thus, the normal function of IgG4 appears to be an anti-inflammatory effect, particularly on Type 2 inflammation. For example, IgG4 antibodies have been found to represent 50–95% of anti-filarial IgG antibodies [25]. Nevertheless, there is one inflammatory and enigmatic disorder which is linked to excessive local production of IgG4: IgG4-related disease [37], an entity that will be described in detail elsewhere in this volume (Chap. 15).

In concert with its antigen binding functions, IgG carries out a complex array of effector functions through its Fc domain which, in addition to the activation of complement by three of the four subclasses (Table 3.1), are mediated in part by a group of receptors belonging to the immunoglobulin superfamily (FcγR1, FcγRIIA, FcγRIIB, FcγRIIIA), two of which (FcgRIIB and FcgRIII) have isoforms that add a further degree of complexity. A second class of receptors are C-type lectins (CD23 and CD209/DC-SIGN). Although IgG has the lowest percentage of glycosylation of any of the five isotypes, the relative affinities for different IgG subclasses of both of these groups of receptors is modulated by the nature and extent of Fc glycosylation, particularly fucosylation and sialylation, which can vary considerably among different individuals [38]. FcRn is an MHC class I–related Fc-receptor for IgG that performs a similar function to that of the pIgR with IgA and IgM, transporting IgG across epithelial boundaries and, by continuously recycling IgG, extending the half-life of the different isotypes [39, 40]. FcRn binds to no other isotypes except IgG and is expressed in placenta and lung but not in the gastrointestinal tract [39]. A further discussion of these receptor-mediated effector functions is outside the scope of this chapter.

IgM, together with IgD, serves as the surface receptor for nascent and mature B cells and without IgD for "switched" and memory IgM B cells. With the deletion by alternate splicing of the exon coding for the transmembrane domain, secreted soluble IgM is produced [41]. Because IgM antibodies are the first isotype of immunoglobulin produced during an immune response, they are often useful in the diagnosis of acute infections. IgM antibodies typically have relatively low affinity, but because of their polymeric structure they have relatively high avidity. Similarly, because of the inherent proximity of the C1q binding regions of the Fc domains, activation of complement through the classical pathway by IgM antibodies is robust. Because pentameric IgM molecules contain the J chain, like IgA they are transported across mucosal borders by the pIgR. However, IgM plasma cells are typically much less abundant along mucosal surfaces, and thus by far the larger amount of immunoglobulin secreted into the mucosal lumen is IgA. A receptor for IgM has been described and is expressed on T and B lymphocytes where it has been reported to modulate T cell function and affect T-B cell interactions [42].

IgA, the third isotype to be described, has primarily an anti-inflammatory role in controlling interactions with the environment through its dominant presence in the mucosal secretions. It does not activate complement and serves to block microbial and antigen interactions with the mucosal immune system, limiting pathogen invasion and antigen-mediated sensitization. Although only a minor component of serum immunoglobulin (10–15%), IgA comprises the bulk of immunoglobulin produced daily by the immune system, some 3 g per day in the adult human, more than all the other immunoglobulin isotypes combined [43]. Two thirds of the IgA produced daily is dimeric or tetrameric and is transported across mucosal surfaces into the secretions by the pIgR. Although the basic structure of the two IgA subclasses in humans is similar, there are differences in the location and extent of N- and O-linked glycosylation, in the specificity for certain types of antigens, and in effector functions [22, 44]. The relative proportion of IgA in different mucosal sites varies considerably. In the gastrointestinal tract, the largest proportion of immunoglobulin is IgA, with some IgM and virtually no IgG while the respiratory tract contains equivalent amounts of IgA and IgG with some IgM and IgD. As mentioned previously, the transport of IgG into the respiratory secretions occurs via FcRn, which is present in the lung mucosa but not in the gut [39]. IgA1 comprises about 85% of serum IgA, and the majority of IgA in secretions, except the colon and the vagina, is also IgA1 [44]. Serum IgA is derived principally from IgA plasma cells in the bone marrow, while mucosal IgA is secreted by IgA plasma cells in the mucosae. The relatively low serum IgA concentration is a function of its relatively short half-life (4–9 days) compared to IgG (generally about 21 days) (Table 3.1).

IgD, the fourth immunoglobulin isotype to be identified, remains the most enigmatic of the five. Produced by alternative splicing of the common RNA precursor that also includes IgM, it is present on the surface of naive B cells. Antigen-induced antibody responses are intact in IgD-deficient mice but careful scrutiny reveals that they have less efficient affinity maturation, the process that generates higher affinity antibody in germinal centers through somatic hypermutation of the portion of the variable domain that forms the antigen binding site [45]. Despite the fact that IgD is highly expressed on mature naive B cells, secreted IgD antibody makes up only a small fraction of the serum immunoglobulin (0.25%) compared to IgG (75%), IgA (10–15%), IgM (5–10%), and IgE (0.002%) [31]. Intriguingly, IgM-IgD+ B cells utilize the lambda light chain, suggesting that there is a yet to be defined differentiation pathway in which they are selected from IgM+IgD+lambda+ precursors [45]. IgD does not activate complement, and there is no clear evidence that the Fc portion of the molecule has an effector function although there is some functional evidence that IgD can bind to T-cells, basophils, monocytes, and mast cells, suggesting that a specialized receptor may exist [46]. It seems clear that the full importance of this immunoglobulin isotype has yet to be defined because it has been conserved throughout the history of vertebrate evolution from the cartilaginous fish through mammals [45].

IgE, the last of the immunoglobulin isotypes to be identified, can also be detected in respiratory and gastrointestinal secretions, particularly in the presence of allergy or parasitic infections. It seems clear that the principal evolutionary function of IgE and Type 2 immune responses lies in host defense against parasitic infestation. Isotype switching to IgE is dependent on IL-4/IL-13. A considerable body of clinical and experimental evidence exists concerning the details of how IgE functions in binding to the multimeric high affinity Fc receptor, FcεRI, primarily on mast cells and basophils, and how aggregation of that receptor by antigen augments Type 2 immune responses. Like IgM, IgE differs from the other immunoglobulin isotypes in possessing a fourth heavy chain constant domain (Fig. 3.1). IgE is the most heavily glycosylated of all the isotypes and although the low affinity receptor CD23 is a member of the C-type lectin family, binding of CD23 to IgE does not involve carbohydrate. Instead CD23 binds to amino acids in the region between the third and fourth heavy chain constant domains where it sterically inhibits binding by FcεRI [39]. While the function of the high affinity receptor is to augment Type 2 immune responses by inducing activation of cells bearing the receptor and the release of Type 2 mediators, the function of CD23 is at least partly to down-regulate IgE production by B cells [47].

The kappa and lambda light chains, which are covalently linked by disulfide bonds to the first heavy chain constant domain, form the other half of the antigen binding site through their rearranged variable domains. As occurs with heavy chain rearrangement, expression of light chain genes is sequential, regulated, and exhibits a distinctive process known as allelic exclusion, in which only one allele among several possible is translated to form a functional gene product. The other allele continues to be transcribed but does not form a functional protein because of lack of or incomplete rearrangement [48]. This exclusion of other alleles is essential in order for the B cell to maintain monospecificity of its antigen receptor and secreted immunoglobulin product, a property characterized by the "one B cell – one antibody" rule inherent in Burnet's clonal selection theory of the adaptive immune system [49]. Following successful rearrangement of the μ heavy chain, the heavy chain forms a complex with two surrogate light chain proteins encoded within the Igλ locus at chromosome 22q11.2 (λ5 and V_{preB}), which together possess substantial homology to λ light chains and cover the hypervariable HCDR3 region on the heavy chain, thus preventing antigen-driven clonal selection before light chain rearrangement occurs [50]. Rearrangement of the Igκ locus on chromosome 2p11.2 proceeds first, and if a successful rearrangement of either allele that can pair with the μ heavy chain does not occur, the cell switches to rearrangement of the Igλ genes [48]. Ultimately, if the cell is unable to undergo a productive rearrangement of heavy and light chain genes to create a functional B cell receptor, it undergoes apoptosis.

Conclusion

Immunoglobulins represent the humoral arm of the adaptive immune response. Defects in the process of B cell differentiation and selection to produce protective immunoglobulins of the appropriate isotypes for host defense are responsible for a wide array of diseases. Deficiency of specific antibody production is the most common manifestation of primary immune deficiency while production of autoreactive antibodies is a common mechanism for autoimmunity. The protean manifestations of disease caused by unregulated production of immunoglobulins by neoplastic B cells and plasma cells comprise a vast and complex area of medicine and will be the focus of the remainder of this book.

References

1. Black CA. A brief history of the discovery of the immunoglobulins and the origin of the modern immunoglobulin nomenclature. Immunol Cell Biol. 1997;75:65–8. [PMID: 9046436].
2. Klein J. Immunology, the science of self-nonself discrimination. New York: Wiley; 1982. 687 p.
3. Kaufmann SH. Remembering Emil von Behring: from tetanus treatment to antibody cooperation with phagocytes. mBio. 2017;8:e00117. [PMID: 28246359].
4. Valent P, Groner B, Schumacher U, et al. Paul Ehrlich (1854-1915) and his contributions to the foundation and birth of translational medicine. J Innate Immun. 2016;8:111–20. [PMID: 26845587].
5. Cohen SG, Zelaya-Quesada M. Prausnitz and Küstner phenomenon: the P-K reaction. J Allergy Clin Immunol. 2004;114:705–10. [PMID: 15356578].
6. Marrack JR. The chemistry of antigens and antibodies. London: Medical Research Council; 1934.
7. Tiselius A, Kabat EA. Electrophoresis of immune serum. Science. 1938;87:416–7. [PMID: 17829941].
8. Kyle RA, Shampo MA. Theodor Svedberg and the ultracentrifuge. Mayo Clin Proc. 1997;72:830. [PMID: 9294529].
9. Waldenstrom J. Incipient myleomatosis or 'essential' hyperglobulinemia with fibrinogenopenia—a new syndrome? Acta Med Scand. 1944;67:216–47.

10. Wallenius G, Trautman R, Kunkel HG, Franklin EC. Ultracentrifugal studies of major non-lipide electrophoretic components of normal human serum. J Biol Chem. 1957;225:253–67. [PMID: 13416235].
11. Grabar P, Williams CA. [Method permitting the combined study of the electrophoretic and the immunochemical properties of protein mixtures; application to blood serum]. Biochim Biophys Acta. 1953;10:193–4. [PMID: 13041735].
12. Heremans JF. Immunochemical studies on protein pathology. The immunoglobulin concept. Clin Chim Acta. 1959;4:639–46. [PMID: 14401240].
13. Heremans JF, Heremans MT, Schultze HE. Isolation and description of a few properties of the beta 2A-globulin of human serum. Clin Chim Acta. 1959;4:96–102. [PMID: 13629856].
14. Rowe DS, Fahey JL. A new class of human immunoglobulins. II. Normal serum IgD. J Exp Med. 1965;121:185–99. [PMID: 14253483].
15. Ishizaka K, Ishizaka T, Hornbrook MM. Physico-chemical properties of human reaginic antibody. IV. Presence of a unique immunoglobulin as a carrier of reaginic activity. J Immunol. 1966;97:75–85. [PMID: 4162440].
16. Ishizaka K, Ishizaka T, Hornbrook MM. Physicochemical properties of reaginic antibody. V. Correlation of reaginic activity with gamma-E-globulin antibody. J Immunol. 1966;97:840–53. [PMID: 4163008].
17. Johansson SG, Bennich H. Immunological studies of an atypical (myeloma) immunoglobulin. Immunology. 1967;13:381–94. [PMID: 4168094].
18. Pauling L. A theory of the structure and process of formation of antibodies. J Am Chem Soc. 1940;62:2643–57.
19. Gearhart PJ. The birth of molecular immunology. J Immunol. 2004;173:4259. [PMID: 15383552].
20. Hozumi N, Tonegawa S. Evidence for somatic rearrangement of immunoglobulin genes coding for variable and constant regions. 1976 [classical article]. J Immunol. 2004;173:4260–4. [PMID: 15383553].
21. Pancer Z, Amemiya CT, Ehrhardt GR, et al. Somatic diversification of variable lymphocyte receptors in the agnathan sea lamprey. Nature. 2004;430:174–80. [PMID: 15241406].
22. Arnold JN, Wormald MR, Sim RB, et al. The impact of glycosylation on the biological function and structure of human immunoglobulins. Annu Rev Immunol. 2007;25:21–50. [PMID: 17029568].
23. Barclay AN. Membrane proteins with immunoglobulin-like domains—a master superfamily of interaction molecules. Semin Immunol. 2003;15:215–23. [PMID: 14690046].
24. Madej T, Lanczycki CJ, Zhang D, et al. MMDB and VAST+: tracking structural similarities between macromolecular complexes. Nucleic Acids Res. 2014;42:D297–303. [PMID: 24319143].
25. Furtado PB, Whitty PW, Robertson A, et al. Solution structure determination of monomeric human IgA2 by X-ray and neutron scattering, analytical ultracentrifugation and constrained modelling: a comparison with monomeric human IgA1. J Mol Biol. 2004;338:921–41. [PMID: 15111057].
26. Jelinek DF, Li JT. Immunoglobulin structure and function. In: Adkinson NF, Bochner BS, Burks AW, et al., editors. Middleton's allergy : principles and practice. 8th ed. Philadelphia: Elsevier/Saunders; 2014. p. 30–44.
27. Morell A, Skvaril F, Noseda G, Barandun S. Metabolic properties of human IgA subclasses. Clin Exp Immunol. 1973;13:521–8. [PMID: 4717094].
28. Morell A, Terry WD, Waldmann TA. Metabolic properties of IgG subclasses in man. J Clin Invest. 1970;49:673–80. [PMID: 5443170].
29. Muller-Eberhard HJ, Kunkel HG. Ultracentrifugal characteristics and carbohydrate content of macromolecular gamma-globulins. Clin Chim Acta. 1959;4:252–8. [PMID: 13639270].
30. Cohen S, Porter RB. Structure and biological activity of immunoglobulins. Adv Immunol. 1964;27:287–349. [PMID: 14333020].
31. Wei H, Wang JY. Role of polymeric immunoglobulin receptor in IgA and IgM transcytosis. Int J Mol Sci. 2021;22. [PMID: 33668983].

32. Snapper CM, Finkelman FD, Paul WE. Differential regulation of IgG1 and IgE synthesis by interleukin 4. J Exp Med. 1988;167:183–96.
33. Snapper CM, Peschel C, Paul WE. IFN-gamma stimulates IgG2a secretion by murine B cells stimulated with bacterial lipopolysaccharide. J Immunol. 1988;140:2121–7. [PMID: 3127461].
34. Aalberse RC, Stapel SO, Schuurman J, Rispens T. Immunoglobulin G4: an odd antibody. Clin Exp Allergy. 2009;39:469–77. [PMID: 19222496].
35. Agresti A, Vercelli D. Analysis of gamma4 germline transcription in human B cells. Int Arch Allergy Immunol. 1999;118:279–81. [PMID: 10224410].
36. van der Neut KM, Schuurman J, Losen M, et al. Anti-inflammatory activity of human IgG4 antibodies by dynamic Fab arm exchange. Science. 2007;317:1554–7. [PMID: 17872445].
37. Stone JH. What do the IgG4-related disease (IgG4-RD) classification criteria tell us about the nature of IgG4-RD? Presse Med. 2020;49:104020. [PMID: 32229230].
38. Wang TT, Ravetch JV. Functional diversification of IgGs through Fc glycosylation. J Clin Invest. 2019;129:3492–8. [PMID: 31478910].
39. Spiekermann GM, Finn PW, Ward ES, et al. Receptor-mediated immunoglobulin G transport across mucosal barriers in adult life: functional expression of FcRn in the mammalian lung. J Exp Med. 2002;196:303–10. [PMID: 12163559].
40. Patel DD, Bussel JB. Neonatal Fc receptor in human immunity: function and role in therapeutic intervention. J Allergy Clin Immunol. 2020;146:467–78. [PMID: 32896307].
41. Yabas M, Elliott H, Hoyne GF. The role of alternative splicing in the control of immune homeostasis and cellular differentiation. Int J Mol Sci. 2015;17:3. [PMID: 26703587].
42. Meryk A, Pangrazzi L, Hagen M, et al. Fcμ receptor as a costimulatory molecule for T cells. Cell Rep. 2019;26:2681–91.e5. [PMID: 30840890].
43. Kaetzel CS, Mestecky J, Johansen FE. Two cells, one antibody: the discovery of the cellular origins and transport of secretory IgA. J Immunol. 2017;198:1765–7. [PMID: 28223403].
44. Mestecky J. Antibody-dependent passive protection of mucosal surfaces. Hum Vaccin Immunother. 2022;18:1899549. [PMID: 33939589].
45. Chen K, Cerutti A. The function and regulation of immunoglobulin D. Curr Opin Immunol. 2011;23:345–52. [PMID: 21353515].
46. Nguyen TG. The therapeutic implications of activated immune responses via the enigmatic immunoglobulin D. Int Rev Immunol. 2022;41:107–22. [PMID: 33410368].
47. Engeroff P, Vogel M. The role of CD23 in the regulation of allergic responses. Allergy. 2021;76:1981–9. [PMID: 33378583].
48. Vettermann C, Schlissel MS. Allelic exclusion of immunoglobulin genes: models and mechanisms. Immunol Rev. 2010;237:22–42. [PMID: 20727027].
49. Burnet FM. A modification of Jerne's theory of antibody production using the concept of clonal selection. Aust J Sci. 1957;20:67–9.
50. Schroeder HW Jr, Cavacini L. Structure and function of immunoglobulins. J Allergy Clin Immunol. 2010;125:S41–52. [PMID: 20176268].

Chapter 4
The Bone Marrow as a Hotbed for Plasma Cell Activation

Aikaterini Poulaki, Stavroula Giannouli, and Michael Voulgarelis

Abbreviations

Ab	Antibody
Ag	Antigen
APRIL	A proliferation inducing ligand
APS	Antiphospholipid syndrome
ASC	Antibody secreting cell
ATP	Adenosine triphosphate
BAFF	B cell activating factor
BCL2	B-cell lymphoma 2
BCL6	B-cell lymphoma 6
BCMA	B-cell maturation antigen/tumor necrosis factor receptor superfamily member 17
BCR	B cell receptor
Blimp1	B-lymphocyte-induced maturation protein 1
BM	Bone marrow
BMSC	Bone marrow stromal cell
CD138	Cluster of differentiation 138

A. Poulaki · M. Voulgarelis (✉)
Department of Pathophysiology, School of Medicine, National and Kapodistrian University of Athens, Athens, Greece
e-mail: mvoulgar@med.uoa.gr

S. Giannouli
2nd Department of Internal Medicine, School of Medicine, National and Kapodistrian University of Athens, Athens, Greece
e-mail: stgiannouli@gail.com

© The Author(s), under exclusive license to Springer Nature Switzerland AG 2022
G. Ragab et al. (eds.), *Paraproteinemia and Related Disorders*,
https://doi.org/10.1007/978-3-031-10131-1_4

CD19	Cluster of differentiation 19
CD20	Cluster of differentiation 20
CD27	Cluster of differentiation 27
CD28	Cluster of differentiation 28
CD38	Cluster of differentiation 38
CD80	Cluster of differentiation 80
CD86	Cluster of differentiation 86
CXCL12	C-X-C motif chemokine ligand 12
CXCR4	C-X-C motif chemokine receptor 4
DC	Dendritic cell
ENPP1	Ectonucleotide pyrophosphatase/phosphodiesterase 1
ER	Endoplasmic reticulum
FN-1	Fibronectin
GC	Germinal center
GLUT	Glucose transporter
HSC	Hematopoietic stem cell
ICAM	Intercellular adhesion molecule
IDO	Indoleamine-pyrrole 2,3-dioxygenase
IgE	Immunoglobulin E
IL6	Interleukin 6
IRF4	Interferon regulatory factor 4
IRF8	Interferon regulatory factor 8
LLPC	Long lived plasma cell
LPS	Lipopolysaccharide
MBC	Memory B cell
Mcl1	Myeloid cell leukemia-1
MGUS	Monoclonal gammopathy of undetermined significance
MHC II	Major histocompatibility complex II
MM	Multiple myeloma
mTOR	Mammalian target of rapamycin
mTORC1	Mammalian target of rapamycin complex 1
NF-κB	nuclear factor kappa-light-chain-enhancer of activated B cells
OXPHOS	Oxidative phosphorylation
Pax5	Paired box 5
Pb	Plasmablast
PC	Plasma cell
PD1	Programmed death 1
PDL1	Programmed death-ligand 1
PI3K	Phosphoinositide 3-kinase
rMSC	Reticula mesenchymal stromal cell
ROS	Reactive oxygen species
SLE	Systemic lupus erythematosus
Slp76	Lymphocyte cytosolic protein 2 or SH2 domain containing leukocyte protein of 76 kDa
SLPC	Short lived plasma cell

STAT3	Signal transducer and activator of transcription 3
TCA	Tricarboxylic acid cycle
TNF-a	Tumor necrosis factor alpha
UPR	Unfolded protein response
VCAM	Vascular cell adhesion protein 1
XBP1	X-box binding protein 1
YWHAZ	14-3-3 protein zeta/delta

Introduction

Apart from its role as the primary lymphoid organ, the bone marrow (BM) also functions as a secondary one. Thus, aside from hematopoiesis and conditional initial priming of the hematopoietic stem cell (HSC) towards the lymphoid and thereafter the B-cell lineage, the effects of homing of the B-lymphocytes within it expand much further [1, 2]. Primarily affected from this interaction are the terminally differentiated B cells, both memory B cells (MBCs) yet most importantly plasma cells (PCs). For the latter, homing within the BM might eventually change the fate of a newly developed plasmablast (Pb) and instead of it forming a short-lived plasma cell (SLPC) guides it towards a long-lived phenotype with a subsequent dependency on the BM microenvironment for longevity and survival [3]. The foundation for this dependency lies on the ability of the BM microenvironment to attract the precursor cell subset, the Pb, allowing the PC differentiation to be complete and most importantly facilitate its long-term survival [3, 4]. On the other hand, the newly formed and thereafter BM residing long-lived plasma cells (LLPC) themselves interact with their surrounding niche and this ambiguous relationship eventually allows for a terminally differentiated otherwise transient cell to survive without dividing, for even decades in acquired quiescence [5–7].

Apart from homing the BM micro-niche which offers essential trophic signals and confers extensive bioenergetic reprogramming, the prerequisites for B cell to LLPC differentiation remain largely unknown [8]. According to the established knowledge, only Pbs that have differentiated through the germinal center (GC) reaction, namely against a T-dependent antigen are capable of homing the BM and becoming LLPCs [9]. Although scattered evidence exists that extra-GC Pbs against T-independent stimuli are capable of long-term survival, no solid experimental work has been until now published either confirming or dismissing this theory [10–12]. It is also unclear if there exists a differential ability of longevity dependent on the type of antigen (Ag) against which the Pb is specialized. It has been proposed that monovalent Ags such as single proteins, for example, tetanus toxoid, elicit shorter term longevity in PCs than multivalent Ags, for instance [13, 14]. Theoretically, given that most self-antigens are monovalent such an evolutionary advantage would offer an extra protective hindrance against autoimmunity so that if autoreactive Pbs were to form they would be extremely transient. The theory could also explain the necessity of repeated vaccinations for tetanus and the impressive longevity of anti-measles LLPC against the structurally complex viral for longer than lifetime [15]. Besides, LLPC formation happens at the very late stages of the GC reaction long after memory B cells have formed in order for the maximum specificity of the secreted Ab to be achieved [16, 17].

While in its infancy, research around the BM microenvironmental niches has already made a great impact on the way we consider physiology, pathophysiology, and therapeutics. The potentials though of such microenvironmental influence and especially that of the BM on the residing cells particularly the PCs are only now starting to be investigated. Moreover, it is now clear that such relationships which develop between pathogenic PC and their niche increase their resistance to therapeutic interventions hindering effective treatment of all PC-mediated diseases [18]. In this chapter, we aim to summarize and critically present the acquired knowledge surrounding the relatively novel and expanding field of the effects of a healthy BM microenvironment on the PC fate, the components of the LLPC niche as well as the biological processes allowing for the BM to function as a selective/supportive "hotbed" for long-term PC survival and immunologic memory. Special tribute will be paid to the recycling of LLPCs during infection and the ability of the LLPC pool to adapt to newly acquired antigens expanding their antibody (Ab) repertoire. We will also briefly discuss the importance of the BM PC niche with regard to the major PC-driven diseases, monoclonal gammopathy of undetermined significance (MGUS), multiple myeloma (MM), and antibody-mediated autoimmune diseases, including systemic lupus erythematosus (SLE).

The Bone Marrow as a "Hotbed" for Plasma Cells in Health. The LLPC Niche

LLPC are responsible for the baseline Ab titers of immune humans and do not need constant antigenic stimulation to survive [19, 20]. They are terminally differentiated Ab-secreting $CD19^{-}$ $CD38^{high}CD138^{+}$ BM residing PCs. Their surface B-cell receptors (BCRs) and major histocompatibility complexes type II (MHCII) are both downregulated [21], hence they are practically insensitive to external Ags.

Cellular Components of the LLPC Niche. Attracting and Maintaining the LLPCs

The first step in understanding the BM PC niche is to describe its cellular components. To begin with, no single factor has been established as absolutely essential for LLPCs survival, thus the idea of their niche should be considered as a whole of cells and soluble factors. Many different stromal and hematopoietic cells along with their secretome cooperate to initially attract, then engage and thereafter retain the Pbs that will eventually transform into LLPCs, constantly offering them an essential mixture of survival intermediates [22]. The general principle governing niche organization is work allotment. A stable meshwork of specialized bone marrow stromal cells (BMSCs) and the reticular mesenchymal stromal cells (rMSCs) attract the circulating CXCR4+ Pbs by expressing and secreting a mixture of chemokines, including but not limited to the CXCR4 ligand, CXCL12 [23]. Interestingly, contrary to their secretome these CXCL12/VCAM+ MSCs proved not to be essential for PC longevity but instead create a docking site for circulating Pbs to attach to [24]. In this process, several other integrins collaborate with CXCR4+/CXCL12 to stabilize the BMSC-PC interaction [8, 23].

Out of the rMSC secretome both activating, for example, APRIL, as well as binding, fibronectin (FN-1) along with metabolic modifiers and antiapoptotic mediators such as the protein YWHAZ regulate the fate of adjacent PCs [22, 25]. Of note, YWHAZ is a 4–3-3ζ/δ cytoplasmic protein with complex action that favors longevity of LLPCs through an mTORC1-dependent reshaping of their bioenergetic state. It thus induces prosurvival signaling through the BCL2 family member Mcl1 [25]. Such a high level of cooperation exists that LLPCs have, for instance, upregulated the surface marker CD138 (cluster of differentiation 138) to bind the rMSCs-secreted FN-1 and anchor them in close proximity to rMSCs [26]. In fact, it is now established that rMSCs' numerical limitation, comprising approximately 0.001–0.1% of nucleated stromal cells, limits the healthy BM LLPC capacity [25, 27]. It is suggested that cohabitation with the rMSCs allows the LLPCs to receive their secretory feedback and quiescently survive in the massive BM span something otherwise impossible given the confined number of both populations. The intrinsic cellular requirements of such quiescence and the contribution of the BM microniche for the Pb to LLPC metamorphosis will be further analyzed in the next section.

Aside from the BMSCs, a variety of accessory transient hematopoietic cells support the extended LLPC life span. To name the most important of them, eosinophils, megakaryocytes, and myeloid progenitors which under normal conditions secrete APRIL and IL-6 [8, 22]. APRIL from both the BMSCs and the hematopoietic cells along with BAFF and to a much lesser extent in the healthy state TNF-alpha are all differentially secreted by niche components. They all stimulate the surface PC receptor, BCMA adding to the prosurvival effect of the niche [23, 28]. Moreover, in the case of APRIL, it is proved to cross activate the LLPCs CD138 receptor through interaction with its side chains and therefore increase the prosurvival (Mcl1 mediated) signal it transduces [26, 28, 29]. LLPCs have a profound dependency on Mcl1 for survival [30]. Out of all accessory niche cells, eosinophils are most vital for LLPC maintenance likely through production of the largest amounts of IL-6 and APRIL [22]. Given their transient nature though, it is not surprising that even eosinophils are not indispensable for memory plasma cell quiescence. Impressively enough combined deprivation of both IL-6 and the BCMA ligands, APRIL with or without BAFF/TNFa, can severely compromise the in vitro survival ability of human memory plasma cells [22, 24, 25, 31]. Such essential combinations are continuously being identified and their description will contribute to novel therapeutic target identification against the LLPC-driven pathologies.

The list of LLPC trophic agents/pathways is rapidly expanding. Several interactions that improve the life span and Ab production of either human or mouse LLPCs are being described. Maybe the most ambitious of them is the CD28-CD80/CD86 interaction and the CD28-induced PC intracellular reprogramming. Engagement of the CD28 receptor on Pbs with the CD80/CD86 receptor of bystander niche dendritic cells (DCs) is essential for their bioenergetic reshaping that culminates in the LLPC phenotype. Activation of the CD28-induced pathways impressively increases the effect of CD28-CD80/CD86 interaction on PCs while causing upregulation of the latter receptors on the niche DCs, kind of a self-stimulatory loop. Moreover, SLPCs seem incapable of unlocking the CD28-induced profile being in a way unable to unlock niche beneficial program, which makes the CD28-CD80/CD86 a turning point for the LLPC fate [32]. Ectonucleotide pyrophosphatase/phosphodiesterase 1 (ENPP1), a transmembrane glycoprotein with ATP degrading activity has also been identified to positively affect the ASC to LLPC transition in that its deficiency markedly increases SLPC numbers at the expense of BM LLPCs in mice [33]. The exact mechanism by which ATP degradation by ENPP1 promotes LLPC survival remains elusive. One possibility is that PPi produced through ATP hydrolysis inhibits bone mineralization preserving the niche space. ENPP1 is also known to regulate glucose metabolism in pancreatic cells. Enhancement of glycolysis and reduction of exogenous ATP-induced oxygen consumption in LPS-induced Pbs has also been associated with ENPP1 and leads to the LLPC phenotype [3, 33, 34].

To sum it up, it is now more than ever evident that the biology of LLPCs is tightly interwoven with the BM microenvironmental niche and that the niche itself is a balanced medley of transient cellular components with overlapping secretomes. This type of organization ensures maximal efficiency as no specific ingredient is absolutely indispensable for LLPC maintenance and can be substituted by bystander cellular presence and function. The question arising at this point is the etiology of this uniqueness of the BM to form the LLPC micro-niche. It is likely that apart from the niche itself, the oxygenation and nutritional state of the BM per se largely impact the LLPC longevity. The cellular components of the BM micro-niche along with the major interactions regulating the LLPC inside it are summarized in Fig. 4.1.

Intrinsic Cellular Requirements for Longevity. The LLPC Niche Reshapes the PC Bioenergetic Profile

The life span of an LLPC extends from months in vitro and in vivo mouse models to several years or even decades in stochastic human models while their short-lived counterparts, SLPCs, are known to survive for a mere 3–5 days [15]. This remarkable difference between two cell populations that are or at least seem similar yet possess profound different capabilities is achieved through extensive intracellular reprogramming. In order to better understand the requirements for such longevity, we will briefly assess the Pb to either SLPC or LLPC differentiation process. In this

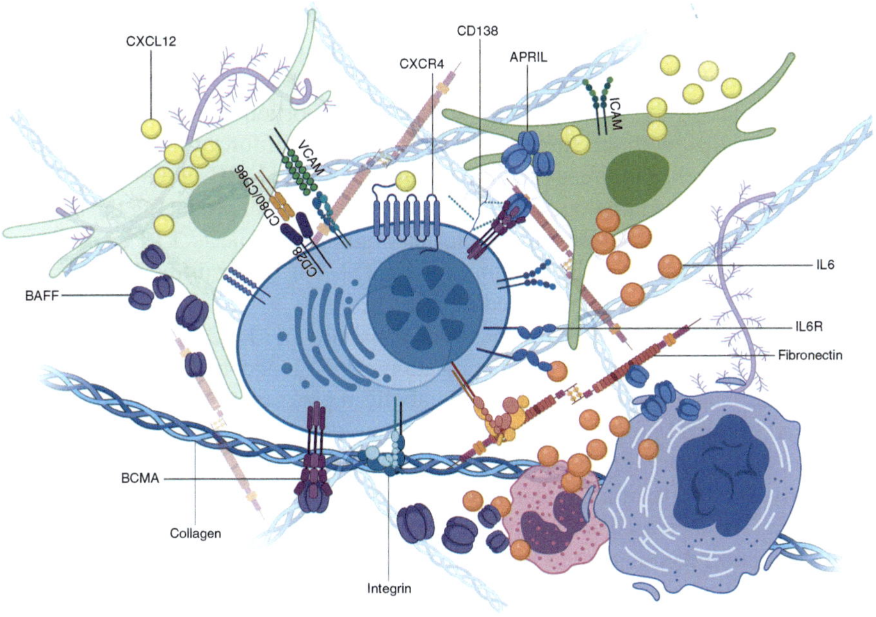

Fig. 4.1 Cellular component of the LLPC BM niche. Several cells contribute to the homing, retention, and survival of LLPCs in the BM niche. Stromal cells provide the adequate docking site for passing Pbs both through secretion of chemokines (CXCL12) and extracellular matrix (Fibronectin-FN-1/collagen) as well as directly through VCAM-ICAM and integrins. Transient components of the niche, mostly eosinophils and megakaryocytes along with the niche stromal cells ensure survival of the attracted PC through secretion of the BCMA ligands APRIL/BAFF and IL6. Of course, the niche, through these and many more signals confers extensive intracellular reprogramming of the PCs to achieve their longevity. The figure was created with BioRender.com

section, we will pay special tribute to the intracellular transitions that allow for such a massive antibody secretion to occur and comment on the impressive ability of LLPC to deal with the imposed stress in order to survive.

Following the GC reaction to a T-cell-dependent antigen, two distinct transcription programs arise in the differentiating B-cell population. The one, dominated by Pax5, IRF8, and BCL6 drives terminal B-cell fate and eventual memory B-cell formation [11]. A portion of the newly formed MBCs exits lymph nodes and the spleen and following chemokine gradients migrate to the BM where they reside in silence [23]. For their survival, a constant level of specific minor antigen stimulation is required [35]. The other population which undergoes extensive GC maturation is driven by the transcriptional program induced by IRF4, Blimp1, and XBP1 and marks the antibody-secreting phenotype [36]. The B cell to antibody-secreting cell (ASCs) transition coincides with a profound metabolic change governed by mitochondrial respiration and its related tricarboxylic acid cycle (TCA) [37]. This metabolic adaptation that is largely governed by the mTORC1 complex is needed for rapid energy and metabolite production in order for the large quantities of Abs to be synthesized [38, 39]. As anticipated, most ASCs that are produced will die in

3–5 days. Overwhelmed by the consequent stress, a mere portion of them however will undergo extensive intracellular reprogramming and following chemokine signals from the future LLPC niche will be home to the BM where they reside for years [14, 40]. Impressively, this terminally differentiated portion will continue antibody secretion and deal with the stress that comes with it until forced to leave the niche [27, 41]. These cells, as already mentioned, in contrast to MBCs are not in need for a constant antigen stimulation to survive and are in charge of producing the baseline antibody titers that are detected in the plasma of immune subjects. LLPCs are therefore a vital part of the acquired immunity [11, 15]. The major differences between the SLPCs and LLPCs are visualized in Fig. 4.2.

Two intrinsic cell programs that facilitate the ability of LLPC to meet the requirements for constant antibody production along with longevity distinguish LLPC from SLPC, autophagy and a global metabolic reprogramming dominated by an optimized unfolded protein response (UPR) coupled with an impressively efficient mitochondrial respiration [5, 42, 43].

Briefly, the ability of a GC-derived Pb for longevity is judged from its bioenergetic state. The increased ability to import glucose and highly functional mitochondrial respiration dominate their metabolism [44, 45]. The active mTOR axis drives intracellular glucose towards oxidation into pyruvate and subsequent import into mitochondria [3, 46]. Because of mTOR activity, pyruvate is not further oxidized to

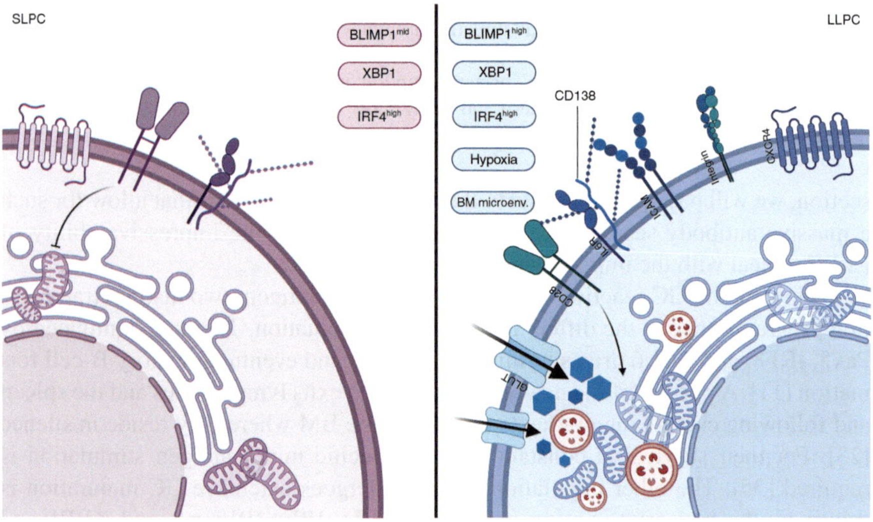

Fig. 4.2 Major differences between the SLPC and the LLPC. Apart from differences in surface receptors that allow LLPC BM homing and binding (ICAM/integrins), SLPC and LLPC share the rest of their surface receptors. The major difference that eventually regulates the LLPC fate is the ability of the cell to import glucose (through GLUT glucose transporters) and unlock a CD28-mediated bioenergetic reprogramming after stimulation from the hypoxic BM microenvironment. In this novel bioenergetic state, autophagy and mitochondrial respiration/metabolism are predominantly featured. The figure was created with BioRender.com

lactate despite BM microenvironmental hypoxia [37, 46]. Although one would anticipate that in order to maintain longevity mitochondrial respiration should be silenced to avoid reactive oxygen species (ROS) release, LLPCs seem to do things quite differently. In fact, contrary to most stem cells in which protecting the genome from ROS attack is essential for quiescence, LLPCs are a terminally differentiated cell in which a balanced amount of ROS seems to play a rather unexpected role [32]. ROS act as mediators to reshape and in a way train the LLPC to effectively regulate the increased stress it deals with [25, 32, 47].

The abundant pyruvate is used to feed TCA with resultant production of lipid intermediates. Lipids that eventually form expand and/or replenish the endoplasmic reticulum that is being consumed in the process of antibody making through the UPR [39, 45, 48, 49]. The UPR is a complex intracellular reflex to increased ER stress such as that exists in PCs due to increased presence of intra-ER unfolded Ab or Ab fragments. Excessive UPR leads to apoptotic death. To this end, balance is ensured through a negative UPR regulator, X-box-binding protein 1 (XBP1) which was impressively enriched in the LLPC transcriptome and proteome [22, 48]. A detailed review regarding the UPR and its necessity for PC function are beyond the purpose of this chapter yet the reader can refer to the following documents for further information [48, 50].

UPR is indispensable for PC fate as it allows for the ASCs to survive the extreme ER stress elicited by the massive Ab production [39]. While the ability to unlock UPR thus dictates the ASC fate, it does not suffice to sustain longevity [51]. The downstream effector of UPR though, autophagy does [51]. The initiation and maintenance of balanced autophagic levels is a prerequisite for the LLPCs lifestyle [3]. Apart from participating in the UPR, autophagy serves a double role in LLPCs, which is unique and essential for their persistence, (a) mitochondrial quality control and (b) limitation of ER expansion [51, 52]. While the former has an obvious positive effect on cellular fate, the latter requires further explanation. PCs are massively secretory cells, their ERs continuously expanded to adjust to the Ab production needs. Trimming the ER through autophagy confines the Abs produced and thus regulates both the ER stress and the amount of energy consumed in this process. Accordingly, recycling of the unfolded proteins released from the ER as autophagosomes does not seem to play a vital role in healthy LLPCs reflecting their ability to self-maintain a balanced Ab release [3, 5, 22]. To this end, BMSC-LLPC cellular contact is shown to directly prevent overt mitochondrial and ER stress that would lead to caspase-mediated apoptotic death in PI3K-dependent way [28]. Besides, mitochondrial and ER-stress responses in LLPCs, namely the proteasome, the UPR, and the autophagic response largely intersect to regulate cellular survival in the heavily functioning Ab factory [52, 53].

The hypoxic BM environment is likely to allow the described bioenergetic adaptation. Hypoxia was an independent positive factor for LLPC longevity [25]. It is established that moderate hypoxia can act to optimize mitochondrial electron transport instead of increasing ROS release [54]. Moreover, although mitochondrial exchange has been established as a crucial factor in MM cell survival and drug resistance in a CD38-driven way, and it is now generally accepted that the LLPC is the physiologic analog of the MM cell, a direct proof of mitochondrial transfer in the healthy BM has yet to be established and can only be hypothesized [18]. Besides, the hypoxic BM microenvironment could also regulate the degree of OXPHOS and thus the amount of glucose in the form of pyruvate being shunted for mitochondrial respiration and TCA, leaving adequate amounts of sugars for the glycosylation of produced Abs [43]. Of course, this whole metabolic adaptation is achieved through continuous LLPC-BM stroma feedback. Several pathways on LLPC have been shown to facilitate this reprogramming by communicating one way or another extracellular signals to the intracellular compartment. It is noteworthy to mention the most important two, the CD27-slp70- and the CD38-induced pathways [25, 32]. Detailed ascription of those lies beyond the scope of this chapter.

Eventually, the LLPC-BM interaction succeeds in making a terminally differentiated heavy duty-secreting cell, with increased ER stress to acquire quiescent features in the BM hypoxic "hotbed." The summary of the LLPC bioenergetic reprogramming described in this section is shown in Fig. 4.3.

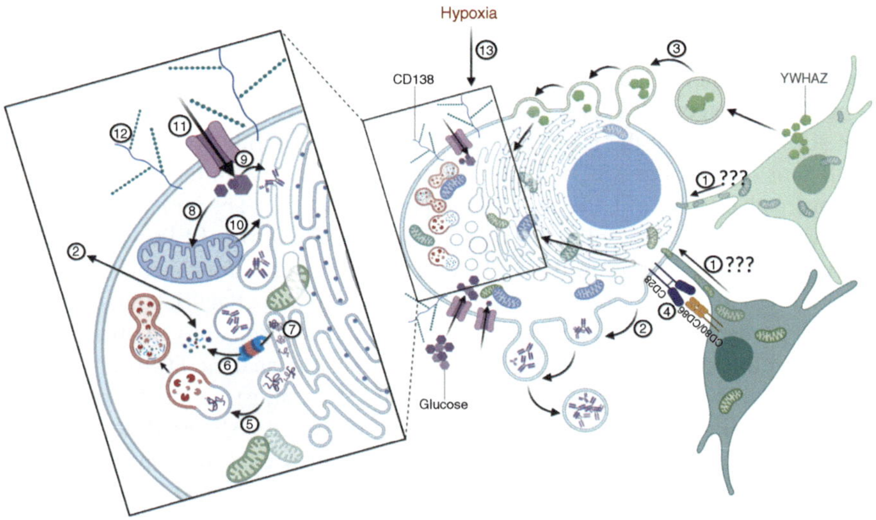

Fig. 4.3 Overview of the LLPC bioenergetic reprogramming. (1) Mitochondrial transport from adjacent stromal cells has been established in MM, suggested in healthy LLPCs but not yet established. (2) The exocytic pathway of the LLPCs, or otherwise described, Ab secretion. (3) The endocytic pathway where exosomal release from the surrounding niche stromal regulates LLPC intrinsic reprogramming. (4) CD28/CD80-CD86 interaction is a major determinant of the LLPC fate decision through modulation of the cellular bioenergetic state. (5) Autophagic degradation of misfolded Abs is a part of the LLPC intrinsic survival program with subsequent ER trimming. (6, 7) Proteasomal degradation of unfolded Abs and the UPR. (8–11) Glucose import [11] with subsequent mitochondrial metabolism [8] or Ab glycosylation [9] is vital for effective Ab production and replenishment of the ER that is consumed during autophagy-UPR [10] accordingly. (11) CD138 is essential in communicating extracellular signals to the LLPC intracellular compartment. The figure was created with BioRender.com

The LLPC Niche in Disease

LLPCs have a complex biology that, as elaborately explained, relies on and subsequently affects the BM micro-niche. In the following paragraphs, we will briefly discuss current knowledge regarding the LLPC in several pathologic conditions.

The LLPC Niche in Infection/Vaccination

LLPCs maintain the baseline Ab titers that are detected in the plasma of immune humans. Their physiologic role is as vital for immunity as that of classical MBCs. Contrary to the MBCs' B-cell receptor (BCR), the LLPCs' ontogeny has provided them with the highest affinity Ab. Thus, maximal binding to Ags is ensured while reactivity to self-antigens is minimized [16]. During the GC reaction, two chronologically distinct B -cell producing phases can be identified [17]. The first phase corresponds to the production of MBCs. These are polyclonal semi-mature B-cell subsets that have BCRs with partial and variable specificity for the targeted antigen. Upon antigen re-exposure, these poorly specific B cells can reenter a GC reaction, undergo further BCR modification, and eventually produce PCs with highly specific class switched Abs that will enter either the short ASC pool or enrich the LLPC repertoire by homing to the BM [17]. The second phase in the GC maturation is marked by a switch towards the ABS phenotype either short- or long-lived. These cells possess BCRs which are specialized to recognize the antigen that eluted the GC reaction. In fact, the more the GC matures, the higher the specificity is [5]. BM LLPCs are enriched in such maximal specificity ABSs [55]. It thus seems that a prerequisite for an LLPCs formation is the achievement of maximal Ab-Ag specificity couples [13, 14]. The question that arises though is, if LLPC depends on the niche to survive, and there is limited niche availability, how can the LLPC pool renew to adapt to the newly met Ags?

It has been shown that upon encountering new Ags, following the GC reaction and Pbs BM homing, these classes switched newly formed Pbs antagonize with the resident LLPCs for niche access [27, 56]. Some newcomers succeed in supplanting the old residents of the niche and settle. Of course, senescence and death of old BM LLPCs can free vital niche space that will thereafter be co-opted by young plasmablast and be their home afterwards [57]. The experimental data supporting both hypotheses are miniscule but exist. Mobilization of BM LLPCs has been hypothesized due to disruption of the niche cellular meshwork under cytokine pressure due to infection/inflammation possibly weakening the old LLPC-stromal interaction [56]. Further research is required to describe the kinetics of the LLPC pool upon inflammation, yet the immunophenotypic similarity of activated LLPCs to the infection induced newly formed SLPCs hinders a detailed pathophysiological description.

The LLPC Niche in Antibody-Mediated Autoimmune Diseases

Antibody-mediated autoimmune diseases including but not limited to SLE, antiphospholipid syndrome (APS), rheumatoid arthritis, myasthenia gravis, etc. pose a therapeutic challenge for all clinician at least at some point during their medical career. The mainstay of therapeutic approach is B-cell depletion using, for instance, the nitrogen mustard cyclophosphamide or targeted anti-CD20 approaches, or even combinations of several agents. Despite the aggressive nature of the established therapeutic algorithms, refractoriness with variable duration of remissions circumscribes the clinical course of such diseases [19, 58]. The pathophysiological background of this autoimmune category is summarized as an aberrant T-helper 2 immune response against self-antigens with subsequent B involvement. B cells mature through GC reactions and produce both self-reactive SLPC and memory B cells. The Abs that are produced thereafter drive the main pathology of the disease [59].

For many years, this established GC-mediated Ab-driven pathophysiology has shaped the therapeutic armamentarium and algorithms. The subsequent B-cell depletion though does not always suffice to clear autoreactive Ab titers and prevent exacerbations as anticipated. In an effort to explain such a therapeutic failure, the global scientific community paid more attention to the primary pathologic structure of the disease(s), the GC itself [60].

One inevitable consequence of the GC B-cell maturation is the generation of Pbs with long-lived potential. It has been proved, especially in SLE and APS, that LLPCs against self-antigens not only exist in BM of autoimmune patients but most likely have preexisted years before clinical eruption [58]. Moreover, multiple independent teams worldwide have proved that upon chronic inflammation, such as in autoimmunity, peripheral organs like the spleen, or the kidney in SLE can in a way support long-term survival for the infiltrating Pbs transformation into peripheral LLPC niches [61]. These do not have the impressive structure and stability of the BM micro-niche but due to continuous cytokine stimulation they express many of the vital homing, CXCL12/integrins and survival, APRIL, TNF-a, BAFF, IL-6, etc. Factors that are able to sustain prolonged ASC survival [9]. Therefore, a vital need arises that these autoreactive LLPCs are taken into account in the establishment of therapeutic approaches. Indeed, the extinction of such autoreactive LLPCs that are notoriously refractory to B-cell depleting agents has led recently to a revised therapeutic strategy involving PC depleting agents through proteasome inhibition [62]. Bortezomib has now proven efficacy against multirefractory autoimmune thrombocytopenia, autoimmune anemia, and Evan's syndrome [63]. Bortezomib in combination with B-cell depletion with, for example, cyclophosphamide has yielded promising results in refractory SLE nephritis and the list is continuously expanding [62]. The pathophysiology and therapeutics of Ab-mediated autoimmunity are being extensively analyzed in corresponding chapters. Besides, IgE producing LLPCs have been extensively described in the BM of allergic patients upon constant/repeated allergen exposure [64].

A last aspect of the Ab-mediated autoimmune pathobiology that merits further notice is the possible implication of LLPCs in the autoimmunity-associated immunosuppression [65]. If we accept the theory of LLPC-Pb antagonism for vital BM niche homing, given the continuous production of autoreactive LLPCs during the disease course, along with the niche disruption due to ongoing inflammation, it is logical to hypothesize that protective LLPCs that confer Ag immunity may crowded out by invading autoreactive PBs. Of course, more extensive work addressing these subjects is yet to come.

The LLPC Niche in PC Malignancies. MM and MGUS (Fig. 4.4)

LLPCs have long been considered the healthy analog of MGUS and MM PCs [9]. Several pieces of evidence point towards this consensus, the most obvious one being the dependency of malignant PC on the BM microenvironment. Moreover, several signaling pathways vital for normal LLPC survival have also been proven to have a positive effect on the MM PC fate [66]. To name a few, the IL6/STA3 and BCMA/

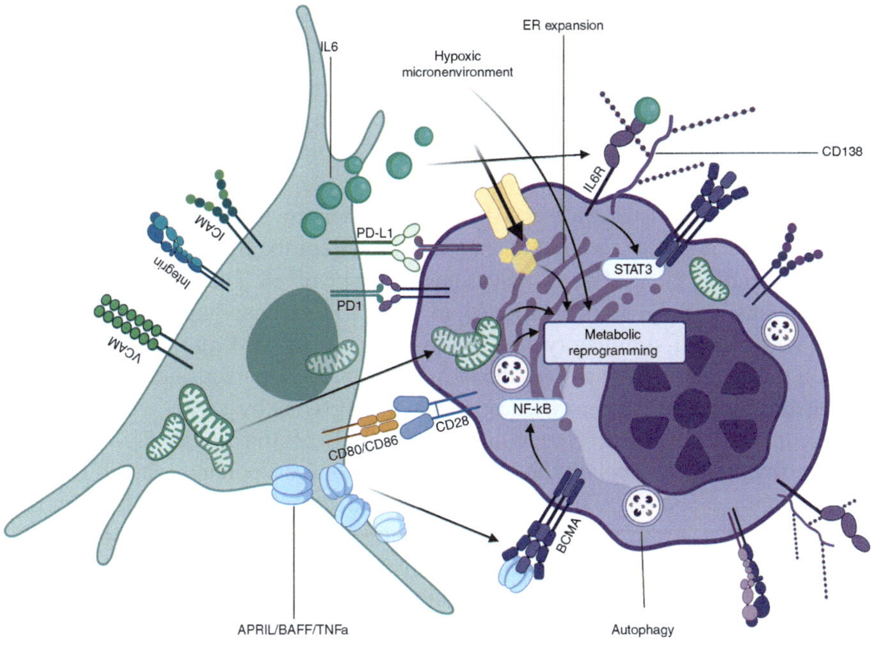

Fig. 4.4 The MM BM Niche. MM cells are considered the malignant analog of LLPCs. In this figure, we summarize the interactions of the malignant PC with its BM microenvironment that facilitate survival and drug resistance. The figure was created with BioRender.com

NF-κB pathways, along with the upregulated CD138 protein the basis for anti-MM effects of the monoclonal antibody daratumumab [25, 67]. Bioenergetically, MM cells show upregulated autophagic drive and increased glucose consumption with preserved OXPHOS and mitochondrial function [24, 68]. This metabolic profile matches that of LLPC. Starting from this beneficial metabolic state, several adaptations are observed as the tumor cells become more malignant [69]. Therapy-resistant MM PCs have been documented to heavily rely on glycolysis and pentose phosphate pathway to produce adequate reducing power and nucleotides for the upcoming divisions accordingly [69]. It has also been documented that in such circumstances, mitochondrial function is sustained through glutaminolysis providing the cell with adequate lipid intermediates for ER synthesis and ATP [35, 69]. This kind of metabolic adaptation which is a common model observed in malignancy, reshapes the surrounding BM microenvironment into a disease permissive niche. Extracellular space acidosis mostly due to lactate export and glutaminolysis stimulates the surrounding BMSCs [67]. Indeed, mitochondrial transfer through tunneling nanotubes from adjacent stromal cells along with their exosomal release have both been established in MM and proven essential for disease progression and chemo-resistance [18, 70–74]. Besides, manipulation of the tumor microenvironment for malignant cell survival and progression is now a common feature among all hematological malignancies [75, 76].

The dependency of MGUS/MM PCs on autophagy is another common aspect they share with LLPCs. Several autophagy inhibitors have been studied in the process of MM drug discovery either alone or in combination with proteasome inhibitors [77]. Results were variable but, in most cases, promising. Given the great variability of the disease and the intersecting autophagic and proteasomal pathways caution is needed when evaluating the potential and thereafter the in vivo efficiency of such approaches.

Another aspect of the MGUS/MM PC-BM microenvironment interactions that merits further notice is the immunosuppressive effect the malignant cells have on their surrounding niche. Two pathways have been involved. The CD28-CD80/CD86 pathway has already been mentioned in the LLPC bioenergetic metamorphosis along with its self-stimulatory nature [78]. In case of MM and most likely also MGUS though, it further involves the immunosuppressive effects the of ectoenzyme indoleamine-pyrrole 2,3-dioxygenase (IDO) and IL6 that bystander DCs are forced to produce and that negatively regulate bystander T-cell functions [67]. The second noteworthy pathway involves the PD1/PDL1 axis and the potential role of CD38, a transmembrane protein abundant in LLPCs and in MGUS/MM cells. Although PD1/PDL1 is active in the MM microenvironment its therapeutic manipulation is promising in multirefractory or primary resistant cases. Much more studies are on the way to establish such immunomodulators in the mainstay of MM therapeutics [72, 79]. Increasing manipulation of the BM microenvironment from the malignant PC translates to MGUS clonal expansion and diversion towards MM [80]. To this end, mobilization of multiple BM residing cell subsets including HSCs and myeloid progenitors marks this transition as the malignant PCs antagonize with physiologic

BM residents for access to the survival niche [41]. Although the pathways underlying such phenomena remain greatly elusive, they most likely include vital space acquisition through expansion and thus usage of BM stromal components for self-proliferation.

Conclusion

LLPCs are an indispensable component of acquired immunity and an exceptional paradigm of the magnificence and complexity of cellular–microenvironmental interactions. Many discoveries about this unique, highly specific B-cell minority have been made, but many more are still to be made. Research around their normal physiology will shed light on many dark spots in the human immune response. The acquired and now expanding knowledge has immediate applications in vaccination response improvement, autoimmune disease treatment optimization yet also in MM drug discovery and therapeutic algorithm design.

References

1. Bixel MG, Kusumbe AP, Ramasamy SK, Sivaraj KK, Butz S, Vestweber D, et al. Flow dynamics and HSPC homing in bone marrow microvessels. Cell Rep. 2017;18(7):1804–16.
2. Pabst R. The bone marrow is not only a primary lymphoid organ: the critical role for T lymphocyte migration and housing of long-term memory plasma cells. Eur J Immunol. 2018;48(7):1096–100.
3. Lightman SM, Utley A, Lee KP. Survival of long-lived plasma cells (LLPC): piecing together the puzzle. Front Immunol. 2019;10:965.
4. Minges Wols HA, Ippolito JA, Yu Z, Palmer JL, White FA, Le PT, et al. The effects of microenvironment and internal programming on plasma cell survival. Int Immunol. 2007;19(7): 837–46.
5. Nguyen DC, Joyner CJ, Sanz I, Lee FE. Factors affecting early antibody secreting cell maturation into long-lived plasma cells. Front Immunol. 2019;10:2138.
6. Pioli PD, Casero D, Montecino-Rodriguez E, Morrison SL, Dorshkind K. Plasma cells are obligate effectors of enhanced myelopoiesis in aging bone marrow. Immunity. 2019;51(2):351–66.e6.
7. Tarlinton D. Do plasma cells contribute to the determination of their lifespan? Immunol Cell Biol. 2020;98(6):449–55.
8. Lindquist RL, Niesner RA, Hauser AE. In the right place, at the right time: spatiotemporal conditions determining plasma cell survival and function. Front Immunol. 2019;10:788.
9. O'Connor BP, Gleeson MW, Noelle RJ, Erickson LD. The rise and fall of long-lived humoral immunity: terminal differentiation of plasma cells in health and disease. Immunol Rev. 2003;194:61–76.
10. Bortnick A, Allman D. What is and what should always have been: long-lived plasma cells induced by T cell-independent antigens. J Immunol. 2013;190(12):5913–8.
11. Palm AE, Henry C. Remembrance of things past: long-term B cell memory after infection and vaccination. Front Immunol. 2019;10:1787.

12. Bortnick A, Chernova I, Quinn WJ 3rd, Mugnier M, Cancro MP, Allman D. Long-lived bone marrow plasma cells are induced early in response to T cell-independent or T cell-dependent antigens. J Immunol. 2012;188(11):5389–96.
13. Chackerian B, Peabody DS. Factors that govern the induction of long-lived antibody responses. Viruses. 2020;12(1):74.
14. Slifka MK, Amanna IJ. Role of multivalency and antigenic threshold in generating protective antibody responses. Front Immunol. 2019;10:956.
15. Slifka MK, Antia R, Whitmire JK, Ahmed R. Humoral immunity due to long-lived plasma cells. Immunity. 1998;8(3):363–72.
16. Weisel FJ, Zuccarino-Catania GV, Chikina M, Shlomchik MJ. A temporal switch in the germinal center determines differential output of memory B and plasma cells. Immunity. 2016;44(1):116–30.
17. Viant C, Weymar GHJ, Escolano A, Chen S, Hartweger H, Cipolla M, et al. Antibody affinity shapes the choice between memory and germinal center B cell fates. Cell. 2020;183(5):1298–311.e11.
18. Boise LH, Shanmugam M. Stromal support of metabolic function through mitochondrial transfer in multiple myeloma. Cancer Res. 2019;79(9):2102–3.
19. DiLillo DJ, Hamaguchi Y, Ueda Y, Yang K, Uchida J, Haas KM, et al. Maintenance of long-lived plasma cells and serological memory despite mature and memory B cell depletion during CD20 immunotherapy in mice. J Immunol. 2008;180(1):361–71.
20. Hammarlund E, Thomas A, Amanna IJ, Holden LA, Slayden OD, Park B, et al. Plasma cell survival in the absence of B cell memory. Nat Commun. 2017;8(1):1781.
21. Halliley JL, Tipton CM, Liesveld J, Rosenberg AF, Darce J, Gregoretti IV, et al. Long-lived plasma cells are contained within the CD19(−)CD38(hi)CD138(+) subset in human bone marrow. Immunity. 2015;43(1):132–45.
22. Khodadadi L, Cheng Q, Radbruch A, Hiepe F. The maintenance of memory plasma cells. Front Immunol. 2019;10:721.
23. Tokoyoda K, Hauser AE, Nakayama T, Radbruch A. Organization of immunological memory by bone marrow stroma. Nat Rev Immunol. 2010;10(3):193–200.
24. Nguyen DC, Garimalla S, Xiao H, Kyu S, Albizua I, Galipeau J, et al. Factors of the bone marrow microniche that support human plasma cell survival and immunoglobulin secretion. Nat Commun. 2018;9(1):3698.
25. Nguyen DC, Lewis HC, Joyner C, Warren V, Xiao H, Kissick HT, et al. Extracellular vesicles from bone marrow-derived mesenchymal stromal cells support ex vivo survival of human antibody secreting cells. J Extracell Vesicles. 2018;7(1):1463778.
26. Utley A, Lipchick B, Lee KP, Nikiforov MA. Targeting multiple myeloma through the biology of long-lived plasma cells. Cancers (Basel). 2020;12(8):2117.
27. Radbruch A, Muehlinghaus G, Luger EO, Inamine A, Smith KG, Dorner T, et al. Competence and competition: the challenge of becoming a long-lived plasma cell. Nat Rev Immunol. 2006;6(10):741–50.
28. Cornelis R, Hahne S, Taddeo A, Petkau G, Malko D, Durek P, et al. Stromal cell-contact dependent PI3K and APRIL induced NF-kappaB signaling prevent mitochondrial- and ER stress induced death of memory plasma cells. Cell Rep. 2020;32(5):107982.
29. Papatriantafyllou M. B cells: secrets to plasma cell longevity. Nat Rev Immunol. 2013;13(3):156–7.
30. Peperzak V, Vikstrom I, Walker J, Glaser SP, LePage M, Coquery CM, et al. Mcl-1 is essential for the survival of plasma cells. Nat Immunol. 2013;14(3):290–7.
31. O'Connor BP, Raman VS, Erickson LD, Cook WJ, Weaver LK, Ahonen C, et al. BCMA is essential for the survival of long-lived bone marrow plasma cells. J Exp Med. 2004;199(1):91–8.
32. Utley A, Chavel C, Lightman S, Holling GA, Cooper J, Peng P, et al. CD28 regulates metabolic fitness for long-lived plasma cell survival. Cell Rep. 2020;31(12):107815.
33. Wang H, Gonzalez-Garcia I, Traba J, Jain S, Conteh S, Shin DM, et al. ATP-degrading ENPP1 is required for survival (or persistence) of long-lived plasma cells. Sci Rep. 2017;7(1):17867.

34. Di Paola R, Caporarello N, Marucci A, Dimatteo C, Iadicicco C, Del Guerra S, et al. ENPP1 affects insulin action and secretion: evidences from in vitro studies. PLoS One. 2011;6(5):e19462.
35. Akkaya M, Kwak K, Pierce SK. B cell memory: building two walls of protection against pathogens. Nat Rev Immunol. 2020;20(4):229–38.
36. Radtke D, Bannard O. Expression of the plasma cell transcriptional regulator Blimp-1 by dark zone germinal center B cells during periods of proliferation. Front Immunol. 2018;9:3106.
37. Lam WY, Becker AM, Kennerly KM, Wong R, Curtis JD, Llufrio EM, et al. Mitochondrial pyruvate import promotes long-term survival of antibody-secreting plasma cells. Immunity. 2016;45(1):60–73.
38. Bertolotti M, Yim SH, Garcia-Manteiga JM, Masciarelli S, Kim YJ, Kang MH, et al. B- to plasma-cell terminal differentiation entails oxidative stress and profound reshaping of the anti-oxidant responses. Antioxid Redox Signal. 2010;13(8):1133–44.
39. Gaudette BT, Jones DD, Bortnick A, Argon Y, Allman D. mTORC1 coordinates an immediate unfolded protein response-related transcriptome in activated B cells preceding antibody secretion. Nat Commun. 2020;11(1):723.
40. Hargreaves DC, Hyman PL, Lu TT, Ngo VN, Bidgol A, Suzuki G, et al. A coordinated change in chemokine responsiveness guides plasma cell movements. J Exp Med. 2001;194(1):45–56.
41. Paiva B, Perez-Andres M, Vidriales MB, Almeida J, de las Heras N, Mateos MV, et al. Competition between clonal plasma cells and normal cells for potentially overlapping bone marrow niches is associated with a progressively altered cellular distribution in MGUS vs myeloma. Leukemia. 2011;25(4):697–706.
42. Cenci S. Autophagy, a new determinant of plasma cell differentiation and antibody responses. Mol Immunol. 2014;62(2):289–95.
43. Lam WY, Bhattacharya D. Metabolic links between plasma cell survival, secretion, and stress. Trends Immunol. 2018;39(1):19–27.
44. Corcoran LM, Nutt SL. Long-lived plasma cells have a sweet tooth. Immunity. 2016;45(1):3–5.
45. Price MJ, Patterson DG, Scharer CD, Boss JM. Progressive upregulation of oxidative metabolism facilitates plasmablast differentiation to a T-independent antigen. Cell Rep. 2018;23(11):3152–9.
46. Mao Z, Zhang W. Role of mTOR in glucose and lipid metabolism. Int J Mol Sci. 2018;19(7):2043.
47. Sena LA, Chandel NS. Physiological roles of mitochondrial reactive oxygen species. Mol Cell. 2012;48(2):158–67.
48. Hetz C. The unfolded protein response: controlling cell fate decisions under ER stress and beyond. Nat Rev Mol Cell Biol. 2012;13(2):89–102.
49. Masciarelli S, Sitia R. Building and operating an antibody factory: redox control during B to plasma cell terminal differentiation. Biochim Biophys Acta. 2008;1783(4):578–88.
50. Brewer JW, Hendershot LM. Building an antibody factory: a job for the unfolded protein response. Nat Immunol. 2005;6(1):23–9.
51. Kroemer G, Marino G, Levine B. Autophagy and the integrated stress response. Mol Cell. 2010;40(2):280–93.
52. Xiong S, Chng WJ, Zhou J. Crosstalk between endoplasmic reticulum stress and oxidative stress: a dynamic duo in multiple myeloma. Cell Mol Life Sci. 2021;78(8):3883–906.
53. Milan E, Fabbri M, Cenci S. Autophagy in plasma cell ontogeny and malignancy. J Clin Immunol. 2016;36(Suppl 1):18–24.
54. Fuhrmann DC, Brune B. Mitochondrial composition and function under the control of hypoxia. Redox Biol. 2017;12:208–15.
55. Fink K. Origin and function of circulating plasmablasts during acute viral infections. Front Immunol. 2012;3:78.
56. Lemke A, Kraft M, Roth K, Riedel R, Lammerding D, Hauser AE. Long-lived plasma cells are generated in mucosal immune responses and contribute to the bone marrow plasma cell pool in mice. Mucosal Immunol. 2016;9(1):83–97.

57. Siegrist CA, Aspinall R. B-cell responses to vaccination at the extremes of age. Nat Rev Immunol. 2009;9(3):185–94.
58. Taddeo A, Khodadadi L, Voigt C, Mumtaz IM, Cheng Q, Moser K, et al. Long-lived plasma cells are early and constantly generated in New Zealand Black/New Zealand White F1 mice and their therapeutic depletion requires a combined targeting of autoreactive plasma cells and their precursors. Arthritis Res Ther. 2015;17:39.
59. Hoyer BF, Moser K, Hauser AE, Peddinghaus A, Voigt C, Eilat D, et al. Short-lived plasmablasts and long-lived plasma cells contribute to chronic humoral autoimmunity in NZB/W mice. J Exp Med. 2004;199(11):1577–84.
60. Hiepe F, Dorner T, Hauser AE, Hoyer BF, Mei H, Radbruch A. Long-lived autoreactive plasma cells drive persistent autoimmune inflammation. Nat Rev Rheumatol. 2011;7(3):170–8.
61. Winter O, Dame C, Jundt F, Hiepe F. Pathogenic long-lived plasma cells and their survival niches in autoimmunity, malignancy, and allergy. J Immunol. 2012;189(11):5105–11.
62. Alexander T, Cheng Q, Klotsche J, Khodadadi L, Waka A, Biesen R, et al. Proteasome inhibition with bortezomib induces a therapeutically relevant depletion of plasma cells in SLE but does not target their precursors. Eur J Immunol. 2018;48(9):1573–9.
63. Kohler S, Marschenz S, Grittner U, Alexander T, Hiepe F, Meisel A. Bortezomib in antibody-mediated autoimmune diseases (TAVAB): study protocol for a unicentric, non-randomised, non-placebo controlled trial. BMJ Open. 2019;9(1):e024523.
64. Asrat S, Kaur N, Liu X, Ben LH, Kajimura D, Murphy AJ, et al. Chronic allergen exposure drives accumulation of long-lived IgE plasma cells in the bone marrow, giving rise to serological memory. Sci Immunol. 2020;5(43):eaav8402.
65. Grammatikos AP, Tsokos GC. Immunodeficiency and autoimmunity: lessons from systemic lupus erythematosus. Trends Mol Med. 2012;18(2):101–8.
66. Paiva B, Puig N, Cedena MT, de Jong BG, Ruiz Y, Rapado I, et al. Differentiation stage of myeloma plasma cells: biological and clinical significance. Leukemia. 2017;31(2):382–92.
67. Garcia-Ortiz A, Rodriguez-Garcia Y, Encinas J, Maroto-Martin E, Castellano E, Teixido J, et al. The role of tumor microenvironment in multiple myeloma development and progression. Cancers (Basel). 2021;13(2):217.
68. Hoang B, Benavides A, Shi Y, Frost P, Lichtenstein A. Effect of autophagy on multiple myeloma cell viability. Mol Cancer Ther. 2009;8(7):1974–84.
69. Rizzieri D, Paul B, Kang Y. Metabolic alterations and the potential for targeting metabolic pathways in the treatment of multiple myeloma. J Cancer Metastasis Treat. 2019;5:26.
70. Noll JE, Williams SA, Tong CM, Wang H, Quach JM, Purton LE, et al. Myeloma plasma cells alter the bone marrow microenvironment by stimulating the proliferation of mesenchymal stromal cells. Haematologica. 2014;99(1):163–71.
71. Wang J, Hendrix A, Hernot S, Lemaire M, De Bruyne E, Van Valckenborgh E, et al. Bone marrow stromal cell-derived exosomes as communicators in drug resistance in multiple myeloma cells. Blood. 2014;124(4):555–66.
72. Marlein CR, Piddock RE, Mistry JJ, Zaitseva L, Hellmich C, Horton RH, et al. CD38-driven mitochondrial trafficking promotes bioenergetic plasticity in multiple myeloma. Cancer Res. 2019;79(9):2285–97.
73. Roccaro AM, Sacco A, Maiso P, Azab AK, Tai YT, Reagan M, et al. BM mesenchymal stromal cell-derived exosomes facilitate multiple myeloma progression. J Clin Invest. 2013;123(4):1542–55.
74. Umezu T, Imanishi S, Yoshizawa S, Kawana C, Ohyashiki JH, Ohyashiki K. Induction of multiple myeloma bone marrow stromal cell apoptosis by inhibiting extracellular vesicle miR-10a secretion. Blood Adv. 2019;3(21):3228–40.
75. Kumar B, Garcia M, Weng L, Jung X, Murakami JL, Hu X, McDonald T, Lin A, Kumar AR, DiGiusto DL, Stein AS, Pullarkat VA, Hui SK, Carlesso N, Kuo YH, Bhatia R, Marcucci G, Chen CC. Acute myeloid leukemia transforms the bone marrow niche into a leukemia-permissive microenvironment through exosome secretion. Leukemia. 2018;32(3):575–87.

76. de Jong MME, Kellermayer Z, Papazian N, Tahri S, Hofste Op Bruinink D, Hoogenboezem R, Sanders MA, van de Woestijne PC, Bos PK, Khandanpour C, Vermeulen J, Moreau P, van Duin M, Broijl A, Sonneveld P, Cupedo T. The multiple myeloma microenvironment is defined by an inflammatory stromal cell landscape. Nat Immunol. 2021;22(6):769–80.
77. Yun Z, Zhichao J, Hao Y, Ou J, Ran Y, Wen D, et al. Targeting autophagy in multiple myeloma. Leuk Res. 2017;59:97–104.
78. Nair JR, Carlson LM, Koorella C, Rozanski CH, Byrne GE, Bergsagel PL, et al. CD28 expressed on malignant plasma cells induces a prosurvival and immunosuppressive microenvironment. J Immunol. 2011;187(3):1243–53.
79. Costa F, Marchica V, Storti P, Malavasi F, Giuliani N. PD-L1/PD-1 axis in multiple myeloma microenvironment and a possible link with CD38-mediated immune-suppression. Cancers (Basel). 2021;13(2):164.
80. Zingone A, Kuehl WM. Pathogenesis of monoclonal gammopathy of undetermined significance and progression to multiple myeloma. Semin Hematol. 2011;48(1):4–12.

Chapter 5
Animal Models in Monoclonal Immunoglobulin-Related Diseases

Steven D. Shnyder, Suchit K. Chatterji, and Sherif El-Khamisy

Abbreviations

AH	Primary heavy chain amyloidosis
AHL	Light and heavy chain amyloidosis
AL	Primary light chain amyloidosis
BMM	Bone marrow microenvironment
Cav1	Caveolin 1
DLBCL	Diffuse large B-cell lymphoma
FS	Fanconi Syndrome
HC	Heavy chain
HCDD	Heavy chain deposition disease
HDAC	Histone deacetylase
Ig	Immunoglobulin
LC	Light chain
LCDD	Light chain deposition disease
LMP2A	Latent membrane protein 2A
LPL	Lymphoplasmacytic lymphoma
MCN	Myeloma cast nephropathy
MGRS	Monoclonal gammopathy of renal significance
MGUS	Monoclonal gammopathy of undetermined significance
MIDD	Monoclonal immunoglobulin deposition disease
MM	Multiple myeloma
MPGN	Membranoproliferative glomerulonephritis

S. D. Shnyder (✉) · S. K. Chatterji · S. El-Khamisy
Institute of Cancer Therapeutics, University of Bradford, Bradford, West Yorkshire, UK
e-mail: S.D.Shnyder@Bradford.ac.uk; s.k.chatterji@bradford.ac.uk; S.El-Khamisy@bradford.ac.uk

© The Author(s), under exclusive license to Springer Nature Switzerland AG 2022

G. Ragab et al. (eds.), *Paraproteinemia and Related Disorders*,
https://doi.org/10.1007/978-3-031-10131-1_5

NAS	Nonsense-associated altered splicing
NHL	Non-Hodgkin lymphoma
NSG	NOD/SCID gamma null
RAG-2	Recombinase-activating gene-2
SCID	Severe combined immunodeficient
V	Variable
ZOL	Zoledronic acid

Introduction

The term "paraproteinemias" or "plasma cell dyscrasias" is used to describe a group of clinically distinct disorders that commonly include immunoproliferative disorders like multiple myeloma (MM), lymphoplasmacytic lymphoma (LPL), B-cell non-Hodgkin lymphoma (NHL), primary light chain amyloidosis (AL), and plasmacytoma.

Paraproteinemias are usually associated with the deposition of components of, or entire immunoglobulin (Ig) molecules in major organs, with accumulation usually associated with damage and compromised functioning of the affected organs. This is observed mainly in the kidneys where damage to all anatomically distinct areas including the tubular, glomerular, and vascular areas can be seen. Glomerular damage is Ig deposition related and commonly causes immunotactoid glomerulopathy, Ig amyloidosis, and monoclonal Ig deposition disease as well as Types 1 and 2 cryoglobulin-linked cryoglobulinemic glomerulonephritis. Renal injury also occurs by complement deposition, as seen in C3 glomerulopathy (as a result of complement cascade activation), as well as by cytokine/growth factor-induced thrombotic microangiopathy [1–3].

Another associated condition has previously been called "Monoclonal Gammopathy of Undetermined Significance (MGUS)." MGUS is a monoclonal gammopathy where the clonal proliferation is not sufficiently extensive to be considered malignant [4–6]. MGUS was previously thought to be a clinically benign entity because it transforms to a full-blown MM or a lymphoma at a rate of less than 1% per year; however, recent studies show that vital organ damage occurs in this setting as well [4, 5]. Renal damage has recently been described to occur secondary to MGUS, and this entity is now called "Monoclonal Gammopathy of Renal Significance (MGRS)" [1, 4, 7]. In addition, other pathologies such as specific types of neuropathies, including demyelinating ones, dermopathies like Monoclonal Ig Cryoglobulinemia (Type 1 and Type 2) associated petechiae and purpura, and ocular conditions like crystalline keratopathy (due to light-chain crystal deposition in the epithelial and stromal areas of the cornea) have also been reported.

A clear understanding of the pathogenesis of paraproteinemias is central to the development of effective strategies for the management of these diseases, and preclinical animal models play a significant role in this. In this chapter, we review both the animal models available for studying monoclonal Ig-related diseases, and their resultant pathologies in the kidney and other organs.

Animal Models Investigating Specific Paraproteinemias

Table 5.1 summarizes the animal models used for these disease entities.

The MM Family of Disease Entities (Including Lymphoplasmacytic Lymphoma, Plasmacytoma, Primary Light Chain Amyloidosis and Non-proliferative Monoclonal Gammopathy)

It is interesting to note that despite the clinically distinct entities described in the previous section, due to the shared pathogenesis there is extensive overlap in utilization of animal models. Therefore, in the following sections, MM will indicate multiple diseases of the MM "family" as described previously.

In MM, a vicious circle is created where bone cells are stimulated by the proliferating monoclonal plasma cells that in turn stimulate growth of bone. Animal models help in understanding this complex interaction between the proliferating plasma cells and the bone cells at the tissue, cellular and molecular levels. At present, most model work in this respect is done in mouse models focusing on pathogenesis of MM and the effect on remodeling of bone, and in the evaluation of novel potential therapies which have anti-osteoblastic/anti-tumor activity [9].

The most commonly used mouse MM models come under one of three categories: induced, cell transplantation, or transgenic models.

Table 5.1 The common animal model types used for investigating the paraproteinemias

Disorder	Model type	Genetic modification (where applicable)	References
Multiple myeloma	Induced		[8]
	Cell transplantation		[8–19]
	Transgenic	*KalwRij*	[20–24]
		RAG-2	[6]
		IL-6	[25–31]
		v-abl	[32, 33]
		XBP-1	[34–38]
		c-MAF	[39, 40]
		BCL-2 family	[41–44]
B-cell non-Hodgkin's lymphoma	Cell transplantation		[45–47]
	Transgenic	*myc*	[31, 48–50]
		NFS.V	[51]
		IL-14α	[52]
		HCV	[53]

Induced Models

First reported in 1969, plasmacytoma growth can be stimulated by intraperitoneal injection of the mineral oil Pristane into BALB/c mice, with plasmacytomas evident 16 weeks after injection [9]. These cells can subsequently be passed into other Pristane pre-treated mice for further studies. This model is well suited for studying genetic involvement in the disease, and has been especially useful in determining the role of c-myc and IL-6 in MM development [9]. It has also played a key role in the development of drugs implicated in controlling growth of plasmacytomas such as zoledronic acid (ZOL) [9]. This drug is the most potent third-generation bisphosphonate and is currently in use to treat human MM, having demonstrated its ability in controlling skeletal events in human MM [9]. Reduced plasmacytoma production and increased longevity was seen in pristane injected BALB/c mice who had received ZOL [9].

The main drawback in using the induced model is that unlike human MM where IgG is the main antibody type secreted, the plasmacytomas induced here only secrete monoclonal IgA. Also, the characteristic bone lesions of MM are not seen in this model, with growth only in the peritoneum, which limits its use in pathophysiological studies of systemic disease for human MM [9].

Cell Transplantation Models

The most common cell transplantation model used to study MM is to transplant human plasma cells into immunodeficient mouse strains, with severe combined immunodeficient (SCID) mice the host of choice due to their very limited innate immunity which reduces the chances of graft rejection. These models are well suited for studying bone colonization of malignant plasma cells (in the marrow cavity), and osteolytic lesions are formed in a similar fashion to human MM [9]. In addition, as with human MM, a monoclonal protein is secreted that can be quantified in serum [9]. The model has also been frequently used for screening drug candidates, such as Ibandronate, as well as antisense MIP-1α and the recombinant RANK antagonist, RANK-Fc tested using the ARH77 cell line [6, 9]. One limitation of these models is the EBV-positive status of the majority of the immortalized cell lines used [6, 9].

"Modified" SCID Models

The SCID model has undergone further modifications over time to enhance the mimicry of specialized aspects of the human disease, with elements of their tissue microenvironment replaced by elements from other species created to study the bone marrow microenvironment (BMM) and MM plasma cell "Interactome" [8]. For MM-specific models, this is done by implantation of bone from a different animal, for example, rabbit, within the flanks of mice followed by subsequent seeding with MM cell lines or fresh explanted cells from the primary bone marrow of the initial donor species [6]. This allows for the study of MM cells in a species-specific environment [8, 10–12].

1. *SCID-hu.* A piece of human fetal bone is inserted in the mouse. The implanted MM cells choose this implant over parent mouse bone for colonization. The human bone develops human MM-like lesions (increased osteoclastic activity with neoangiogenic responses) and monoclonal protein can be detected in mouse sera. Vital signaling pathways for MM propagation, like p38 MAPK, have been discovered using this model, and it has been reported that ZOL limits bone destruction in this model. The main disadvantage of this model is that fetal BMM is not the same as mature adult human BMM where classical MM is usually seen [8, 10–12].
2. *SCID-rab.* Adult rabbit bone is inserted, and MM cells colonize the rabbit bone and proliferate. This model has been used for studying the bone building activity of the proteasome inhibitor bortezomib [8]. The drawback of this model is that while there is ontogenic similarity, rabbit and adult human bones are not the same, and any finding still has to be translated to human models [8, 13, 14].
3. *SCID-synth-hu.* This is a step closer to the simulation of the human MM micro-environment. Here a three-dimensional synthetic scaffold made of polyε-caprolactone polymers and human trabeculae, within which MM cells/primary PCs can be inserted, is implanted subcutaneously in the flanks of SCID mice [6]. This model has been used to demonstrate the anti-myeloma activity of bortezomib in combination with dexamethasone [8, 15, 16].
4. *NOD/SCID gamma null (NSG).* This mouse strain lacks the IL-2 gamma chain which results in a total absence of B-cell/T-cell/NK-cell function and severe deficiencies of antigen-presenting cell function and complement system defects [8]. Post-radiation intravenous introduction of MM cells in these mice has demonstrated homing of MM cells to the murine bone marrow with the subsequent development of classic MM bone lesions. The main drawback of this model is the large load of extramedullary disease and a phenotype closer to a plasma cell leukemia than the typical indolent MM [8]. NSG studies have shown that ZOL can control bone disease but not reduce tumor burden, and that the proteasome inhibitor Carfilzomib decreased tumor load and stimulated anabolism in MM [8, 17–19].

Transgenic Models

Transgenic models take another step closer to simulating MM, as since the tumors form in a syngeneic background, the influence of the tumor microenvironment can also be considered, and this aids in identifying proteins that promote tumorigenesis.

1. *5TMM model (Radl model).* This C57BL/KalwRij mouse model was developed in 1978 by Radl et al. [23]. It spontaneously develops MM and following intravenous transplantation of bone marrow cells from these mice into syngeneic donors, multiple phenotypically distinct cell lines have been created and assigned nomencla-

ture with a root of "5TMM" [6, 9, 20–23, 54]. Some of these derived cell line models are well suited for pathophysiological and pharmacotherapeutic studies due to the pathophysiological similarities (of some popular subtypes) with human MM [6]. They are also a good model for bone microenvironment studies as further genetic manipulation can be done by breeding mice with specific genetic traits, with the RAG-2 model, described below, as a good example of this [6, 8, 9, 21]. However, some differences exist with typical human MM, as renal lesions due to light chain deposits are not observed. In addition, some cell lines, such as 5T2MM, behave very aggressively and non-hematopoietic organ involvement is seen [9].

Bisphosphonates, the current standard therapy of human MM due to their anti-osteoclastic action (promotion of apoptosis in osteoclasts), have been tested extensively in 5TMM models. Drugs tested include oral pamidronate (tested in 5T2MM models), ibandronate (in both 5T2MM and 5T3MM models), and newer bisphosphonates like ZOL or apomine (in 5T2MM models) [9]. The proteasome, a physiological mechanism for degrading proteins in eukaryotes, was identified as having key involvement in the pathogenesis of MM where it regulates the RANK/RANKL biosystem. Proteasome inhibitor drugs (e.g., bortezomid) which are currently used in the treatment of human MM, have been studied extensively in the 5T3MM model [9, 54].

2. *RAG-2 model.* Developed with the express goal of making a mouse MM model suitable for host microenvironment studies. C57BL/6 mice were made with aberrant B- and T-cell development that was stimulated by a Recombinase-activating gene-2 (RAG-2)-immunodeficiency. This produced a myeloma-permissive mouse model. Inoculating RAG-2-deficient mice with GFP-tagged 5TGM1 plasma cells produced similar MM features to the 5TMM Radl model [6, 8]. The model is classified by some as a modified 5TMM Radl model while some consider it as a distinct entity [8]. This model is useful for host microenvironment studies since the RAG-2-deficiency is non-lethal and hence mice can grow to maturity [8].
3. *IL-6 model.* IL-6 has been shown to be central to MM development [8], and IL-6 transgenic mice developed large polyclonal plasmacytomas that when transplanted into mineral oil-treated BALB/c mice produced monoclonal IgA plasmacytomas that also had c-myc and t(12;15) gene rearrangements. These early studies confirmed the central role of IL-6 in MM [8, 24–27].
4. *v-abl model.* Several studies have indicated that the *myc* locus is involved in the transition from a MGUS to overt MM (refs). A complex genetic manipulation activates the *myc* locus and stimulates giant cell reaction and monoclonal plasma cell proliferation within bone marrow and at extramedullary sites, thus accurately mimicking MM disease. These clonal plasma cells when inserted into syngeneic mice produce an MGUS like state with monoclonal protein production in the recipient mice. This model, interestingly, accurately recapitulates the slow progression of typical human MM disease and is thus suitable to study MM pathogenesis. It has been used to test MM therapeutic candidates such as proteasome inhibitors as well as histone deacetylase (HDAC) inhibitors [8, 28, 32].
5. *XBP-1 model.* XBP-1 is needed for normal plasma cell differentiation. There is a rapid XBP-1 upregulation in B cells upon exposure to stimuli that bring about

plasma cell differentiation, and mice lacking XBP-1 retain normal B-cell activity but show very low levels of antibodies in the absence of plasma cell differentiation [8]. XBP-1 transgenic mice with increased expression of XBP-1 develop MM after 2 years with typical kidney and bone lesions [8]. This model has been used to identify molecular pathways involved in MM such as upregulation of chaperone protein gp96 in MM [8, 33–37].

6. *c-MAF model.* The c-MAF proto-oncogene shows overexpression in MM in the presence of a specific translocation, t(14:16). Transgenic mice with overexpression of c-MAF develop high proliferation of plasma cells in the bone marrow, and renal disease along with monoclonal gammopathy. The tumors produced here are, however, phenotypically closer to plasma cell lymphomas than typical MM [8, 38, 39].
7. *BCL-2 model.* BCL-2 promotes plasma cell survival by its anti-apoptotic action. Transgenic mice for both BCL-XL and Bcl-B have been studied [8]. The BCL-XL transgenic mouse has no M-protein spike, but extramedullary plasma cell deposits are seen and MM-like renal cast nephropathy. Bone marrow disease is rare [8, 40–42].

   Previously, BCL-B was shown to be overexpressed in overt MM but not in MGUS. BCL-B transgenic mice demonstrated bone marrow plasmacytosis (that was reversed by MM drugs), anemia, and M-protein spike in serum. These findings demonstrate the promise of this model to test future MM drugs [8, 43].
8. *IL-6 "Knock-in" humanized mouse model.* A recent model where the MM-promoting cytokine IL-6 human gene has replaced its mouse counterpart [8]. On bone marrow injection of MM cells into the mice [8], they grew preferentially in the bone marrow like human MM without infiltrating extramedullary sites like the spleen. However, the tumors showed genomic variability possibly linked to new sub-clones [8, 29, 30, 44].

B-Cell NHL

B-cell NHL covers a series of pathologies. Around 50% are of the diffuse large B-cell variety, with the others belonging to a heterogeneous group made up of marginal zone lymphomas, follicular lymphomas, Burkitt's type lymphomas and B-cell mediastinal lymphomas [31]. The most common NHL models come under one of two categories: cell transplantation or transgenic models.

Cell Transplantation Models

These models have formed the cornerstone of development of novel therapies for NHL and fall into four subtypes; (1): Purely syngeneic models; (2): Syngeneic models containing murine tumor cells that express human antigens; (3): Xenogeneic type of models; (4): "Humanized" models. These can be inoculated with either human(h) or murine(m) cells [31].

Examples of these include: (1) Syngeneic: immunocompetent mice strains such as BALB/c that have been inoculated by murine cells like with Pi-BCL1 (m) or FL5.12 transfected Bcl2 (m), A20 (m) 4TOO (m) or BCL1 (m). Inoculation can be intravenous, as in the above cases, intrasplenic (A20 (m)), intraperitoneal (CH44 (m) BCL1 (m) 38C13 (m)), subcutaneous (LY-ar or LY-as (m)), intramuscular (MSV-MuLV-M induced) or even intracerebral (A20.IIA-GFP (m)). (2) Syngeneic expressing human antigens: immunocompetent strains such as C3H/HeN expressing antigens like 38C13 Her2/neu (m) through intravenous inoculation or 38C13 Her2/neu (m) through subcutaneous inoculation. (3) Xenogenic: immunodeficient SCID mice expressing human cells like Z138 (h), BJAB (h), and SU-DHL-4 (h), all inoculated intravenously, or Ramos (h), BJAB (h), and SC-1 (h) cells, all inoculated subcutaneously. (4) Humanized: SCID/beige mice with "partially rebuilt" immunity with Daudi (h) or Jijoye (h) cells are introduced subcutaneously [31, 45, 46].

Rituximab, a key therapeutic for NHL, was mainly developed through utilizing xenogeneic type models [31]. The SCID model was used to study rituximab against Diffuse Large B-Cell Lymphoma (DLBCL SU-DHL4) and Burkitt Lymphoma where rituximab successfully controlled the NHL [47, 55]. The success of these studies led to analyses of newer monoclonal antibody drugs like humanized GA101 or EMAB-6 on induced lymphoma models comprising human SUDHL4 tumor cells that were introduced into SCID/beige mice [45, 46].

The main drawback of many of these experimental models is that they involve immunodeficient mice that do not possess the adaptive type of immunity found in the tumor microenvironment of human tumors, and thus they do not accurately represent the complex interactions seen in human disease [31].

Transgenic Models

1. *myc* models. Models centered around manipulation of the *myc* oncogene are frequently used for studying B-cell NHL, with the *myc* oncogene frequently implicated in these diseases [56]. There are two phenotypically distinct subtypes of this transgenic mouse model. The first subtype develops early and is made up of immature B cells, which has a Burkitt's lymphoma-like phenotype. The second subtype develops later, after at least a year, and is primarily made up of mature B cells, having a diffuse large B-cell lymphoma-like phenotype [31, 48, 56]. This transgenic mouse model of lymphoma has been found to have genetically distinct subtypes that display the full spectrum of aggressive human B-cell neoplasia [48]. The most common model, the Eμ-*myc* model, has a translocation that is located behind an enhancer/promoter area that is B-cell specific inside the IgH locus [31, 56]. B-cell lymphomas invariably develop over a time interval that ranges from a month to almost 2 years. This variability in speed of formation is also seen in human NHL [31, 56].

   Many studies have identified genes that not only change the onset of this lymphoma but also influence how it responds to single-agent chemotherapeutic drugs. This model has also been used as a genetic screening test to identify genes that influence response to doxorubicin therapy [48].

A disease like human Burkitt's Lymphoma could be established in the mouse if the *myc* gene was inserted under the enhancer region area of the Ig light chain genes [31, 49]. It was found that *myc* derangement, at least in some cases, was insufficient for oncogenesis, however oncogenic virus exposure can be a trigger. Lymphoma development, for example, was also found to be accelerated in *myc* altered mice by concurrent infection with oncogenic viruses like murine Moloney Leukemia virus [31]. The tumor microenvironment is also important in producing a malignant phenotype. Studies focused on the role of Bcl-2 overexpression in follicular B-cell lymphomagenesis found that CD4+ T cells were vital in stimulating the proliferation germinal center B cells and thus in promoting follicular B-cell lymphomas [31].

2. Other transgenic models. Many other models exist that are beyond the scope of this chapter, and we would recommend the review by Donnou et al. [31] which covers these in great detail. What is abundantly clear, however, is that the diversity of these models makes it very difficult to draw definitive conclusions about the influence of specific characteristics on the creation of very specific lymphomas in experimental animals and to extrapolate these findings on human B-cell lymphomas [31].

   Examples of popular (and successful) models in this category are the NFS.V mouse model for marginal zone lymphomas [50], the mantle cell lymphoma (blastoid variant) murine model [51], and the recent model where HCV transgenic mice that expressed the full HCV genome in B cells (RzCD19Cre mice) show a high incidence of diffuse large B-cell NHL [52].

Models for the Pathologies Resulting from the Paraproteinemias

The pathologies can be divided into those associated with deposition of single light or heavy chains, and deposition of complete Ig molecules. Given that many animal models can act as a surrogate for the pathologies associated with paraproteinemias, the general model types for the single chain or complete molecules will be discussed before progressing to describe the models for specific pathologies. Table 5.2 summarizes the animal models used for these disease entities.

Models of Diseases Caused by Deposition of Single Ig Chains

Two general approaches have been taken to model these diseases: light chain injection and transgenic models, and these have been utilized for modeling specific diseases as described below.

Table 5.2 Common animal models used in investigating pathologies arising from the paraproteinemias

Disorder	Model type	Genetic modification (where applicable)	References
Monoclonal LC-induced proximal tubulopathy associated with renal Fanconi syndrome	Induced		[57–59]
	Cell transplantation		[60]
	Transgenic	*VκJκ*	[61–63]
Amyloidosis	Induced		[64, 65]
	Transgenic	*λ6LC*	[66, 67]
Randall-type MIDD	Induced		[68]
	Transgenic	*VκIV*	[69]
		γHC	[62]
Myeloma cast nephropathy	Induced		[70, 71]
MGUS/MGRS	Transgenic	*κLC*	[72]
Type I and type II Cryoglobulinemias	Cell transplantation		[73–77]

Purified Human Ig Light Chain Injection Models

Ig light chains for these mouse models are obtained either by purifying patient urine (by salt precipitation, column purification, or dialysis) or by recombinant protein production techniques (using cloned monoclonal Ig genes from patients that are expressed in *E. Coli* or mammalian cell lines). These have been introduced to the mouse by injection into the tail vein, intraperitoneally or into the penile vein (a technique that was found to deliver the maximum light chain load to the kidneys) [53, 69, 78, 79]. The technical challenges of these models are that they present low light chain levels which do not accurately mimic human pathology. This is further exacerbated by the short half-life of these light chains which necessitates repeated injections to maintain load.

Zebrafish and *C. Elegans* have been successfully used as alternative hosts [57, 60, 80]. *C. Elegans* has been used as a model to evaluate the heart damage by AL light chain heart amyloidosis. Studying the pharynx (the equivalent of the vertebrate heart), it was seen that pharyngeal function was reduced significantly by exposure to light chains of AL patients with cardiomyopathy. It was also demonstrated that exposure to human amyloid-producing light chains caused cardiac dysfunction related to early death in Zebrafish [57, 60, 80].

Transgenic Models

Hybridoma Cells Engineered to Secrete Ig Fragments

SP2/0 non-producing hybridoma cells from BALB/c mice were stably transfected with a gene that encoded a human monoclonal Ig fragment and cultured in vitro. The most competent clones were then introduced into immunocompetent BALB/c mice intravenously (tail vein) and as the tumors grew over weeks, retroperitoneally, they secreted human pathological Igs. Immunofluorescence studies revealed deposits of human κ chain determinants in the basement membranes in the tumors as well as in the liver, kidneys, spleen, heart, and ovaries [79].

The key advantage of these models is continuous Ig production, mimicking human disease, and in addition, mutation analyses can also be undertaken to study the contribution of individual residues in the variable (V) domain in light chain deposition/aggregation. The main drawback of this model is that animals die quickly due to rapid progression to advanced disease, and this prevents not only detailed disease studies but also studies of potential therapeutic drugs [69, 79].

Direct Plasma Cell Engineering

Initial efforts have focused on inserting the light chain gene flanked by the main regulatory areas of the IgH locus to induce "physiological" production of the pathological Igs by the plasma cell population. While this was seen ex vivo, in the mouse free light chains were only produced in small amounts, and mostly the human light chains joined with mouse heavy chains making hybrid Igs which failed to form deposits [81].

LMP2A Transgenic Models

In this knock-in transgenic mouse model, the gene encoding latent membrane protein 2A (LMP2A), sourced from Epstein–Barr virus, replaced the JH segments in the IgH locus. As a result, since the viral-sourced LMP2A efficiently replaces B-cell receptor signaling, complete B-cell development occurs in the absence of Ig heavy chains. LMP2A mice have an increased plasma cell population and thus can produce a large quantity of free light chains without having any hematological pathology. As a result, after crossing these LMP2A mice with human κlight chain knock-in mice, circulating human light chains are of quantities that exceed the circulating light chain quantities in the humans from whom the light chains were originally isolated, and hence this improves upon the models described above [82, 83]. More recent studies using this model have shown that aberrant Ig chains deficient in V domains can be made post non-sense-associated altered splicing (NAS) events. Expression of these shortened Ig polypeptides increases endoplasmic reticulum stress and reduces plasma cell life span. V domain exon skipping appears to be coupled to transcription and this only increases as plasma cell differentiation proceeds [84].

Subsequently transgenic models have been constructed for specific conditions as described in the section below with varying amounts of success.

Monoclonal Light Chain-Induced Proximal Tubulopathy

The light chain-induced tubulopathy has a varied clinical presentation and the exact pathogenesis of this entity remains poorly understood [60, 85]. It is associated with renal Fanconi Syndrome (FS) where low molecular weight protein is found in the urine, and osteomalacia and a slowly progressive renal failure occurs; light chains accumulate here within the lysosomes in the cells of the proximal convoluted tubules [58, 86].

FS can be modeled through exposure of mouse renal tubules to human monoclonal light chains through injection of Bence-Jones protein, with a reduced proximal tubular uptake of glucose and amino acids observed [60, 86, 87]. SP2/0 hybridoma grafts also led to the development of the first human FS mouse model which displayed proximal tubular lesions that closely resembled the human lesions [69]. However as mentioned previously, the rapid onset of progressive disease limits these models for any therapeutic studies.

In a successful FS transgenic mouse model, the mouse Jκ cluster was replaced by a human VκJκ rearranged gene that was cloned from a patient with smouldering myeloma related FS [59]. The V region here was of the VκI subgroup, a V segment that was linked to FS with light-chain crystallization in many myeloma patients. This marriage of the human VκI domain with the mouse κ constant domain in the transgenic animal produced nephrotoxicity that closely resembled human FS, thus proving that the nephrotoxic abilities of the monoclonal FS Light Chains were linked to the V domain [59, 61, 62].

AL and Related Diseases

Ig amyloidosis is the most frequent and the most aggressive form of amyloidosis. It is a systemic disease that affects the heart and liver as well as the kidneys. Most commonly light chains (AL Amyloidosis) are deposited, but sometimes heavy chain deposition (AH Amyloidosis) in combination with light chain deposits (AHL Amyloidosis) also occurs. Deposits are usually extracellular and in toxic Ig fibril form though unstable oligomers of these amyloidogenic proteins are also deposited. Invasion of the extracellular space of vital organs by these toxic fibrils ultimately leads to functional compromise and can potentially precipitate organ failure [63, 88–91].

Initial models injected large quantities of Bence-Jones protein in mice and found Congo Red-positive deposits in mouse organs. This model had some major problems in that multiple doses were usually needed for deposits to occur, and mouse deposits only occurred in samples from patients with high serum creatinine levels, exceeding 168 μmol/L [64, 92]. Engineered hybridoma models, as detailed in Sect. 5.3.1.2.1, consisting of SP2/0 cells that expressed AL amyloidosis light chains within BALB/c mice, or grafts made up of human AL amyloidosis plasma cells in the immunodeficient mouse, had very disappointing results. Animals died quickly due to fulminant disease which prevented detailed targeted studies of not only the pathogenesis of the disease but also the role of potential drugs [60]. A partially successful model is where the ubiquitous expression of human λ6 light chains (CMVλ6) has produced a few (Ig) amyloid deposits within the gastric glands [60]. Light chain production is strictly localized with levels of circulating human light chains in the transgenic mice below the detection limit, and no deposits in other organs. This model has been important for establishing doxycycline as a therapeutic for this disease [65, 66].

Randall-Type Monoclonal Immunoglobulin Deposition Disease (MIDD)

In Randall-type MIDD extracellular deposits of a non-amyloid variety comprising monoclonal Ig fragments are observed which have an amorphous ultrastructure. Deposits are both renal and extra-renal (hepatic and cardiac). Renal lesions are typically linear depositions of Ig in tubules and the glomerular basement membranes; nodular glomerulosclerosis typically ensues, ultimately causing a progressive kidney failure [67, 93, 94]. Commonly, light chains are deposited but heavy chain deposition has also been described [60, 95–97].

Unlike in AL Amyloidosis, the general models described in Sect. 5.3.1 above have been successful in recreating Randall-Type MIDD. Penile dorsal vein/renal artery injection of light chains from a biopsy of confirmed human Light Chain Deposit Disease (LCDD) into mice reproduced the typical renal features of Randall-type MIDD nephropathy. It was seen that when these light chains were injected into Caveolin 1 (Cav1)-knockout mice, they escaped developing the renal lesions thus signifying the importance of Cav1 in the genesis of MIDD nephropathy [98].

In another study, transgenic mouse models were made to evaluate alterations to κ L chain sequences (of human origin), comparing a somatically mutated chain (LCDD) with a related control κ chain, both encoded by the distinctive VκIV gene. Mice that secreted the LCDD but not the control chain developed deposits that were similar to those found in human MIDD [79].

Randall-type heavy chain deposition disease (HCDD) is a variant where amorphous renal (glomerular/peritubular) deposits of truncated monoclonal Ig heavy chains (HC) with a deletion in the first constant domain (CH1) are seen. A transgenic mouse model of MIDD (HCDD) was made by insertion of a (MIDD patient-sourced) human HC in the Ig κ locus. This led to significant expression of the human heavy chains in the mouse B cells and plasma cells. Conditional deletion of the CH1 domain here closely recreated human MIDD (HCDD), with marked reduction of HC levels in the serum. Histopathological analyses showed renal lesions commonly seen in typical Randall-type nephropathy which were not seen in mice that expressed the complete human HC. Treatment with bortezomib reduced the renal deposition. Thus, this model appeared to suggest that MIDD (HCDD) nephropathy is promoted by the presence of isolated truncated HC, that, when coupled with the absence of an LC partner, aggregates readily, even at very low serum levels [61].

Myeloma Cast Nephropathy (MCN) Models

In MCN, toxic monoclonal light chains damage the kidney by release of proinflammatory cytokines in the proximal tubule epithelium. In addition, some light chains undergo precipitation with uromodulin in the distal convoluted tubule, leading to tubular blockade and renal interstitial inflammation, conditions that can precipitate renal failure [60, 85].

Injection of large amounts of purified Bence-Jones proteins into the mice efficiently recreated human MCN [68, 70]. Light chains were found to precipitate with uromodulin when they exceeded a threshold level, helped by triggering factors such as furosemide, low pH, high salt concentrations, and application of contrast agents [85].

MGUS/MGRS

During clinical MM, the large number of light chains filtered by the glomerulus is far in excess of the absorptive capacity of the processing receptors cubilin and megalin in the proximal convoluted tubule, and this leads to AL. Even small accumulations of light chains can lead to damage of the affected organs. This resulted in the re-classification of MGUS in this condition to MGRS, as discussed previously [60, 71, 99].

A recent transgenic model used site-directed insertion of the variable domain area of a disease-producing human light chain gene into the Ig κ locus of a mouse to ensure its production by all mouse plasma cells. High levels of free light chains were obtained after backcrossing with mice that had increased levels of plasma cell differentiation but absence of heavy chain production [100].

Models of Disorders Involving Deposition of Complete Monoclonal Ig Molecules (Two Heavy Chains and Two Light Chains)

Three disorders fall into this category, and as discussed below, there is a lack of successful models for investigating two of these disorders.

In the cryoglobulinemias abnormal Igs (called cryoglobulins) in the serum precipitate at lower temperatures but redissolve on warming. These cryoglobulins can be made up of monoclonal Igs (Simple Type I cryoglobulinemias), monoclonal Igs attached to polyclonal Igs (Mixed Type II cryoglobulinemias), or may be composed entirely of polyclonal Igs (Mixed Type III cryoglobulinemias).

In the paraproteinemia context, only Type 1 and Type 2 are significant. Type I cryoglobulinemia presents clinically with symptoms and signs that are often related to intravascular obstruction, whereas for Type 2 the precipitates result in immune complex-mediated vasculitis with purpura and skin ulcers. The peripheral nerves and joints are also affected. Renal effects are seen as cryoglobulinemic glomerulonephritis, which is a membranoproliferative glomerulonephritis (MPGN). The glomerulus shows a blockade of the peripheral capillary lumens by numerous infiltrating cells of monocytic lineage, and pink immune thrombi, made up of cryoglobulin deposits, are observed [72, 101]. The renal damage seen in this disorder has been successfully modeled [73–76, 102], and an example is discussed here:

Murine Ig3 Hybridoma Model

This model is induced by infusion of murine hybridoma cells that secrete monoclonal IgG3, which stimulates a Type I cryoglobulinemia [75]. These mice have cutaneous leukocytoclastic vasculitis in addition to glomerular injury. Glomerular involvement produces sclerosis and crescents in addition to the membranoproliferative glomerulonephritis that is typically associated with cryoglobulinemia. Around a third of mice also show necrotizing arteritis in the skeletal musculature and the kidneys [75]. Further investigation demonstrated that the kidney and skin lesions occur via distinctly different pathways [77].

Immunotactoid Glomerulopathy

Considered today as distinct from amyloidosis and common paraproteinemias due to its composition ("immuno") and polymeric glomerular deposits ("tactoid"). Deposits are mainly mesangial and appear ultrastructurally as parallel microtubules or random fibrils which comprise C3 and IgG. Unlike AL, deposits are negative for Congo Red and Thioflavin T. These patients do not have systemic manifestations, unlike other diseases commonly linked to deposition of organized IgG [103–105].

There are currently no well-characterized animal models for immunotactoid glomerulopathy; however, a group in Japan have reported spontaneous renal lesions pathologically similar to immunotactoid glomerulopathy (global fibrillary and microtubular subendothelial glomerular deposits of IgG, IgM, IgA, and C3 that were amorphous, eosinophilic, and Congo Red negative) in young female mice of the ddY strain which is maintained as a closed colony with only one repository [106]. Models for other renal diseases have been derived from the ddY strain such as the HIGA mice model for IgA nephritis [107], and thus it may be that new derivatives from the ddY strain have the potential to model for immunotactoid nephropathy.

Proliferative Glomerulonephritis with Monoclonal Ig Deposits

A monoclonal gammopathy seen in the kidneys that closely mimics immune-complex glomerulonephritis, and has a poor renal prognosis, with progression to end-stage disease in around a quarter of patients in 3 years. Histologically, most cases show a predominantly membranoproliferative pattern while other patients have endocapillary proliferation with membranous features. Immunofluorescence studies show glomerular deposition of granular deposits consisting of a solitary light-chain isotype with a single heavy chain subtype, commonly IgG3κ [108, 109]. No experimental animal model has yet been established for this distinct disease entity.

Conclusions

Animal models are an essential tool to investigate paraproteinemias since they offer a platform to study not only the disease itself, but also prospective therapeutic compounds in a whole-body system that closely mimics human physiology, allowing detailed study of interactions between different cell types, which is not afforded in the more basic in vitro models.

Given the heterogeneity of the paraproteinemias, multiple models exist, which cover both the diseases themselves, and the pathological conditions that arise. Each model has its own advantages and disadvantages, and careful consideration must be taken to ensure that a specific model has the desired characteristics which mimic the facet of the disease under investigation to ensure meaningful correlation of the results with the clinical situation.

While significant improvements in transgenic technology and "humanized" models have been made over time, no one animal model can truly represent the complexity of a paraproteinemia, and therefore further advancements are still required in this area.

References

1. Leung N, Drosou ME, Nasr SH. Dysproteinemias and glomerular disease. Clin J Am Soc Nephrol. 2018;13(1):128–39.
2. Wells JV, Fudenberg HH. Paraproteinemias. Disease-a-Month. 1974;20(2):1–45.
3. Kanzaki G, Okabayashi Y, Nagahama K, Ohashi R, Tsuboi N, Yokoo T, et al. Monoclonal Ig deposition disease and related diseases. J Nippon Med Sch. 2019;86(1):2–9.
4. Glavey SV, Leung N. Monoclonal gammopathy: the good, the bad and the ugly. Blood Rev. 2016;30(3):223–31.
5. Merlini G, Stone MJ. Dangerous small B-cell clones. Blood. 2006;108(8):2520–30.
6. Lwin ST, Edwards CM, Silbermann R. Preclinical animal models of multiple myeloma. Bonekey Rep. 2016;5:772.
7. Leung N, Bridoux F, Batuman V, Chaidos A, Cockwell P, D'Agati VD, et al. The evaluation of monoclonal gammopathy of renal significance: a consensus report of the International Kidney and Monoclonal Gammopathy Research Group. Nat Rev Nephrol. 2019;15(1):45–59.
8. Rossi M, Botta C, Arbitrio M, Grembiale RD, Tagliaferri P, Tassone P. Mouse models of multiple myeloma: technologic platforms and perspectives. Oncotarget. 2018;9(28):20119–33.
9. Libouban H. The use of animal models in multiple myeloma. Morphologie. 2015;99(325):63–72.
10. Tassone P, Neri P, Carrasco DR, Burger R, Goldmacher VS, Fram R, et al. A clinically relevant SCID-hu in vivo model of human multiple myeloma. Blood. 2005;106(2):713–6.
11. Urashima M, Chen BP, Chen S, Pinkus GS, Bronson RT, Dedera DA, et al. The development of a model for the homing of multiple myeloma cells to human bone marrow. Blood. 1997;90(2):754–65.
12. Yaccoby S, Barlogie B, Epstein J. Primary myeloma cells growing in SCID-hu mice: a model for studying the biology and treatment of myeloma and its manifestations. Blood. 1998;92(8):2908–13.

13. Yaccoby S, Ling W, Zhan F, Walker R, Barlogie B, Shaughnessy JD Jr. Antibody-based inhibition of DKK1 suppresses tumor-induced bone resorption and multiple myeloma growth in vivo. Blood. 2007;109(5):2106–11.
14. Yata K, Yaccoby S. The SCID-rab model: a novel in vivo system for primary human myeloma demonstrating growth of CD138-expressing malignant cells. Leukemia. 2004;18(11):1891–7.
15. Calimeri T, Battista E, Conforti F, Neri P, Di Martino MT, Rossi M, et al. A unique three-dimensional SCID-polymeric scaffold (SCID-synth-hu) model for in vivo expansion of human primary multiple myeloma cells. Leukemia. 2011;25(4):707–11.
16. Zhu D, Wang Z, Zhao JJ, Calimeri T, Meng J, Hideshima T, et al. The Cyclophilin A-CD147 complex promotes the proliferation and homing of multiple myeloma cells. Nat Med. 2015;21(6):572–80.
17. Lawson MA, Paton-Hough JM, Evans HR, Walker RE, Harris W, Ratnabalan D, et al. NOD/SCID-GAMMA mice are an ideal strain to assess the efficacy of therapeutic agents used in the treatment of myeloma bone disease. PLoS One. 2015;10(3):e0119546.
18. Miyakawa Y, Ohnishi Y, Tomisawa M, Monnai M, Kohmura K, Ueyama Y, et al. Establishment of a new model of human multiple myeloma using NOD/SCID/gammac(null) (NOG) mice. Biochem Biophys Res Commun. 2004;313(2):258–62.
19. Ito M, Hiramatsu H, Kobayashi K, Suzue K, Kawahata M, Hioki K, et al. NOD/SCID/gamma(c)(null) mouse: an excellent recipient mouse model for engraftment of human cells. Blood. 2002;100(9):3175–82.
20. Manning LS, Berger JD, O'Donoghue HL, Sheridan GN, Claringbold PG, Turner JH. A model of multiple myeloma: culture of 5T33 murine myeloma cells and evaluation of tumorigenicity in the C57BL/KaLwRij mouse. Br J Cancer. 1992;66(6):1088–93.
21. Radl J. Animal model of human disease. Benign monoclonal gammopathy (idiopathic paraproteinemia). Am J Pathol. 1981;105(1):91–3.
22. Radl J. Differences among the three major categories of paraproteinaemias in aging man and the mouse. A minireview. Mech Ageing Dev. 1984;28(2):167–70.
23. Radl J, Hollander CF, van den Berg P, de Glopper E. Idiopathic paraproteinaemia. I. Studies in an animal model—the ageing C57BL/KaLwRij mouse. Clin Exp Immunol. 1978;33(3):395–402.
24. Hilbert DM, Kopf M, Mock BA, Köhler G, Rudikoff S. Interleukin 6 is essential for in vivo development of B lineage neoplasms. J Exp Med. 1995;182(1):243–8.
25. Kovalchuk AL, Kim JS, Park SS, Coleman AE, Ward JM, Morse HC 3rd, et al. IL-6 transgenic mouse model for extraosseous plasmacytoma. Proc Natl Acad Sci U S A. 2002;99(3):1509–14.
26. Rosean TR, Tompkins VS, Tricot G, Holman CJ, Olivier AK, Zhan F, et al. Preclinical validation of interleukin 6 as a therapeutic target in multiple myeloma. Immunol Res. 2014;59(1–3):188–202.
27. Nordan RP, Potter M. A macrophage-derived factor required by plasmacytomas for survival and proliferation in vitro. Science. 1986;233(4763):566–9.
28. Vandenberg CJ, Waring P, Strasser A, Cory S. Plasmacytomagenesis in Eμ-v-abl transgenic mice is accelerated when apoptosis is restrained. Blood. 2014;124(7):1099–109.
29. Rongvaux A, Willinger T, Martinek J, Strowig T, Gearty SV, Teichmann LL, et al. Corrigendum: development and function of human innate immune cells in a humanized mouse model. Nat Biotechnol. 2017;35(12):1211.
30. Rongvaux A, Takizawa H, Strowig T, Willinger T, Eynon EE, Flavell RA, et al. Human hemato-lymphoid system mice: current use and future potential for medicine. Annu Rev Immunol. 2013;31:635–74.
31. Donnou S, Galand C, Touitou V, Sautès-Fridman C, Fabry Z, Fisson S. Murine models of B-cell lymphomas: promising tools for designing cancer therapies. Adv Hematol. 2012;2012:701704.
32. Rosenbaum H, Harris AW, Bath ML, McNeall J, Webb E, Adams JM, et al. An E mu-v-abl transgene elicits plasmacytomas in concert with an activated myc gene. EMBO J. 1990;9(3):897–905.

33. Shaffer AL, Shapiro-Shelef M, Iwakoshi NN, Lee AH, Qian SB, Zhao H, et al. XBP1, downstream of Blimp-1, expands the secretory apparatus and other organelles, and increases protein synthesis in plasma cell differentiation. Immunity. 2004;21(1):81–93.
34. Reimold AM, Iwakoshi NN, Manis J, Vallabhajosyula P, Szomolanyi-Tsuda E, Gravallese EM, et al. Plasma cell differentiation requires the transcription factor XBP-1. Nature. 2001;412(6844):300–7.
35. Carrasco DR, Sukhdeo K, Protopopova M, Sinha R, Enos M, Carrasco DE, et al. The differentiation and stress response factor XBP-1 drives multiple myeloma pathogenesis. Cancer Cell. 2007;11(4):349–60.
36. Hua Y, White-Gilbertson S, Kellner J, Rachidi S, Usmani SZ, Chiosis G, et al. Molecular chaperone gp96 is a novel therapeutic target of multiple myeloma. Clin Cancer Res. 2013;19(22):6242–51.
37. Iwakoshi NN, Lee AH, Vallabhajosyula P, Otipoby KL, Rajewsky K, Glimcher LH. Plasma cell differentiation and the unfolded protein response intersect at the transcription factor XBP-1. Nat Immunol. 2003;4(4):321–9.
38. Morito N, Yoh K, Fujioka Y, Nakano T, Shimohata H, Hashimoto Y, et al. Overexpression of c-Maf contributes to T-cell lymphoma in both mice and human. Cancer Res. 2006;66(2):812–9.
39. Chesi M, Bergsagel PL, Shonukan OO, Martelli ML, Brents LA, Chen T, et al. Frequent dysregulation of the c-maf proto-oncogene at 16q23 by translocation to an Ig locus in multiple myeloma. Blood. 1998;91(12):4457–63.
40. Boylan KL, Gosse MA, Staggs SE, Janz S, Grindle S, Kansas GS, et al. A transgenic mouse model of plasma cell malignancy shows phenotypic, cytogenetic, and gene expression heterogeneity similar to human multiple myeloma. Cancer Res. 2007;67(9):4069–78.
41. Linden M, Kirchhof N, Carlson C, Van Ness B. Targeted overexpression of Bcl-XL in B-lymphoid cells results in lymphoproliferative disease and plasma cell malignancies. Blood. 2004;103(7):2779–86.
42. Spets H, Strömberg T, Georgii-Hemming P, Siljason J, Nilsson K, Jernberg-Wiklund H. Expression of the bcl-2 family of pro- and anti-apoptotic genes in multiple myeloma and normal plasma cells: regulation during interleukin-6(IL-6)-induced growth and survival. Eur J Haematol. 2002;69(2):76–89.
43. Hamouda MA, Jacquel A, Robert G, Puissant A, Richez V, Cassel R, et al. BCL-B (BCL2L10) is overexpressed in patients suffering from multiple myeloma (MM) and drives an MM-like disease in transgenic mice. J Exp Med. 2016;213(9):1705–22.
44. Das R, Strowig T, Verma R, Koduru S, Hafemann A, Hopf S, et al. Microenvironment-dependent growth of preneoplastic and malignant plasma cells in humanized mice. Nat Med. 2016;22(11):1351–7.
45. de Romeuf C, Dutertre CA, Le Garff-Tavernier M, Fournier N, Gaucher C, Glacet A, et al. Chronic lymphocytic leukaemia cells are efficiently killed by an anti-CD20 monoclonal antibody selected for improved engagement of FcgammaRIIIA/CD16. Br J Haematol. 2008;140(6):635–43.
46. Mössner E, Brünker P, Moser S, Püntener U, Schmidt C, Herter S, et al. Increasing the efficacy of CD20 antibody therapy through the engineering of a new type II anti-CD20 antibody with enhanced direct and immune effector cell-mediated B-cell cytotoxicity. Blood. 2010;115(22):4393–402.
47. Yan JS, Chen XY, Li WP, Yang Y, Song ZL. Establishing SCID mouse models of B-cell non-Hodgkin's lymphoma. Ai Zheng. 2009;28(2):181–3.
48. Rempel RE, Jiang X, Fullerton P, Tan TZ, Ye J, Lau JA, et al. Utilization of the Eμ-Myc mouse to model heterogeneity of therapeutic response. Mol Cancer Ther. 2014;13(12):3219.
49. Kovalchuk AL, Qi CF, Torrey TA, Taddesse-Heath L, Feigenbaum L, Park SS, et al. Burkitt lymphoma in the mouse. J Exp Med. 2000;192(8):1183–90.
50. Fredrickson TN, Lennert K, Chattopadhyay SK, Morse HC 3rd, Hartley JW. Splenic marginal zone lymphomas of mice. Am J Pathol. 1999;154(3):805–12.

51. Ford RJ, Shen L, Lin-Lee YC, Pham LV, Multani A, Zhou HJ, et al. Development of a murine model for blastoid variant mantle-cell lymphoma. Blood. 2007;109(11):4899–906.
52. Kasama Y, Sekiguchi S, Saito M, et al. Persistent expression of the full genome of hepatitis C virus in B cells induces spontaneous development of B-cell lymphomas in vivo. Blood. 2010;116(23):4926–4933. Blood. 2011;117(21):5782–3.
53. Teng J, Turbat-Herrera EA, Herrera GA. An animal model of glomerular light-chain-associated amyloidogenesis depicts the crucial role of lysosomes. Kidney Int. 2014;86(4):738–46.
54. Fowler JA, Mundy GR, Lwin ST, Lynch CC, Edwards CM. A murine model of myeloma that allows genetic manipulation of the host microenvironment. Dis Model Mech. 2009;2(11–12):604–11.
55. Hernandez-Ilizaliturri FJ, Jupudy V, Ostberg J, Oflazoglu E, Huberman A, Repasky E, et al. Neutrophils contribute to the biological antitumor activity of rituximab in a non-Hodgkin's lymphoma severe combined immunodeficiency mouse model. Clin Cancer Res. 2003;9(16):5866.
56. Mori S, Rempel RE, Chang JT, Yao G, Lagoo AS, Potti A, et al. Utilization of pathway signatures to reveal distinct types of B lymphoma in the Emicro-myc model and human diffuse large B-cell lymphoma. Cancer Res. 2008;68(20):8525–34.
57. Diomede L, Rognoni P, Lavatelli F, Romeo M, del Favero E, Cantù L, et al. A Caenorhabditis elegans-based assay recognizes Ig light chains causing heart amyloidosis. Blood. 2014;123(23):3543–52.
58. Maldonado JE, Velosa JA, Kyle RA, Wagoner RD, Holley KE, Salassa RM. Fanconi syndrome in adults. A manifestation of a latent form of myeloma. Am J Med. 1975;58(3):354–64.
59. Sirac C, Bridoux F, Carrion C, Devuyst O, Fernandez B, Goujon JM, et al. Role of the monoclonal kappa chain V domain and reversibility of renal damage in a transgenic model of acquired Fanconi syndrome. Blood. 2006;108(2):536–43.
60. Sirac C, Herrera GA, Sanders PW, Batuman V, Bender S, Ayala MV, et al. Animal models of monoclonal Ig-related renal diseases. Nat Rev Nephrol. 2018;14(4):246–64.
61. Bonaud A, Bender S, Touchard G, Lacombe C, Srour N, Delpy L, et al. A mouse model recapitulating human monoclonal heavy chain deposition disease evidences the relevance of proteasome inhibitor therapy. Blood. 2015;126(6):757–65.
62. Sirac C, Bender S, Jaccard A, Bridoux F, Lacombe C, Touchard G, et al. Strategies to model AL amyloidosis in mice. Amyloid. 2011;18(Suppl 1):45–7.
63. Liao R, Jain M, Teller P, Connors LH, Ngoy S, Skinner M, et al. Infusion of light chains from patients with cardiac amyloidosis causes diastolic dysfunction in isolated mouse hearts. Circulation. 2001;104(14):1594–7.
64. Solomon A, Weiss DT, Kattine AA. Nephrotoxic potential of Bence Jones proteins. N Engl J Med. 1991;324(26):1845–51.
65. Ward JE, Ren R, Toraldo G, SooHoo P, Guan J, O'Hara C, et al. Doxycycline reduces fibril formation in a transgenic mouse model of AL amyloidosis. Blood. 2011;118(25):6610–7.
66. Wechalekar AD, Whelan C. Encouraging impact of doxycycline on early mortality in cardiac light chain (AL) amyloidosis. Blood Cancer J. 2017;7(3):e546.
67. Cohen C, Javaugue V, Joly F, Arnulf B, Fermand JP, Jaccard A, et al. [Randall-type monoclonal Ig deposition disease: from diagnosis to treatment]. Nephrol Ther. 2016;12(3):131–9.
68. Weiss JH, Williams RH, Galla JH, Gottschall JL, Rees ED, Bhathena D, et al. Pathophysiology of acute Bence-Jones protein nephrotoxicity in the rat. Kidney Int. 1981;20(2):198–210.
69. Decourt C, Rocca A, Bridoux F, Vrtovsnik F, Preud'homme JL, Cogné M, et al. Mutational analysis in murine models for myeloma-associated Fanconi's syndrome or cast myeloma nephropathy. Blood. 1999;94(10):3559–66.
70. Koss MN, Pirani CL, Osserman EF. Experimental Bence Jones cast nephropathy. Lab Invest. 1976;34(6):579–91.
71. Christensen EI, Birn H, Storm T, Weyer K, Nielsen R. Endocytic receptors in the renal proximal tubule. Physiology (Bethesda). 2012;27(4):223–36.
72. Muchtar E, Magen H, Gertz MA. How I treat cryoglobulinemia. Blood. 2017;129(3):289–98.

73. Vernon KA, Pickering MC, Cook T. Experimental models of membranoproliferative glomerulonephritis, including dense deposit disease. Contrib Nephrol. 2011;169:198–210.
74. Berney T, Shibata T, Izui S. Murine cryoglobulinemia: pathogenic and protective IgG3 self-associating antibodies. J Immunol. 1991;147(10):3331–5.
75. Gyotoku Y, Abdelmoula M, Spertini F, Izui S, Lambert PH. Cryoglobulinemia induced by monoclonal Ig G rheumatoid factors derived from autoimmune MRL/MpJ-lpr/lpr mice. J Immunol. 1987;138(11):3785.
76. Taneda S, Segerer S, Hudkins KL, Cui Y, Wen M, Segerer M, et al. Cryoglobulinemic glomerulonephritis in thymic stromal lymphopoietin transgenic mice. Am J Pathol. 2001;159(6):2355–69.
77. Reininger L, Berney T, Shibata T, Spertini F, Merino R, Izui S. Cryoglobulinemia induced by a murine IgG3 rheumatoid factor: skin vasculitis and glomerulonephritis arise from distinct pathogenic mechanisms. Proc Natl Acad Sci U S A. 1990;87(24):10038–42.
78. Rognoni P, Lavatelli F, Casarini S, Palladini G, Verga L, Pedrazzoli P, et al. A strategy for synthesis of pathogenic human Ig free light chains in E. coli. PLoS One. 2013;8(9):e76022.
79. Khamlichi AA, Rocca A, Touchard G, Aucouturier P, Preud'homme JL, Cogné M. Role of light chain variable region in myeloma with light chain deposition disease: evidence from an experimental model. Blood. 1995;86(10):3655–9.
80. Mishra S, Guan J, Plovie E, Seldin DC, Connors LH, Merlini G, et al. Human amyloidogenic light chain proteins result in cardiac dysfunction, cell death, and early mortality in zebrafish. Am J Physiol Heart Circ Physiol. 2013;305(1):H95–H103.
81. Chauveau C, Decourt C, Cogné M. Insertion of the IgH locus 3′ regulatory palindrome in expression vectors warrants sure and efficient expression in stable B cell transfectants. Gene. 1998;222(2):279–85.
82. Lechouane F, Bonaud A, Delpy L, Casola S, Oruc Z, Chemin G, et al. B-cell receptor signal strength influences terminal differentiation. Eur J Immunol. 2013;43(3):619–28.
83. Casola S, Otipoby KL, Alimzhanov M, Humme S, Uyttersprot N, Kutok JL, et al. B cell receptor signal strength determines B cell fate. Nat Immunol. 2004;5(3):317–27.
84. Ashi MO, Srour N, Lambert J-M, Marchalot A, Martin O, Le Noir S, et al. Physiological and druggable skipping of Ig variable exons in plasma cells. Cell Mol Immunol. 2019;16(10):810–9.
85. Hutchison CA, Batuman V, Behrens J, Bridoux F, Sirac C, Dispenzieri A, et al. The pathogenesis and diagnosis of acute kidney injury in multiple myeloma. Nat Rev Nephrol. 2011;8(1):43–51.
86. Messiaen T, Deret S, Mougenot B, Bridoux F, Dequiedt P, Dion JJ, et al. Adult Fanconi syndrome secondary to light chain gammopathy. Clinicopathologic heterogeneity and unusual features in 11 patients. Medicine (Baltimore). 2000;79(3):135–54.
87. Batuman V, Sastrasinh M, Sastrasinh S. Light chain effects on alanine and glucose uptake by renal brush border membranes. Kidney Int. 1986;30(5):662–5.
88. Palladini G, Lavatelli F, Russo P, Perlini S, Perfetti V, Bosoni T, et al. Circulating amyloidogenic free light chains and serum N-terminal natriuretic peptide type B decrease simultaneously in association with improvement of survival in AL. Blood. 2006;107(10):3854–8.
89. Brenner DA, Jain M, Pimentel DR, Wang B, Connors LH, Skinner M, et al. Human amyloidogenic light chains directly impair cardiomyocyte function through an increase in cellular oxidant stress. Circ Res. 2004;94(8):1008–10.
90. Desport E, Bridoux F, Sirac C, Delbes S, Bender S, Fernandez B, et al. AL amyloidosis. Orphanet J Rare Dis. 2012;7:54.
91. Pepys MB. Amyloidosis. Annu Rev Med. 2006;57:223–41.
92. Solomon A, Weiss DT, Pepys MB. Induction in mice of human light-chain-associated amyloidosis. Am J Pathol. 1992;140(3):629–37.
93. Lin J, Markowitz GS, Valeri AM, Kambham N, Sherman WH, Appel GB, et al. Renal monoclonal Ig deposition disease: the disease spectrum. J Am Soc Nephrol. 2001;12(7):1482–92.

94. Buxbaum J, Gallo G. Nonamyloidotic monoclonal Ig deposition disease. Light-chain, heavy-chain, and light- and heavy-chain deposition diseases. Hematol Oncol Clin North Am. 1999;13(6):1235–48.
95. Bridoux F, Javaugue V, Bender S, Leroy F, Aucouturier P, Debiais-Delpech C, et al. Unravelling the immunopathological mechanisms of heavy chain deposition disease with implications for clinical management. Kidney Int. 2017;91(2):423–34.
96. Kambham N, Markowitz GS, Appel GB, Kleiner MJ, Aucouturier P, D'Agati VD. Heavy chain deposition disease: the disease spectrum. Am J Kidney Dis. 1999;33(5):954–62.
97. Aucouturier P, Khamlichi AA, Touchard G, Justrabo E, Cogne M, Chauffert B, et al. Brief report: heavy-chain deposition disease. N Engl J Med. 1993;329(19):1389–93.
98. Herrera GA, Turbat-Herrera EA, Teng J. Animal models of light chain deposition disease provide a better understanding of nodular glomerulosclerosis. Nephron. 2016;132(2):119–36.
99. Batuman V, Verroust PJ, Navar GL, Kaysen JH, Goda FO, Campbell WC, et al. Myeloma light chains are ligands for cubilin (gp280). Am J Physiol. 1998;275(2):F246–54.
100. Bender S, Ayala MV, Bonaud A, Javaugue V, Carrion C, Oblet C, et al. Ig light-chain toxicity in a mouse model of monoclonal Ig light-chain deposition disease. Blood. 2020;136(14):1645–56.
101. Desbois AC, Cacoub P, Saadoun D. Cryoglobulinemia: an update in 2019. Joint Bone Spine. 2019;86(6):707–13.
102. Kowalewska J. Cryoglobulinemic glomerulonephritis—lessons from animal models. Folia Histochem Cytobiol. 2011;49(4):537–46.
103. Schwartz MM, Korbet SM, Lewis EJ. Immunotactoid glomerulopathy. J Am Soc Nephrol. 2002;13(5):1390–7.
104. Korbet SM, Schwartz MM, Lewis EJ. Immuotactoid glomerulopathy (fibrillary glomerulonephritis). Clin J Am Soc Nephrol. 2006;1(6):1351.
105. Haas M. Glomerular disease pathology in the era of proteomics: from pattern to pathogenesis. J Am Soc Nephrol. 2018;29(1):2.
106. Kouchi M, Toyosawa K, Matsumoto I, Michimae Y, Tochitani T, Koujitani T, et al. Hyaline Glomerulopathy with Tubulo-fibrillary deposits in young ddY mice. Toxicol Pathol. 2011;39(6):975–9.
107. Yamazaki T, Kishimoto K, Ezaki O. The ddY mouse: a model of postprandial hypertriglyceridemia in response to dietary fat. J Lipid Res. 2012;53(10):2024–37.
108. Miller P, Xiao AY, Kung VL, Sibley RK, Higgins JP, Kambham N, et al. Progression of proliferative glomerulonephritis with monoclonal IgG deposits in pediatric patients. Pediatr Nephrol. 2021;36(4):927–37.
109. Nasr SH, Satoskar A, Markowitz GS, Valeri AM, Appel GB, Stokes MB, et al. Proliferative glomerulonephritis with monoclonal IgG deposits. J Am Soc Nephrol. 2009;20(9):2055–64.

Chapter 6
An Approach to the Diagnosis of Paraproteinemia

Mohamed Tharwat Hegazy, Ayman Abdel-Monem Ahmed Mahmoud, Hend Attia, and Gaafar Ragab

Abbreviations

AL	Light-chain amyloid
BCSH	British Committee for Standards in Haematology
BM	Bone marrow
CBC	Complete blood count
Del	Deletions
EBV	Epstein–Barr virus
EHA	European Hematology Association
ESMO	European Society for Medical Oncology
ESR	Erythrocyte sedimentation rate
FDG PET-CT	Fluorodeoxyglucose Positron Emission Tomography-Computed Tomography
FISH	Fluorescence in situ hybridization
GGT	Gamma-glutamyl transferase

M. T. Hegazy · G. Ragab (✉)
Rheumatology and Clinical Immunology Unit, Internal Medicine Department, Faculty of Medicine, Cairo University, Cairo, Egypt

School of Medicine, Newgiza University (NGU), Giza, Egypt
e-mail: Dr_moh_tharwat@kasralainy.edu.eg

A. A.-M. A. Mahmoud
Internal Medicine Department, Rheumatology, and Clinical Immunology Unit, Faculty of Medicine, Cairo University, Cairo, Egypt

H. Attia
School of Medicine, Newgiza University (NGU), Giza, Egypt
e-mail: Hend.mokhtar@ngu.edu.eg

© The Author(s), under exclusive license to Springer Nature Switzerland AG 2022
G. Ragab et al. (eds.), *Paraproteinemia and Related Disorders*,
https://doi.org/10.1007/978-3-031-10131-1_6

HLC	Heavy/light chain
IFE	Immunofixation
Ig	Immunoglobulin
IKMG	International Kidney and Monoclonal Gammopathy Research Group
IMWG	International Myeloma Working Group
ISE	Immunosubtraction electrophoresis
ISH	In situ hybridization
ISS	International Staging System
MG	Monoclonal gammopathy
MGCS	Monoclonal gammopathy of clinical significance
MGNS	Monoclonal gammopathy of neurological significance
MGRS	Monoclonal gammopathy of renal significance
MGUS	Monoclonal gammopathy of undetermined significance
MIDD	Monoclonal immunoglobulin deposition disease
Mig	Monoclonal immunoglobulin
MM	Multiple myeloma
MRD	Minimal residual disease
NCCN	National Comprehensive Cancer Network
NDMM	Newly diagnosed MM
NHS	National Health Service
NXG	Necrobiotic xanthogranuloma
OS	Overall survival
PP	Paraproteinemia
R-ISS	Revised-International Staging System
SFLC	Serum free light chain
SMM	Smoldering multiple myeloma
SPEP	Serum protein electrophoresis
T	Translocations
WBLDCT	Whole-body low-dose computed tomography
WM	Waldenstrom macroglobulinemia
β2M	Beta 2 microglobulin

Introduction

Paraproteinemia (PP), also known as "monoclonal gammopathy" (MG) is the term used to describe the presence of excessive amounts of a single clone of gamma globulin or paraprotein in the blood. This phenomenon can be encountered in many disorders including autoimmune, autoinflammatory, infectious, neoplastic, and many other miscellaneous disorders [1]. It has been described even in healthy individuals, especially the elderly group, and its prevalence cannot be considered insignificant [2]. The diagnosis and the identification of paraproteinemia can thus be a challenging task for the clinician.

PP may be reached for, purposefully, as an imperative step in the context of a suspected disease entity like multiple myeloma (MM) or it may be present surreptitiously in association with another disorder. In both situations, they should be detected, specified, and quantified for a complete diagnosis and a proper management.

The physician should be alert to the presence of certain patterns or clusters of findings that can provide important clues. These can be gathered from medical history, physical examination, laboratory investigations, imaging modalities, and tissue biopsies. A high index of suspicion is mandatory otherwise the diagnosis will be missed.

In this chapter, we plan to present some of the patterns or clusters that have been studied and reported, highlighting the important investigative procedures that can be helpful in our endeavor. Once PP has been detected, systematic investigation should proceed to characterize and quantify the PP.

When to Suspect the Presence of Monoclonal Gammopathy

During a standard meticulous clinical examination, the physician should be alert to certain renal, neurological, cutaneous and ophthalmological findings, or specific patterns of combinations or clusters. This also applies to the existence of certain findings or phenomena that may be encountered when interpreting laboratory results or imaging reports.

Clusters of Clinical Symptoms that Can Provide Clues to MG Diagnosis

Hypercalcemia, renal impairment, anemia, and bony lesions are given the acronym CRAB, and can point to MM [3].

The presence of bleeding, dizziness, headache, visual, or auditory involvement will betray the presence of hyperviscosity and **Waldenstrom macroglobulinemia (WM)** [3] **or cryoglobulinemia type 1** [4].

The classic triad of hyperviscosity comprises mucosal bleeding, visual disturbance, and manifestations of nervous system disorder. Also, headache, lightheadedness, and hearing loss may be present, but the most dreaded ophthalmological outcome of hyperviscosity is central retinal vein occlusion. Blood viscosity is at its maximum in small venules which can cause wall tearing when tissue support is inadequate. This is most likely to take place in the nasal mucosa, the gum, the retina, and the alimentary tract, as well as the brain surface.

Cardiac, renal, and peripheral nerve symptoms should raise suspicion of amyloid light-chain (AL) amyloidosis [5].

The important clusters and their attribution to major organ involvement are summarized in Table 6.1.

The eye can be very helpful as a clue. Symptoms such as transient or progressive diminution of vision or even complete blindness may be present [14]. Examination may reveal conjunctival, corneal deposits, myositis, and proptosis. Eleven distinct types of MGUS-related paraproteinemic keratopathies have been identified [15, 16].

Fundoscopy is indispensable and can unmask increased viscosity or hypertension.

Table 6.1 Important clusters and major organ involvement

Category	Specific diseases and disorders
Monoclonal gammopathy of neurological significance [6, 7]	• AL amyloidosis • POEMS syndrome • Cryoglobulinemia • CANOMAD • DADS-M
Monoclonal gammopathy of renal significance [6, 8, 9]	Includes: • C3 glomerulopathy with MG and thrombotic microangiopathy • The nonorganized deposits include – MIDD – Proliferative GN with monoclonal immune deposits • Organized deposits: – Fibrillar deposits, which include AL amyloidosis (nephrotic syndrome) Monoclonal fibrillary GN – Microtubular deposits, which include Immunotactoid GN Cryoglobulinemia GN – Inclusions or crystalline deposits, which include LC proximal tubulopathy Crystal-storing histiocytosis Cryocrystalglobulin
Monoclonal gammopathy of cutaneous significance [10, 11]	• Schnitzler syndrome • Scleromyxedema • NXG • TEMPI syndrome • Cryoglobulinemia • SCLS • POEMS syndrome
Muscles [12, 13]	• Sporadic late onset nemaline myopathy

AL Amyloid light-chain, *POEMS* polyradiculoneuropathy, organomegaly, endocrinopathy, monoclonal plasma cell disorder, and skin changes, *CANOMAD* chronic ataxic neuropathy, ophthalmoplegia, immunoglobulin M [IgM] paraprotein, cold agglutinins, and disialosyl ganglioside antibodies, *DADS-M* distal acquired demyelinating symmetric neuropathy with M protein, *MIDD* Monoclonal immunoglobulin deposition disease, *GN* glomerulonephritis, *LC* light chain, *NXG* Necrobiotic xanthogranuloma, *TEMPI* telangiectasias, elevated erythropoietin and erythropoiesis, monoclonal gammopathy, perinephric fluid, intrapulmonary shunting, *SCLS* Systemic capillary leak syndrome

Fundoscopic Examination May Detect the Following

1. Acute or chronic uveitis [17]
2. Maculopathy, foveolar drusen [18, 19], Doyne retinal dystrophy [20]
3. Exudative macular detachment, retinal hemorrhage, or cotton-wool spots
4. Papilledema, distended and tortuous retinal veins, and hemorrhages
5. Central retinal artery or vein occlusion [21]

Moreover, there are areas in medical practice where we are more likely to encounter MG. These include autoimmune diseases with severe activity, specific types of autoinflammatory diseases, certain infections like Epstein–Barr virus, and malignancies (refer to Chaps. 17–20).

Imaging Findings that Can Help to Suspect Paraproteinemia

The detection of certain findings, even if inadvertently discovered in radiological images and other imaging modalities can be extremely helpful.

1. Plain radiography
   Multiple round punched out lytic lesions affecting skull, vertebrae, ribs, pelvis, and less commonly long bones appear in MM. However, when a solitary lesion is found, it is called plasmacytoma [22]. Evidence of pulmonary infiltrates, effusions, and congestive heart failure in the absence of lytic bony lesions are present in WM. Osteosclerosis, hyperostosis, and periosteal reaction may be found in Schnitzler syndrome usually affecting distal femur, proximal tibia (hot knees sign), and iliac bones [23].
2. Computerized tomography (CT)
   CT scan showing cortical involvement and diffuse osteopenia may be indicators of MM involvement even before discrete lesions become conspicuous. CT scan of the chest, abdomen, and pelvis provide evidence of lymphadenopathy and hepatosplenomegaly which are more common in WM, IgG and IgM heavy chain diseases and amyloidosis.
3. Magnetic resonance imaging (MRI)
   MRI is useful in detecting thoracic and lumbar spine lesions, paraspinal involvement, and early cold compressions. In this regard, it is more sensitive than plain radiography and can detect as many as 40% of spinal abnormalities in patients with asymptomatic gammopathy whose radiographic studies might be normal [24].
4. Ultrasonography
   Can reveal organ enlargement like hepatomegaly, splenomegaly, and lymphadenopathy in lymphoma or WM. It can also detect pancreatic masses, for example, IgG4-related disease [25].

Laboratory Findings that Raise Suspicion of MG if Unexplained by Other Causes [26–28]

These include the following abnormalities, particularly if more than one abnormality is reported: normocytic normochromic anemia, rouleaux formation of erythrocytes, pancytopenia, renal impairment, proteinuria, hypercalcemia, hyperuricemia, elevated erythrocyte sedimentation rate (ESR), and C-reactive protein, elevated total protein and globulin, hypoalbuminemia combined with elevated globulin.

Proceed Further Towards Establishing Complete Diagnosis

Once PP is detected, there will be a need to obtain a full description of its characteristics as well as those of its related disease.

In PP, the released proteins are used as diagnostic markers as well as quantitative measures during the follow-up of disease progression [27]. There is no single laboratory test considered to be diagnostic. A panel of tests is customarily used to establish the diagnosis and/or monitor the course of illness [28].

We derived a great deal of our knowledge in the field of PP from the medical experience with MM. This influenced our diagnostic approach to similar diseases associated with PP. There exist clinical practice guidelines stating the obligatory laboratory tests in MM investigations.

We refer the reader to five internationally recognized recommendations for such tests. These are recommendations of the Myeloma Canada Research Network Consensus Guideline Consortium [4], the International Myeloma Working Group (IMWG) guidelines [29], the National Comprehensive Cancer Network (NCCN) Guidelines: Multiple Myeloma [30], the European Hematology Association (EHA), and the European Society for Medical Oncology (ESMO) guidelines [3]. Figure 6.1 represents an algorithmas a practical guide to approach a case of PP based on internationally acknowledged guidelines and recommendations [3, 4, 35, 42].

Imaging for a Suspected Case with Paraproteinemia

Similarly, there are recommendations concerning the imaging modalities in cases suspected of having PP.

1. Skeletal survey

   Plain radiography is usually requested once MM is considered. It usually shows lytic lesions in myeloma [22]. However, the NHS and BCSH consider skeletal survey by plain radiography for evaluation of MGUS or MM obsolete, they recommend whole-body low-dose CT scan (WBLDCT), whole-body MRI or positron emission tomography-CT scan PET-CT scan [29]. Whole-body low-

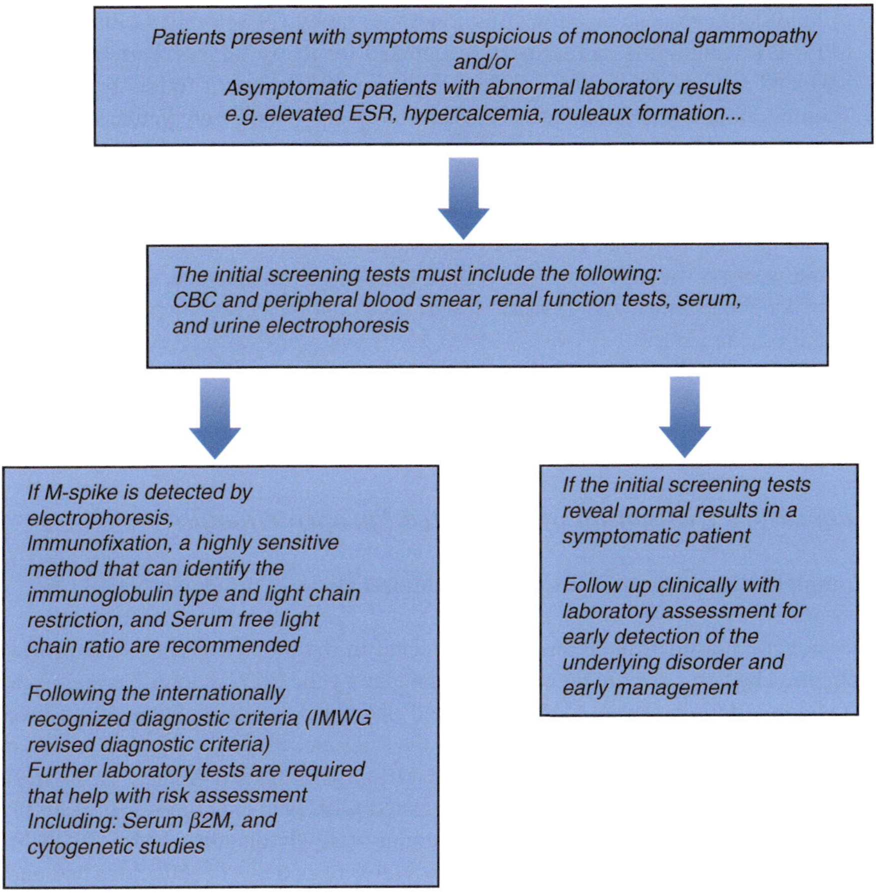

Fig. 6.1 Algorithm to Approach a case of paraproteinemia: This algorithm follows the internationally recognized guidelines and recommendations for laboratory evaluation of paraproteinemia. *β2M* Beta 2 microglobulin, *CBC* Complete blood count, *ESR* Erythrocyte sedimentation rate, *IMWG* International Myeloma Working Group

dose computed tomography has successfully replaced skeletal survey as the recent standard imaging modality in MM to assess bone involvement. It has approximately 70% sensitivity and 90% specificity making it more accurate than skeletal surveys, having a low dose of radiation exposure, amounting to only 1–2x the radiation dose of skeletal survey.

2. Whole-body MRI

   This can yield more accurate data in MGUS, smoldering multiple myeloma (SMM), and MM. MRI also is the gold standard modality to detect bone marrow (BM) involvement [24]. MRI can also delineate CNS involvement in Bing-Neel syndrome, a rare complication in WM, where it shows diffuse thickening and increased enhancement of the meninges and cranial nerves [30].

3. Fluorodeoxyglucose positron emission tomography-CT scan (FDG PET-CT)
   PET-CT scanning is increasingly recognized for its usefulness. It is superior to skeletal survey and useful also for prognosis and treatment follow-up [31]. Its combination with MRI increases its sensitivity and positive predictive value [32] since it describes the disease extent more accurately.
4. Bone scan
   Technetium bone scan may be a cost-effective test for Schnitzler syndrome [23]. It should not, however, be used in the evaluation of myeloma because the cytokines secreted by myeloma cells suppress the osteoblasts; hence, there will be no uptake enhancement. More than 50% of bone involvement may pass undetected on this scan [33].
5. Bone densitometry by dual energy X-ray absorptiometry
   This may show osteopenia or osteoporosis and can assess fracture risk.

Laboratory Evaluation of Suspected Paraproteinemia

Complete Blood Count (CBC) and Blood Smear

Normocytic normochromic anemia is detected in the blood count of 75% of MM patients. The latest criteria for end-organ damage by the IMWG describes anemia as a myeloma-defining event. MM-associated anemia describes a hemoglobin level >20 g/L (2 g/dL) below the lower limit of the reference range for age and sex, or an absolute hemoglobin level below 100 g/L (10 g/dL) [34–36]. Anemia is the most prevalent complication of MM. It is associated with poor outcomes [36]. Lanting and his group (2020) reported the blood count of newly diagnosed MM (NDMM) patients (n = 1363) and demonstrated that 84.4% of patients (1150/1363) had anemia (Hgb < 120 g/L) at the time of diagnosis regardless of their gender. In the same study, 55.2% (753/1363) of patients manifested with moderate (90–120 g/L) or severe anemia (60–90 g/L) at diagnosis [37].

The patients who had the lower figures of hemoglobin reveal an advanced stage disease both in the DS (Durie–Salmon) staging system (80.1 ± 0.8 g/L in DS stage III) and in the Revised International Staging System (RISS) (84.3 ± 1.6 g/L in RISS stage III). Hemoglobin figures in MM are in negative correlation with BM myeloma cells infiltration ($r = -0.1545$, $p < 0.0001$) [37].

Thrombocytopenia occurs less frequently [38]. Morphological examination of peripheral smear, however, may occasionally reveal circulating plasma cells and leukoerythroblastic reaction. The increased background staining, a bluish tinge to the blood film, is due to increased PP. This bluish background can be detected in MM while non-secretory MM (NSMM) lacks this feature [36].

Pathological rouleaux formation of red cells in peripheral blood smear is evident in PP. Rouleaux formation describes aggregation of red blood cells giving a "stack of coins" like appearance [38, 39]. In pathological states, the high level of plasma proteins (e.g., fibrinogen and globulins) coats the red blood cells. This renders the red cells "sticky" and results in rouleaux formation [39]. Rouleaux formation is associated with any condition that results in an increase of plasma proteins including acute and chronic inflammatory conditions, plasma cell myeloma, and polyclonal or monoclonal hyperglobulinemia [40, 41]. In MM and WM rouleaux formation is always detected [40]. This also explains the abnormally elevated ESR in paraproteinemias including MM which may exceed 100 mm in one third of cases [38].

Blood Chemistry Tests

- ***Calcium***
  As previously stated, the acronym CRAB comprises a high calcium level. Diagnosis of MM requires the presence of end-organ damage criteria, high Calcium level, Renal impairment, Anemia, and Osteolytic Bone lesions (CRAB) [42].
  The new definition of active MM describes CRAB features and myeloma-defining events that include hypercalcemia with a calcium level of >0.25 mmol/L (>1 mg/dL) higher than the upper limit of the normal reference range or a calcium level of >2.75 mmol/L (>11 mg/dL) [42].
  Hypercalcemia, most of the time, is explained by the cytokines that are expressed in MM or secreted locally by the myeloma cells. Hypercalcemia can be explained by the increased receptor activator of nuclear factor-kappa B ligand (RANKL), macrophage inflammatory protein (MIP)-1α, and tumor necrosis factors (TNFs). These cytokines increase osteoclastic activity causing bone resorption. Hypercalcemia manifests later during the course of MM [43, 44].
- ***Renal Function Tests***
  The revised IMWG Diagnostic Criteria for MM have changed and so the criteria of renal failure with inclusion of creatinine clearance <40 mL/min as a myeloma-defining event. Renal insufficiency with creatinine clearance less than 40 mL/min or serum creatinine level of more than 177 mmol/L (>2 mg/dL) is also described [34, 42, 45].
  Light chain cast nephropathy (biopsy proven or presumptive) renal failure is the described myeloma-defining event. SFLC >500 mg/L is suggestive of cast nephropathy [34, 45].
  In 2012, the term monoclonal gammopathy of renal significance (MGRS) was coined by the International Kidney and Monoclonal Gammopathy Research Group (IKMG). After the IKMG meeting in April 2017, the updated diagnostic criteria for MGRS-related diseases describe any B cell or plasma cell clonal lymphoproliferation with both of the following characteristics:
  - The presence of one or more kidney lesions related to monoclonal immunoglobulin
  - The underlying B cell or plasma cell clone not causing any current hematological criteria with the absence of any tumor complications [8, 46].
  - MGRS was introduced to describe the associated paraprotein as a nephrotoxic protein which may cause progressive renal pathology independent of the clonal size and with no increase in the paraprotein concentration. This allows early treatment and preservation of renal function [8].

- ***Liver Function Tests***
  A minority of patients with MM may show mild elevation of liver enzymes. Patients with hepatic involvement may manifest hepatomegaly, ascites, and jaundice. Although this is uncommon, it is still possible. MM patients with hepatic amyloid deposition may present with jaundice. Liver function tests should include total and direct bilirubin, alanine aminotransferase, aspartate aminotransferase, gamma-glutamyl transferase, and alkaline phosphatase which has been described in sporadic cases of amyloid liver to be elevated. Prothrombin time is also part of the hepatic evaluation tests in this condition [47].

Protein Electrophoresis and Immunofixation

In PP, the full laboratory workup at any stage includes serum protein electrophoresis (SPEP), serum immunofixation (SIFE), immunoturbidimetric or immunonephelometric quantification of serum Igs, routine urinalysis, as well as protein electrophoresis and immunofixation of collected 24-h urine sample [37, 48]. The M-protein appears as a sharp restricted band in the electrophoresis migration pattern (Fig. 6.2). Igs make up the gamma fraction. The IgG and IgM Igs usually migrate in the gamma region, while the IgA immunoglobulin can migrate in the beta-gamma and beta fractions. However, M-proteins can be detected anywhere from alpha-2 to gamma regions [27].

Although rarely a false-positive result, all patients with localized band or non-homogeneous distribution of the gamma region on SPEP require additional IFE or capillary zone immunosubtraction electrophoresis (ISE) tests to confirm and identify the isotype of the Ig heavy and light chains (Fig. 6.3) [27, 48]. IFE is highly sensitive and can detect small bands with ~ten-fold more sensitivity [34, 48].

The precise and accurate interpretation of EP and IFE, following the published diagnostic criteria, is important to approach the diagnosis. For example, the MGUS is defined as serum monoclonal protein (non-IgM) level < 30 g/L and urinary monoclonal protein level < 500 mg/24 h while SMM is defined as a serum M-protein (IgG or IgA) level of >30 g/L and/or urinary M-protein level of >500 mg/24 h [27].

In patients with oligo-secretory disease, such as light-chain MM, SPEP, and SIFE may not be able to detect the light-chain aberrations. Serum free light chains (FLC) have a rapid renal clearance because they have low molecular weight. The oligo-secretory disease reveals low serum gamma globulins, while a simultaneous 24-h urine collection shows a large light chain peak (Bence Jones protein). In such cases, a 24-h urine collection to measure the monoclonal band, or a serum sample, is collected for automated SFLC immunoassay which is characterized by a higher sensitivity in detection and quantification of the involved light chain [27].

An investigator should be cautious since M-protein may exist in spite of reporting all other fractions to be within the reference range. The M-protein could be hidden in other serum fractions on the gel. The IFE must be requested, even in the context of a normal SPEP, since the latter is not as sensitive as IFE particularly if MM is suspected [4].

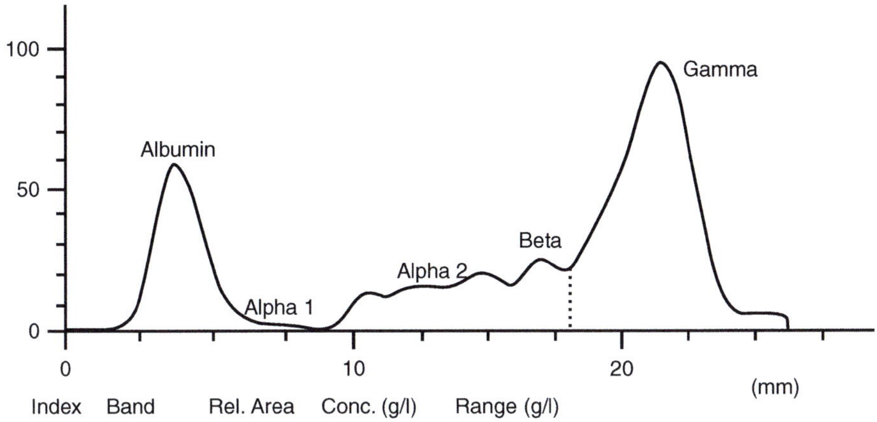

Index	Band	Rel. Area	Conc. (g/l)	Range (g/l)
1	Albumin	*18.50%*	*20.90 L*	*32.00...50.00*
2	Alpha1	0.31%	0.35 L	1.00...4.00
3	Alpha 2	8.44%	9.54	5.00...11.00
4	Beta	14.78%	16.70 H	6.00...13.00
5	Gamma	57.78%	65.51 H	7.00...15.00
Total			113.00	

Fig. 6.2 SPEP graph of a patient with monoclonal gammopathy showing a typical M spike in the gamma region

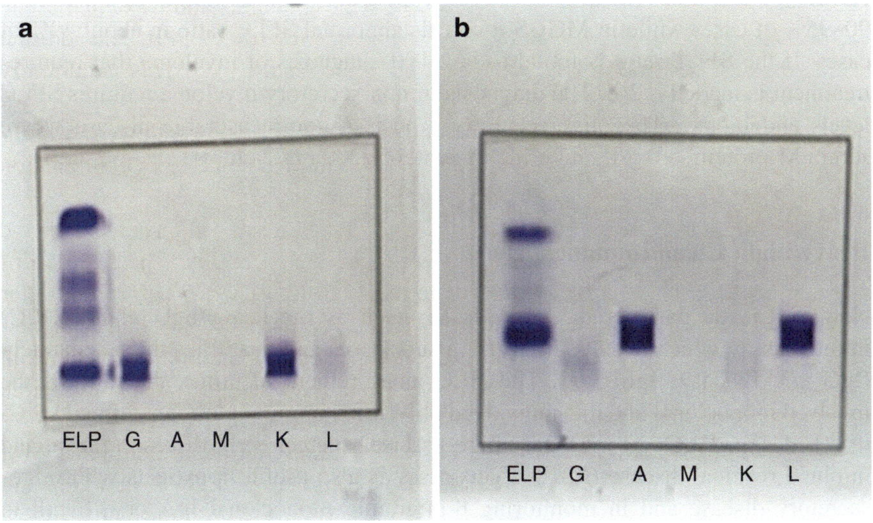

Fig. 6.3 Immunofixation strips. (**a**): The type of the M-band is IgG with kappa light chain restriction. (**b**): The type of the M-band is IgA with lambda light chain restriction

The IMWG recommends performing serum and urinary EP, IFE as well as SFLC assay to diagnose monoclonal plasma cell disorders [34].

Mass Spectrometry-Based Methods

The various heavy chains and the light chain isotypes when combined with nanobody-immuno-enrichment possess distinct unique molecular mass signatures. Such a characteristic feature is exploited in this assay to produce information-rich spectra which can identify isotype and quantify M-proteins. This has the potential to substitute IFE, M-protein quantitation, and heavy/light chain (HLC) measurements [27].

If the initial workup is abnormal, pursue additional investigations. These include serum beta 2 macroglobulin, lactate dehydrogenase, SFLC, and bone marrow (BM) examination.

Serum Free Light Chain Ratio

The principle of the FLC assays depends on the addition of antisera which are directed against light chain epitopes that are exposed only when the light chains are free (unbound to heavy chain) in solution. The ratio of kappa to lambda FLC concentrations can thus reveal unbalanced light chain synthesis and confirm clonality. The normal ratio ranges from 0.26 to 1.65. The ratio may be as high as 3.5 in the context of renal failure not due to gammopathy as the optimal range is 0.82–3.6 for eGFR $\leq$55 mL/min/1.73 m^2 [49]. In MM, the test reveals abnormal SFLC ratio in 90–95% of cases while in MGUS it reveals abnormal SFLC ratio in about 40% of cases. If the SFLC ratio is found to be >100, diagnosis of myeloma that requires treatment is made [7, 26]. The diagnosis of non-secretory myeloma requires SFLC levels and biopsy. The oligo-secretory type is a non-measurable disease where serum M-protein <10 g/L and urine M-protein <200 mg/24 h [4].

Heavy/Light Chain Immunoassay

New diagnostic parameters are assessed, such as the heavy/light chain (HLC) immunoassay which detects different Ig subclasses and quantifies them separately (IgG κ/λ, IgA κ/λ, IgM κ/λ). The HLC measurement identifies the ratio of the involved monoclonal and the uninvolved polyclonal immunoglobulin, termed HLC-matched pair. HLC κ/λ-ratio can more precisely detect early disease relapse and minimal residual disease (MRD). This assay is also useful in patients with oligo-secretory disease and in monitoring ß-migrating monoclonal IgA or difficult to detect IgM monoclonal protein by EP [50].

The results of Greil et al. in 2016 verified the close association between both HLC values and HLC κ/λ-ratios with standard MM diagnostics, as well as with disease staging and remission status [50].

Quantitative Total Immunoglobulin Testing

For quantitative Total Ig testing nephelometry is the method of choice, especially when M-spike >30 g/L. Ig testing is mainly used in diagnosing concomitant hypogammaglobulinemia and monitoring monoclonal proteins that cannot be accurately quantified on SPEP such as IgAs [4].

Western Blot Analysis

The spectrum of monoclonal gammopathy of clinical significance (MGCS) manifest as a result of deposition of all or part of the monoclonal immunoglobulin (MIg) in the form of aggregates, amorphous, crystalline, microtubular, or fibrillar forms in different organs. MGCS includes an organized type like AL amyloidosis and a nonorganized type known as monoclonal immunoglobulin deposition disease (MIDD). MIDD deposits contain the LC deposition disease (LCDD), sometimes the heavy chain deposition disease (HCDD), or the combination of both (LHCDD). MIDD is characterized by HCDD which could be a truncated HC only (mostly γ1 and γ3) or LHCDD with LC plus truncated HC. It remains to be determined whether HC truncation in HCDD is attributed to a defective LC production or other factors. Western blot analysis performed on serum samples at the time of disease diagnosis could confirm that a truncated chain corresponding to the deposited HC is present [51].

Serum Viscosity

The increased circulating Igs results in increased serum viscosity. Serum viscosity evaluation is recommended in patients with suspicious clinical manifestations. IgM levels >40 g/L, IgA > 50 g/L, IgG > 60 g/L are indications of hyperviscosity [4]. WM is commonly associated with hyperviscosity (10–30% of patients). In MM, it is reported in 2–6% of cases [52]. Viscosity can be measured in centipoise (cP), or in relative terms in comparison to water (0.894 cP). The normal serum viscosity equals 1.5 cP [52, 53].

Serum β2M and LDH Levels

In MM, β2M level correlates with the tumor burden and evaluates response to therapy. It is one of the key features of the International Staging System (ISS) as well as the more recent revised ISS (R-ISS). β2M is considered a biomarker for kidney diseases [54]. It accumulates in cases with renal disease. They can precipitate as hemodialysis-related amyloidosis. So β2M loses its significance in renal impairment with MM but remains a prognostic marker for MM. Albumin and lactic dehydrogenase (LDH) are important baseline laboratory tests in MM. Baseline

LDH is an important risk stratification factor. LDH is part of the R-ISS, and in itself may correlate with aggressive disease or plasma cell leukemia. Albuminuria indicates glomerular disease which is a feature of AL amyloidosis and MGRS conditions [4].

Bone Marrow Examination

BM aspiration and core biopsy are required for the quantification of plasma cells (Fig. 6.4) and are mandatory components of MM investigation. Clonality is determined by in situ hybridization (ISH) for kappa/lambda LC, mRNAs or less accurately with immunocytochemistry, on the core (trephine) biopsies [4]. Revised IMWG for MGUS, SMM, and MM include lymphoplasmacytic infiltration of BM with <10% in MGUS, 10–60% in SMM, and ≥60% in MM [42].

Flow Cytometry

Flow cytometry identifies aberrant immune profiles of the plasma cell. It is not needed for the diagnosis when BM biopsy is done [4]. In 2016, the IMWG updated MM response categories. It defined MRD-negative responses assessed by next-generation flow cytometry or next-generation sequencing both in and outside the bone marrow [55].

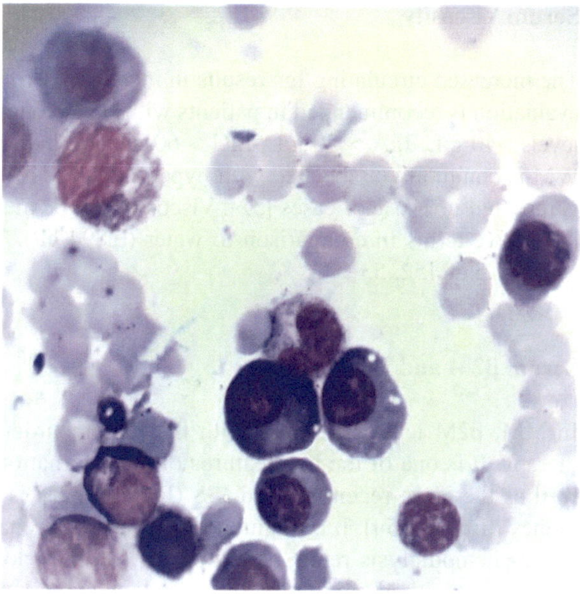

Fig. 6.4 Bone marrow Leishman-stained smear showing plasma cells; plasma cells appear as ovoid cells with abundant deep blue cytoplasm. The cytoplasm of plasma cells has a clear or pale perinuclear zone or hollow corresponding to the cytoplasmic organelle, Golgi apparatus. The nucleus is eccentric with coarse chromatin arranged in a clock face (cartwheel appearance) pattern

Cytogenetic Analysis and Risk Stratification

Myeloma cells divide slowly, hence they may go undetected by standard cytogenetics. The chromosomal aberrations that can be detected in MM cases include deletions (del), translocations (t), and amplifications (gain) [4].

Myeloma-associated translocations are not detected by G-banding karyotyping [4]. The G-banding technique is used to detect myeloma-associated chromosomal aberrations. This includes detection of numerical chromosomal 13 aberrations, monosomy, or interstitial deletion with a high sensitivity [56].

MM diagnostic criteria do not include chromosomal aberrations; however, cytogenetic evaluations by FISH are needed for all new MM cases as they are helpful for prognostication including remission duration and overall survival (OS). The IMWG presented a high-risk MM model designated by its cytogenetic aberrations where one or more of the following, as detected by FISH is present: del17p, t(4;14), or t(14;16) [57].

It has been shown that the association of any of these aberrations results in a lower OS [55]. Moreover, high-risk MM patients were reported to have the following cytogenetic aberrations: gain (1q) with R-ISS III, with or without del(1p), and t(14;20) [58]. Some of these genomic aberrations are included in the R-ISS for MM [58].

FISH technique is considered the standard technique for chromosomal aberrations analysis in MM [4]. Other techniques that have been introduced to detect chromosomal aberrations are not routinely used in clinical settings. They include single-nucleotide polymorphism, comparative genomic hybridization, and gene expression profiling, but they are not incorporated in clinical practice [4].

Tissue Biopsy and Histopathological Examination

Some disease entities will further necessitate tissue sampling for histopathological examination. Biopsies can be obtained for amyloidosis by fat pad aspiration or biopsy from periumbilical subcutaneous tissues, the rectum, or the kidney [5]. In IgG4-related disease, a biopsy may be obtained from salivary or lacrimal glands, but it may be more tedious to obtain it in case of presenting with retroperitoneal fibrosis.

The use of certain stains is important and helps in the differentiation between disease entities. Congo red stain will be positive in amyloidosis, but it will always be negative in MIDD [59].

Microscopic examination can be performed employing polarized microscopy as in amyloidosis [60]. Fluorescent microscopy is beneficial in LCDD [61]. Electron microscopy proved to be of great value in MIDD [59, 62]. Other microscopic techniques have been introduced. These include light microscopy immunohistochemistry and immunoelectron microscopy [63].

Other Modalities

The list of investigative techniques is incessantly expanding and includes highly sophisticated procedures like molecular genetic testing [64], proteomics, and mass spectrometry [65].

(For a deeper understanding of these techniques, we refer our reader to Chaps. 7 through 21 which discuss individual diseases and disorders in more detail.)

Conclusion

Paraproteinemia is a phenomenon that can be encountered in many disorders and has been described even in healthy individuals.

Awareness of its existence demands maintaining a high index of suspicion by all medical practitioners. The clinician should be highly attentive while obtaining the symptoms and signs. On the other hand, the laboratory investigator and the radiologist should deal with their data very meticulously.

Once identified it is imperative to proceed further to investigate the paraprotein. This is usually directed by guidelines and recommendations that are internationally acknowledged.

A systematic approach will be extremely productive in the assessment of both the paraproteinemia and its associated disorder.

References

1. Tate JR. The paraprotein—an enduring biomarker. Clin Biochem Rev. 2019;40:5.
2. Cook L, Macdonald DHC. Management of paraproteinaemia. Postgrad Med J. 2007;83:217.
3. Dimopoulos MA, Moreau P, Terpos E, et al. Multiple myeloma: EHA-ESMO clinical practice guidelines for diagnosis, treatment and follow-up. Hemasphere. 2021;5:e528. https://doi.org/10.1097/HS9.0000000000000528.
4. Bergstrom DJ, Kotb R, Louzada ML, et al. Consensus guidelines on the diagnosis of multiple myeloma and related disorders: recommendations of the Myeloma Canada Research Network consensus guideline consortium. Clin Lymphoma Myeloma Leuk. 2020;20:e352–67.
5. Vaxman I, Gertz M. When to suspect a diagnosis of amyloidosis. Acta Haematol. 2020;143:304–11.
6. Castillo JJ, Callander NS, Baljevic M, Sborov DW, Kumar S. The evaluation and management of monoclonal gammopathy of renal significance and monoclonal gammopathy of neurological significance. Am J Hematol. 2021;96:846–53.
7. Mani AM, Devasia AJ, Nair A, Benjamin RN, Prabhakar AT, Sivadasan A, Mathew V, Aaron S, George B, Alexander M. Monoclonal gammopathies of "neurological significance": paraproteinemic neuropathies. Can J Neurol Sci. 2021;48:616–25.
8. Bridoux F, Leung N, Hutchison CA, et al. Diagnosis of monoclonal gammopathy of renal significance. Kidney Int. 2015;87:698–711.
9. Li JP, Du YT, Li S, Rao XR. Monoclonal gammopathy of renal significance (MGRS): prospects for treatment in integrated Chinese and Western medicine. Chin J Integr Med. 2021;27:643–8.

10. Lipsker D. Monoclonal gammopathy of cutaneous significance: review of a relevant concept. J Eur Acad Dermatol Venereol. 2017;31:45–52.
11. Fermand JP, Bridoux F, Dispenzieri A, Jaccard A, Kyle RA, Leung N, Merlini G. Monoclonal gammopathy of clinical significance: a novel concept with therapeutic implications. Blood. 2018;132:1478–85.
12. Schnitzler LJ, Schreckenbach T, Nadaj-Pakleza A, et al. Sporadic late-onset nemaline myopathy: clinico-pathological characteristics and review of 76 cases. Orphanet J Rare Dis. 2017;12:86. https://doi.org/10.1186/S13023-017-0640-2.
13. Kotchetkov R, Susman D, Buadi F, Dispenzieri A. Sporadic late-onset nemaline myopathy with monoclonal paraprotein as a malignancy rather than disimmunity and treatment with chemotherapy-based approach. J Clin Oncol. 2020;38:8545. https://doi.org/10.1200/JCO20203815_suppl.8545.
14. Kormányos K, Kovács K, Németh O, et al. Ocular signs and ocular comorbidities in monoclonal Gammopathy: analysis of 80 subjects. J Ophthalmol. 2021;2021:9982875. https://doi.org/10.1155/2021/9982875.
15. Lisch W, Saikia P, Pitz S, Pleyer U, Lisch C, Jaeger M, Rohrbach JM. Chameleon-like appearance of immunotactoid keratopathy. Cornea. 2012;31:55–8.
16. Nakazawa T, Yamaguchi K, … YN-NGG, 2004 undefined Two cases of orbital myositis with monoclonal gammopathy of undetermined significance. europepmc.org
17. Milman T, Kao AA, Chu D, et al. Paraproteinemic keratopathy. Ophthalmology. 2015;122:1748–56.
18. Balderman SR, Lichtman MA. Unusual manifestations of monoclonal gammopathy: I. Ocular disease. Rambam Maimonides Med J. 2015;6:e0026.
19. Smith SJ, Johnson MW, Ober MD, Comer GM, Smith BD. Maculopathy in patients with monoclonal gammopathy of undetermined significance. Ophthalmol Retina. 2020;4:300–9.
20. Munteanu G. [Doyne's macular heredodystrophy and benign monoclonal gammopathy. Genetic and pathogenetic correlations (author's transl)]. J Fr Ophtalmol.1980;3:753–758.
21. Agorogiannis E, Hippokratia VK. 2015 undefined Paraproteinemia and central retinal vein occlusion. ncbi.nlm.nih.gov
22. Dimopoulos M, Terpos E, Comenzo RL, et al. International myeloma working group consensus statement and guidelines regarding the current role of imaging techniques in the diagnosis and monitoring of multiple myeloma. Leukemia. 2009;23:1545–56.
23. Niederhauser BD, Dingli D, Kyle RA, Ringler MD. Imaging findings in 22 cases of Schnitzler syndrome: characteristic para-articular osteosclerosis, and the "hot knees" sign differential diagnosis. Skeletal Radiol. 2014;43:905–15.
24. Zamagni E, Cavo M, Fakhri B, Vij R, Roodman D. Bones in multiple myeloma: imaging and therapy. Am Soc Clin Oncol Educ. 2018;38:638–46.
25. Yoo BW, Song JJ, Park YB, Lee SW. 2019 American College of Rheumatology/European League Against Rheumatism classification criteria for IgG4-related disease by Wallace et al. Ann Rheum Dis. 2020;72(1):7–19. https://doi.org/10.1136/ANNRHEUMDIS-2020-217086.
26. Willrich MAV, Katzmann JA. Laboratory testing requirements for diagnosis and follow-up of multiple myeloma and related plasma cell dyscrasias. Clin Chem Lab Med. 2016;54:907–19.
27. Willrich MAV, Murray DL, Kyle RA. Laboratory testing for monoclonal gammopathies: focus on monoclonal gammopathy of undetermined significance and smoldering multiple myeloma. Clin Biochem. 2018;51:38–47.
28. Katzmann JA, Kyle RA, Benson J, Larson DR, Snyder MR, Lust JA, Rajkumar SV, Dispenzieri A. Screening panels for detection of monoclonal gammopathies. Clin Chem. 2009;55:1517–22.
29. Sive J, Cuthill K, Hunter H, Kazmi M, Pratt G, Smith D. Guidelines on the diagnosis, investigation and initial treatment of myeloma: a British Society for Haematology/UK myeloma forum guideline. Br J Haematol. 2021;193:245–68.
30. Thomas R, Braschi-Amir Farzan M, Laferriere SL, Jagannathan JP. Imaging of Waldenström macroglobulinemia: a comprehensive review for the radiologist in the era of personalized medicine. AJR Am J Roentgenol. 2019;213:W248–56.

31. Chantry A, Kazmi M, Barrington S, Goh V, Mulholland N, Streetly M, Lai M, Pratt G. Guidelines for the use of imaging in the management of patients with myeloma. Br J Haematol. 2017;178:380–93.
32. Shortt CP, Gleeson TG, Breen KA, McHugh J, O'Connell MJ, O'Gorman PJ, Eustace SJ. Whole-body MRI versus PET in assessment of multiple myeloma disease activity. AJR Am J Roentgenol. 2009;192:980–6.
33. Ludwig H, Kumpan W, Sinzinger H. Radiography and bone scintigraphy in multiple myeloma: a comparative analysis. Br J Radiol. 1982;55:173–81.
34. Genzen JR, Murray DL, Abel G, et al. Screening and diagnosis of monoclonal gammopathies: an international survey of laboratory practice. Arch Pathol Lab Med. 2018;142:507–15.
35. Kumar SK, Callander NS, Adekola K, et al. Multiple myeloma, version 3.2021, NCCN clinical practice guidelines in oncology. J Natl Compr Cancer Netw. 2020;18:1685–717.
36. Siegel RL, Miller KD, Jemal A. Cancer statistics, 2020. CA Cancer J Clin. 2020;70:7–30.
37. Liu L, Yu Z, Cheng H, et al. Multiple myeloma hinders erythropoiesis and causes anaemia owing to high levels of CCL3 in the bone marrow microenvironment. Sci Rep. 2020;101(10):1–14.
38. Kyle RA, Gertz MA, Witzig TE, et al. Review of 1027 patients with newly diagnosed multiple myeloma. Mayo Clin Proc. 2003;78:21–33.
39. Jones KW. 2009 undefined Evaluation of cell morphology and introduction to platelet and white blood cell morphology. fondation-merieux.org
40. Landis-Piwowar K, Landis J, Keila P. The complete blood count and peripheral blood smear evaluation. Clin Lab Hematol. 3rd ed. New Jersey: Pearson; 2015. p. 154–177.
41. Rodak BF, Carr JH. Variations in shape and distribution of erythrocytes. Clin Hematol Atlas. 5th ed. St Louis: Elsevier Inc; 2017. p. 93–106.
42. Rajkumar SV, Dimopoulos MA, Palumbo A, et al. International myeloma working group updated criteria for the diagnosis of multiple myeloma. Lancet Oncol. 2014;15:e538–48.
43. Oyajobi BO. Multiple myeloma/hypercalcemia. Arthritis Res Ther. 2007;9:1–6.
44. Scheuer C, Boot E, Carse N, et al. Pathophysiology of myeloma bone disease. Phys Educ Sport Child Youth with Spec Needs Res Best Pract Situat; 2004. p. 74–88.
45. Leung N, Barnidge DR, Hutchison CA. Laboratory testing in monoclonal gammopathy of renal significance (MGRS). Clin Chem Lab Med. 2016;54:929–37.
46. Dimopoulos MA, Sonneveld P, Leung N, et al. International myeloma working group recommendations for the diagnosis and management of myeloma-related renal impairment. J Clin Oncol. 2016;34:1544–57.
47. Khan Y, Mansour I, Ong E, Shrestha M. Obstructive jaundice as initial presentation of multiple myeloma: case presentation and literature review. Case Rep Med. 2015;2015:686210. https://doi.org/10.1155/2015/686210.
48. Jenner E. Serum free light chains in clinical laboratory diagnostics. Clin Chim Acta. 2014;427:15–20.
49. Molina-Andújar A, Robles P, Cibeira MT, Montagud-Marrahi E, Guillen E, Xipell M, Blasco M, Poch E, Rosiñol L, Bladé J, Quintana LF. The renal range of the κ/λ sFLC ratio: best strategy to evaluate multiple myeloma in patients with chronic kidney disease. BMC Nephrol. 2020;21(1):111. https://doi.org/10.1186/s12882-020-01771-3.
50. Greil C, Ihorst G, Gaiser F, Salzer U, Bisse E, Kastritis E, Ludwig H, Wäsch R, Engelhardt M. The serum heavy/light chain immunoassay: a valuable tool for sensitive paraprotein assessment, risk, and disease monitoring in monoclonal gammopathies. Eur J Haematol. 2017;99:449–58.
51. Bender S, Ayala MV, Javaugue V, Bonaud A, Cogné M, Touchard G, Jaccard A, Bridoux F, Sirac C. Comprehensive molecular characterization of a heavy chain deposition disease case. Haematologica. 2018;103:e557–60.
52. Weaver A, Rubinstein S, Cornell RF. Hyperviscosity syndrome in paraprotein secreting conditions including Waldenstrom macroglobulinemia. Front Oncol. 2020;10:815.
53. Riccardi A, Gobbi PG, Ucci G, Bertoloni D, Luoni R, Rutigliano L, Ascari E. Changing clinical presentation of multiple myeloma. Eur J Cancer. 1991;27:1401–5.

54. Argyropoulos CP, Chen SS, Ng YH, Roumelioti ME, Shaffi K, Singh PP, Tzamaloukas AH. Rediscovering beta-2 microglobulin as a biomarker across the spectrum of kidney diseases. Front Med. 2017;4:73. https://doi.org/10.3389/fmed.2017.00073.
55. Kumar S, Paiva B, Anderson KC, et al. International myeloma working group consensus criteria for response and minimal residual disease assessment in multiple myeloma. Lancet Oncol. 2016;17:e328–46.
56. Fonseca R, Barlogie B, Bataille R, et al. Genetics and cytogenetics of multiple myeloma: a workshop report. Cancer Res. 2004;64:1546–58.
57. Fonseca R, Bergsagel PL, Drach J, et al. International myeloma working group molecular classification of multiple myeloma: spotlight review. Leukemia. 2009;23:2210–21.
58. Ross FM, Chiecchio L, Dagrada G, Protheroe RKM, Stockley DM, Harrison CJ, Cross NC, Szubert AJ, Drayson MT, Morgan GJ. The t(14;20) is a poor prognostic factor in myeloma but is associated with long-term stable disease in monoclonal gammopathies of undetermined significance. Haematologica. 2010;95:1221–5.
59. Herrera GA. Renal lesions associated with plasma cell dyscrasias: practical approach to diagnosis, new concepts, and challenges. Arch Pathol Lab Med. 2009;133:249.
60. Dhingra S, Krishnani N, Kumari N, Pandey R. Evaluation of abdominal fat pad aspiration cytology and grading for detection in systemic amyloidosis. Acta Cytol. 2007;51(6):860–4.
61. Markowitz GS. Dysproteinemia and the kidney. Adv Anat Pathol. 2004;11:49.
62. Herrera GA. The contributions of electron microscopy to the understanding and diagnosis of plasma cell dyscrasia-related renal lesions. Med Electron Microsc. 2001;34:1.
63. Fernández de Larrea C, Verga L, Morbini P, Klersy C, Lavatelli F, Foli A, et al. A practical approach to the diagnosis of systemic amyloidoses. Blood. 2015;125(14):2239–44.
64. Obici L, Kuks JB, Buades J, et al.; European Network for TTR-FAP (ATTReuNET). Recommendations for presymptomatic genetic testing and management of individuals at risk for hereditary transthyretin amyloidosis. Curr Opin Neurol. 2016;29:S27–S35.
65. Picken MM. Proteomics and mass spectrometry in the diagnosis of renal amyloidosis. Clin Kidney J. 2015;8(6):665–72.

Part II
Diseases and Disorders

Chapter 7
Amyloidosis: Pathogenesis, Types, and Diagnosis

Shereef Elmoamly and Laura Obici

Abbreviations

DPD	^{99m}Tc-labeled 3,3-diphosphono-1,2-propanodicarboxylic acid
FLC	Free light chains
FMF	Familial Mediterranean fever
HSPG	Heparan sulphate proteoglycan
IEM	Immunoelectron microscopy
IHC	Immunohistochemistry
ISA	International Society of Amyloidosis
LCM-MS	Laser capture microdissection and mass spectrometry
NAC	National Amyloidosis Centre
NGS	Next-generation sequencing
PYP	^{99m}Tc-labeled pyrophosphate
SAP	Serum amyloid P

The original version of the chapter has been revised. A correction to this chapter can be found at https://doi.org/10.1007/978-3-031-10131-1_24

S. Elmoamly (✉)
Internal Medicine and Haematology Department, Kasr Alainy Faculty of Medicine, Cairo University, Cairo, Egypt
e-mail: shereefasaad@kasralainy.edu.eg

L. Obici
Amyloidosis Research and Treatment Centre, IRCCS Fondazione Policlinico San Matteo, Pavia, Italy
e-mail: l.obici@smatteo.pv.it

© The Author(s), under exclusive license to Springer Nature Switzerland AG 2022, corrected publication 2022

G. Ragab et al. (eds.), *Paraproteinemia and Related Disorders*,
https://doi.org/10.1007/978-3-031-10131-1_7

Introduction

Amyloidoses are heterogeneous pathological conditions characterized by the extracellular deposition of insoluble protein fibrils that cause progressive organ damage. Amyloidosis may be a systemic disorder, resulting in a spectrum of clinical presentations, or a localized disease associated with single tissue or organ involvement. The term amyloid was first adopted by Rudolph Virchow in 1854 to describe the deposition of a starch-like material with hyaline appearance under light microscopy [1]. The fibrillar nature of amyloid was revealed only in the second half of the twentieth century and the first amyloid protein, namely a fragment of a monoclonal light chain, was isolated from natural amyloid deposits in 1970 [2].

Amyloid has a pathognomonic microscopic appearance, showing apple-green birefringence under polarized light after Congo red staining. Amyloidosis may be hereditary or acquired. The latter also includes an iatrogenic form such as β2-microglobulin amyloidosis occurring in patients on chronic haemodialysis.

Pathogenesis

Amyloid fibrils are derived from globular precursor proteins that undergo misfolding and aggregation into a highly ordered structure. Under electron microscopy amyloid fibrils are rigid, non-branching and around 8–12 nm in diameter (Fig. 7.1) [3]. X-ray diffraction demonstrates a crossed beta-sheet structure.

In vitro studies indicate that the fibrillogenesis process involves protein misfolding, generation of partially unfolded intermediates, aggregation into oligomeric species and/or protofibrils, and ultimately formation of mature, crossed beta-sheet fibril structures. Fibril formation is accelerated in the presence of amyloid seeds, according to nucleation kinetics [4].

Several mechanisms, often acting in combination, are known to play a role in promoting *in vivo* amyloidogenesis. These include a persistent increase in the concentration of the circulating precursor, mutations that perturb the stability of the native structure, an intrinsic misfolding propensity of the protein in its wild-type form and/or proteolytic remodelling leading to the generation of amyloidogenic fragments [5, 6]. In hereditary amyloidosis, fibrillogenesis is promoted by a genetic variant, mostly consisting of a point mutation leading to single amino acid substitution or a premature stop codon. Amyloidogenic mutations result in protein structural changes that destabilize the native conformation. Acquired forms of amyloidosis associated with increased or abnormal production of the precursor include, for example, AA amyloidosis secondary to chronic inflammation and AL amyloidosis resulting from underlying plasma cell dyscrasia.

Moreover, amyloidogenesis is favoured when the proteostasis system, that targets misfolded and aggregated proteins to degradation in the cellular and extracellular compartments, is overwhelmed and/or reduced in its capacity by ageing [7].

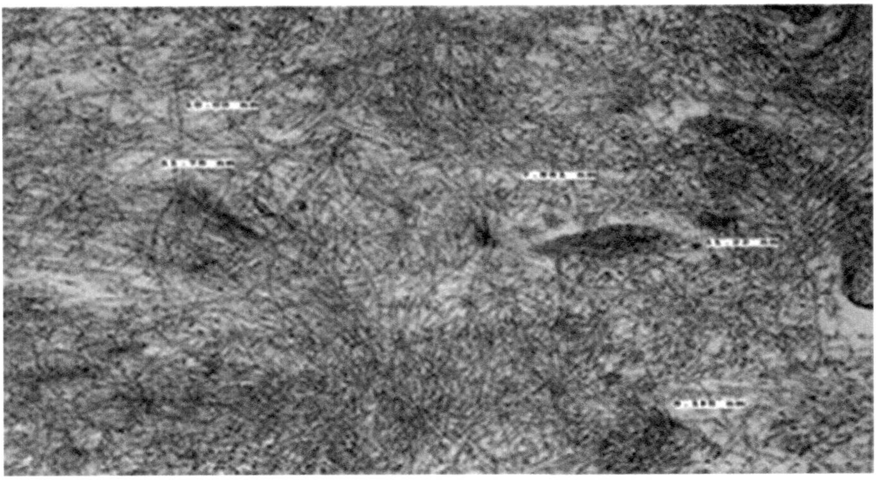

Fig. 7.1 Electron microscopy appearance of amyloid (in renal amyloidosis). Photo courtesy of Dr. B Vydianath, University Hospitals Birmingham NHS Foundation Trust

Amyloid deposits not only consist of one key precursor protein among those indicated in Table 7.1 but also contain additional constituents including heparan sulphate proteoglycan (HSPG), serum amyloid P component (SAP), apolipoprotein E, and vitronectin. These components, that are invariably present, serve as universal amyloid signatures [8]. The pathological roles of these additional molecules in amyloidogenesis are not fully clarified although there is evidence that glycosaminoglycans may act as scaffold for amyloid aggregation and SAP inhibits fibril degradation [9].

Whereas systemic forms of amyloidosis are caused by circulating precursor proteins, in localized amyloidosis, such as AL amyloidosis involving the lungs, the skin, or the genitourinary tract the precursor immunoglobulin light chain is synthesized and processed at affected local sites [10, 11].

Amyloid Protein Nomenclature and Classification

According to the International Society of Amyloidosis (ISA) nomenclature, all amyloid fibril proteins are named protein A together with the specific protein name as a suffix, for example, AL (L for immunoglobulin light chain), ATTR (TTR for transthyretin), or AFib (Fib for fibrinogen alpha chain). The protein name may be further specified, for example, ATTRwt or ATTRv (wt for wild type and v for variant). Hereditary amyloidosis protein variants are named according to the mature protein substitution or deletion, with the amino acid involved and the change position listed, for example, ATTRV30M (methionine replacing valine). The main

Table 7.1 Amyloid fibril proteins and their precursors in human [8]

Fibril protein	Precursor protein	Systemic and/or localized	Acquired or hereditary	Target organs
AL	Immunoglobulin light chain	S, L	A, H	All organs, usually except CNS
AH	Immunoglobulin heavy chain	S, L	A	All organs except CNS
AA	(Apo) serum amyloid A	S	A	All organs except CNS
ATTR	Transthyretin, wild type	S	A	Heart mainly in males, lung, ligaments, tenosynovium
	Transthyretin, variants	S	H	PNS, ANS, heart, eye, leptomeninges
Ab2M	b2-microglobulin, wild type	S	A	Musculoskeletal system
	b2-microglobulin, variants	S	H	ANS
AApoAI	Apolipoprotein A I, variants	S	H	Heart, liver, kidney, PNS, testis, larynx (C terminal variants), skin (C terminal variants)
AApoAII	Apolipoprotein A II, variants	S	H	Kidney
AApoAIV	Apolipoprotein A IV, wild type	S	A	Kidney medulla and systemic
AApoCII	Apolipoprotein C II, variants	S	H	Kidney
AApoCIII	Apolipoprotein C III, variants	S	H	Kidney
AGel	Gelsolin, variants	S	H	Kidney, PNS, cornea
ALys	Lysozyme, variants	S	H	Kidney
ALECT2	Leukocyte chemotactic factor-2	S	A	Kidney, primarily
AFib	Fibrinogen a, variants	S	H	Kidney, primarily
ACys	Cystatin C, variants	S	H	CNS, PNS, skin
ABri	ABriPP, variants	S	H	CNS
ADan	ADanPP, variants	L	H	CNS
Ab	Ab protein precursor, wild type	L	A	CNS
	Ab protein precursor, variant	L	H	CNS
AaSyn	a-Synuclein	L	A	CNS
ATau	Tau	L	A	CNS
APrP	Prion protein, wild type	L	A	CJD, fatal insomnia
	Prion protein variants	L	H	CJD, GSS syndrome, fatal insomnia
	Prion protein variant	S	H	PNS

Table 7.1 (continued)

Fibril protein	Precursor protein	Systemic and/or localized	Acquired or hereditary	Target organs
ACal	(Pro)calcitonin	L	A	C-cell thyroid tumours
		S	A	Kidney
AIAPP	Islet amyloid polypeptide[c]	L	A	Islets of Langerhans, insulinomas
AANF	Atrial natriuretic factor	L	A	Cardiac atria
APro	Prolactin	L	A	Pituitary prolactinomas, ageing pituitary
AIns	Insulin	L	A	Iatrogenic, local injection
ASPC	Lung surfactant protein	L	A	Lung
ACor	Corneodesmosin	L	A	Cornified epithelia, hair follicles
AMed	Lactadherin	L	A	Senile aortic, media
AKer	Kerato-epithelin	L	A	Cornea, hereditary
ALac	Lactoferrin	L	A	Cornea
AOAAP	Odontogenic ameloblast-associated protein	L	A	Odontogenic tumours
ASem1	Semenogelin 1	L	A	Vesicula seminalis
AEnf	Enfurvitide	L	A	Iatrogenic
ACatK	Cathepsin K	L	A	Tumour associated
AEFEMP1	EGF-containing fibulin-like extracellular matrix protein 1 (EFEMP1)	L	A	Portal veins Ageing associated

clinical presentation may be added to the amyloidosis name, for example, ATTRv cardiomyopathy or ATTR polyneuropathy [8].

To date, at least 36 proteins have been identified that form amyloid deposits in humans. As mentioned before, amyloid deposits may be systemic, affecting various organs and tissues throughout the body, or localized, with deposits being formed in a single organ or tissue.

Exclusively localized amyloid deposits have been associated with 22 proteins, while 18 proteins (and many more variants) are classified to be associated with systemic amyloidosis. Interestingly, some protein types (most notably AL/AH, amyloidosis derived from immunoglobulin light or heavy chain, respectively, and amyloidosis derived from prion protein) can occur as either localized or systemic forms (Table 7.1). This list is periodically updated. In addition, novel potential amyloidogenic precursor proteins are currently under investigation [8].

Certain amyloid proteins have specific target organs resulting in typical clinical manifestations. In general, however, systemic amyloidoses are clinically heterogeneous, with considerable overlap in presenting features. The potential contribution of genetic and/or environmental factors to the phenotypic variability that characterizes these diseases has been suggested, particularly in hereditary transthyretin amyloidosis and in AL amyloidosis [7].

Fifteen inherited amyloid types are known that are caused by genetic variants of the precursor proteins, mostly represented by missense mutations. Genetic variants result in protein products more amyloidogenic than their wild-type counterparts [12]. Some polymorphisms are also associated with increased amyloid risk, such as certain alleles of the apolipoprotein E gene in acquired cerebral amyloid angiopathy [13] and some specific isoforms of serum amyloid A protein in systemic AA amyloidosis [14]. Moreover, hereditary autoinflammatory disorders such as familial Mediterranean fever (FMF) or cryopyrinopathies may result in chronic inflammation and development of AA amyloidosis [15].

Epidemiology

Amyloidosis is a rare disorder for which it is still difficult to obtain a reliable estimate of incidence and prevalence [16]. In 2013, the UK National Amyloidosis Centre (NAC) reported that the estimated incidence of systemic amyloidosis was exceeding 8.0 per million inhabitants per year with around one third diagnosed with AL amyloidosis [17]. In the developed world, AL amyloidosis has long been the most prevalent with significant increases in diagnosis in the last decade [18]. Moreover, wild-type ATTR amyloidosis, which typically affects male subjects over the age of 60, is more and more recognized nowadays, with a prevalence that increases according to age. On the contrary, AA amyloidosis is more frequent in developing countries where endemic infectious diseases (e.g. tuberculosis or leprosy) and/or autoinflammatory diseases are relatively frequent (e.g. familial Mediterranean fever in the Mediterranean countries) [19]. Hereditary amyloidoses are much rarer, constituting approximately 10% of all systemic forms. However, their prevalence is still likely underestimated due to lack of clinical suspicion and insufficient detection of genetic mutations [20]. ATTRv is the most common hereditary amyloidosis worldwide.

Diagnosis

Diagnosis of systemic amyloidosis relies on the critical combination of clinical findings, histopathological evidence, genetic results, and imaging studies. Family history may guide towards an inherited form, leading to further investigations.

Histologic demonstration of amyloid deposits and characterization of the amyloid precursor protein in tissue is the cornerstone for a definitive and accurate diagnosis (Fig. 7.2). First, a tissue sample should be examined by polarized light microscopy after Congo red staining in order to detect the presence of amyloid (Figs. 7.3 and 7.4). Biopsies can be initially obtained from abdominal fat, minor salivary glands, skin, or rectal mucosa. If negative, an affected organ (e.g. kidney, heart) should be investigated to definitively confirm or exclude the diagnostic suspicion.

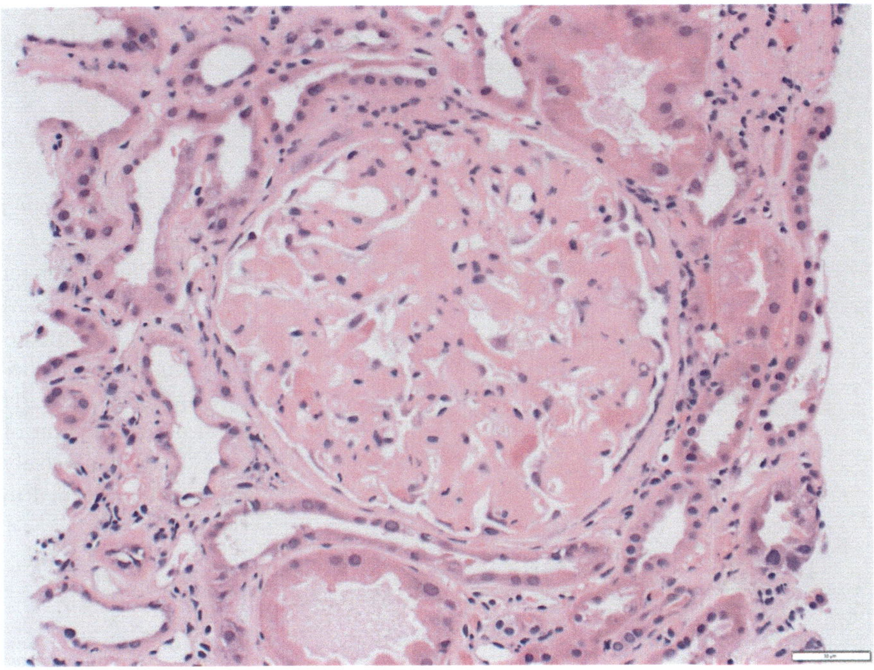

Fig. 7.2 Amyloid deposition in a renal glomerulus as seen on Haematoxylin and Eosin stain. Original magnification x 200, Photo courtesy of Dr. Y Hock, University Hospitals Birmingham NHS Foundation Trust

Subcutaneous fat pad aspiration or biopsy is suggested as a good initial sampling source as it's a safe, rapid, simple, and cheap procedure with no risk of serious bleeding. Congo red staining and examination using polarizing microscopy of subcutaneous fat pad aspiration or biopsy has an overall sensitivity of 57–85% and a specificity of 92–100% for light chain (AL) and secondary (AA) amyloidosis [21–23]. Single organ involvement may yield lower sensitivity of fat pad aspiration or biopsy [24]. Other potential sites of biopsy have variable degrees of sensitivity, rectal biopsy reported to be 84% sensitive in one large series. The sensitivity of kidney, liver, and carpal ligament biopsies were 90% or more in the same cohort (Fig. 7.4) [25].

When a positive biopsy is identified, the second step is to define the amyloidogenic protein in order to unequivocally establish the type of amyloidosis, as this guides its specific treatment. Amyloid typing can be performed by light microscopy immunohistochemistry (IHC), immunoelectron microscopy (IEM) characterization or proteomics, the latter being now considered the gold standard.

IHC involves the use of antibodies for a panel of amyloidogenic proteins. It is not expensive, and it is potentially widely available. However, due to its low specificity and sensitivity, it needs to be performed by a highly specialized pathologist usually

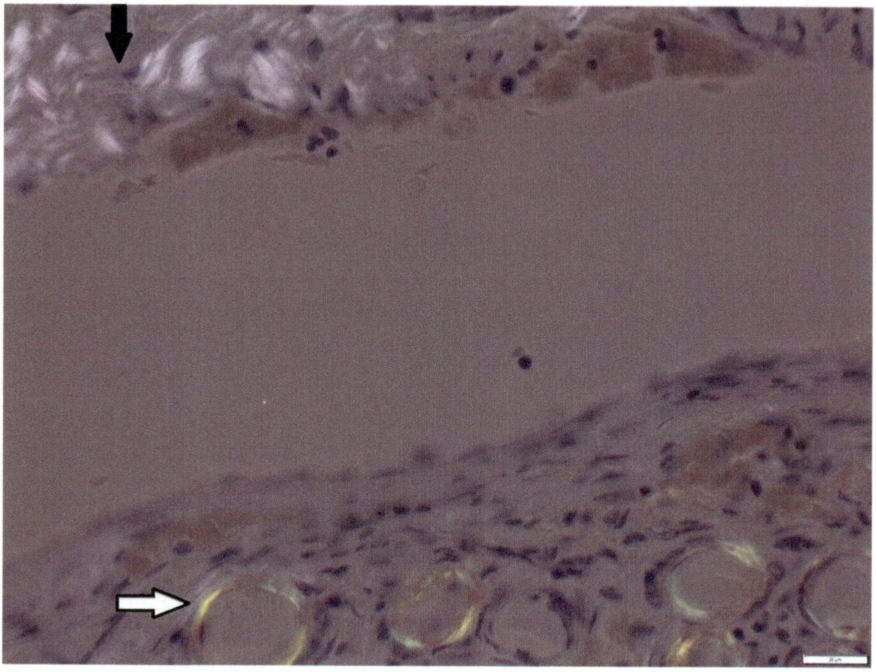

Fig. 7.3 Abundant amyloid deposition in renal blood vessels as seen by Congo red staining (with polarization). Apple green birefringence of amyloid in blood vessels can be seen in the lower part (white arrow) with non-birefringent collagen fibres in the upper part for comparison (black arrow). Original magnification x 200, Photo courtesy of Dr. Y Hock, University Hospitals Birmingham NHS Foundation Trust

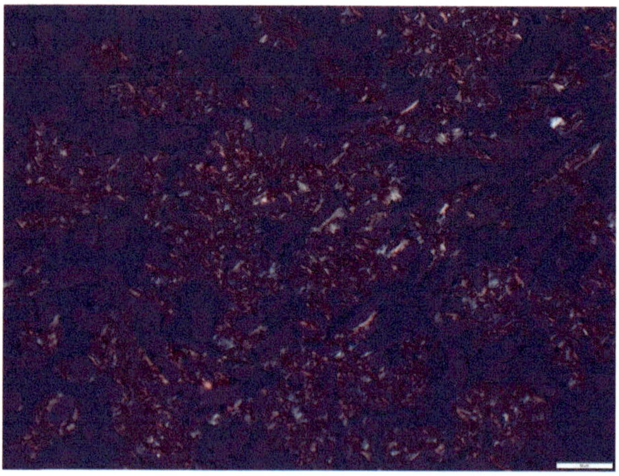

Fig. 7.4 Abundant amyloid deposition in liver as seen on Congo red stain (with polarization demonstrating apple green birefringence). Original magnification x 200, Photo courtesy of Dr. Y Hock, University Hospitals Birmingham NHS Foundation Trust

in expert centres. It is mandatory to use antibodies specifically developed for the recognition of amyloidogenic proteins to avoid false-positive or false-negative results.

In a study conducted by the national amyloidosis centre in the UK, IHC was diagnostic in 76%, and showed 100% concordance with the results of laser capture microdissection and mass spectrometry (LCM-MS) performed on the same samples [26]. The rate of false positives and negatives may be unacceptably high without using a validated panel of antibodies and proper methods. Background staining may occur due to non-immunological binding or to the presence of normal proteins containing epitopes targeted by the antibody in the extracellular space, such as normal immunoglobulins, resulting in false-positive results [27].

IEM is a technique available in few referral centres that combines immunohistochemistry and electron microscopy. Using gold-labelled secondary antibodies, IEM can co-localize the protein within amyloid fibrils and greatly reduce background staining, increasing accuracy. In an Italian study, IEM was equally sensitive (75–80%) but significantly more specific (100% vs 80%; $P < 0.001$) in diagnosing the type of systemic amyloidosis compared to light microscopy [28].

In cases where IHC is equivocal and not decisive or additional information is considered useful for clinical or diagnostic purposes, samples should be analysed by mass spectrometry-based proteomics. This approach relies on laser microdissection of Congo red positive amyloid deposits followed by mass spectrometry of digested proteins (LMD-LC-MS/MS), a sophisticated and highly accurate approach to determine the amyloid fibril type based on accurate measurement of the molecular mass of the more abundant peptides. This technique requires accurate sample preparation, mass spectrometry analysis, and protein identification by bioinformatics tools [29]. It is highly effective in recognizing all amyloid types in a single assay, increasing the diagnostic accuracy from 76 to 94% compared to IHC [26, 30]. Limitations include costs, accessibility, the need for experience and longer turnaround time [29].

In parallel with histological investigation and tissue amyloid typing, the corresponding protein precursor should be identified and quantified in blood by means of biochemical and/or genetic tests. The presence of a monoclonal protein in patients with suspected or biopsy-proved AL amyloidosis should always be investigated by serum and urinary immunofixation coupled with measurement of monoclonal free light chains (FLC). Only the combination of these tests allows detecting and quantifying the culprit monoclonal protein in 100% of cases.

Molecular genetic testing is essential for the diagnosis of hereditary amyloidosis. This is usually performed by Sanger sequencing of selected genes but next-generation sequencing (NGS) is becoming an increasingly available tool to test a panel of potentially involved genes at the same time.

Diagnosis of ATTRv amyloidosis, the most common form of hereditary amyloidosis worldwide, still takes several months or years from symptom onset in people with no known family history from non-endemic regions. This is still mostly due to limited disease awareness and/or misdiagnosis with other more common diseases. However, once an index patient has been identified in a family, genetic counselling and pre-symptomatic testing in at-risk relatives can be undertaken to identify possible mutation carriers, ensuring close monitoring and early diagnosis [31].

Bone tracer scintigraphy, particularly ^{99m}Tc-labelled 3,3-diphosphono-1,2-propanodicarboxylic acid (DPD) and ^{99m}Tc-labelled pyrophosphate (PYP), is now a well-acknowledged tool for the diagnosis of cardiac transthyretin amyloidosis and has substantially contributed to increasingly identify this disease in the past few years. The mechanisms underlying the specific tropism of these tracers for ATTR amyloid deposits are still elusive but a positive DPD or PYP scan can permit a non-invasive diagnosis of TTR amyloidosis according to validated diagnostic algorithms, avoiding the need for a positive biopsy. Briefly, a positive scan defined by a Perugini score higher than 1, in the absence of a monoclonal protein, is diagnostic for cardiac transthyretin amyloidosis [32]. As wild-type ATTR is not distinguished from hereditary ATTR based on this tool, genetic analysis is ultimately always needed to accurately differentiate acquired from hereditary TTR amyloidosis.

Scintigraphy using radioisotope-labelled serum amyloid P component (SAP) can demonstrate the presence of amyloid within some organs and provide an estimate of amyloid burden [33]. This procedure is however available only in a few centres. It is safe and can be repeated every 6–12 months to monitor the course of the disease, particularly in patients with secondary AA amyloidosis, therefore guiding treatment strategy. Sensitivity of SAP Scintigraphy is higher in AA and AL amyloid (90%) compared to 48% for hereditary transthyretin-related (ATTR) amyloidosis, with 93% specificity in all these conditions [34].

References

1. Kyle RA. Amyloidosis: a convoluted story. Br J Haematol. 2001;114:529.
2. Kisilevsky R, Raimondi S, Bellotti V. Historical and current concepts of fibrillogenesis and *in vivo* amyloidogenesis: implications of amyloid tissue targeting. Front Mol Biosci. 3:17. https://doi.org/10.3389/fmolb.2016.00017.
3. Benson MD, Buxbaum JN, Eisenberg DS, Merlini G, Saraiva MJ, Sekijima Y, et al. Amyloid nomenclature 2018: recommendations by the International Society of Amyloidosis (ISA) nomenclature committee. Amyloid. 2018;25(4):215–9.
4. Arosio P, Knowles TP, Linse S. On the lag phase in amyloid fibril formation. Phys Chem Chem Phys. 2015;17:7606.
5. Chiti F, Dobson CM. Protein misfolding, amyloid formation, and human disease: a summary of Progress over the last decade. Annu Rev Biochem. 2017;86(1):27–68.
6. Misra P, Blancas-Mejia LM, Ramirez-Alvarado M. Mechanistic insights into the early events in the aggregation of immunoglobulin light chains. Biochemistry. 2019;58(29):3155–68.
7. Picken MM. The pathology of amyloidosis in classification: a review. Acta Haematol. 2020;143:322–34.
8. Benson MD, Buxbaum JN, Eisenberg DS, Merlini G, Saraiva MJM, Sekijima Y, Sipe JD, Westermark P. Amyloid nomenclature 2020: update and recommendations by the International Society of Amyloidosis (ISA) nomenclature committee. Amyloid. 2020;27(4):217–22.

9. Bodin K, Ellmerich S, Kahan MC, et al. Antibodies to human serum amyloid P component eliminate visceral amyloid deposits. Nature. 2010;468:93–7.
10. Hamidi Asl K, Liepnieks JJ, Nakamura M, Benson MD. Organ-specific (localized) synthesis of Ig light chain amyloid. J Immunol. 1999;162:5556.
11. Westermark P. Localized AL amyloidosis: a suicidal neoplasm? Ups J Med Sci. 2012;117:244.
12. Calero M, Pawlik M, Soto C, et al. Distinct properties of wild-type and the amyloidogenic human cystatin C variant of hereditary cerebral haemorrhage with amyloidosis, Icelandic type. J Neurochem. 2001;77:628.
13. Seripa D, D'Onofrio G, Panza F, Cascavilla L, Masullo C, Pilotto A. The genetics of the human APOE polymorphism. Rejuvenation Res. 2011;14(5):491–500. https://doi.org/10.1089/rej.2011.1169. Epub 2011 Sep 29.
14. Migita K, Agematsu K, Masumoto J, et al. The contribution of SAA1 polymorphisms to familial Mediterranean fever susceptibility in the Japanese population. PLoS One. 2013;8:e55227.
15. De Torre-Minguela C, Mesa Del Castillo P, Pelegrín P. The NLRP3 and pyrin inflammasomes: implications in the pathophysiology of autoinflammatory diseases. Front Immunol. 2017;8:43. https://doi.org/10.3389/fimmu.2017.00043. PMID: 28191008; PMCID: PMC5271383.
16. Kyle RA, Linos A, Beard CM, Linke RP, Gertz MA, O'Fallon WM, Kurland LT. Incidence and natural history of primary systemic amyloidosis in Olmsted County, Minnesota, 1950 through 1989. Blood. 1992;79:1817–22.
17. Pinney JH, Smith CJ, Taube JB, Lachmann HJ, Venner CP, Gibbs SD, Dungu J, Banypersad SM, Wechalekar AD, Whelan CJ, Hawkins PN, Gillmore JD. Systemic amyloidosis in England: an epidemiological study. Br J Haematol. 2013;161:525–32.
18. Quock TP, Yan T, Chang E, Guthrie S, Broder MS. Epidemiology of AL amyloidosis: a real-world study using US claims data. Blood Adv. 2018;2(10):1046–53.
19. Nienhuis HL, Bijzet J, Hazenberg BP. The prevalence and management of systemic amyloidosis in Western countries. Kidney Dis (Basel). 2016;2:10–9.
20. Benson MD. The hereditary amyloidoses. In: Picken MM, Herrera GA, Dogan A, editors. Amyloid and related disorders—surgical pathology and clinical correlations. 2nd ed. Totowa: Humana Press; 2015. p. 65–80.
21. Duston MA, Skinner M, Meenan RF, Cohen AS. Sensitivity, specificity, and predictive value of abdominal fat aspiration for the diagnosis of amyloidosis. Arthritis Rheum. 1989;32:82.
22. van Gameren II, Hazenberg BP, Bijzet J, van Rijswijk MH. Diagnostic accuracy of subcutaneous abdominal fat tissue aspiration for detecting systemic amyloidosis and its utility in clinical practice. Arthritis Rheum. 2006;54:2015.
23. Dhingra S, Krishnani N, Kumari N, Pandey R. Evaluation of abdominal fat pad aspiration cytology and grading for detection in systemic amyloidosis. Acta Cytol. 2007;51:860.
24. Andrews TR, Colon-Otero G, Calamia KT, et al. Utility of subcutaneous fat aspiration for diagnosing amyloidosis in patients with isolated peripheral neuropathy. Mayo Clin Proc. 2002;77:1287.
25. Kyle RA, Bayrd ED. Amyloidosis: review of 236 cases. Medicine (Baltimore). 1975;54:271.
26. Gilbertson JA, Theis JD, Vrana JA, Lachmann H, Wechalekar A, Whelan C, et al. A comparison of immunohistochemistry and mass spectrometry for determining the amyloid fibril protein from formalin-fixed biopsy tissue. J Clin Pathol. 2015;68(4):314–7.
27. Kebbel A, Röcken C. Immunohistochemical classification of amyloid in surgical pathology revisited. Am J Surg Pathol. 2006;30(6):673–83.
28. Fernández de Larrea C, Verga L, Morbini P, Klersy C, Lavatelli F, Foli A, et al. A practical approach to the diagnosis of systemic amyloidoses. Blood. 2015;125(14):2239–44.
29. Picken MM. Proteomics and mass spectrometry in the diagnosis of renal amyloidosis. Clin Kidney J. 2015;8(6):665–72.
30. Dasari S, Theis JD, Vrana JA, Rech KL, Dao LN, Howard MT, Dispenzieri A, Gertz MA, Hasadsri L, Highsmith WE, Kurtin PJ, McPhail ED. Amyloid typing by mass spectrom-

etry in clinical practice: a comprehensive review of 16,175 samples. Mayo Clin Proc. 2020;95(9):1852–64. https://doi.org/10.1016/j.mayocp.2020.06.029. PMID: 32861330.
31. Obici L, Kuks JB, Buades J, et al.; European Network for TTR-FAP (ATTReuNET). Recommendations for presymptomatic genetic testing and management of individuals at risk for hereditary transthyretin amyloidosis. Curr Opin Neurol. 2016;29:S27–S35.
32. Gillmore JD, Maurer MS, Falk RH, Merlini G, Damy T, Dispenzieri A, et al. Nonbiopsy diagnosis of cardiac transthyretin amyloidosis. Circulation. 2016;133(24):2404–12.
33. Hawkins PN. Serum amyloid P component scintigraphy for diagnosis and monitoring amyloidosis. Curr Opin Nephrol Hypertens. 2002;11:649.
34. Hazenberg BP, van Rijswijk MH, Piers DA, et al. Diagnostic performance of 123I-labeled serum amyloid P component scintigraphy in patients with amyloidosis. Am J Med. 2006;119:355.e15.

Chapter 8
Amyloidosis: Clinical Manifestations and Treatment

Ahmed Abdulhameed Abdulgawad, Matthew Nicholson, and Hadi Goubran

Abbreviations

AA	AA amyloidosis
AL	AL amyloidosis
ASCT	Autologous stem cell transplantation
ATTR amyloidosis	Transthyretin amyloidosis
BNP	Brain natriuretic peptide
CAA	Cerebral amyloid angiopathy
CIDP	Chronic inflammatory demyelinating polyradiculoneuropathy
CR	Complete remission
cTnT	Cardiac troponin T
dFLC	Difference between involved minus uninvolved serum free light chains
DRA	Dialysis-related amyloidosis

A. A. Abdulgawad (✉)
Manchester Royal Infirmary, Manchester, UK

Faculty of Medicine, Cairo University, Cairo, Egypt
e-mail: aahameed@kasralainy.edu.eg

M. Nicholson · H. Goubran
Saskatoon Cancer Centre and College of Medicine, University of Saskatchewan, Saskatoon, SK, Canada
e-mail: Matthew.Nicholson@saskcancer.ca; hadi.goubranmessiha@saskcancer.ca

© The Author(s), under exclusive license to Springer Nature Switzerland AG 2022

G. Ragab et al. (eds.), *Paraproteinemia and Related Disorders*,
https://doi.org/10.1007/978-3-031-10131-1_8

ESRD	End-stage renal disease
FLC	Free light chain
FMF	Familial Mediterranean fever
MGUS	Monoclonal gammopathy of undetermined significance
MM	Multiple myeloma
MRI	Magnetic resonance imaging
NT-pro-BNP	N-terminal fragment of the pro-brain natriuretic peptide
PLCA	Primary localized cutaneous amyloidosis
PN	Polyneuropathy
RA	Rheumatoid arthritis
SAA	Serum amyloid A
SAP	Serum amyloid protein
TFNEs	Transient Focal Neurological Episodes
VCD	Velcade-cyclophosphamide-dexamethasone
VD	Velcade-dexamethasone
VMP	Velcade-melphalan-prednisone

Introduction

Amyloidosis comprises a group of disorders characterized by the deposition of abnormal extracellular protein material. It can involve multiple organs (systemic amyloidosis) or, less commonly, deposits in a single organ (organ-specific amyloidosis). These extracellular proteins deposit in tissues aggregated in ß-pleated sheets arranged in an antiparallel fashion and distort the tissue architecture and function [1].

Clinical presentation depends on the site and rate of deposition of amyloid fibrils. This deposition is governed by several factors, including amyloid protein precursor type, genetic and ethnic variations. More than 30 amyloid proteins have been identified [2]. AL amyloidosis is the most common type in developed countries [3]. The AA subtype is more common in developing countries [4].

Diagnosis and management of common amyloidosis types are discussed below: types and pathogenesis are discussed in Chap. 7.

Clinical Presentation

Amyloidosis is usually a multisystem disease with variable amyloid fibril deposition in various organs. Usually, multiple organs are affected to varying degrees, and one or two organs dominate the clinical presentation.

Systemic Amyloidosis

Systemic amyloidosis is the most common presentation of amyloidosis, with circulating amyloid precursors depositing in various organs in the form of insoluble amyloid fibrils. Clinical presentation depends on the nature of the amyloid protein and the site and rate of deposition. The clinical presentation is often due to effects on a single organ or a pair of organ systems although other organs/tissues might be affected on a subclinical level. Affected organ systems include:

- Renal

  The kidney is a principal target for amyloid deposition in the commoner types of systemic amyloidosis, namely AL and AA. However, it can be part of any systemic amyloid presentation.

  Renal involvement can have variable presentations. Proteinuria reaching a nephrotic range is by far the most common presentation. Patients can exhibit severe proteinuria, exceeding 20 g per day. Renal function is usually preserved initially. Gradual decline in renal function progresses to reach end-stage renal disease (ESRD) in one-fifth of patients. Progressive renal disease is a poor prognostic marker. This is true for AL amyloidosis [5] and AA amyloidosis [6].

  Less commonly, renal amyloidosis can present with progressive renal failure with mild or no proteinuria, renal tubular defect, or acute renal failure depending on the site of amyloid deposition (glomerular, vascular, tubular, or interstitial) as well as on the rate of deposition [7].
- Cardiovascular myocardial infiltration with amyloid fibrils can occur with most systemic amyloidosis subtypes. Cardiac disease is the primary determinant of prognosis in AL amyloidosis as advanced cardiac amyloidosis is generally irreversible and carries a poor prognosis.

  The most common pathology is restrictive cardiomyopathy resulting from myocardial infiltration. It usually presents with diastolic dysfunction with limited effect on the ejection fraction. Patients typically present with manifestations of systemic volume overload and generalized edema. Amyloid deposition interferes with the heart's conduction system as well, with both brady- and tachyarrhythmias [8]. Syncope and postural hypotension are common, though in some cases, these are related to autonomic neuropathy rather than direct cardiac effects. Systemic thromboembolism is a common presentation of cardiac amyloidosis partly due to a higher incidence of arrhythmias often coupled with atrial and ventricular amyloid deposits [9]. Ischemic heart disease, however, is uncommon in cardiac amyloid disease. In an autopsy study on 108 patients published in 1976 with cardiac amyloidosis, 5 (4.6%) only had severe occlusive amyloid deposits in intramyocardial arteries [10].

  The age of presentation varies depending on the amyloid subtype. AL amyloidosis presents at a wide range of ages, but nearly all patients are >40 years of age. Transthyretin amyloidosis (ATTR amyloidosis) is a "protein misfolding disorder." Transthyretin is a protein made by the liver that helps carry thyroid hormone and vitamin A in the blood. In ATTR amyloidosis, the protein becomes unstable. It gets fragmented and deposited in the heart and/or the nerves and other organs and tissues.

Patients with ATTR-mutated amyloidosis are typically older (>60–70 years of age) and much older still in ATTR wild-type amyloidosis. Of the 266 patients diagnosed with hereditary ATTR amyloidosis, a pathogenic mutation could be identified in 206; the most common mutation was Thr60Ala (68 patients [25%]). The median age at diagnosis was 63.3 years [11]. The type of presentation also varies according to the amyloid fibril subtype. More cardiomyopathies are reported with AL amyloidosis in contrast to arrhythmias, the salient feature of ATTR amyloidosis. Other extra-cardiac manifestations also vary depending on the amyloidosis syndrome [11].

- GIT/Liver

  Amyloidosis can affect any part of the gastrointestinal tract. Symptoms are attributable to one or more of the following mechanisms [12]:

  - Amyloid fibril deposition involves any part of the GIT and the liver, pancreas, and gallbladder. This can lead to dysmotility, bleeding, and malabsorption.
  - Associated autonomic neuropathy with its effect mainly on GIT motility.
  - Associated etiological factors as inflammatory bowel disease (IBD), chronic infections, and rheumatologic diseases affecting GIT.
  - Adverse effects from amyloidosis medications, for example, combination chemotherapy for AL amyloidosis.
  - Hepatic and splenic infiltrations commonly present with clinical hepatosplenomegaly. Although isolated reports described obstructive jaundice, elevated alkaline phosphatase and giant hepatomegaly with portal hypertension, liver functions are usually preserved in the majority of patients [13–16].

  AL amyloidosis is the most common cause of GIT amyloidosis; however, AA, ATTR, and dialysis-related amyloidosis (DRA) can lead to GIT involvement.

- Hematological

  Bleeding is the most prominent hematological symptom in amyloidosis. Many components of the hemostatic system can be affected in systemic amyloidosis [17]:

  - Impaired vascular integrity as a direct consequence of amyloid fibril deposition.
  - Thrombocytopenia occurring as a result of splenomegaly, associated myeloma or chemotherapy.
  - Low levels of coagulation factors. Factor X deficiency has a direct interaction with amyloid fibrils in the liver. The impaired hepatic synthetic function also contributes to coagulopathy.

  Bruising around the ocular orbits (raccoon eyes) without a history of trauma is generally considered pathognomonic for AL amyloidosis. Other foci of cutaneous and visceral bleeding are common.

  Anemia, and less commonly, neutropenia, can occur due to bone marrow infiltration in AL amyloidosis or result from hypersplenism or associated myeloma.

- Neurological

  Peripheral nerve involvement is a relatively common feature in systemic amyloidosis [18]. Manifestations include:

  - Sensorimotor peripheral neuropathy with classical clinical features of paresthesias and less commonly motor weakness.
  - Entrapment neuropathy with external compression on peripheral nerves as in carpal tunnel syndrome.
  - Autonomic neuropathy causing postural dizziness and syncope and GI and urinary tract dysmotility.

  ATTR amyloidosis with polyneuropathy (PN) is a progressive, debilitating, systemic disease wherein transthyretin protein misfolds to form amyloid deposits in the endoneurium. Symptoms may be mistakenly attributed to other conditions such as chronic inflammatory demyelinating polyradiculoneuropathy (CIDP), idiopathic axonal polyneuropathy, lumbar spinal stenosis, and, more rarely, diabetic neuropathy and AL amyloidosis.

  Central nervous system involvement in the most common systemic amyloidosis subtypes (AL and AA) is infrequent.

  Cerebral amyloid angiopathy (CAA) is a spectrum of clinical presentations caused by amyloid fibril deposition in small- and medium-sized cerebral arteries [19]. The few mutations identified in CAA are linked to the younger age of presentation and worse outcomes. Patients can present with any of the following:

  - Acute, recurrent, or chronic cerebral lobar bleeds. Identification is essential as the risk of recurrence is higher than many other causes of a cerebral hemorrhage. Patients can remain asymptomatic with incidental findings of microbleeds being picked up on MRI imaging performed for unrelated conditions.
  - Transient focal neurological episodes (TFNEs). These are recurrent, focal, reversible stereotyped neurological deficits. TFNEs are thought to happen due to cerebral irritation by microbleeds and chronic siderosis caused by CAA. History, gradual onset, MRI can help to differentiate it from other focal neurological syndromes like migraine, epilepsy, and TIAs [20].

  Associated atherosclerosis exhibits a similar incidence as in the general population with similar risk factors (diabetes, hypertension, etc.). Atheroembolic disease remains a common cause of CNS events in amyloidosis patients.

- Musculoskeletal

  - Muscle involvement

    In systemic AL amyloidosis, amyloid fibrils can deposit in skeletal muscles. It is usually asymptomatic, but can lead to numerous presentations ranging from myalgia, pseudohypertrophy, macroglossia, proximal myopathy, or myositis [21].

  - Amyloid arthropathy

    Amyloid deposition in the synovial membrane of shoulders, knees, wrists, and small hand joints is not uncommon. Arthropathy as a presenting symptom is uncommon. Joint involvement is usually very gradual, with little to no inflammatory features compared to rheumatoid arthritis (RA).

DRA leads to erosive and destructive osteoarthropathy, mainly involving the shoulders, the hips, and carpal bones. It resembles inflammatory arthritis with juxta-articular soft tissue swelling, mild periarticular osteoporosis, and juxta-articular and subchondral cystic lesions (geodes), usually with well-defined sclerotic margins [22].

  - Bone disease

    Amyloid deposition in bone-forming bone cysts has been described. Lytic bone lesions can be seen in AL amyloidosis associated with multiple myeloma (MM) [23].

- Pulmonary

  Pulmonary amyloidosis can occur in virtually all types of systemic and localized amyloidosis [24]. Clinical features are heterogeneous and include:

  - Pulmonary infiltration with amyloid fibrils can affect the tracheobronchial tree causing hoarseness, stridor, and obstruction.
  - It can also affect pulmonary parenchyma or pleura, causing pulmonary nodules or pleural effusion, respectively. The most common presentation is pleural effusion as part of generalized anasarca due to cardiac amyloidosis and can be difficult to distinguish clinically from primary amyloid deposition.

- Skin

  Skin infiltration is common, and subcutaneous fat biopsy is one of the most common sites for initial histopathologic sampling. Amyloid skin disease may be localized (see below) or comprise part of systemic amyloidosis. Deposition can have the shape of macules, nodules, or vesicles. In the absence of thrombocytopenia or platelet dysfunction, bruises are relatively common in AL amyloidosis with the pathognomonic raccoon eyes. AL amyloidosis is the most likely to exhibit cutaneous manifestations [25]. However, AA, ATTR, and DRA can rarely present with cutaneous manifestations.

Localized Amyloidosis

In contrast to systemic amyloidosis, amyloid fibril deposition can be confined to only one organ due to the light chain amyloid fibrils produced by tissue-specific plasma cells. This is not associated with systemic clonal plasma cell disorders. Bone marrow is not infiltrated with clonal plasma cells. The following are few examples of localized organ-specific amyloidosis:

- Cutaneous amyloidosis: As previously mentioned, subcutaneous deposition of amyloid fibrils occurs in many systemic amyloidosis syndromes. Isolated skin infiltration can be a localized process. Primary localized cutaneous amyloidosis (PLCA) is characterized by the extracellular deposition of heterogenic amyloid

proteins in the skin without systemic involvement. Lichen amyloidosis, macular amyloidosis, and (primary localized cutaneous) nodular amyloidosis are different subtypes of PLCA [26].
- CNS infiltration with amyloid fibrils is implicated in familial and sporadic forms of Alzheimer's disease [27].

Diagnosis

A high index of clinical suspicion is required due to disease rarity.

1. **Clinical context**

   Typical organ involvement (renal, cardiac, neurological) in an appropriate clinical context is suggestive. For example:

   - AL amyloidosis should be suspected in myeloma, monoclonal gammopathy of undetermined significance (MGUS) and lymphoma patients with:
     - Generalized edema, nephrotic range of proteinuria
     - Unexplained cardiac failure
     - Progressive neuropathy
     - Hepatosplenomegaly
   - AA amyloidosis should be looked for in RA, IBD, bronchiectasis, and periodic fever patients with:
     - Nephrotic syndrome, renal failure
     - Gastrointestinal and hepatic manifestations
     - Biventricular hypertrophy or diastolic cardiac failure
   - ATTR amyloidosis in patients with positive family history and one or more of the clinical amyloidosis presentations. Family history might be missing, and this should not exclude the diagnosis completely.
   - DRA in dialysis patients with musculoskeletal manifestations, including shoulder arthropathy. DRA-related hospitalizations decreased over ten-fold from 1998 to 2018 with the use of high-flux hemodialysis. Serum β2 microglobulin, the precursor of amyloid fibrils, remains positively associated with mortality, even in the current era [28].

2. **Laboratory Evaluation**

   (a) **Initial lab tests and imaging**

   These will help assess organ functions and exclude other etiologies but will not confirm a diagnosis of amyloidosis. They include:

   - Urine analysis: A bland sediment is expected in renal amyloidosis. A nephrotic range of proteinuria is a common finding.
   - Renal functions are usually preserved until late in the disease process. However, patients may less commonly proceed quickly to end-stage renal

disease. Others may present with acute kidney injury with or without proteinuria.

- Deranged liver functions.
- Anemia, thrombocytopenia, or pancytopenia are generally rare. They may be the result of splenomegaly or associated myeloma in AL amyloidosis.
- Troponin and NT-ProBNP are very sensitive markers of cardiac amyloidosis of any etiology, and normal values largely exclude significant cardiac amyloidosis. They are also used to risk-stratify amyloidosis and can guide treatment decisions.
- Imaging studies:
  - Echocardiography and cardiac magnetic resonance imaging (MRI)
  - Abdominal ultrasound
- Nerve conduction studies
- The presence of clonal free light chains (usually lambda) should not be the sole evidence of AL amyloidosis. Even in the presence of histopathological evidence of amyloidosis MGUS can co-exist with other forms of amyloidosis.

(b) **Tissue biopsy:**

- The hallmark of amyloid diagnosis is the histological demonstration of amyloid fibril deposition with its characteristic appearance.
  - Homogenous structureless eosinophilic deposition in Hematoxylin and Eosin prepared sections.
  - Apple-green birefringence under polarized light microscopy when stained with Congo-red.
  - Intense yellow-green fluorescence with thioflavin T.
- The clinical presentation should always be considered to determine where to biopsy. However, classic locations of biopsies include:
  - Abdominal fat biopsy: This safe site for biopsy is a relatively straightforward outpatient procedure. However, sample processing needs an experienced histopathologist.
  - Rectal snip: This is an accessible site of biopsy with a relatively high yield.
  - Bone marrow trephine biopsy: This will also detect the presence of clonal plasma cells in AL amyloidosis. Fluorescence in situ hybridization (FISH) has prognostic value in untreated AL amyloidosis and may guide therapeutic decisions. Often the amyloidogenic clone is characterized by chromosomal abnormalities [29]. The most frequent genetic abnormalities in AL amyloidosis are t(11; 14) (50%) [30], monosomy 13/del(13q) (36%), and trisomies (26%) [30].
  - Renal, hepatic, or cardiac biopsies: In AL amyloidosis, the risk of bleeding associated with renal biopsy is significant. Choosing an alternate biopsy site can successfully demonstrate the deposits sparing the patients' bleeding risks [31].

(c) **SAP (serum amyloid P component) scanning**

Serum amyloid P component scanning is a noninvasive, accurate scintigraphic diagnosis of amyloidosis [32].

Advantages
- Allows for quantification and hence follow-up of disease progression and response to therapy.
- Relatively quick with the whole procedure completed in less than one hour.
- Relatively safe with minimal radiation exposure.

Disadvantages:
- Not widely available worldwide.
- The substrate of the scan (SAP protein) is derived from donors with the potential of transmitting infections.
- Not sensitive to cardiac amyloidosis and a different modality is needed.

Treatment

(a) **General approach**

Amyloidosis clinical manifestations depend on the degree and sites of amyloid deposition. Unlike other proteins, amyloid degradation is prolonged, leading to its accumulation in tissues.

Traditionally, treatment efforts were directed towards slowing progression and supportive measures since amyloidosis was deemed incurable.

It has been shown that halting or slowing down further amyloid deposition in tissues allows the slow degradation of amyloid deposits to reduce amyloid burden, leading to histopathological and clinical improvement. It depends mainly on the etiology of amyloidosis and patient characteristics, and treatment has to be individualized and tailored to the patient's general condition and organ reserve.

Given the disease's rarity and complexity, management should be provided in tertiary centers and whenever available in a dedicated amyloidosis management center. This will allow for:

- Expert patient management.
- A multidisciplinary approach with the much-needed input from various medical teams, including hematology, nephrology, cardiology, and pathology, to help with supportive management.
- Data collection will feed into current and future research with a better understanding of the disease dynamics and future management.
- Availability of newer treatment options from clinical trials.

Treatment will include specific measures to halt disease progression, depending on the relevant amyloidosis subtype pathogenesis (specific management) and organ support to manage target organ affection by amyloid deposition (supportive management).

(b) **Specific Management**

1. **AL Amyloidosis**

   Specific treatment of AL amyloidosis is usually directed towards clonal plasma cells. This is primarily inspired by the multiple myeloma chemotherapy protocols tailored to amyloidosis patients. Both conditions can co-exist, and the treatment then would depend on the predominant features and comorbidities. On the other hand, MM and amyloidosis can manifest sequentially along the course of MM; the reverse is rare. This is discussed in detail in Chap. 9.

2. **AA Amyloidosis**

   Treatment of AA amyloidosis is primarily directed towards treating the cause. This will control the rate of SAA production back to an average level. This will stabilize the disease and gradually might cause regression.

   Treatment would differ depending on the etiology. However, treating a chronic septic focus, refractory bronchiectasis, Familial FMF, or advanced RA is usually challenging.

   Cytokine-directed therapy

   Cytokine-directed therapy is showing an increasing success in controlling AA amyloidosis secondary to RA [33], Seronegative arthropathies [34], Periodic fever syndromes [35] and Crohn's disease [36].

   TNF antagonists' efficacy seems to correlate with the degree of primary disease control. IL-1 receptor antagonist anakinra seems to directly improve AA amyloidosis independent of the primary disease with marked reduction of SAA level [37]. The IL-6 antagonist tocilizumab equally showed clinical improvement (delayed progression to dialysis, improved renal functions) and normalization of SAA levels [38, 39].

   Some success in controlling AA amyloidosis could also be achieved using colchicine, commonly used in autoinflammatory conditions [40].

3. **ATTR Amyloidosis**

   Like other types, treatment relies on reducing the rate of amyloid deposition allowing for the natural slow process of amyloid degradation to reduce amyloid burden, stabilize and eventually improve clinical manifestations.

   These types are even less common than AL and AA amyloidosis, with even less available high-quality evidence.

   Since ATTR amyloidosis is caused by the production of abnormal TTR protein (in ATTRmut) or excessive production of structurally normal TTR protein (ATTR wild type), the diagnosis should include DNA testing for mutations, biopsy, and amyloid typing [41]. In both conditions, the target would be to interfere with hepatic production of TTR as follows:

   Genetic modifiers:

   The RNA-interfering agent patisiran was effective in improving neuropathy and quality of life in ATTRmut patients. No significant side effects have been reported, and the drug was generally well tolerated [42]. The antisense oligonucleotide agent inotersen has demonstrated similar results [43].

Neutralizing agents:

Tafamidis is a new drug that binds to TTR to reduce its ability to form amyloid fibrils. It showed promising results in ATTR presenting with both neuropathy and cardiomyopathy [44].

Conclusions

Amyloidosis comprises a heterogeneous group of disorders characterized by the deposition of abnormal extracellular protein material. This deposition is governed by several factors, including amyloid protein precursor type, genetic and ethnic variations. It can involve multiple organs (systemic amyloidosis) or, less commonly, deposits in a single organ (organ-specific amyloidosis). These extracellular proteins deposit in tissues aggregated in ß-pleated that distort tissue architecture and function.

Clinical presentation depends on the site and rate of deposition of amyloid fibrils. It is crucial to identify the type of deposits and the extent of organ damage before considering the different treatment options.

For AL-amyloidosis, treatment is primarily inspired by the multiple myeloma chemotherapy protocols tailored to amyloidosis patients based on their organ reserve. In AA amyloidosis, on the other hand, where inflammation is the driver for the process, the use of cytokine-based therapy is more appropriate. For ATTR RNA-interfering agents, antisense oligonucleotide or neutralizing agents can be offered.

References

1. Dahiya DS, Kichloo A, Singh J, Albosta M, Wani F. Gastrointestinal amyloidosis: a focused review. World J Gastrointest Endosc. 2021;13(1):1–12. https://doi.org/10.4253/wjge.v13.i1.1. PMID: 33520102.
2. Sipe JD, Benson MD, Buxbaum JN, et al. Nomenclature 2014: amyloid fibril proteins and clinical classification of the amyloidosis. Amyloid. 2014;21:221–4.
3. Wechalekar AD, Gillmore JD, Hawkins PN. Systemic amyloidosis. Lancet. 2016;387:2641–54.
4. Westermark P, Westermark GT. Review. Reflections on amyloidosis in Papua New Guinea. Philos Trans R Soc Lond B Biol Sci. 2008;363:3701–5.
5. Palladini G, Merlini G. Current treatment of AL amyloidosis. Haematologica. 2009;94:1044–8.
6. Uda H, Yokota A, Kobayashi K, et al. Two distinct clinical courses of renal involvement in rheumatoid patients with AA amyloidosis. J Rheumatol. 2006;33(8):1482–7.
7. Khalighi MA, Wallace WD, Palma-Diaz MF. Amyloid nephropathy. Clin Kidney J. 2014;7(2):97–106. Published online 2014 Mar 13. PMCID: PMC4377792. https://doi.org/10.1093/ckj/sfu021.
8. Mathew V, Olson LJ, Gertz MA, Hayes DL. Symptomatic conduction system disease in cardiac amyloidosis. Am J Cardiol. 1997;80:1491–2. https://doi.org/10.1016/S0002-9149(97)82785-3.
9. Martinez-Naharro A, Gonzalez-Lopez E, Corovic A, et al. High prevalence of intracardiac thrombi in cardiac amyloidosis. J Am Coll Cardiol. 2019;73:1733–4.

10. Smith RR, Hutchins GM. Ischemic heart disease secondary to amyloidosis of intramyocardial arteries. Am J Cardiol. 1979;44(3):413–7. https://doi.org/10.1016/0002-9149(79)90389-8. PMID: 157693.
11. Swiecicki PL, Zhen DB, Mauermann ML, Kyle RA, Zeldenrust SR, Grogan M, Dispenzieri A, Gertz MA. Hereditary ATTR amyloidosis: a single-institution experience with 266 patients. Amyloid. 2015;22(2):123–31. https://doi.org/10.3109/13506129.2015.1019610. Epub 2015 May 27. PMID: 26017327.
12. Rowe K, Pankow J, Nehme F, Salyers W. Gastrointestinal amyloidosis: review of the literature. Cureus. 2017;9(5):e1228. https://doi.org/10.7759/cureus.1228.
13. Levy M, Fryd CH, Eliakim M. Intrahepatic obstructive jaundice due to amyloidosis of the liver. A case report and review of the literature. Gastroenterology. 1971;61(2):234–8. PMID: 5314952.
14. Carey E, Plesec T, Menon KV. Elevated alkaline phosphatase in a man with ascites. Gastroenterology. 2013;144(3):e5–6. https://doi.org/10.1053/j.gastro.2012.09.044. Epub 2013 Feb 1. PMID: 23380945.
15. Serra L, Poppi MC, Criscuolo M, Zandomeneghi R. Primary systemic amyloidosis with giant hepatomegaly and portal hypertension: a case report and a review of the literature. Ital J Gastroenterol. 1993;25(8):435–8. PMID: 8286779.
16. Takayasu V, Laborda LS, Bernardelli R, Pinesi HT, Silva MP, Chiavelli V, Simões AB, Felipe-Silva A. Amyloidosis: an unusual cause of portal hypertension. Autops Case Rep. 2016;6(2):9–18. https://doi.org/10.4322/acr.2016.035. eCollection 2016 Apr-Jun. PMID: 27547738.
17. Sucker C, Hetzel GR, Grabensee B, et al. Amyloidosis and bleeding: pathophysiology, diagnosis, and therapy. Am J Kidney Dis. 2006;47:947–55.
18. Shin SC, Robinson-Papp J. Amyloid neuropathies. Mt Sinai J Med. 2012;79:733–48. https://doi.org/10.1002/msj.21352.
19. Van Etten ES, Gurol ME, Van Der Grond J, et al. Recurrent hemorrhage risk and mortality in hereditary and sporadic cerebral amyloid angiopathy. Neurology. 2016;87:1482–7. https://doi.org/10.1212/WNL.0000000000003181.
20. Charidimou A, Peeters A, Fox Z, et al. Spectrum of transient focal neurological episodes in cerebral amyloid angiopathy: multicentre magnetic resonance imaging cohort study and meta-analysis. Stroke. 2012;43:2324–30.
21. Muchtar E, Derudas D, Mauermann M, et al. Systemic immunoglobulin light chain amyloidosis–associated myopathy: presentation, diagnostic pitfalls, and outcome. Mayo Clin Proc. 2016;91:1354–61. https://doi.org/10.1016/j.mayocp.2016.06.027.
22. Prokaeva T, Spencer B, Kaut M, et al. Soft tissue, joint, and bone manifestations of AL amyloidosis: clinical presentation, molecular features, and survival. Arthritis Rheum. 2007;56:3858–68. https://doi.org/10.1002/art.22959.
23. Healy CF, Murray JG, Eustace SJ, Madewell J, O'Gorman PJ, O'Sullivan P. Multiple myeloma: a review of imaging features and radiological techniques. Bone Marrow Res. 2011;2011:583439. Published online 2011 Aug 8. PMCID: PMC3200072. https://doi.org/10.1155/2011/583439.
24. Utz JP, Swensen SJ, Gertz MA. Pulmonary amyloidosis: the Mayo Clinic experience from 1980 to 1993. Ann Intern Med. 1996;124:407–13. https://doi.org/10.7326/0003-4819-124-4-199602150-00004.
25. Silverstein SR. Primary, systemic amyloidosis and the dermatologist: where classic skin lesions may provide the clue for early diagnosis. Dermatol Online J. 2005;11(1):5. PMID: 15748546.
26. Weidner T, Illing T, Elsner P. Primary localized cutaneous amyloidosis: a systematic treatment review. Am J Clin Dermatol. 2017;18(5):629–42. https://doi.org/10.1007/s40257-017-0278-9. PMID: 28342017.
27. Morris GP, Clark IA, Vissel B. Questions concerning the role of amyloid-β in the definition, aetiology and diagnosis of Alzheimer's disease. Acta Neuropathol. 2018;136(5):663–89. Published online 2018 Oct 22. PMCID: PMC6208728. https://doi.org/10.1007/s00401-018-1918-8.

28. Kanda E, Muenz D, Bieber B, Cases A, Locatelli A, Port FK, Pecoits-Filho R, Robinson BM, Perl J. Beta-2 microglobulin and all-cause mortality in the era of high-flux hemodialysis: results from the dialysis outcomes and practice patterns study. Clin Kidney J. 2021;14(5):1436–42. Published online 2020 Oct 27. PMCID: PMC8087125. https://doi.org/10.1093/ckj/sfaa155.
29. Bochtler T, Hegenbart U, Cremer FW, Heiss C, Benner A, Hose D, et al. Evaluation of the cytogenetic aberration pattern in amyloid light chain amyloidosis as compared with monoclonal gammopathy of undetermined significance reveals common pathways of karyotypic instability. Blood. 2008;111(9):4700–5.
30. Muchtar E, Dispenzieri A, Kumar SK, Ketterling RP, Dingli D, Lacy MQ, et al. Interphase fluorescence in situ hybridization in untreated AL amyloidosis has an independent prognostic impact by abnormality type and treatment category. Leukemia. 2017;31(7):1562–9.
31. Merlini G, Wechalekar AD, Palladini G. Systemic light chain amyloidosis: an update for treating physicians. Blood. 2013;121(26):5124–30.
32. Hawkins PN, Pepys MB. Imaging amyloidosis with radiolabelled SAP. Eur J Nucl Med. 1995;22(7):595–9. https://doi.org/10.1007/BF01254559. PMID: 7498219.
33. Dispenzieri A, Gertz MA, Kyle RA, et al. Serum cardiac troponins and N-terminal pro-brain natriuretic peptide: a staging system for primary systemic amyloidosis. J Clin Oncol. 2004;22:3751–7. https://doi.org/10.1200/JCO.2004.03.029.
34. Palladini G, Sachchithanantham S, Milani P, et al. A European collaborative study of cyclophosphamide, bortezomib, and dexamethasone in upfront treatment of systemic AL amyloidosis. Blood. 2015;126:612–5. https://doi.org/10.1182/blood-2015-01-620302.
35. Gattorno M, Pelagatti MA, Meini A, et al. Persistent efficacy of anakinra in patients with tumor necrosis factor receptor-associated periodic syndrome. Arthritis Rheum. 2008;58:1516–20. https://doi.org/10.1002/art.23475.
36. Yoon KP, Dong SH, Chang SE. Systemic amyloidosis with Crohn's disease treated with infliximab. Inflamm Bowel Dis. 2008;14:431–2.
37. Lane T, Wechalekar AD, Gillmore JD, et al. Safety and efficacy of empirical interleukin-1 inhibition using anakinra in AA amyloidosis of uncertain aetiology. Amyloid. 2017;24:189–93. https://doi.org/10.1080/13506129.2017.1352503.
38. Inui K, Sawa N, Suwabe T, Mizuno H, Yamanouchi M, Hiramatsu R, Hayami N, Hoshino J, Kinowaki K, Fujii T, Ohashi K, Ubara Y. Long term administration of tocilizumab improves renal amyloid A (AA) amyloidosis deposition in familial Mediterranean fever. Mod Rheumatol Case Rep. 2020;4(2):310–1. https://doi.org/10.1080/24725625.2020.1739193. Epub 2020 Mar 19. PMID: 33087008.
39. Courties A, Grateau G, Philippe P, Flipo RM, Astudillo L, Aubry-Rozier B, Fabreguet I, Fahd W, Fain O, Guggenbuhl P, Hachulla E, Papo T, Richez C, Sibilia J, Morel J, Berenbaum F, Sellam J, Club Rhumatismes Inflammation and the REGATE Registry. AA amyloidosis treated with tocilizumab: case series and updated literature review. Amyloid. 2015;22(2):84–92. https://doi.org/10.3109/13506129.2014.1002031. Epub 2015 Jan. PMID: 25585627.
40. Meneses CF, Egües CA, Uriarte M, Belzunegui J, Rezola M. Colchicine use in isolated renal AA amyloidosis. Reumatol Clin. 2015;11(4):242–3. https://doi.org/10.1016/j.reuma.2014.09.007. Epub 2014 Nov 14. PMID: 25453598.
41. Adams D, Ando Y, Beirão JM, Coelho T, Gertz MA, Gillmore JD, Hawkins PN, Lousada I, Suhr OB, Merlini G. Expert consensus recommendations to improve diagnosis of ATTR amyloidosis with polyneuropathy. J Neurol. 2021;268(6):2109–22. https://doi.org/10.1007/s00415-019-09688-0. Epub 2020 Jan 6. PMID: 31907599.
42. Adams D, Gonzalez-Duarte A, O'Riordan WD, et al. Patisiran, an RNAi therapeutic, for hereditary transthyretin amyloidosis. N Engl J Med. 2018;379:11–21. https://doi.org/10.1056/nejmoa1716153.
43. Benson MD, Waddington-Cruz M, Berk JL, et al. Inotersen treatment for patients with hereditary transthyretin amyloidosis. N Engl J Med. 2018;379:22–31. https://doi.org/10.1056/nejmoa1716793.
44. Maurer MS, Schwartz JH, Gundapaneni B, et al. Tafamidis treatment for patients with transthyretin amyloid cardiomyopathy. N Engl J Med. 2018;379:1007–16. https://doi.org/10.1056/nejmoa1805689.

Chapter 9
Primary Light Chain (AL) Amyloidosis

Ashutosh D. Wechalekar

Introduction

The deposition of misfolded proteins causes systemic amyloidosis as interstitial fibrillar deposits (amyloid deposits) and direct cellular proteotoxicity from the pre-fibrillary oligomers [1]. Progressive multiorgan dysfunction results from the ongoing accumulation of protein fibrils that are remarkably resistant to proteolysis. About 35 different proteins have been reported to cause human amyloidoses. Of these, systemic AL amyloidosis (AL) due to the deposition of misfolded immunoglobulin light chains and wild-type transthyretin amyloidosis (wtATTR), due to misfolded native transthyretin deposition, are the two commonest types [2]. AL was considered the commonest, but wtATTR is set to overtake AL as the globally commonest type of amyloidosis. Cardiac involvement remains the common cause of morbidity and mortality in patients with systemic AL amyloidosis. AL has an incidence of 8–10 cases per million person-years, the median age at diagnosis of 63, and is a rapidly fatal disease if untreated. Secondary amyloidosis (AA) is becoming rarer in developed countries. Still, it occurs with autoimmune or inflammatory conditions such as multicentric Castleman's disease, renal cell cancer, autoimmune disorders, and chronic infections due to bronchiectasis or osteomyelitis. Leucocyte chemotactic factor 2 (LECT2) amyloidosis [3], seen in countries like Mexico, India, Egypt, is becoming another frequently recognized acquired amyloidosis.

Amyloidosis is a rare diagnosis. The presenting symptoms, however, are prevalent in the affected age group leading to a delay in diagnosis. In this chapter, we will review the steps to AL amyloid diagnosis, investigations, and approach to its management.

A. D. Wechalekar (✉)
National Amyloidosis Centre, University College London, Royal Free Campus, London, UK
e-mail: a.wechalekar@ucl.ac.uk

© The Author(s), under exclusive license to Springer Nature Switzerland AG 2022

G. Ragab et al. (eds.), *Paraproteinemia and Related Disorders*,
https://doi.org/10.1007/978-3-031-10131-1_9

Diagnosis

The heart and kidneys are the two commonest organs affected by amyloidosis. Symptoms due to dysfunction of these organs underpin the clinical presentation—fatigue, breathlessness, and edema. Figure 9.1 gives the organ involvement in AL amyloidosis. In AL, soft tissue involvement leading to macroglossia, with typical stiff enlarged tongue with teeth indentation, is a pathognomonic feature. Periorbital purpura (the so-called panda eyes) in a patient with monoclonal gammopathy puts amyloidosis at the top of the differential unless proven otherwise. Involvement of peripheral or autonomic nerves is seen in 20–30% of patients with AL amyloidosis. Unexplained weight loss, diarrhea, erectile dysfunction, and painful/painless peripheral neuropathy may also underlie gastrointestinal, autonomic, and peripheral nerve damage, respectively, in these patients. While some clinical presentations may be very typical of AL amyloidosis, most often, clinical manifestations are similar for all types of systemic amyloidosis and often not specific enough to distinguish amyloid fibril type clinically. Table 9.1 gives the distribution of organ involvement in various kinds of amyloidosis.

With the increasing recognition of wild-type transthyretin amyloidosis in the elderly, a population group where monoclonal gammopathy of uncertain significance is also common, the potential for two amyloid-forming precursor proteins in a single patient is an increasingly frequent situation in clinical practice [4], leading to a critical need for accurate amyloid typing. This is especially the case in older men with an African background where gammopathies are commoner, and 4% of the population carry a mutation in the TTR gene (V122I), which also predisposes to amyloidosis [5].

In the majority of patients with systemic amyloidosis, a tissue diagnosis is required to confirm amyloid deposition and to obtain material for confirming the protein type in amyloid fibrils. Biopsy of the affected organ has the highest chance

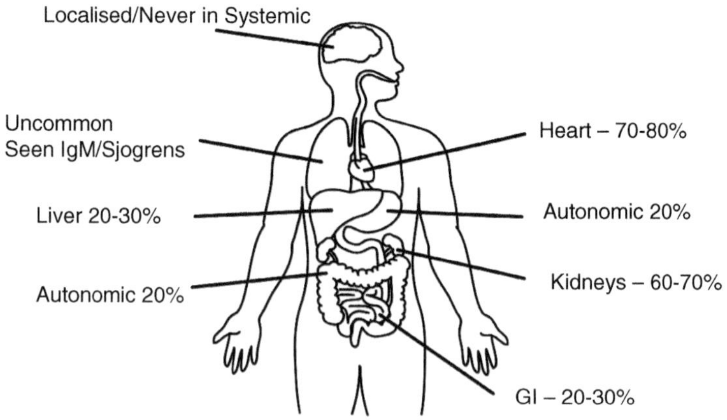

Fig. 9.1 Organ involvement in AL amyloidosis

Table 9.1 Presentation in different types of amyloidosis

Type	Heart	Kidneys	Liver	Nerves	Soft tissue
AL	+++	+++	+	+	+
AA	–	+++	+	–	–
ALECT2	–	+++	++	–	–
ATTRm	+/–	–	–	+++	–
ATTRwt	+++	–	–	–	Carpal tunnel/Spinal stenosis only
AFib	–	+++	–	–	–
AApoA1	+	++	++	+/–	–
ALys	–	+	+++	–	GI tract

AL Immunoglobulin light-chain, *AA* Secondary amyloidosis, *ALECT2* Leucocyte chemotactic factor 2 amyloidosis, *ATTRm* Mutant transthyretin, *ATTRwt* Wild-type transthyretin, *AFib* Fibrinogen A-α, *AApoA1* Apolipoprotein A1, *ALys* Lysozyme
Very common +++; Common ++; can occur +; not involved –

of yielding a positive result but may be fraught with risks such as bleeding; hence, abdominal fat or bone marrow biopsies may be a lower risk alternative. The combination of abdominal fat and bone marrow biopsies is likely to yield a positive result in 87% of cases with probable AL amyloidosis [6]. Demonstration amyloid deposition by classic Congo red staining remains the gold standard. False-negative or false-positive results with Congo red-stained biopsy preparations can occur, and all such results must be interpreted keeping the clinical context in the background [7, 8]. Once amyloid deposition has been confirmed by Congo red staining, in most of the cases, the next step is confirmatory fibril typing. Immunohistochemistry has been used for many years as a confirmatory technique. However, false positives and false negatives are common, especially in AL. Laser capture with mass spectrometry (LCMS) has become a gold standard due to its high sensitivity and specificity. In LCMS, Congo red-positive areas dissected from slides, digested and analyzed [9]. All amyloid deposits contain Apo E and serum amyloid P protein, which are considered amyloid signature proteins. After mass spectrometry, using protein reference databases, amyloid fibril protein can be reliably identified in the vast majority of the cases where adequate tissue samples are available. DNA sequencing of genes related to hereditary variants is also essential for confirming proteomic findings and family screening when appropriate [4].

Once a biopsy has demonstrated amyloidosis, subsequent workup involves a detailed assessment to identify the monoclonal protein (in AL) and define the extent of organ involvement. Testing for a monoclonal gammopathy is performed with serum and urine protein studies. The serum free light chain assay is critical for evaluating and monitoring patients with AL. Serum and urine immunofixation are also needed as patients may have modestly abnormal serum free light chains, particularly when renal function is impaired [10, 11]. All patients will require a bone marrow biopsy to confirm the presence of clonal plasma cells. In 6–9% of cases, the amyloid-forming light chain is produced by a low-grade lymphoproliferative disorder, and therapy then should be tailored to treat the underlying B cell disorder [12, 13]. Cytogenetic analysis of the bone marrow is becoming increasingly important to identify chromosome translocations, such as t(11;14). This has a poorer prognostic significance for targeted treatments. The so-called high-risk abnormalities for multiple myelomas, such as del13 by cytogenetics or t (4;14) or del17p, are uncommon in amyloidosis.

Staging and Risk Assessment

The prognosis and treatment of patients with amyloidosis depend on the disease stage and the risk assessment. Following diagnosis, the next key step is accurate staging. The use of cardiac biomarkers, NTpro-BNP, and troponin T continues to remain the cornerstone of staging as defined by the Mayo Clinic group. Patients with both biomarkers within the normal range while considered to have stage one disease, either one of the biomarkers being abnormal (NTpro-BNP > 332 ng/L or troponin T > 0.035 μg/L) is stage two, and both biomarkers being abnormal is classed stage three; with progressively decreasing median survival. NT-proBNP levels >8500 ng/L identify an especially high subgroup with a 50–60% risk of early mortality [14]. In addition to the heart, assessment of other organs is also essential. The International Society of amyloidosis has criteria for the assessment of organ involvement at baseline (Table 9.2).

Imaging of amyloid deposits is complex but, when possible, may give important information about the extent of the disease. Imaging is also becoming important in assessing the prognosis for patients with amyloidosis. Echocardiogram with measurement of global longitudinal strain is a widely available tool that can be used in

Table 9.2 Organ response and progression criteria in AL

Organ	Response	Progression
Heart	NT-proBNP response (>30% and >300 ng/L decrease in patients with baseline NT-proBNP ≥650 ng/L) OR NYHA class response (≥2 class decrease in subjects with baseline NYHA class 3 or 4)	NT-proBNP progression (>30% and >300 ng/L increase in presence of stable creatinine) OR cTn progression (≥33% increase) OR Ejection fraction progression (≥10% decrease)
Kidney	50% decrease (at least 0.5 g/day) of 24-h urine protein (urine protein must be >0.5 g/day pretreatment). Creatinine and creatinine clearance must not worsen by 25% over baseline	50% increase (at least 1 g/day) of 24-h urine protein to greater than 1 g/day or 25% worsening of serum creatinine or creatinine clearance
Liver	50% decrease in abnormal alkaline phosphatase value Decrease in liver size radiographically at least 2 cm	50% increase of alkaline phosphatase above the lowest value
Peripheral nervous system	Improvement in electromyogram nerve conduction velocity (rare)	Progressive neuropathy by electromyography or nerve conduction velocity

routine clinical practice [15]. Cardiac magnetic resonance imaging can give detailed structural information about the amyloid heart and provide additional prognostic information. However, it has limitations as it cannot be done in patients with implanted devices or impaired renal function. Radionuclide imaging using ^{123}I labeled serum amyloid P component scintigraphy [16] can serially monitor changes in the total body amyloid load—and can act as a helpful guide to therapy. However, this is not widely available. PET scans using tracers such as Florbetapir or Florbetaben appear to be highly sensitive and specific for cardiac imaging in AL and may well become a new standard of care [17]. Imaging with ^{99m}Tc-labeled DPD/PYP, bone scanning agents, are helpful non-invasive tools to differentiate between cardiac AL and ATTR amyloidosis [18].

Response Assessment

Response assessment in amyloidosis involves measuring changes in the precursor protein (the monoclonal protein in AL or inflammatory markers in AA) and changes in the end-organ function affected by amyloidosis. Hence, in a patient with systemic AL amyloidosis, there is a definition of hematologic response and organ response. As currently available therapies only target the precursor protein, the hematologic response is a critical surrogate for outcomes in patients with AL amyloidosis. Achievement of a hematologic response remains the crucial variable for predicting organ improvement and prolonged survival [19]. The goal of treatment is complete or near-complete elimination of the monoclonal protein, which is associated with the best long-term outcomes. Criteria for scoring hematologic response based partly on reductions in the difference between involved and uninvolved FLC (the dFLC) have been validated in a large international case series [20]. Response categories include complete (CR), very good partial (VGPR), partial (PR), and no response (NR).

Table 9.2 gives the agreed criteria for response assessment following treatment in the patient with their amyloidosis. Cardiac biomarkers are important in assessing cardiac response. Echocardiographic improvement in global longitudinal strain will give additional information. In patients with cardiac involvement, a > 30% reduction and a > 300 ng/L decrease in the NT-proBNP level from baseline correlate with improved overall survival. In contrast, increases of that magnitude correlate with progression and worse survival [21].

Management

Systemic AL is a complex multi-system disease. Management requires a multidisciplinary approach with involvement from cardiologists, nephrologists, neurologists, and hematologists. Stringent supportive therapy is key, including careful fluid balance and patient education in monitoring blood pressure and fluid status. In AL amyloidosis, chemotherapy directed at the underlying plasma cell clone remains the mainstay of treatment.

Treatment for AL amyloidosis was underpinned by data from small prospective trials and several large registry-based retrospective analyses. Recently, a phase three clinical trial using daratumumab has been completed leading to a new milestone in AL treatment: daratumumab and cyclophosphamide bortezomib dexamethasone have become the first licensed treatment for systemic AL amyloidosis. Figure 9.2 gives an approach to the treatment of AL amyloidosis.

Bortezomib has been a mainstay of upfront treatment in AL for the last decade. The benefit of bortezomib-melphalan-dexamethasone was clearly demonstrated in a recent randomized phase III trial of 100 newly diagnosed patients with AL amyloidosis, improving CR/VGPR rates from 28 to 53% [22]. The most widely used regimen is CyBorD (combination of cyclophosphamide, bortezomib, and dexamethasone). A European collaborative study of 230 patients demonstrated the efficacy of CyBorD, reporting hematologic, renal, and cardiac response rates of 60%, 25%, and 17%, respectively [23]. We have recently reported the outcomes of 915 patients with hematologic, renal, and cardiac response rates of 65%, 15.4%, and 32.5%, respectively [24]. A rapid response with bortezomib-based therapy can significantly improve outcomes even in advanced cardiac patients (median OS improving from 5 to 26 m in patients achieving a CR/VGPR by the end of one month [25]).

In the recently published report of the ANDROMEDA clinical trial comparing daratumumab/placebo with CyBorD, [26] in 388 patients who underwent randomization, at a median follow-up of 11.4 months, the percentage of patients who had a complete hematologic response was significantly higher in the daratumumab group than in the control group (53.3% vs. 18.1%) (relative risk ratio, 2.9; 95% confidence interval [CI], 2.1–4.1; $P < 0.001$). Survival free from major organ deterioration or hematologic progression favored the daratumumab group (hazard ratio for major

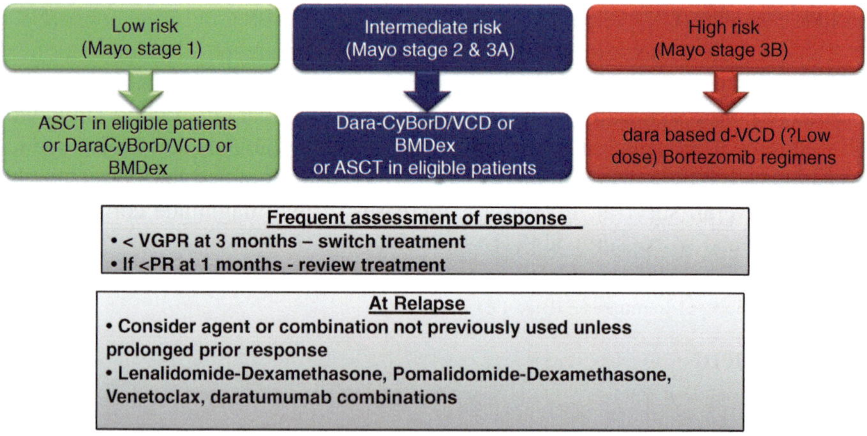

Fig. 9.2 Treatment approach to patient with systemic AL amyloidosis (*CyBorD* cyclophosphamide, bortezomib, dexamethasone, *ASCT* autologous stem cell transplantation, *VGRP* very good partial response, *PR* partial response)

organ deterioration, hematologic progression, or death, 0.58; 95% CI, 0.36–0.93; $P = 0.02$). At 6 months, more cardiac and renal responses occurred in the daratumumab group than in the control group (41.5% vs. 22.2% and 53.0% vs. 23.9%, respectively). The four most common grade 3 or 4 adverse events were lymphopenia (13.0% in the daratumumab group and 10.1% in the control group), pneumonia (7.8% and 4.3%, respectively), cardiac failure (6.2% and 4.8%), and diarrhea (5.7% and 3.7%). Systemic administration-related reactions to daratumumab occurred in 7.3% of the patients. A total of 56 patients died (27 in the daratumumab group and 29 in the control group), most due to amyloidosis-related cardiomyopathy. The authors concluded that the addition of daratumumab to bortezomib, cyclophosphamide, and dexamethasone was associated with higher frequencies of hematologic complete response and survival free from major organ deterioration or hematologic progression. The results of this study led to the licensing of daratumumab-CyBorD for front-line treatment of AL amyloidosis.

Alkylator-based chemotherapy regimens were the mainstay for many years but have been superseded by combined novel agent-based chemotherapy. Oral melphalan and dexamethasone (MDex) induced a hematologic response rate of 67%, a CR rate of 33%, and an organ response rate of 48% in a phase II study of 45 patients [27]. An update of this cohort with a 5-year follow-up showed an impressive median progression-free survival (PFS) of 3.8 years and a median OS of 5.1 years [28]. It still continues to have a role in selected patients who are not candidates for novel agent chemotherapy.

High-dose melphalan with autologous stem cell transplant (ASCT) is beneficial initial therapy for up to 20% of newly diagnosed patients [29]. High rates of hematologic and organ response are reported, and median survival is nearly a decade in ASCT patients achieving a complete response. Patient selection for ASCT remains the key due to the high treatment-related mortality (TRM) that stays around 10% even at experienced centers [30]. Eighty percent of patients achieving a complete hematologic response experience organ response; half of all patients surviving one year after SCT experience organ responses [29]. However, the excellent response is seen with bortezomib-based treatment regimens in AL, especially with the addition of daratumumab, which have led to questions about the utility of autologous stem cell transplantation in this disease. We recently reported a matched comparison of CyBorD versus stem cell transplantation in amyloidosis, showing no significant survival benefit for patients treated with autologous stem cell transplantation. This remains a question to be answered in a prospective clinical trial.

Immunomodulatory drugs such as lenalidomide, pomalidomide, and thalidomide have been used to treat amyloidosis for many years. Thalidomide-based treatments are no longer considered appropriate for patients with amyloidosis due to high toxicity. Lenalidomide and pomalidomide are useful for patients in the treatment of relapsed disease. In phase II trials, full-dose lenalidomide had significant toxicity requiring dose reductions or discontinuation. It was better tolerated at 15 mg/day in combination with weekly dexamethasone (LenDex), with hematologic response rates of 40–50% [21, 31]. Single-agent lenalidomide has limited efficacy and is not recommended. In a retrospective study in relapsed AL treated with

LenDex, there was a 49% hematologic response rate with 16% CR, median OS of about 2 years, and in those achieving CR, a PFS of over 3 years [32]. In a preliminary report on a phase II study of pomalidomide with weekly dexamethasone, over 30% of relapsed AL patients achieved a complete response, highlighting the promise of this potent immunomodulatory (IMiD) therapy [33]. More recently, we reported good responses (VGPR or better in 40%) with 27 months (95% confidence interval 15.7–38.1 month) and median progression-free survival (PFS) was 15 months (95% confidence interval 6.24–23.77) in multiple relapsed AL patients treated with pomalidomide [34].

Translocation t (11;14) is seen in 45% of patients with AL amyloidosis. This is a potential for targeted therapy due to the specific activation of cyclin D1. Venetoclax is one such agent which has been used in the treatment of multiple myeloma. We recently reported a retrospective international collaborative study showing high response rates in patients treated with Venetoclax in patients with relapsed AL amyloidosis [35]. Amongst 43 patients reports, the hematologic response rate for all patients was 68%; 63% achieved VGPR/CR. Patients with t(11;14) had higher hematologic response (81% vs. 40%) and higher VGPR/CR rate (78% vs. 30%, odds ratio: 0.12, 95% CI 0.02–0.62) than non-t(11;14) patients. The toxicities appeared to be modest, and the deep response rates were striking. This agent, or similar agents, needs to be investigated in prospective trials in AL.

Direct Anti-Amyloid Therapies

Accelerating the removal of amyloid deposits has remained challenging. It is well documented that macrophage-mediated processes clear amyloid deposits. Accelerating this clearance by the use of monoclonal antibodies has been appealing. Several small molecules such as doxycycline may reduce the amyloid formation and are potentially appealing but have not been proven in prospective clinical trials. Clinical trials with monoclonal antibodies directed at proteins on the amyloid deposits (serum amyloid P component) and anti-fibril antibodies NEO001D were performed but proved unsuccessful. Lately, a novel anti-fibril antibody (CAEL101) has been reported in phase 1 clinical trial to show rapid improvement in cardiac and renal function [36]. Fifteen of 24 patients (63%) who manifested cardiac, renal, hepatic, gastrointestinal, or soft tissue involvement had a therapeutic response to mAb CAEL-101 with a median time to response of 3 weeks. Two phase III clinical trials with CAEL-101/placebo are ongoing in patients with cardiac AL amyloidosis.

Supportive Care

Cardiac amyloid causes restrictive cardiomyopathy with reduced cardiac output and, when combined with autonomic dysfunction and nephrotic syndrome, makes management challenging. Loop diuretics such as furosemide or bumetanide are standard therapy, but they may compromise cardiac output [37]. Close clinical monitoring with frequent adjustments of dose are mandatory. Patients must be taught to limit their salt intake and weigh themselves daily. Beta-blockers and angiotensin-converting enzyme inhibitors or angiotensin receptor blockers should be avoided due to poor tolerance.

In patients with severe nephrotic syndrome and low serum album, intravenous salt poor albumin infusion given once or twice weekly are often very useful, especially during chemotherapy, to allow adequate diuresis. Two-thirds of patients presenting with advanced renal impairment or severe proteinuria will develop end-stage renal failure with amyloidosis. In selected cases without severe cardiac involvement, particularly for patients in a complete hematologic response, renal transplant outcomes appear to be excellent, and patients should be referred appropriately.

Gastrointestinal symptoms in amyloidosis may either be due to direct amyloid infiltration (rare) or due to autonomic involvement (commoner). Patients can have intractable nausea and vomiting and often do not respond to enteral feeding or pharmacologic interventions. The most common presenting symptoms of bowel involvement are persistent severe diarrhea. The diarrhea of amyloid is challenging to treat [38]. Loperamide and codeine may help many patients. Somatostatin analogous (octreotide or lanreotide) are helpful when opioids fail to control diarrhea. There is a risk for GI bleeding in patients who undergo ASCT [39] or with high-dose corticosteroids, which need close monitoring.

Superficial cutaneous bruising is very common in amyloidosis. Severe bleeding due to clotting factor deficiencies is well recognized but uncommon. Acquired factor X deficiency (seen in ~5% of patients) is a typical feature. The majority of these patients have significant amyloid deposits in the liver and spleen. The management of factor X deficiency has included splenectomy and the use of recombinant human factor VIIa. [19] Highly purified factor X concentrate is available in some countries and may have a role in these cases. Paradoxically, patients with AL amyloidosis may also be significantly prothrombotic, particularly in the presence of the nephrotic syndrome. Management of thrombosis, or indeed thromboprophylaxis, in these patients, is challenging because of competing risks of bleeding from amyloid deposition in the gut/liver. Immunomodulatory agents will increase thrombotic risk.

Conclusions

Amyloidosis is an increasingly recognized disease. AL amyloidosis remains the commonest amyloid type, but wild-type transthyretin amyloidosis is likely to overtake this in the near future. Delays in diagnosis remain, and most patients still present with advanced disease. Recognizing disease manifestations is critical. Education of physicians in all specialties to understand the amyloid symptom complex, the recognition that although uncommon, amyloid is not as rare as commonly considered, is important. This would allow early consideration of this disease in the differential diagnosis. Risk stratification of amyloidosis is well evolved, and accurate treatment can be chosen based on the nature and degree of organ damage. Treatment outcomes and survival have substantially improved, with over half the patients with AL likely to survive more than 5 years from diagnosis. Daratumumab (with CyBorD) has now become the first licensed treatment for AL amyloidosis. Attention to supportive care remains crucial to managing patients with multiorgan involvement in multidisciplinary settings. Reversal of end-organ damage remains a limitation in amyloid therapy. Monoclonal antibody-based approaches to accelerate amyloid removal show promise.

References

1. Merlini G. AL amyloidosis: from molecular mechanisms to targeted therapies. Hematology Am Soc Hematol Educ Program. 2017;2017(1):1–12.
2. Ravichandran S, Lachmann HJ, Wechalekar AD. Epidemiologic and survival trends in amyloidosis, 1987-2019. N Engl J Med. 2020;382(16):1567–8.
3. Rezk T, Gilbertson JA, Rowczenio D, Bass P, Lachmann HJ, Wechalekar AD, et al. Diagnosis, pathogenesis and outcome in leucocyte chemotactic factor 2 (ALECT2) amyloidosis. Nephrol Dial Transplant. 2018;33(2):241–7.
4. Comenzo RL, Zhou P, Fleisher M, Clark B, Teruya-Feldstein J. Seeking confidence in the diagnosis of systemic AL (Ig light-chain) amyloidosis: patients can have both monoclonal gammopathies and hereditary amyloid proteins. Blood. 2006;107(9):3489–91.
5. Jacobson DR, Pastore RD, Yaghoubian R, Kane I, Gallo G, Buck FS, et al. Variant-sequence transthyretin (isoleucine 122) in late-onset cardiac amyloidosis in Black Americans. N Engl J Med. 1997;336(7):466–73.
6. Cohen OC, Sharpley F, Gilbertson JA, Wechalekar AD, Sachchithanantham S, Mahmood S, et al. The value of screening biopsies in light-chain (AL) and transthyretin (ATTR) amyloidosis. Eur J Haematol. 2020;105(3):352–6.
7. Bely M, Makovitzky J. Sensitivity and specificity of Congo red staining according to Romhanyi. Comparison with Puchtler's or Bennhold's methods. Acta Histochem. 2006;108(3):175–80.
8. Giorgadze TA, Shiina N, Baloch ZW, Tomaszewski JE, Gupta PK. Improved detection of amyloid in fat pad aspiration: an evaluation of Congo red stain by fluorescent microscopy. Diagn Cytopathol. 2004;31(5):300–6.
9. Vrana JA, Gamez JD, Madden BJ, Theis JD, Bergen HR 3rd, Dogan A. Classification of amyloidosis by laser microdissection and mass spectrometry-based proteomic analysis in clinical biopsy specimens. Blood. 2009;114(24):4957–9.
10. Dispenzieri A, Kyle R, Merlini G, Miguel JS, Ludwig H, Hajek R, et al. International myeloma working group guidelines for serum-free light chain analysis in multiple myeloma and related disorders. Leukemia. 2009;23(2):215–24.
11. Bochtler T, Hegenbart U, Heiss C, Benner A, Cremer F, Volkmann M, et al. Evaluation of the serum-free light chain test in untreated patients with AL amyloidosis. Haematologica. 2008;93(3):459–62.
12. Cohen AD, Zhou P, Xiao Q, Fleisher M, Kalakonda N, Akhurst T, et al. Systemic AL amyloidosis due to non-Hodgkin's lymphoma: an unusual clinicopathologic association. Br J Haematol. 2004;124(3):309–14.
13. Palladini G, Foli A, Russo P, Milani P, Obici L, Lavatelli F, et al. Treatment of IgM-associated AL amyloidosis with the combination of rituximab, bortezomib, and dexamethasone. Clin Lymphoma Myeloma Leuk. 2011;11(1):143–5.
14. Wechalekar AD, Schonland SO, Kastritis E, Gillmore JD, Dimopoulos MA, Lane T, et al. A European collaborative study of treatment outcomes in 346 patients with cardiac stage III AL amyloidosis. Blood. 2013;121(17):3420–7.

15. Cohen OC, Ismael A, Pawarova B, Manwani R, Ravichandran S, Law S, et al. Longitudinal strain is an independent predictor of survival and response to therapy in patients with systemic AL amyloidosis. Eur Heart J. 2022;43(4):333–41.
16. Hawkins PN, Lavender JP, Pepys MB. Evaluation of systemic amyloidosis by scintigraphy with ^{123}I-labeled serum amyloid P component. N Engl J Med. 1990;323:508–13.
17. Varga C, Dorbala S, Lousada I, Polydefkis MJ, Wechalekar A, Maurer MS, et al. The diagnostic challenges of cardiac amyloidosis: a practical approach to the two main types. Blood Rev. 2021;45:100720.
18. Gillmore JD, Maurer MS, Falk RH, Merlini G, Damy T, Dispenzieri A, et al. Nonbiopsy diagnosis of cardiac transthyretin amyloidosis. Circulation. 2016;133(24):2404–12.
19. Cohen AD, Zhou P, Chou J, Teruya-Feldstein J, Reich L, Hassoun H, et al. Risk-adapted autologous stem cell transplantation with adjuvant dexamethasone +/− thalidomide for systemic light-chain amyloidosis: results of a phase II trial. Br J Haematol. 2007;139(2):224–33.
20. Palladini G, Dispenzieri A, Gertz MA, Kumar S, Wechalekar A, Hawkins PN, Schönland S, Hegenbart U, Comenzo R, Kastritis E, Dimopoulos MA, Jaccard A, Klersy C, Merlini G. Identification of the criteria for response to treatment in AL amyloidosis based on survival outcomes. J Clin Oncol. 2011.
21. Sanchorawala V, Wright DG, Rosenzweig M, Finn KT, Fennessey S, Zeldis JB, et al. Lenalidomide and dexamethasone in the treatment of AL amyloidosis: results of a phase 2 trial. Blood. 2007;109(2):492–6.
22. Kastritis E, Leleu X, Arnulf B, Zamagni E, Cibeira MT, Kwok F, et al. A randomized phase III trial of Melphalan and dexamethasone (MDex) versus Bortezomib, Melphalan and dexamethasone (BMDex) for untreated patients with AL amyloidosis. Blood. 2016;128(22):646.
23. Palladini G, Sachchithanantham S, Milani P, Gillmore J, Foli A, Lachmann H, et al. A European collaborative study of cyclophosphamide, bortezomib, and dexamethasone in upfront treatment of systemic AL amyloidosis. Blood. 2015;126(5):612–5.
24. Manwani R, Cohen O, Sharpley F, Mahmood S, Sachchithanantham S, Foard D, et al. A prospective observational study of 915 patients with systemic AL amyloidosis treated with upfront bortezomib. Blood. 2019;134(25):2271–80.
25. Manwani R, Foard D, Mahmood S, Sachchithanantham S, Lane T, Quarta C, et al. Rapid hematologic responses improve outcomes in patients with very advanced (stage IIIb) cardiac immunoglobulin light chain amyloidosis. Haematologica. 2018;103(4):e165–8.
26. Kastritis E, Palladini G, Minnema MC, Wechalekar AD, Jaccard A, Lee HC, et al. Daratumumab-based treatment for immunoglobulin light-chain amyloidosis. N Engl J Med. 2021;385(1):46–58.
27. Palladini G, Perfetti V, Obici L, Caccialanza R, Semino A, Adami F, et al. Association of melphalan and high-dose dexamethasone is effective and well tolerated in patients with AL (primary) amyloidosis who are ineligible for stem cell transplantation. Blood. 2004;103(8):2936–8.
28. Palladini G, Russo P, Nuvolone M, Lavatelli F, Perfetti V, Obici L, et al. Treatment with oral melphalan plus dexamethasone produces long-term remissions in AL amyloidosis. Blood. 2007;110(2):787–8.
29. Cibeira MT, Sanchorawala V, Seldin DC, Quillen K, Berk JL, Dember LM, et al. Outcome of AL amyloidosis after high-dose melphalan and autologous stem cell transplantation: long-term results in a series of 421 patients. Blood. 2011;118(16):4346–52.
30. Gertz MA, Blood E, Vesole DH, Abonour R, Lazarus HM, Greipp PR. A multicenter phase 2 trial of stem cell transplantation for immunoglobulin light-chain amyloidosis (E4A97): an Eastern Cooperative Oncology Group Study. Bone Marrow Transplant. 2004;34(2):149–54.
31. Dispenzieri A, Lacy MQ, Zeldenrust SR, Hayman SR, Kumar SK, Geyer SM, et al. The activity of lenalidomide with or without dexamethasone in patients with primary systemic amyloidosis. Blood. 2007;109(2):465–70.
32. Sanchorawala V, Finn KT, Fennessey S, Shelton A, Doros G, Zeldis JB, et al. Durable hematologic complete responses can be achieved with lenalidomide in AL amyloidosis. Blood. 2010;116(11):1990–1.

33. Dispenzieri A, Gertz M, Hayman SR, Buadi F, Kumar SK, Reeder C, Zeldenrust SR, Rajkumar SV, Detweiler-Short K, Lust JA, Witzig TE, Kyle RA, Greipp PR, Russell SJ, Dingli D, Allred JB, Laumann K, Thompson M, Fonseca R, Bergsagel L, Stewart K, Mikhael J, Roy V, Lacy MQ. Pomalidomide and dexamethasone for previously treated AL: a phase 2 study. Amyloid. 2010;17:87a.
34. Sharpley FA, Manwani R, Mahmood S, Sachchithanantham S, Lachmann H, Gilmore J, et al. Real world outcomes of pomalidomide for treatment of relapsed light chain amyloidosis. Br J Haematol. 2018;183(4):557–63.
35. Premkumar VJ, Lentzsch S, Pan S, Bhutani D, Richter J, Jagannath S, et al. Venetoclax induces deep hematologic remissions in t(11;14) relapsed/refractory AL amyloidosis. Blood Cancer J. 2021;11(1):10.
36. Edwards CV, Rao N, Bhutani D, Mapara MY, Radhakrishnan J, Shames S, et al. Phase 1a/b study of monoclonal antibody CAEL-101 (11-1F4) in patients with AL amyloidosis. Blood. 2021;138(25):2632–41.
37. Sack FU, Kristen A, Goldschmidt H, Schnabel PA, Dengler T, Koch A, et al. Treatment options for severe cardiac amyloidosis: heart transplantation combined with chemotherapy and stem cell transplantation for patients with AL-amyloidosis and heart and liver transplantation for patients with ATTR-amyloidosis. Eur J Cardiothorac Surg. 2008;33(2):257–62.
38. Guirl MJ, Hogenauer C, Santa Ana CA, Porter JL, Little KH, Stone MJ, et al. Rapid intestinal transit as a primary cause of severe chronic diarrhea in patients with amyloidosis. Am J Gastroenterol. 2003;98(10):2219–25.
39. Kumar S, Dispenzieri A, Lacy MQ, Litzow MR, Gertz MA. High incidence of gastrointestinal tract bleeding after autologous stem cell transplant for primary systemic amyloidosis. Bone Marrow Transplant. 2001;28(4):381–5.

Chapter 10
Monoclonal Immunoglobulin Deposition Disease

Marco Allinovi, Fiammetta Ravaglia, Gianmarco Lugli, Francesco Pegoraro, and Augusto Vaglio

Introduction

Monoclonal immunoglobulin deposition disease (MIDD) is a systemic disease characterized by the abnormal clonal production and tissue deposition of monoclonal immunoglobulins (mIg) by plasma cells or other B cells. The mIg production in MIDD may be malignant or non-malignant, but always results in the tissue deposition of mIg proteins as amorphous, non-congophilic material in a non-fibrillar state.

Three subtypes of MIDD have been reported based on the composition of the deposits. Light chain deposition disease (LCDD), the most common subtype, is a systemic disorder characterized by the deposition of monotypic immunoglobulin light chains in the kidney and other organs. As LCDD was first described as a

M. Allinovi
Nephrology, Dialysis and Transplantation Unit, Careggi University Hospital, Florence, Italy

F. Ravaglia
Nephrology and Dialysis Unit, Santo Stefano Hospital, Prato, Italy

G. Lugli
Department of Biomedical, Experimental and Clinical Sciences, University of Firenze, Florence, Italy

F. Pegoraro
Department of Health Science, University of Firenze, Florence, Italy

A. Vaglio (✉)
Department of Biomedical, Experimental and Clinical Sciences, University of Firenze, Florence, Italy

Nephrology and Dialysis Unit, Meyer Children's Hospital, Florence, Italy
e-mail: augusto.vaglio@unifi.it

© The Author(s), under exclusive license to Springer Nature Switzerland AG 2022
G. Ragab et al. (eds.), *Paraproteinemia and Related Disorders*,
https://doi.org/10.1007/978-3-031-10131-1_10

Table 10.1 Definitions

Terms	Definition
MIDD	Monoclonal immunoglobulin deposition disease: a type of monoclonal gammopathy of renal significance (MGRS) characterized by non-organized monoclonal light, heavy, or both chains which deposit along the glomerular basement membrane and the tubular basement membrane
LCDD	Light chain deposition disease: a MIDD with light chain deposition on kidney biopsy
HCDD	Heavy-chain deposition disease: a MIDD with heavy chain deposition on kidney biopsy
LHCDD	Light- and heavy-chain deposition disease: a MIDD with both light and heavy chain deposition on kidney biopsy
PGNMID	Proliferative glomerulonephritis with monoclonal immunoglobulin deposits: a type of MGRS characterized by non-organized monoclonal immunoglobulin deposits consisting of an intact immunoglobulin deposited in the glomeruli

systemic disease by Randall et al. in the 1970s [1], the term "Randall-type MIDD" is widely accepted for LCDD. Less frequently, the intact monoclonal protein (light and heavy chains), or the truncated heavy chain alone, deposits both in the renal basement membranes and in other organs, defining two other subtypes of MIDD, light- and heavy-chain deposition disease (LHCDD), and heavy-chain deposition disease (HCDD), respectively (Table 10.1).

MIDDs are part of a large and heterogeneous group of diseases identified as paraprotein-associated disorders or monoclonal Ig-related renal diseases, that also include light-chain (AL) amyloidosis, myeloma cast nephropathy, light-chain proximal tubulopathy, and cryoglobulinemic glomerulonephritis.

Multiple paraprotein tests can be used for MIDD diagnosis. The serum free light chain (FLC) assay is the most sensitive available technique, proving abnormal in almost all patients with LCDD [2–4]. However, no technique alone is sufficient [5]. When used together immunofixation electrophoresis, serum protein electrophoresis, Bence-Jones proteinuria, and serum free light chains can result in higher sensitivity rates.

The clinical picture of MIDD is typically driven by renal involvement. Although the disease primarily affects the glomeruli (the glomerular basement membranes and the glomerular mesangium), involvement of tubules, interstitium, and arteries is often described. The deposition of light chains along the tubular and glomerular basement membranes at immunofluorescence (IF), and the presence of "powdery" electron-dense deposits on electron microscopy, are essential for the diagnosis. The affinity for basement membrane components is thought to be due to the peculiar structural features of the involved pathogenic chain.

Severe proteinuria (consisting of light chains and other plasma proteins) and renal dysfunction are the most common clinical presentations of MIDD [3, 6–8] (Table 10.2). Kidney function is already compromised at onset in most cases, with features of acute or chronic renal failure. In a minority of cases, the disease presents with slowly progressive CKD without significant proteinuria, leading to a

Table 10.2 Clinical manifestations and hematologic features at diagnosis in patients with monoclonal immunoglobulin deposition disease

	All patients	HCDD	LHCDD	Pure LCDD	LCDD + cast nephropathy
Frequency among MIDD cases (%)	100	10	7	63	20
Hematological diagnosis (%)					
MGUS	66	90	95	80	0
Symptomatic MM	32	10	5	16	100
Other malignant neoplasms	2	0	0	4	0
dFLC (mg/L)	440	150	600	1500	5400
Renal function					
eGFR (mg/dL)	25	42	27	23	<10
CKD $\geq$ 4 (%)	50	30	50	60	0
AKI (%)	23	0	0	0	100
Dialysis (%)	20	5	10	3	90
Mean serum albumin (g/L)	33	28	30	33	35
Mean 24 h proteinuria (g)	2.8	3.8	3.2	2.8	2
Nephrotic-range proteinuria (%)	45	80	55	40	15
Full-blown nephrotic syndrome (%)	22	60	30	25	5
Extra-renal involvement (%)	30	15	10	40	10

MIDD monoclonal immunoglobulin deposition disease, *MGUS* monoclonal gammopathy of undetermined significance, *MM* multiple myeloma, *dFLC* difference between the involved and the uninvolved free light chains, *eGFR* estimated glomerular filtration rate, *CKD* chronic kidney disease, *AKI* acute kidney failure
Table based on the following references: [2–4, 9–13]

diagnostic delay. In these patients, glomerulosclerosis is uncommon, and deposits are prevalent in the renal vascular and tubular compartments [2, 14].

Immunoglobulins can deposit in different organs, resulting in a variety of clinical presentations. Extra-renal involvement is described in one third of patients with LCDD [9, 13]. The most commonly involved organs include the heart, the lungs, the liver, and the peripheral nerves [15, 16]. The specific pattern of organ involvement is determined by molecular characteristics of the pathogenic mIg, rather than by the tumoral extension [9]. Recognition of extra-renal involvement is essential for the diagnosis of MIDD, especially in those patients (around 20%) who rapidly progress to advanced CKD [2–4] without performing renal biopsy.

The natural history and prognosis of MIDD depend on the severity of renal failure at diagnosis, the presence of an underlying multiple myeloma (MM), and the delay in the hematologic response to chemotherapy. Additionally, LCDD patients with cardiac involvement have poorer survival and a significantly higher risk of treatment-related mortality after autologous stem cell transplantation (ASCT), compared with those without cardiac involvement [13].

Current treatment strategies are targeted at reducing the production of mIg, and mainly consist of high-dose melphalan followed by autologous stem cell transplantation (HDM/ASCT) or bortezomib-based regimens. The hematological response is a crucial prognostic factor in MIDD.

Pathology

The mIg can deposit in virtually every organ, but the kidneys are involved in most cases. The renal deposition of mIg occurs primarily along the glomerular and tubular basement membranes (Fig. 10.1b, c, d). However, as the disease progresses, massive deposits accumulate in the mesangium, leading to nodular glomerulosclerosis, which is the most characteristic expression of MIDD identifiable by light microscopy, especially in the clinically overt disease. In fact, light or heavy chain deposition typically spares the glomeruli in early phases, being detectable only in the tubulointerstitial and vascular compartments. Careful differential diagnosis with diabetic nephropathy, amyloidosis, or other types of nodular glomerulosclerosis (obesity, hypertension, smoking) is mandatory.

MIDD diagnosis requires the demonstration of monoclonal light or heavy chain deposition by IF. Additionally, electron microscopy helps assessing the nature of the deposition, further defining the location of deposits, and eventually ruling out the

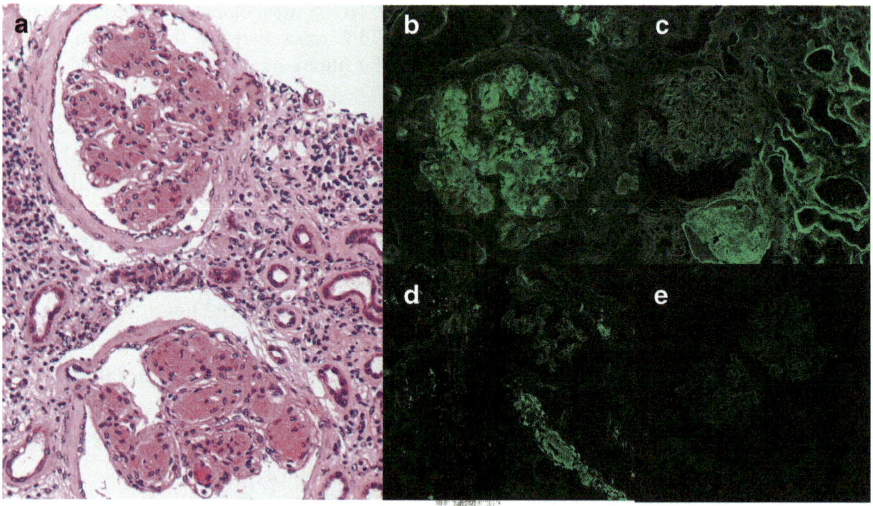

Fig. 10.1 Pathology findings in MIDD (**a**) Nodular mesangial glomerulosclerosis in LCDD (H&E 40×); (**b**) mesangial and peripheral glomerular capillary wall staining for kappa light chains; (**c**) diffuse linear tubular basement membrane staining for kappa light chains; (**d**) linear vessel wall staining for kappa light chain (**b**, **c**, **d** direct IF for kappa light chain, Fluorescein 40×); (**e**) negative lambda staining of the same patient shown in **b**, **c**, and **d** (direct IF for lambda light chain, Fluorescein 40×)

Table 10.3 Clinical and pathological characteristics of disorders associated with paraproteinemias with non-organized Ig deposits

	Light microscopy	Immunofluorescence	Electron microscopy
LCDD	Nodular glomerulosclerosis Thickened tubular basement membranes Thickened vessel walls Hyperplastic vasculopathy	Linear deposits along tubular basement membranes, glomerular basement membranes, and vessel walls (mostly kappa)	Punctate, to floccular, to granular, to powdery deposits in tubular basement membranes, glomerular basement membranes, mesangium, Bowman's capsule, and arteriolar walls
HCDD	Nodular glomerulosclerosis with/without crescents Thickened tubular basement membranes Thickened vessel walls	Linear deposits along tubular basement membranes, glomerular basement membranes, and vessel walls Truncated heavy chain (mostly IgG, C3, C1q)	Similar to LCDD Fibrils in fibrillary variant
LHCDD	Nodular glomerulosclerosis with/without crescents Thickened tubular basement membranes Thickened vessel walls	Linear deposits along tubular basement membranes, glomerular basement membranes, and vessel walls Light chain (mostly kappa) + truncated heavy chain	Similar to LCDD
PGNMID	Membranoproliferative, membranous, or mesangial proliferative pattern	Granular deposits in mesangium Monotypic Ig, mostly IgG3, C3, C1q	Granular deposits in mesangium, subendothelial and subendothelial space
C3G with MN	Membranoproliferative, membranous, or mesangial proliferative pattern	Granular deposits in mesangium and glomerular capillary walls (C3 dominant)	Granular mesangial electron-dense deposits in C3G Sausage-shaped intramembranous electron-dense deposits in DDD

presence of combined deposits. MIDD subtypes are identified on the basis of the immunoglobulin components that deposit in tissue, namely light chains for LCDD, heavy chains for HCDD, or both for LHCDD (Table 10.3).

About one quarter of all LCDD patients show the coexistence of different light chain nephropathy patterns (e.g., AL amyloidosis, cast nephropathy, fibrillary glomerulonephritis, and/or other types of monoclonal gammopathy of renal significance, MGRS) [2, 7, 13, 17, 18]. In most cases—and almost exclusively in patients with MM—the classic lesion of myeloma cast nephropathy is concomitantly present [6–8]. Recently, it has emerged that coexisting light chain diseases are more common than previously reported and confer a worse clinical outcome, emphasizing the need for histopathological evaluation [6, 8, 13, 18].

Light Microscopy

The most characteristic finding of LCDD is nodular glomerulopathy [19]. Unlike in diabetic nephropathy, in LCDD the mesangial nodules are more evenly distributed in the whole glomerulus, especially in advanced disease stages. Moreover, these nodules do not show other typical features of diabetic nephropathy such as capsular drops and hyaline cap lesions. In LCDD, mesangial nodules are PAS-positive, argyrophilic, and composed of extracellular matrix proteins admixed with monotypic light chains (Fig. 10.1a). Mesangial nodules might also show peripheral lamellation by silver staining, and mesangial hypercellularity can be associated with an increase in extracellular matrix. The subendothelial deposition of light chains results in a variable thickening of capillary walls. However, since nodular glomerulopathy is the common end of variable LCDD glomerular patterns in early stages (ranging from minimal change disease to mesangial, membranoproliferative, or rarely crescentic), IF staining for light chains is essential for diagnosis.

Apart from the glomerulus, light chain deposition is invariably observed in tubular basement membranes—typically on the outer aspect—resulting in membrane thickening and tortuosity and requiring IF to distinguish it from diabetic nephropathy. Half of patients with LCDD show thickening of vessel walls, and in some cases the concentric thickening of small- and medium-sized arteries due to light chain deposition leads to hyperplastic vasculopathy. Moreover, also interstitial deposits, appearing as PAS-positive aggregates, can be found, rarely associated with giant-cell reaction.

Similarly, HCDD typically appears as nodular glomerulosclerosis by light microscopy [20], but crescents or intracapillary proliferative glomerulonephritis can also be found. Heavy chain deposition is limited in most cases to the tubular basement membrane, without glomerular or vascular heavy chain deposition. Congo red stain is always negative.

Immunofluorescence

Pattern and intensity of LCDD staining depend on the amount and distribution of light chain deposits. The deposition is monotypic, with a κ to λ ratio of 9:1. Monoclonal light chain deposition is more intense alongside the tubular basement membranes compared to the peripheral capillary walls of the glomeruli (Fig. 10.1b, c). The staining is typically linear and regular though in early stages of the disease it may appear segmental. In a minority of patients, also a granular monotypic mesangial staining or a focal granular interstitium staining can be found together with capillary walls staining (Fig. 10.1d). Staining is negative for immunoglobulin heavy chains, complement fractions, and the non-involved light chain (IgG, IgA, IgM, C3, C1q, C4, and κ or λ) (Fig. 10.1e). Anecdotal cases of LCDD stain positive for complement components. Few cases of combined LCDD and light chain cast nephropathy do not show correspondence of IF deposits in electron microscopy and are therefore referred to as "LCDD by immunofluorescence only" [21]. In LCDD, not all renal deposits can be detected by generic κ- or λ-directed antibodies. Immunogold electron microscopy can increase the sensitivity by labeling the abnormal light chain when generic antibodies are used. Patients with LCDD and concomitant diabetes mellitus require careful analysis, as the glycosylation of abnormal light chains impairs their detection, and the diffuse linear staining of peripheral capillary walls in diabetes hinders the identification of monoclonal light chains.

All patients with renal biopsy findings suggestive of deposition disease with negative stains for κ and λ by IF should be worked up for HCDD. Staining in HCDD is negative for light chains and positive for only one heavy chain class (IgG in cases of γ heavy chain, IgA in cases of α heavy chain, or IgM in cases of μ heavy chain). Among these, γ chain deposits are more frequently described, with a linear pattern along the glomerular and tubular basement membranes, a distribution similar to that of LCDD but less intense. In cases of γ-HCDD, staining for the gamma chain subtypes (1, 2, 3, 4) helps confirming the diagnosis by identifying a single gamma subtype, whereas staining for constant domain antisera (CH1, CH2, and CH3) demonstrates the absence of the constant region of the heavy chain. Signs of complement activation with C3 and C1q deposition by IF, and sometimes serum hypocomplementemia, may be found, usually associated with γ1- and γ3-chains deposition. Extrarenal deposits of heavy chain components have been reported, less frequently than in LCDD, in the pancreas, thyroid, muscle, and liver [7].

LCDD and HCDD may be combined in LHCDD, with γ being the most frequent heavy chain component in these patients. Both κ and λ light chains have been found in the LCDD component. Diagnosis of LHCDD is challenging and requires the integration of light microscopy, IF with the use of specific antisera, and confirmatory evidence of light/heavy chain deposition by electron microscopy.

Electron Microscopy

The mIg deposition is non-organized, differently from amyloidosis and other disorders (e.g., immunotactoid or fibrillary) with organized immunoglobulin deposits associated with paraproteinemias. Light chain deposition can appear as floccular, granular, or powdery electron-dense material, possibly involving any renal compartment, especially in patients with advanced disease and nodular glomerulosclerosis by light microscopy. In the glomerular capillary walls, the deposition of LCDD begins along the lamina rara interna as thin band-like powdery deposits; with disease progression, larger deposits pool in the subendothelial regions. The "powdery" electron-dense deposits generally spread along the outer part of the tubular basement membranes, along the Bowman's capsule or the intima of arterial vessels, and in the interstitium. Electron microscopy is particularly useful in patients with combined MIDD and cast nephropathy, where subtle light microscopic alterations can be found in the glomeruli and in other compartments [11, 22].

HCDD ultrastructural findings are similar to those of LCDD. Deposits range from subtle to massive in the various renal compartments. Few cases with organized deposits have been described, with fibrils ranging from 13 to 18 nm and ultrastructurally different from fibrillary glomerulopathy, suggesting the existence of a fibrillary variant of HCDD.

Other Patterns of Glomerulonephritis Associated with Monoclonal IgG Deposits and Monoclonal Gammopathy of Unknown Significance

Proliferative Glomerulonephritis with Monoclonal IgG Deposits (PGNMID) was first recognized as a specific entity in 2004 [23], with about 100 cases reported so far. By light microscopy the pattern recalls that of membranoproliferative glomerulonephritis type I. By electron microscopy the glomerular electron-dense deposits are granular and non-organized, similar to immune complex-mediated glomerulonephritis, but in PGNMID also activated macrophages and tubular casts can be found. Moreover, IF staining positive only for monoclonal IgG (predominantly IgG3) and monoclonal light chains, either κ or λ, supports the diagnosis. When a membranous pattern is detected, with IgG chain restriction by IF, IgG subclass determination is necessary (typically IgG1). Pronase-digested IF on paraffin sections can increase the diagnostic sensitivity by identifying masked deposits [23].

An association of glomerulonephritis with C3 deposits and monoclonal gammopathy of unknown significance (MGUS) has been reported [26]. In these cases, renal biopsies show a membranoproliferative pattern. No monoclonal chain staining is detected by IF, but only C3 deposits along the peripheral capillary walls and in the mesangium. This pattern is indistinguishable from C3 glomerulopathy and is due to an alternative complement pathway activation rather than to a direct mIg deposition.

Extrarenal Histology

MIDD is a systemic disease. Therefore, deposits may be detected by IF in every organ. Autopsy studies and diagnostic biopsies have demonstrated the presence of linear mIg deposits of the circulating mIg in many sites. In the liver, a linear deposition of light chains along the perisinusoidal space was detected. Few reports of skin manifestations in LCDD revealed a deposition of a homogeneous, eosinophilic, PAS-positive, and Congo red-negative globular material and thioflavin, often localized around the capillaries of the upper dermis. Sparse lymphocytic infiltrates and massive cutaneous hyalinosis due to the deposition of light chains was also present.

Other involved sites included the lung, the heart, the peripheral nerves, the small and large intestine, the thyroid, the prostate, the pancreas, the rectum, the skin, the spleen, and the choroid plexus. Whatever the localization—renal or extrarenal—the light chain deposits are always Congo red negative.

Clinical Presentation and Diagnosis

MIDD are rare diseases (Lin 2011; [3, 8]), with LCDD being much more common than LHCDD and HCDD. MIDD incidence increases with age and is only slightly influenced by gender. In one of the largest series on MIDD, which included 255 patients, the median age at diagnosis was 63.7 years, with a male-to-female ratio of 1.08 [9].

It is often difficult to suspect MIDD in the setting of MGRS; however, the diagnosis of MIDD should always be followed by careful research for clonality.

A summary of the clinical manifestations of MIDD at diagnosis is reported in Table 10.2.

Renal Involvement

The kidney is almost always involved, with a wide spectrum of clinical manifestations. Chronic kidney disease is a key feature in MIDD. Although treatment can have a positive impact in renal survival, around 20–30% of patients already require dialysis at diagnosis. Hypertension and microhematuria—that are uncommon in AL amyloidosis—are common features in MIDD, usually associated with kidney failure [9]. Nephrotic-range proteinuria—with or without overt nephrotic syndrome—is often described, more commonly in HCDD than in LCDD. Moreover, a tubulo-interstitial presentation with subnephrotic proteinuria, leukocyturia, and microhematuria can be found at diagnosis.

A three-phenotype classification has been proposed for LCDD [24]: (a) glomerular disease with severe CKD; (b) mild (<0.5 g/day) or absent proteinuria and progressive CKD, with severe vascular lesions and extensive interstitial fibrosis on kidney biopsy; (c) coexistence of LCDD and myeloma cast nephropathy in patients with symptomatic MM.

MIDD and Hematological Malignancies

There is a strong link between MIDD and hematological conditions, especially with MM. Therefore, screening for MIDD (and other MGRS) when dealing with patients presenting with kidney failure in adult age is mandatory. MM was historically found in about 50% of patients with LCDD or LHCDD and in about 25% of those with HCDD [3] although the frequency is influenced by the definition chosen for MM. Recent case series, reflecting earlier diagnosis of MIDD, suggest that 60–80% of MIDD are associated with an indolent clone [4, 25]. MIDD may occasionally complicate other lymphoid malignancies like Waldenström's macroglobulinemia or chronic lymphocytic leukemia. Interestingly, cases of MIDD occurring in the absence of a detectable malignant process have been described.

Diagnosis

The diagnosis of MIDD requires a careful integration of morphological, clinical, and laboratory findings. The diagnostic mainstay is kidney biopsy, which is the only diagnostic tool that allows a proper assessment and a differential diagnosis [26].

Initial laboratory investigations should include serum protein electrophoresis, urinalysis, assessment of renal function, total proteinuria and albuminuria. However, even taken together, these tests have low sensitivity [5]. Immunofixation can detect any type of mIg in serum or urine. It has a diagnostic and prognostic value and should always be included in the diagnostic investigations [26]. However, a monoclonal protein is detected in patients' serum or urine by electrophoresis/immunofixation in only 65% of cases [2, 4], possibly because the κ chains tend to aggregate not forming a discrete, detectable electrophoretic band.

The serum free light chain (FLC) assays are crucial for MIDD diagnosis. They separately measure κ and λ free light chains and the free κ:λ ratio, the latter posing high suspicion for clonality when markedly altered. An abnormal serum FLC level and ratio is found in most patients with MIDD at diagnosis [24]. Kappa light chains are more commonly associated with LCDD than λ (κ is found in 80% of cases), in contrast to AL amyloidosis where λ light chains are more common. An impaired kidney function should be carefully assessed as it may alter FLC assay results (due to renal FLC clearance reduction). Urine FLC assays have been developed but not still validated: the detection of FLC in urine samples should therefore be performed by electrophoresis (Bence-Jones protein). Interestingly, the percentage of HCDD patients with a positive result on serum immunofixation electrophoresis was significantly lower than for patients with MIDD and other mIg-related nephropathies. Considering that free heavy chains have a high affinity for tissues and do not remain long in circulation, an immunofixation electrophoresis or the FLC ratio cannot be the confirmatory test in patients with HCDD [10]. Conversely, the diagnosis of HCDD can be made by immunoblotting, a technique able to detect the truncated heavy chain [11]. Hypocomplementemia of C3 and/or C4 can be traced in HCDD according to gamma isotypes although γ4-HCDD does not show hypocomplementemia for C3 [10].

Bone marrow aspiration and biopsy should be performed whenever a monoclonal gammopathy or a related disorder is suspected. The morphological assessment should include the quantification of the percentage of plasma cells and the evaluation of deposits. A pathological clone is detected in most patients with MIDD, more frequently than in other diseases of the MGRS spectrum [4]. About two thirds of patients with MIDD have an underlying MGUS. In larger series, around 20–34% of the patients with MIDD have clinical evidence of MM [9, 24]. Conversely, LCDD was detected in approximately 5% of patients with MM in a necropsy study [27]. Only rarely MIDD patients have no detectable paraprotein in serum or urine samples.

In addition, immunohistochemistry, flow cytometric immunophenotyping, and specific fluorescence in situ hybridization (FISH) are essential for the evaluation of the disease burden and for risk stratification [28].

Extrarenal Involvement

MIDD is a systemic disease that can potentially involve any organ. Of them, the liver, the heart, and the lungs are the preferred target for deposition of abnormal proteins, mainly because of the prominent plasma flow to these organs.

Extrarenal manifestations are typical of LCDD: 35–50% of patients with pure LCDD have at least one extrarenal manifestation [9, 10]. Systemic manifestations are less common in HCDD and LHCDD.

A summary of extrarenal manifestations of MIDD is reported in Table 10.4.

Liver

Liver involvement occurs in about 20% of patients with LCDD [9]. Although liver deposits are frequent on ultrastructural analysis, liver abnormalities are usually mild, manifesting with a modest increase in liver enzymes and mild hepatomegaly. However, cases of hepatic insufficiency [29] and cholestatic hepatitis [30] have been described.

Heart

Heart involvement is found in around 10–33% of patients, typically in advanced stages of the disease or in a long-lasting disease, resulting in cardiomegaly and severe heart failure [2, 9, 13, 31]. Diastolic dysfunction, similar to that observed in patients with cardiac AL amyloidosis, strongly impacts the prognosis.

The cardiac deposition of FLC can occur in the interstitium, leading to myocardial edema and myocyte toxicity (likely to cause electric instability and arrhythmias) [37], and in the coronary vasculature, leading in rare cases to myocardial infarction [8, 38].

Cardiac manifestations are variable, ranging from congestive heart failure to arrhythmias and conduction disorders (i.e., atrial fibrillation, sinus bradycardia, or ventricular tachycardia) [13, 32, 39, 40]. Overall, the onset of acute arrhythmias

Table 10.4 Extrarenal manifestations of MIDD

Involved site	Frequency	Clinical manifestations	References
Liver	17–25%	Liver deposits are a constant feature on ultrastructural analysis Modest increase in liver enzymes, mild hepatomegaly, cholestatic jaundice, portal hypertension Hepatic failure (occasionally), fulminant hepatitis (very rare)	[9, 24, 29, 30]
Heart	10–35%	Dyspnea, conduction disorders (atrial fibrillation, prolonged QT interval, sinus bradycardia) Echocardiography findings of hypertrophic cardiomyopathy with restrictive pattern	[9, 13, 16, 24, 31, 32]
Skin	5%	Acquired cutis laxa (mainly HCDD), scleroderma-like induration of the skin, macroglossia, urticarial papules	[46] [9]
PNS	9%	Deposition of Congo red-negative monotypic light chain Thermal-pain sensory impairment, dysautonomia, paresthesia	[9, 33]
Lungs	Rare	Diffuse pattern or cysts and nodules disease with progressive obstructive pulmonary disease Pulmonary vascular disease	[24, 34, 35]
CNS	Rare	Seizures, hemiparesis, weakness, gait instability, and incoordination	[33]
Other	Rare	Gastrointestinal disturbances Amyloid-like arthropathy Sicca syndrome	[36]

LCDD light chain deposition disease, *HCDD* heavy-chain deposition disease, *LHCDD* light- and heavy-chain deposition disease, *PGNMID* proliferative glomerulonephritis with monoclonal immunoglobulin deposits, *C3G* C3 glomerulonephritis, *MN* membranous nephropathy, *DDD* dense deposit disease, *PNS* peripheral nervous system, *CNS* central nervous system

associated with restrictive cardiomyopathy and impaired renal function is highly evocative of LCDD.

The diagnostic workup for cardiac involvement includes ECG, echocardiography, and cardiac MRI. Echocardiographic findings are frequently consistent with left ventricular hypertrophy, a restrictive cardiomyopathy pattern, and normal ejection fraction. Common prognostic markers for cardiac amyloidosis, such as NT-proBNP and troponin, have an unclear role when dealing with LCDD [13], but are frequently increased when the heart is involved [9]. However, the diagnostic mainstay remains myocardial biopsy.

Neuropathy

Peripheral nervous system involvement results in bilateral and symmetric polyneuropathy, affecting both the sensory and motor fibers. It typically starts from the distal end of the nerve, and often the sensory manifestations precede the motor ones, presenting as thermal-pain sensory impairment and dysautonomia [9, 41].

Nerve biopsy can help in the differential diagnosis with AL amyloidosis, showing the immunohistochemical and ultrastructural features typical of MIDD [42].

Lungs

Pulmonary involvement is rare in MIDD. However, LCDD can primarily affect the lungs in anecdotal cases. In patients with lung involvement, a slight decline in ventilation function with small airway dysfunction is detected [34]. Diffuse and nodular or cystic disease, determining progressive obstructive disease, is also described [2, 43]. High-resolution computed tomography (HRCT) can reveal small round cystic airspaces, as found in lymphangioleiomyomatosis, Langerhans cell histiocytosis, and lymphoid interstitial pneumonia. The disease seems to be associated with MALT lymphoma, especially in the setting of Sjögren syndrome [44]. Pulmonary vascular disease can develop owing to deposition of light chain among pulmonary vasculature or following the development of congestive heart failure [35].

Other Localizations

FLC deposition is described in a variety of other peripheral sites. It may be responsible for gastrointestinal disturbances, amyloid-like arthropathy, and sicca syndrome. Of note, isolated central nervous system involvement has been described in LCDD [33, 45]. The clinical presentation can include seizures, hemiparesis, weakness, gait instability, and ataxia.

Extrarenal deposits are less common in patients with HCDD. However, the presence of cutis laxa, an acquired connective tissue disorder characterized by wrinkled inelastic skin, is suggestive of HCDD [46].

Natural History and Prognosis

MIDD is traditionally considered to have poor renal and overall survival [33, 45]. However, the introduction of new drugs and schedules has led to a significant improvement in MIDD survival. Data on the natural history of the disease mostly come from studies on LCDD. In a study of 63 patients, factors that were independently associated with a worse renal prognosis were age and serum creatinine at presentation, thus indicating that a worse CKD stage at diagnosis may predict further kidney function loss. Independent predictors of survival were the age at diagnosis, the coexistence of MM, and extrarenal light chain deposition [8].

No specific criteria have been proposed for hematologic response assessment in MIDD. Thus, the criteria developed in 2012 by the International Society for Amyloidosis for AL amyloidosis are used in common practice also for MIDD [47]. The difference between pathologic and nonpathologic FLC is the most relevant criterion adopted. In a prospective study including 53 patients with LCDD, end-stage kidney disease (ESKD) at last follow-up was more frequent in patients presenting with CKD stage IV or V at diagnosis, emphasizing the role of renal involvement at diagnosis as a marker of kidney failure. Sixty-two percent of patients started renal replacement therapy a median of 5.4 years after diagnosis. Patients receiving hematologic treatment displaying a complete response (CR, defined as a normalization of FLC ratio in the absence of a detectable monoclonal protein by serum and urine immunofixation or electrophoresis) or a very good partial response (VGPR, defined as a decrease in the difference between the involved and uninvolved FLC, dFLC, <40 mg/L) (Fig. 10.2) showed improvement in renal function over time, thus indicating that early detection of LCDD and prompt intervention may prolong renal survival [4]. With respect to extrarenal outcomes, patients with cardiac involvement reaching a CR had a significant drop in NT-proBNP in association with diastolic function improvement.

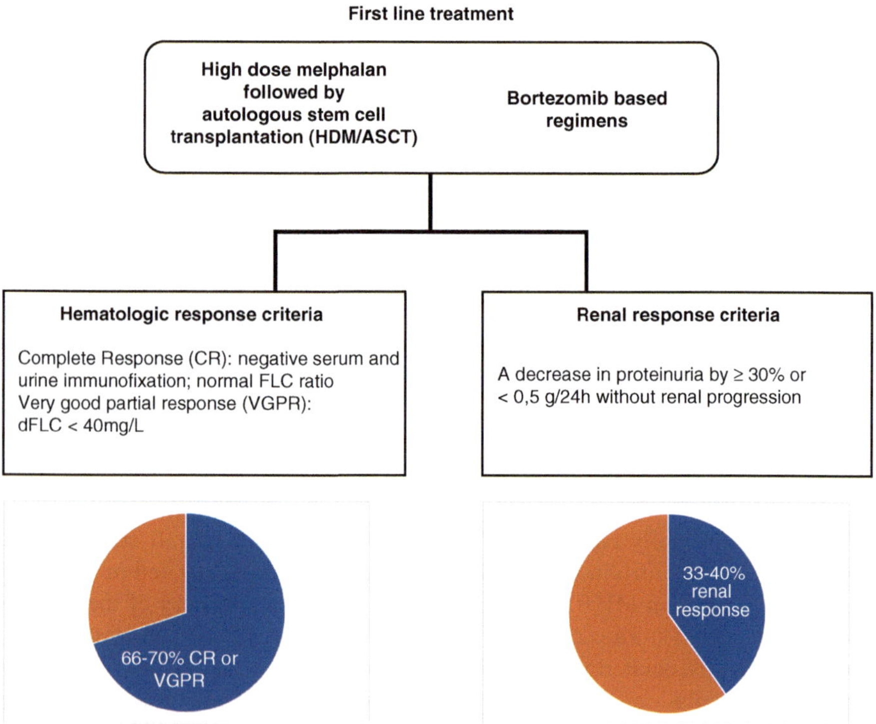

Fig. 10.2 Treatment and Outcome of MIDD. First-line regimens for MIDD include high-dose melphalan followed by HDM/ASCT or bortezomib-based chemotherapy. A complete hematologic response is defined as the disappearance of FLC, whereas a very good partial response as a dFLC of less than 40 mg/L. A hematologic response is obtained in around two thirds of patients treated with first-line regimens. The renal response (defined as a decrease in proteinuria without renal progression) is achieved in around one third of patients treated with first-line regimens

The prognosis of HCDD is generally very poor since it has been estimated that 36–50% of patients require renal replacement therapy within 1 year of follow-up [48]. However, recent findings on a cohort of 25 patients showed that the prevalence of kidney failure at 1 year was 12%, and 5% of patients died during follow-up. Kidney survival was remarkably poorer in the group with no chemotherapy, but there were no significant differences among the different regimens of chemotherapy adopted [10]. As for LCDD, also for HCDD the early diagnosis and treatment are essential to preserve kidney function. In a large french study including 255 patients with MIDD, the achievement of hematological VGPR and the absence of severe interstitial fibrosis on kidney biopsies were associated with prolonged renal survival. Also, the hematologic response was associated with overall survival [9].

MIDD is a model of glomerular and interstitial fibrosis that is induced by a single molecule species. A better understanding of the underlying molecular pathways may also help unravel the pathomechanisms of kidney fibrosis and renal disease progression beyond MIDD [24, 36].

Treatment

Patients with MIDD can benefit from the same chemotherapy protocols used for MM or chronic lymphocytic leukemia, even in case of an underlying MGUS or an isolated renal MIDD with no systemic evidence of plasma cell dyscrasia [49].

The hematologic response is crucial to improve renal and global outcomes in patients with MIDD [12]. As the hematologic response criteria [47] are based on the dFLC (Fig. 10.2), monitoring serum FLCs is necessary to evaluate the hematological response.

A prolonged light chain deposition is associated with progressive organ damage. Thus, the rapid and sustained suppression of FLC production is essential to halt organ damage, and possibly enhance the catabolism of the deposits and the recovery of organ function. A delay in hematologic response results in further deposition of pathologic FLC, which reduces the chances of renal improvement. Therefore, an aggressive treatment might be indicated, especially in high-risk patients (i.e., those with late-referral, high tumor burden, or multi-organ involvement).

Data on long-term outcome of MIDD treatment are scarce and mainly based on small, retrospective case series. This is due to the rarity of the disease and to several different chemotherapeutic regimens attempted over the years. Multidrug chemotherapy with different regimens has been used in MIDD with conflicting results in terms of survival and progression of renal disease.

Before the era of the novel antimyeloma agents, the overall prognosis of MIDD was poor [7]. In particular, thalidomide plus dexamethasone, and VAD regimen (vincristine, adriamycin plus dexamethasone) showed a poor hematological efficacy in patients with MIDD [12]. In historical cohorts, patients who received chemotherapy for MIDD were treated with alkylating agents and prednisone, obtaining slight improvement in survival (70% overall survival at 5 years) [50]. In a recent study on 23 patients, around 70% of patients progressed to ESKD and 40% died after a median follow-up of 8.1 years [49]. Similarly, in another study including 53 patients with MIDD, 53% progressed to ESKD and 36% died after a median follow-up of 6.2 years [4].

The treatment of both MM and AL amyloidosis have dramatically improved with the introduction of bortezomib and autologous stem-cell transplantation (ASCT). Similarly, a parallel shift of administered regimens was undertaken in the treatment of MIDD with promising results in terms of response rates, durability of renal responses, and survival.

Among those patients who received first-line treatment with high-dose melphalan followed by autologous stem cell transplantation (HDM/ASCT) or bortezomib-based regimens, 52–78% achieved at least a VGPR [2, 4, 9, 12, 49]. Response rates in MIDD subtypes were similar to patients with symptomatic MM or MGRS [9]. Bortezomib-based regimens provide rapid, profound, and sustained hematologic responses, resulting in prolonged renal survival. Similarly, HDM/ASCT can induce a high rate of hematologic and renal responses and is well tolerated also in patients with advanced kidney damage. However, ASCT can be proposed only in selected patients: younger than 70 years, with mild to moderate heart involvement (defined based on troponin T and NTproBNP levels, or NYHA class), and no more than two major organs significantly involved. These criteria were adopted from AL amyloidosis excluding those patients with a high disease burden and high risk of post-transplant mortality, but still need to be validated in patients with MIDD.

Recently, targeted anti-plasma cell therapy with anti-CD38 monoclonal antibodies has shown excellent efficacy and tolerability in patients with LCDD and MM [51]. Although data are still scarce, results obtained in AL amyloidosis suggest that anti-CD38 will represent the third therapeutic revolution for patients with MIDD, after bortezomib-based regimens and ASCT.

The renal outcome is often poor. Renal response occurred in about one third (reported range from 22–53%) of patients with MIDD [2, 9, 12, 49], all of whom had achieved hematological response. All patients not receiving chemotherapy inevitably progressed to ESKD [12].

Chemotherapy can improve kidney function regardless of the MIDD subtype, especially if administered at early stages [2, 4, 9, 10]. The main determinant of response to treatment is the severity of kidney dysfunction at chemotherapy initiation. Renal response rates were significantly higher in patients with CKD stages 1–3 at diagnosis than in those with CKD stages 4–5 [2, 13]. However, advanced renal dysfunction is common at diagnosis, with a major impact on long-term renal outcome [4, 9].

Kidney transplantation in patients with MIDD gave discouraging results until the last decade: most patients had early and aggressive post-transplantation recurrence of MIDD [52, 53]. However, as treatments for MIDD have dramatically improved, the achievement of a sustained hematologic response guarantees a longer graft survival [49]. Bortezomib-based regimens followed by HDM/ASCT proved effective in avoiding an early renal MIDD relapse [4, 54]. Considering the high incidence of kidney involvement in MIDD and the delay in diagnosis, many patients progressing to kidney failure require transplantation. Patients should be considered eligible for kidney transplantation only when they have achieved a stable hematologic CR or VGPR (Fig. 10.2) because of their associated longer patient and graft survival compared to those with a partial response or no response.

Extrarenal manifestations also improved in patients who achieved a hematologic response, particularly in those with a CR [55]. The cardiac function improvement is documented by a decrease in NT-proBNP values and a restoration of diastolic function on echocardiography [32]. However, those patients with advanced cardiac disease (documented by highly elevated NT-proBNP and significant changes on echocardiography) may have dismal outcome. A decrease of alkaline phosphatase levels can indicate a hepatic response [4].

Overall, both early diagnosis and prompt treatment with bortezomib or HDM/ASCT-based combinations can improve the prognosis of MIDD, by reducing circulating mIg, preserving renal function, and improving overall survival. The effectiveness of these treatments on renal function is variable, mainly depending on the degree of CKD at diagnosis and the hematologic response.

Conclusions

MIDD is a systemic disease that involves the kidney in most cases. The clinical presentation is variable, but kidney failure requiring dialysis is not uncommon at diagnosis. The severity of kidney failure at presentation and the hematologic response to chemotherapy are the main prognostic factors in MIDD. The presence of an underlying MM and cardiac involvement are also associated with poor prognosis. Current therapeutic strategies targeted at reducing the production of mIg are effective especially if administered at early stages. The exploration of the pathomechanisms of kidney damage, the assessment of new biomarkers, and the integration of new therapies might impact the natural history of the disease.

References

1. Randall RE, Williamson WC Jr, Mullinax F, Tung MY, Still WJ. Manifestations of systemic light chain deposition. Am J Med. 1976;60(2):293–9.
2. Cohen C, Royer B, Javaugue V, et al. Bortezomib produces high hematological response rates with prolonged renal survival in monoclonal immunoglobulin deposition disease. Kidney Int. 2015;88(5):1135–43.
3. Nasr SH, Valeri AM, Cornell LD, et al. Renal monoclonal immunoglobulin deposition disease: a report of 64 patients from a single institution. Clin J Am Soc Nephrol. 2012;7(2):231–9.
4. Sayed RH, Wechalekar AD, Gilbertson JA, et al. Natural history and outcome of light chain deposition disease. Blood. 2015;126(26):2805–10.
5. Katzmann JA, Kyle RA, Benson J, et al. Screening panels for detection of monoclonal gammopathies. Clin Chem. 2009;55(8):1517–22.
6. Buxbaum JN, Chuba JV, Hellman GC, Solomon A, Gallo GR. Monoclonal immunoglobulin deposition disease: light chain and light and heavy chain deposition diseases and their relation

to light chain amyloidosis. Clinical features, immunopathology, and molecular analysis. Ann Intern Med. 1990;112:455–64.
7. Lin J, Markowitz GS, Valeri AM, et al. Renal monoclonal immunoglobulin deposition disease: the disease spectrum. J Am Soc Nephrol. 2001;12(7):1482–92.
8. Pozzi C, D'Amico M, Fogazzi GB, et al. Light chain deposition disease with renal involvement: clinical characteristics and prognostic factors. Am J Kidney Dis. 2003;42(6):1154–63.
9. Joly F, Cohen C, Javaugue V, et al. Randall-type monoclonal immunoglobulin deposition disease: novel insights from a nationwide cohort study. Blood. 2019;133(6):576–87.
10. Zhang Y, Li X, Liang D, et al. Heavy chain deposition disease: clinicopathologic characteristics of a Chinese case series. Am J Kidney Dis. 2020;75(5):736–43.
11. Bridoux F, Javaugue V, Bender S, et al. Unravelling the immunopathological mechanisms of heavy chain deposition disease with implications for clinical management. Kidney Int. 2017;91(2):423–34.
12. Li XM, Rui HC, Liang DD, et al. Clinicopathological characteristics and outcomes of light chain deposition disease: an analysis of 48 patients in a single Chinese center. Ann Hematol. 2016;95(6):901–9.
13. Mohan M, Buros A, Mathur P, et al. Clinical characteristics and prognostic factors in multiple myeloma patients with light chain deposition disease. Am J Hematol. 2017;92(8):739–45.
14. Sicard A, Karras A, Goujon J-M, et al. Light chain deposition disease without glomerular proteinuria: a diagnostic challenge for the nephrologist. Nephrol Dial Transplant. 2014;29(10):1894–902.
15. Buxbaum J, Gallo G. Nonamyloidotic monoclonal immunoglobulin deposition disease. Light-chain, heavy-chain, and light- and heavy-chain deposition diseases. Hematol Oncol Clin North Am. 1999;13(6):1235–48.
16. Buxbaum JN, Genega EM, Lazowski P, et al. Infiltrative nonamyloidotic monoclonal immunoglobulin light chain cardiomyopathy: an underappreciated manifestation of plasma cell dyscrasias. Cardiology. 2000;93(4):220–8.
17. Qian Q, Leung N, Theis JD, Dogan A, Sethi S. Coexistence of myeloma cast nephropathy, light chain deposition disease, and nonamyloid fibrils in a patient with multiple myeloma. Am J Kidney Dis. 2010;56(5):971–6.
18. Zand L, Nasr SH, Gertz MA, et al. Clinical and prognostic differences among patients with light chain deposition disease, myeloma cast nephropathy and both. Leuk Lymphoma. 2015;12:1–8.
19. Herrera GA. Renal lesions associated with plasma cell dyscrasias: practical approach to diagnosis, new concepts, and challenges. Arch Pathol Lab Med. 2009;133:249.
20. Liapis H, Papadakis I, Nakopoulou L. Nodular glomerulosclerosis secondary to μ heavy chain deposits. Hum Pathol. 2000;31:122.
21. Markowitz GS. Dysproteinemia and the kidney. Adv Anat Pathol. 2004;11:49.
22. Herrera GA. The contributions of electron microscopy to the understanding and diagnosis of plasma cell dyscrasia-related renal lesions. Med Electron Microsc. 2001;34:1.
23. Nasr SH, Markowitz GS, Stokes MB, et al. Proliferative glomerulonephritis with monoclonal IgG deposits: a distinct entity mimicking immune-complex glomerulonephritis. Kidney Int. 2004;65:85.
24. Cohen C, Joly F, Sibille A, et al. Randall-type monoclonal immunoglobulin deposition disease: new insights into the pathogenesis. Diagn Manag Diagn. 2021;11(3):420.
25. Kourelis TV, Nasr SH, Dispenzieri A, et al. Outcomes of patients with renal monoclonal immunoglobulin deposition disease. Am J Hematol. 2016;91(11):1123–8.
26. Leung N, Bridoux F, Batuman V, et al. The evaluation of monoclonal gammopathy of renal significance: a consensus report of the international kidney and monoclonal gammopathy research group. Nat Rev Nephrol. 2019;15(1):45–59.
27. Ivanyi B. Frequency of light chain deposition nephropathy relative to renal amyloidosis and Bence Jones cast nephropathy in a necropsy study of patients with myeloma. Arch Pathol Lab Med. 1990;114(9):986–7.

28. Ajise OE, Roshal M, Wang L, et al. Clinical utility of morphology, immunohistochemistry, flow cytometry, and FISH analysis in monitoring of plasma cell neoplasms in the bone marrow. J Hematopathol 2016;9:9–18. https://doi.org/10.1007/s12308-015-0264-1.
29. Samanez C, Domingo A, Cibeira MT, et al. Development of rapidly progressive liver light chain deposition under VAD chemotherapy in multiple myeloma. Eur J Haematol. 2006;76(1):83–5.
30. Brilland B, Sayegh J, Croue A, et al. Recovery from LCDD-associated severe liver cholestasis: a case report and literature review. J Gastrointestin Liver Dis. 2016;25:9–103.
31. Abdallah AOA, Alapat D, Kaur V, Atrash S. Outcomes of autologous stem cell transplant for cardiac AL-amyloidosis and cardiac light chain deposition disease. J Oncol Pharm Pract. 2020;26(5):1128–33.
32. Nakamura M, Satoh M, Kowada S, et al. Reversible restrictive cardiomyopathy due to light-chain deposition disease. Mayo Clin Proc. 2002;77:193–6.
33. Mercado JJ, Markert JM, Meador W, et al. Primary CNS nonamyloidogenic light chain deposition disease: case report and brief review. Int J Surg Pathol. 2017;25(8):755–60.
34. Wei P, Tao R, Liu Y, et al. Pulmonary light chain deposition disease: a case series and literature review. Ann Transl Med. 2020;8(9):588.
35. Rajapreyar I, Joly J, Tallaj J, et al. Pulmonary vascular disease due to plasma cell Dyscrasia. Mayo Clin Proc. 2021;5(1):210–8.
36. Ronco PM, Alyanakian MA, Mougenot B, Aucouturier P. Light chain deposition disease: a model of glomerulosclerosis defined at the molecular level. JASN. 2001;12(7):1558–65.
37. De Lazzari M, Fedrigo M, Migliore F, et al. Nonamyloidotic light chain cardiomyopathy: the Arrhythmogenic magnetic resonance pattern. Circulation. 2016;133(14):1421–3.
38. Peng SK, French WJ, Cohen AH, Fausel RE. Light chain cardiomyopathy associated with small-vessel disease. Arch Pathol Lab Med. 1988;112:844–6.
39. Koopman P, van Dorpe J, Maes B, Dujardin K. Light chain deposition disease as a rare cause of restrictive cardiomyopathy. Acta Cardiol. 2009;64(6):821–4.
40. Toor AA, Ramdane BA, Joseph J, et al. Cardiac nonamyloidotic immunoglobulin deposition disease. Mod Pathol. 2006;19:233–7.
41. Korbet S, Bonsib S. A case of polyneuropathy and proteinuria. CJASN. 2008;3(2):624–36.
42. Grassi MP, Clerici F, Perin C, et al. Light chain deposition disease neuropathy resembling amyloid neuropathy in a multiple myeloma patient. Ital J Neurol Sci. 1998;19(4):229–33.
43. Bhargava P, Rushin JM, Rusnock EJ, et al. Pulmonary light chain deposition disease: report of five cases and review of the literature. Am J Surg Pathol. 2007;31(2):267–76.
44. Arrossi AV, Merzianu M, Farver C, et al. Nodular pulmonary light chain deposition disease: an entity associated with Sjögren syndrome or marginal zone lymphoma. J Clin Pathol. 2016;69(6):490–6.
45. Grainger BT, Issa S, Anderson NE. Primary idiopathic CNS non-amyloidogenic light chain deposition disease complicated by treatment-resistant focal seizure disorder. J Clin Neurosci. 2019;59:313–5.
46. O'Malley JT, D'Agati VD, Sherman WH, Grossman ME. Acquired cutis laxa associated with heavy chain deposition disease involving dermal elastic fibers. JAMA Dermatol. 2014;150(11):1192–6.
47. Palladini G, Dispenzieri A, Gertz MA, et al. New criteria for response to treatment in immunoglobulin light chain amyloidosis based on free light chain measurement and cardiac biomarkers: impact on survival outcomes. J Clin Oncol. 2012;30:4541–9.
48. Oe Y, Soma J, Sato H, Ito S. Heavy chain deposition disease: an overview. Clin Exp Nephrol. 2013;17(6):771–8.
49. Angel-Korman A, Stern L, Angel Y, et al. The role of kidney transplantation in monoclonal Ig deposition disease. Kidney Int Rep. 2020;5(4):485–93.
50. Heilman RL, Velosa JA, Holley KE, Offord KP, Kyle RA. Long- term follow-up and response to chemotherapy in patients with light-chain deposition disease. Am J Kidney Dis. 1992;20(1):34–41.

51. Milani P, Basset M, Curci P, et al. Daratumumab in light chain deposition disease: rapid and profound hematologic response preserves kidney function. Blood Adv. 2020;4:1321–4.
52. Leung N, Lager DJ, Gertz MA, Wilson K, Kanakiriya S, Fervenza FC. Long-term outcome of renal transplantation in light-chain deposition disease. Am J Kidney Dis. 2004;43(1):147–53.
53. Short AK, O'Donoghue DJ, Riad HN, Short CD, Roberts IS. Recurrence of light chain nephropathy in a renal allograft. A case report and review of the literature. Am J Nephrol. 2001;21(3):237–40.
54. Molina-Andújar A, Tovar N, Cuadrado E, et al. Kidney transplantation in monoclonal immunoglobulin deposition disease: a report of 6 cases. Am J Kidney Dis. 2021;78(5):755–9. S0272-6386(21)00576-X.
55. Royer B, Arnulf B, Martinez F, et al. High dose chemotherapy in light chain or light and heavy chain deposition disease. Kidney Int. 2004;65(2):642–8.

Chapter 11
Multiple Myeloma

Rami Kotb, Caroline Hart, and Hadi Goubran

Abbreviations

ASCT	Autologous stem cell transplantation
BJ	Bence Jones
BMPC	Bone marrow plasma cells
CR	Complete response
CRAB	acronym: Hyper Calcemia, Renal failure, Anemia, and Bone disease
CyBorD	Cyclophosphamide, Bortezomib and Dexamethasone
D-RVd	Daratumumab, lenalidomide (Revlimid), bortezomib (Velcade), and dexamethasone
D-VTd	Daratumumab, Velcade (bortezomib), Thalidomide and dexamethasone
ECOG	Eastern Cooperative Oncology Group
IMiDs	Immuno-Modulatory imide Drugs
IMWG	International myeloma working group
MGUS	Monoclonal gammopathy of undetermined significance
MM	Multiple myeloma
NDMM	Newly diagnosed multiple myeloma
PR	Partial response
QoL	Quality of life

R. Kotb (✉)
Department of Medical Oncology and Hematology, CancerCare Manitoba and College of Medicine, University of Manitoba, Winnipeg, MB, Canada
e-mail: rkotb@cancercare.mb.ca

C. Hart (✉) · H. Goubran (✉)
Saskatoon Cancer Centre and College of Medicine, University of Saskatchewan, Saskatoon, SK, Canada
e-mail: Caroline.hart@saskcancer.ca; hadi.goubranmessiha@saskcancer.ca

© The Author(s), under exclusive license to Springer Nature Switzerland AG 2022

G. Ragab et al. (eds.), *Paraproteinemia and Related Disorders*,
https://doi.org/10.1007/978-3-031-10131-1_11

Rd	Lenalidomide (Revlimid) plus dexamethasone
RT	Radiation therapy
RVd	Revlimid (Lenalidomide), Velcade (bortezomib) and dexamethasone
sCR	Stringent complete response
sFLC	Serum free light chains
SLiM	Bone marrow plasma cells at or above 60% (Sixty) of marrow cellularity, serum free light chains (Li) ratio at or above 100, and the presence of more than one focal bone area in MRI (M).
SMM	Smoldering multiple myeloma
VGPR	Very good partial response

Introduction

Multiple myeloma (MM) is a neoplastic disorder of plasma cells. A plasma cell is a differentiated B-lymphocyte at the end stage of maturation, where it can produce antibodies (immunoglobulins) to fight infections. In addition to their uncontrolled proliferation, the malignant plasma cells or myeloma cells usually produce large amounts of monoclonal proteins (paraproteins). These paraproteins could be partial or complete monoclonal immunoglobulins and are generally detectable in the blood before any other disease manifestation.

The proliferation of the myeloma cells can lead to a significant bone marrow infiltration with signs of bone marrow insufficiency, most commonly anemia. These cells can stimulate osteoclasts and inhibit osteoblasts' activity, leading to the typical osteolytic bone disease, decalcification, and hypercalcemia. The paraproteins can impair renal function by different mechanisms. This leads to the cardinal manifestations of myeloma, resumed in the CRAB acronym: Hyper Calcemia, Renal failure, Anemia, and Bone disease. The disease can have a myriad of other non-specific clinical manifestations.

History of Myeloma

Paleopathological data suggest that multiple myeloma existed in ancient Egypt, pre-Columbian Central and South America, and pre-medieval Europe [1]. The earliest reported cases in modern medical literature date back to the mid-nineteenth century [2]. These initial descriptions included the earliest reports of Bence Jones proteinuria (BJ) [3]. It took few decades more to describe the plasma cells. The bone marrow aspiration technique was introduced in 1929, and a year later, the technique of protein electrophoresis [4]. The relation between the monoclonal protein and the Bence Jones proteinuria was later conceptualized [5], and the origin of the BJ proteins was fully described in 1962 [6]. By this era, the disease was almost fully described as it currently is, and the treatment with melphalan and prednisone became a standard of care [7].

The outcome of myeloma did not change much between the early 1960s and the early 1990s, despite different clinical trials. However, From the 1990s, the survival of myeloma patients dramatically improved. This is attributed to the wide use of high-dose chemotherapy [8] and autologous bone marrow/stem cell transplantation, and the addition of different new treatments (immunomodulators, proteasome inhibitors, monoclonal antibodies) [9–11].

Epidemiology

MM is the second most common hematological cancer. It accounts for about 1.8% of all new cancers and 2.1 of all cancer deaths in North America. In Canada, the annual incidence is about 9.6 per 100.000 for men and 6.0 per 100.000 women in 2019.

Recent SEER data suggest that the incidence is slowly increasing over the recent years. The lifetime risk of getting MM is one in 125 (0.8%).

The prevalence of the disease is rapidly increasing, primarily due to treatment improvements and improved survival. About 150.000 people were living with MM in the USA in 2018 [12].

The median age at diagnosis is in North America and Europe in the late 60s. The disease is rare in young adults.

Predisposing Factors

Genetic and hereditary predisposition was suggested by some studies [13], but this is not a significant determinant. There are reports of rare familial cases [14]. The disease is more prevalent in people of African ancestry, and the incidence is lower in people of Asian descent.

While there are no apparent socio-economic differences, there are reports of higher incidence with certain occupations and environmental exposures. Different studies suggest an increased risk with increased body weight [15, 16] and physical inactivity [17].

MGUS-SMM-MM as a Disease Continuum

Different studies showed that almost all cases of symptomatic myeloma are preceded by the presence of MGUS (monoclonal gammopathy of unknown significance) and or smoldering (or asymptomatic) myeloma (SMM).

MGUS is considered a premalignant condition. This is characterized by the presence of a monoclonal protein in the blood, with a normal plasma cell count in the bone marrow and the absence of any related organ damage. MGUS is quite prevalent in the general population, and the prevalence increases with age. MGUS carries the risk of transformation to MM (or related lymphoproliferative diseases) of about 1% per year, and the majority of patients will remain stable over time. Different models were suggested to predict the risk of transformation in MGUS patients, but the risk is still too small in all groups to offer intervention.

Smoldering Myeloma

SMM (or asymptomatic myeloma) was first described in the 1980s and is distinguished from MM (or symptomatic myeloma) by the absence of any detectable myeloma-related organ damage (CRAB signs). SMM is distinguished from MGUS by the increased bone marrow plasma cells to or above the consensual level of 10% of the bone marrow cellularity; and/or the monoclonal protein above a specific cut-off in the blood).

Like MGUS, SMM is often incidentally discovered, and it accounts for about 15% of newly diagnosed MM patients.

Overall, newly diagnosed SMM has a risk of progression of more than 10% per year in the first 3 years. The risk gradually decreases with time. After 10 years from diagnosis, the risk becomes 1% per year, similar to that of MGUS.

This changing risk of progression over time, and the fact that at least one-third of SMM will not progress for 10 or more years after diagnosis, show that SMM is a mixed group of patients, as some have an early malignant disease that will soon develop organ damage, while others have a premalignant condition, like MGUS, that will remain stable for long years, or progress at a very low rate.

Management of SMM

The standard of care for most patients with SMM is still observation. This is based on the lack of clear data to confirm a generalizable overall survival benefit or superior quality of life with early therapy, compared to a delayed intervention. There is also a theoretical concern that early treatment can select resistant clones and worsen the outcome of subsequent treatment lines, as well as the toxicity of therapy in an asymptomatic patient population, and the fact that a good proportion of these patients can be free of progression for many years without any therapy.

The hope is that, with continuous progress in risk stratification of patients with SMM and more effective and less toxic therapies, the percentage of SMM patients who benefit from an early intervention will continue to increase in the near future.

Risk Stratification Studies in SMM

Several studies aimed to identify patients with SMM at high risk of imminent progression so they can receive treatment before end-organ damage. More than one trial showed that each of these predictors: Bone marrow plasma cells (BMPC) ≥ 60%, serum free light chains (sFLC) ratio ≥ 100, or the presence of >1 focal bone lesion on MRI are at such high risk of organ damage in the following months. These criteria are now considered as myeloma defining, expanding the definition of MM (SLiM-CRAB). However, the three predictors are present in only 7–10% of SMM. More data is still needed to identify the high-risk group among SMM.

Several predictive models were developed to risk-stratify patients with SMM. In 2020, the International Myeloma Working Group (IMWG) presented a reproducible and easily applied model (The 20/20/20 score) [18]. This is based on bone marrow clonal plasma cells (more than 20%), sFLC ratio (above 20) and serum monoclonal protein (above 20 g/L), with the presence of high-risk cytogenetics as an additional risk factor (Table 11.1).

Trials of Therapeutic Interventions in SMM

Shortly after the description of SMM as an entity, and as it is uncomfortable for the patient and physicians not to intervene on a premalignant condition and to wait for signs of organ damage (CRAB) to start treatment, at least three trials explored the benefit of melphalan and prednisone in SMM and showed no significant improvement of overall survival compared to observation and treatment at progression [19–21].

Early trials of pamidronate and later with zoledronic acid showed a significant reduction of skeletal-related events compared to observation, however, these trials showed no improvement in overall survival or progression time [22–24].

Table 11.1 IMWG SMM 20/20/20 score. (Adapted from [18]. RP%2Y (Percent risk of progression in 2 years))

PARAMETER	VALUE
Serum M-Protein	>20gm/L
Involved to uninvolved sFLC ratio	>20
Bone marrow Plasma Cell Infiltration	>20%
Additional risk factors: Chromosomal abnormality	t(4:14) t(14:16) +1q Del 13q/ Monosomy 13

RISK	RP%2Y
Low-risk 0	6.0
Low-intermediate 1	22.8
Intermediate-risk 2	45.5
High-risk 3-4	63.1

In SMM patients, a randomized trial explored thalidomide and zoledronic acid versus zoledronic acid alone. Despite initial disease response in the experimental arm, the study showed no significant difference in the time to progression to symptomatic MM or overall survival [25].

QuiRedex trial explored the use of lenalidomide plus dexamethasone versus observation in patients with high-risk smoldering multiple myeloma and concluded that positive results from ongoing trials would support the use of early treatment for patients with the high-risk disease [26]. Despite its limitations, QuiRedex has shown a survival advantage to using lenalidomide and dexamethasone doublet over observation in high-risk SMM [27].

Furthermore, Phase III data from the Spanish Myeloma Group/PETHEMA as well as the Eastern Cooperative Oncology Group (ECOG) E3A06 trial have shown the efficacy of lenalidomide with and without dexamethasone in high-risk SMM in delaying progression to symptomatic disease [28, 29].

Clinical Presentation of Myeloma

The presentation of myeloma can be quite variable and depends on the disease stage and the threshold of suspicion of the medical team. Table 11.2 illustrates the diagnostic criteria and differences between MGUS, SMM, and MM. General nonspecific symptoms such as fatigue are common and often precede the diagnosis. Most patients MM have an unremarkable physical examination at presentation.

Bony pains and/or bone disease are reported in up to 70% of patients at diagnosis using sensitive modalities such as whole-body computed tomography, MRI, or PET/CT scans.

Table 11.2 The diagnostic criteria and differences between MGUS, SMM, and MM

Condition	Diagnostic criteria
MUGS	All of the following: – No myeloma defining events (CRAB) – Clonal plasma cells are less than 10% in the bone marrow – M-protein less than 30 g/L (Light chains MGUS: No M protein, abnormal light chains ratio, less than 500 mg/24 h urine
SMM	– No myeloma-defining events AND at least one of the following: – Clonal plasma cells 10–60% in the bone marrow – Serum M-protein at or above 30 g/L – Urine light chains at or above 500 mg/24 h
MM	Presence of myeloma defining events: CRAB or other MM defining criteria – Elevated serum calcium – Renal involvement – Anemia – Lytic bone lesions – Other MM defining criteria: BMPC at or above 60% of bone marrow cellularity, Serum light chains ratio at/above 100, or the presence of more than one focal bone lesion on MRI

Vertebral fractures are common at diagnosis. Symptomatic and/or radiological spinal disease was reported in about 50% of patients [30]. Spinal cord compression is a rare presentation but could be an indication for an urgent intervention.

Fatigue, altered general condition, and weight loss are also common at presentation. These could be due to anemia, renal insufficiency, or hypercalcemia.

Less common presentations may include hyperviscosity, organ involvement with amyloidosis, peripheral neuropathy, and recurrent infections.

Initial Workup

A detailed history and complete laboratory and radiological investigations are highly important.

The minimal initial investigations of a patient with MM should include routine labs (complete blood count, chemistry, calcium, albumin, total serum protein levels, renal function, and liver functions tests, immunoglobulin levels, serum protein electrophoresis, and serum free light chains) bone imaging (CT scan or x-ray skeletal survey) and bone marrow examination. The serum beta-2 microglobulin and lactate dehydrogenase are of prognostic significance [31].

Bone marrow aspirate and biopsy and histopathological examination is essential to establish the diagnosis and should be complemented by flow cytometry, conventional cytogenetics, and FISH studies. Table 11.3 illustrates the initial workup for myeloma patients (see Chap. 6).

Risk Stratification Tools

There is wide heterogeneity in the way myeloma responds to a specific therapy. Different risk-stratification tools were developed over time. These are of prognostic value but are mainly used to stratify and homogenize patients enrolled in clinical trials, as they can be applied before starting treatment. The different risk stratification tools and staging systems, including the Durie and Salmon classification, the ISS and R-ISS, are summarized in Table 11.4 [32–34].

Table 11.3 Myeloma workup. (Adapted from [31])

Routine labs	• CBC • Chemistry, CrCl, Ca, LFTs, LDH, B2M, Igs levels, SPEP, sFLC
Special labs	• BM aspirate and biopsy • Cytogenetics • Flow cytometry
Imaging tests	• X-ray (or CT) skeletal survey MRI • PET scan (Initial and response evaluation)

Table 11.4 Staging systems for multiple myeloma

Stage	Durie–Salmon	ISS	R-ISS
I	*All of the following*: Hemoglobin above 100 g/L Serum calcium at/below 3 mmol/L Absence of bone disease or solitary plasmacytoma Serum paraprotein below 50 g/L if IgG, 30 g/L if IgA Urinary light chains excretion below 4 g/24 h	Serum beta2 microglobulin below 3.5 mg/L and serum albumin at/above 35 g/L	ISS Stage I and Standard risk cytogenetics (Interphase FISH) and Normal serum LDH
II	Not stage I or III	Not stage I or III	Not stage I or III
III	*Any of the following*: Hemoglobin below 85 g/L Serum calcium above 3 mmol/L More than two lytic lesions Serum paraprotein above 70 g/L if IgG, 50 g/L if IgA Urinary light chains excretion above 12 g/24 h	Serum beta2 microglobulin at/above 5.5 mg/L	ISS Stage III and either: High-risk cytogenetics or High serum LDH

Classification and Risk Stratification Based on Cytogenetics

There are four major subtypes of MM that account for more than 80% of patients with the disease. They include MM with trisomies of one or more odd-numbered chromosomes, t(11;14) MM, t(4;14) MM, and MM with translocations of t(14;16) or t(14;20), referred to as MAF MM [35]. Secondary cytogenetic abnormalities such as deletion 17p, gain 1q, deletion 1p, deletion 13q, or monosomy 13 can occur in any of the primary cytogenetic types of myeloma and can further modify the disease course, response to therapy, and prognosis.

High-risk MM is defined by the presence of t(4;14), t(14;16), t(14;20), deletion 17p, gain 1q, or p53 mutation1. Double-hit MM refers to the presence of any two or more high-risk abnormalities. Triple-hit MM refers to the presence of three or more high-risk abnormalities [36].

Treatment and Goals of Care

When to Treat:

Treatment of myeloma is indicated when there are signs of organ damage or enough presumption that an organ damage is imminent.

With the available treatment tools, myeloma is not a curable disease for most patients. The ultimate goal of a treatment is to obtain disease remission and to maintain it for as long as possible.

For newly diagnosed patients, the presence of any of the cardinal signs of myeloma (CRAB) is an absolute indication to start treatment. The presence of other myeloma-related manifestations (peripheral neuropathy, amyloidosis) is also an indication to start treatment. Different tools were developed to select patients at very high risk of imminent progression in patients with no sign of organ damage. The IMWG guidelines currently include the following additional criteria for treatment-eligible myeloma (SLiM): Bone marrow plasma cells at or above 60% (S) of marrow cellularity, serum free light chains (Li) ratio at or above 100, and the presence of more than one focal bone area in MRI (M).

Although modern treatments can produce deep responses, their aim is still palliative. Some patients, however, can achieve a minimum residual disease (MRD) negative state that reflects on more prolonged progression-free survival and overall survival.

Available Systemic Myeloma-Directed Treatments

Different classes of anti-myeloma therapies are now recognized, including systemic corticosteroids (prednisone or dexamethasone), alkylators (melphalan or cyclophosphamide), proteasome inhibitors (bortezomib, carfilzomib, or ixazomib), immune modulators (IMiDs: thalidomide, lenalidomide, or pomalidomide), and monoclonal antibodies targeting CD38, (daratumumab, isatuximab), whereas elotuzumab targets the SLAMF7 antigen. Other newer agents were recently approved or are currently in development. Panobinostat, a histone deacetylase inhibitor, and selinexor, an inhibitor of exportin-1 (XPO1), are also used in the relapsed refractory setting. Elotuzumab, panobinostat, and selinexor do not seem to have significant single-agent activity but appear to exert their therapeutic effect in combination with other active drugs [36]. Doxorubicin, an anthracycline, is not frequently used but is occasionally incorporated into some multi-agent combination regimens for aggressive or refractory MM.

Therefore, at least seven different classes of approved agents, including alkylators, steroids, proteasome inhibitors, immunomodulatory agents, histone deacetylase inhibitors, monoclonal antibodies, and selective inhibitors of nuclear export, can be combined in doublet, triplet, or even quadruplet regimens and used with or without high-dose therapy and autologous stem cell transplantation (ASCT).

High-dose melphalan is used as the backbone conditioning agent for ASCT. Table 11.5 illustrates the different therapeutic agents used to treat MM.

Chapter 22 covers the novel and experimental clone-directed therapies.

Table 11.5 Main available treatment classes/molecules

Steroids	Alkylators	IMIDs	Proteasome inhibitors	Monoclonal Abs
Prednisone	Melphalan	Thalidomide	Bortezomib	Daratumumab
Dexamethasone	Cyclophosphamide	Lenalidomide	Carfilzomib	Isatuximab
		Pomalidomide	Ixazomib	Elotuzumab

Treatment Algorithm

Therapeutic Approach at Diagnosis

The two main factors that drive the approach to newly diagnosed MM are eligibility for ASCT and risk stratification. In general, eligibility for ASCT is influenced by age, performance status, and comorbidities.

Transplant-eligible patients are usually offered an induction therapy with 3–4 cycles with agents including bortezomib, lenalidomide, dexamethasone, and cyclophosphamide in protocols including the four agents or three of them.

Lenalidomide, bortezomib, and dexamethasone (RVd) followed by autologous stem cell transplantation (ASCT) are commonly used frontline therapy for transplant-eligible patients with newly diagnosed multiple myeloma (NDMM). RVd is a relatively well-tolerated regimen associated with high overall and complete response (CR) rates. In a Southwest Oncology Group (SWOG) randomized trial, treatment with RVd led to superior PFS and OS compared with lenalidomide plus dexamethasone (Rd) [37, 38]. A subsequent randomized trial by the Intergroupe Francophone du Myelome found that the 4-year OS rate with RVd was >80% with or without early ASCT [39]. Bortezomib, Cyclophosphamide, and Dexamethasone (CyBorD) are commonly used regimens with interesting results [40]. The addition of an anti-CD38 to CyBorD seems to improve the results [41]. This is currently evaluated in a prospective Canadian trial [42].

Stem cell collection and cryopreservation are then performed, followed by high-dose melphalan as a conditioning regimen. Lenalidomide alone or in combination (not the standard in all centers) is offered as maintenance.

For high-risk patients and a broader category of patients in certain centers, on the other hand, the addition of monoclonal antibodies is an option. The addition of daratumumab to thalidomide, bortezomib, and steroids (D-Vtd) before and after autologous stem cell transplantation improved the depth of response and progression-free survival with acceptable safety. CASSIOPEIA is the first study showing the clinical benefit of daratumumab plus standard of care in transplant-eligible patients with newly diagnosed multiple myeloma [43].

The addition of daratumumab (D) to RVd (D-RVd) in transplant-eligible NDMM patients was evaluated in the Griffin trial. Daratumumab with RVd induction and consolidation improved depth of response in patients with transplant-eligible NDMM, with no new safety concerns [44].

For transplant-ineligible patients, bortezomib and lenalidomide-based therapies are offered in combination, followed by lenalidomide maintenance or lenalidomide and dexamethasone as offered a single-agent until disease progression [36]. The addition of an anti-CD38 antibody to the first-line therapy significantly improves the outcome.

Optimizing therapy at diagnosis represents a challenge for physicians. However, the therapeutic approaches vary between centers and are often based on drug funding by health authorities and insurance companies.

Therapeutic Approach for Relapsed and Refractory Myeloma

In the relapsed and refractory context, the choice of treatment is influenced by patient-related factors such as patient preference, age, pre-existing toxicities or comorbidities or disease-related factors such as cytogenetic profile and aggressiveness of the relapse. The primary determinant, however, remains the response to previous therapies.

If a patient has disease progression while taking lenalidomide as part of their frontline therapy, a reasonable approach would be to switch the agent class from an immunomodulatory drug to a proteasome inhibitor. Bortezomib plus dexamethasone was the first combination used in this setting, resulting in progression-free survival ranging from 8–10 months [42]. In the CASTOR trial, bortezomib plus dexamethasone was compared with daratumumab plus bortezomib plus dexamethasone in patients with relapsed multiple myeloma who had received at least one previous line of therapy. The triplet combination was associated with significantly longer progression-free survival in all patients [45]. In clinical trials, panobinostat or pomalidomide have been added to bortezomib and dexamethasone in the relapsed refractory setting [46].

Combinations of carfilzomib plus dexamethasone plus anti-CD38 antibodies have also been evaluated in phase 3 studies. Daratumumab plus carfilzomib plus dexamethasone was superior to carfilzomib plus dexamethasone in terms of progression-free survival, both in patients with previous lenalidomide exposure [47, 48].

In patients who have relapsed or became refractory while receiving bortezomib-based frontline therapy without lenalidomide, second-line therapy should be based on lenalidomide and dexamethasone regimens, such as carfilzomib plus lenalidomide plus dexamethasone, daratumumab plus lenalidomide plus dexamethasone, ixazomib plus lenalidomide plus dexamethasone, or elotuzumab plus lenalidomide plus dexamethasone [46] with the most effective combination available in the setting of the first relapse of myeloma not refractory to lenalidomide being daratumumab plus lenalidomide plus dexamethasone [49].

The first relapse in patients progressing on frontline daratumumab-based combinations represents a real challenge as no data exist to date to support the use of daratumumab retreatment at the second line. Salvage therapy with isatuximab in these patients is unlikely to be a suitable option because both antibodies target the same antigen (CD38) [46]. The combination of multiple treatment approaches is being experimented. ASCT salvage may also be offered.

For patients failing two or more lines of therapy, as those patients whose disease has progressed after treatment with bortezomib and lenalidomide, pomalidomide plus dexamethasone has been considered as the standard of care [50].

Isatuximab plus pomalidomide plus dexamethasone was approved by the US Food and Drug Administration and by the European Medicines Agency for adult patients with relapsed and refractory MM who received at least two previous lines of therapies including lenalidomide and a proteasome inhibitor and demonstrated disease progression on the last therapy [51]. Carfilzomib, dexamethasone, and daratumumab have also been used in this context [47].

The approach to patients with refractory and relapsed MM was recently very well highlighted by Moreau et al. in the recommendations from the IMWG [46].

Moreover, next-generation immunotherapies or targeted agents will soon improve the therapeutic armamentarium and are discussed in Chap. 22.

Role of Radiation Therapy

Like most lymphoid cancers, myeloma cells are quite sensitive to radiation therapy (RT). This excellent activity of RT against MM has been known for decades [52].

After an adequate radiation dose to an area, local disease relapse is quite rare.

RT is the standard treatment for localized plasmacytoma.

However, the toxicity of RT is directly related to dose and area of treatment, and the role of RT in MM is limited to rapid local disease control (e.g., spinal disease), often at the time of diagnosis and palliative pain management in relapsed or refractory MM.

Currently, about one-third of MM patients will need RT during the course of their disease [53].

Role of Surgical Interventions

The role of surgical interventions in MM includes diagnostic biopsies (bone marrow or suspicious bone lesions), orthopedic management of bone complications, spinal cord compression, or vertebroplasties.

Response Evaluation

The ultimate goal of systemic therapy is to obtain a durable disease remission and to maintain it for as long as possible.

The IMWG presented response criteria that are widely used to assess the depth of response in clinical trials and clinical practice. Table 11.6 illustrates the different response criteria [54].

Different studies showed a reliable—yet not absolute—correlation between the depth of response and the duration of response.

Myeloma Survivorship

The term "MM survivorship" covers the physical, psychosocial, and economic issues related to MM from diagnosis until the end of life. All of these issues need to be addressed throughout the continuum of care.

Table 11.6 Response evaluation criteria (adapted—IMWG): Adapted from [54]

Response	IMWG criteria
sCR	CR as defined below plus normal FLC ratio and the absence of clonal plasma cells in bone marrow by immunohistochemistry or immunofluorescence
CR	Negative immunofixation on the serum and urine and disappearance of any soft tissue plasmacytomas and <5% plasma cells in bone marrow
VGPR	Serum and urine M-protein detectable by immunofixation but not on electrophoresis or >90% reduction in serum M-protein plus urine M-protein level <100 mg/24 h
PR	>50% reduction of serum M-protein and reduction in 24 h urinary M-protein by >90% or to <200 mg/24 h
No change/ stable disease	Not meeting criteria for CR, VGPR, PR, or progressive disease
Progressive disease	Increase of >25% from the lowest response value in any one or more of the following
Relapse	Clinical relapse requires one or more of: Direct indicators of increasing disease and/or end-organ dysfunction (CRAB features)

sCR Stringent Complete response, *CR* Complete response, *VGPR* Very good partial response, *PR* Partial response

MM is associated with the most significant symptomatic burden and the poorest quality of life (QoL) among the hematologic malignancies and cancer in general. This leads to a substantial impact on patients, their caregivers, and the healthcare system.

Prevention, early detection and prompt management of MM-related manifestations and complications are the cornerstones of improved MM survivorship. If not promptly addressed, long-term sequelae may result. Most patients require long-term or continuous therapies that may be associated with additional side effects (some overlapping with MM-related manifestations and complications) and further affect their QoL [55].

Conclusions

MM is a neoplastic disorder of plasma cells where in addition to their uncontrolled proliferation, the malignant plasma cells often produce monoclonal proteins (paraproteins). The disease is notorious for its target organ damage, and treatment aims at controlling the disease activity. Treatment strategies have changed drastically in the past decade with the incorporation of novel agents into therapeutic strategies. These new drugs, in various combinations, have been added to national and international clinical guidelines and have transformed the approach to the treatment of patients with multiple myeloma, resulting in substantial improvements in the overall survival and quality of life of patients.

References

1. Capasso LL. Antiquity of cancer. Int J Cancer. 2005;113:2–13.
2. Solly S. Remarks on the pathology of mollities ossium with cases. Med Chir Trans. 1844;27:435–61.
3. Bence Jones H. On the new substance occurring in the urine of a patient with mollities ossium. Philos Trans R Soc Lond. 1848;138:55–62.
4. Arinkin MI. Die intravitale Untersuchungsmethodik des Knochenmarks. Folia Haematologie. 1929;38:233–40.
5. Korngold L, Lipari R. Multiple myeloma proteins. III. The antigenic relationship of Bence Jones proteins to normal gammaglobulin and multiple myeloma serum proteins. Cancer. 1956;9:262–72.
6. Edelman GM, Gally JA. The nature of Bence-Jones proteins. Chemical similarities to polypeptide chains of myeloma globulins and normal gamma-globulins. J Exp Med. 1962;116:207–27.
7. Alexanian R, Haut A, Khan AU, Lane M, McKelvey EM, Migliore PJ, Stuckey WJ Jr, Wilson HE. Treatment for multiple myeloma. Combination chemotherapy with different melphalan dose regimens. JAMA. 1969;208:1680–5.
8. McElwain TJ, Powles RL. High-dose intravenous melphalan for plasma-cell leukaemia and myeloma. Lancet. 1983;2:822–4.
9. Singhal S, Mehta J, Desikan R, Ayers D, Roberson P, Eddlemon P, Munshi N, Anaissie E, Wilson C, Dhodapkar M, Zeddis J, Barlogie B. Antitumor activity of thalidomide in refractory multiple myeloma. N Engl J Med. 1999;341:1565–71. [see comment] [erratum appears in N Engl J Med 3 Feb 2000; 342(5):364]
10. Richardson PG, Barlogie B, Berenson J, Singhal S, Jagannath S, Irwin D, Rajkumar SV, Srkalovic G, Alsina M, Alexanian R, Siegel D, Orlowski RZ, Kuter D, Limentani SA, Lee S, Hideshima T, Esseltine DL, Kauffman M, Adams J, Schenkein DP, Anderson KC. A phase 2 study of bortezomib in relapsed, refractory myeloma. N Engl J Med. 2003;348:2609–17.
11. Rajkumar SV, Hayman SR, Lacy MQ, Dispenzieri A, Geyer SM, Kabat B, Zeldenrust SR, Kumar S, Greipp PR, Fonseca R, Lust JA, Russell SJ, Kyle RA, Witzig TE, Gertz MA. Combination therapy with lenalidomide plus dexamethasone (Rev/Dex) for newly diagnosed myeloma. Blood. 2005;106:4050–3.
12. Surveillance, Epidemiology, and End Results Program. SEER stat fact sheets: myeloma. National Cancer Institute. http://seer.cancer.gov/statfacts/html/mulmy.html. Accessed 3 Feb 2021.
13. Landgren O, Weiss B. Patterns of monoclonal gammopathy of undetermined significance and multiple myeloma in various ethnic/racial groups: support for genetic factors in pathogenesis. Leukemia. 2009;23:1691–7. https://doi.org/10.1038/leu.2009.134.
14. Grass S, Preuss K-D, Thome S, Weisenburger DD, Witt V, Lynch J, Zettl F, Trümper L, Fadle N, Regitz E, Lynch H, Pfreundschuh M. Paraproteins of familial MGUS/multiple myeloma target family-typical antigens: hyperphosphorylation of autoantigens is a consistent finding in familial and sporadic MGUS/MM. Blood. 2011;118(3):635–7. https://doi.org/10.1182/blood-2011-01-331454.
15. Alexander D, Mink PJ, Adam HO, Cole P, Mandel JS, Oken MM, Trichopoulos D. Multiple myeloma: a review of the epidemiologic literature. Int J Cancer. 2007;120:40–61.
16. Larsson SC, Wolk A. Body mass index and risk of multiple myeloma: a meta-analysis. Int J Cancer. 2007;121:2512–6.
17. IARC. IARC handbooks of cancer prevention, Weight control and physical activity, vol. 6. Lyon: IARC Press; 2002.
18. Mateos MV, Kumar S, Dimopoulos MA, et al. International myeloma working group risk stratification model for smoldering multiple myeloma (SMM). Blood Cancer J. 2020;10:102. https://doi.org/10.1038/s41408-020-00366-3.

19. Hjorth M, Hellquist L, Holmberg E, Magnusson B, Rödjer S, Westin J, Myeloma Group of Western Sweden. Initial versus deferred melphalan-prednisone therapy for asymptomatic multiple myeloma stage I—a randomized study. Eur J Haematol. 1993;50(2):95–102.
20. Grignani G, Gobbi PG, Formisano R, et al. A prognostic index for multiple myeloma. Br J Cancer. 1996;73(9):1101–7.
21. Riccardi A, Mora O, Tinelli C, et al.; Cooperative Group of Study and Treatment of Multiple Myeloma. Long-term survival of stage I multiple myeloma given chemotherapy just after diagnosis or at progression of the disease: a multicentre randomized study. Br J Cancer. 2000;82(7):1254–1260
22. Martín A, García-Sanz R, Hernández J, et al. Pamidronate induces bone formation in patients with smouldering or indolent myeloma, with no significant anti-tumour effect. Br J Haematol. 2002;118(1):239–42.
23. D'Arena G, Gobbi PG, Broglia C, et al.; Gimema (Gruppo Italiano Malattie Ematologiche Dell'Adulto); Multiple Myeloma Working Party; Gisl (Gruppo Italiano Studio Linfomi) Cooperative Group. Pamidronate versus observation in asymptomatic myeloma: final results with long-term follow-up of a randomized study. Leuk Lymphoma. 2011;52(5):771–775.
24. Musto P, Petrucci MT, Bringhen S, et al.; GIMEMA (Italian Group for Adult Hematologic Diseases)/Multiple Myeloma Working Party and the Italian Myeloma Network. A multicenter, randomized clinical trial comparing zoledronic acid versus observation in patients with asymptomatic myeloma. Cancer. 2008;113(7):1588–1595.
25. Witzig TE, Laumann KM, Lacy MQ, et al. A phase III randomized trial of thalidomide plus zoledronic acid versus zoledronic acid alone in patients with asymptomatic multiple myeloma. Leukemia. 2013;27(1):220–5.
26. Mateos MV, Hernández MT, Giraldo P, de la Rubia J, de Arriba F, Corral LL, Rosiñol L, Paiva B, Palomera L, Bargay J, Oriol A, Prosper F, López J, Arguiñano JM, Quintana N, García JL, Bladé J, Lahuerta JJ, Miguel JS. Lenalidomide plus dexamethasone versus observation in patients with high-risk smouldering multiple myeloma (QuiRedex): long-term follow-up of a randomised, controlled, phase 3 trial. Lancet Oncol. 2016;17(8):1127–36. https://doi.org/10.1016/S1470-2045(16)30124-3.
27. Kapoor P, Rajkumar SV. Smoldering multiple myeloma: to treat or not to treat. Cancer J. 2019;25(1):65–71.
28. Joseph NS, Dhodapkar MV, Lonial S. The role of early intervention in high-risk smoldering myeloma. Am Soc Clin Oncol Educ Book. 2020;40:1–9.
29. Schmidt TM, Callander NS. Progress in the management of smoldering multiple myeloma. Curr Hematol Malig Rep. 2021;16(2):172–82.
30. Sharma AM, Sackett M, Bueddefeld D, Lambert P, Dubey A, Wadhwa V, Kotb R, Ahmed N. Incidence of spinal disease and role of spinal radiotherapy in multiple myeloma. Curr Oncol. 2018;25(6):e539–44.
31. Bergstrom DJ, Kotb R, Louzada ML, Sutherland HJ, Tavoularis S, Venner CP, Myeloma Canada Research Network Consensus Guideline Consortium. Consensus guidelines on the diagnosis of multiple myeloma and related disorders: recommendations of the Myeloma Canada Research Network Consensus Guideline Consortium. Clin Lymphoma Myeloma Leuk. 2020;20(7):e352–67. https://doi.org/10.1016/j.clml.2020.01.017. Epub 2020 Feb 4. PMID: 32249195.
32. Durie BG, Salmon SE. A clinical staging system for multiple myeloma. Correlation of measured myeloma cell mass with presenting clinical features, response to treatment, and survival. Cancer. 1975;36(3):842–54. https://doi.org/10.1002/1097-0142(197509)36:3<842::aid-cncr2820360303>3.0.co;2-u. PMID: 1182674.
33. Greipp PR, San Miguel J, Durie BG, Crowley JJ, Barlogie B, Bladé J, Boccadoro M, Child JA, Avet-Loiseau H, Kyle RA, Lahuerta JJ, Ludwig H, Morgan G, Powles R, Shimizu K, Shustik C, Sonneveld P, Tosi P, Turesson I, Westin J. International staging system for multiple myeloma. J Clin Oncol. 2005;23(15):3412–20. https://doi.org/10.1200/JCO.2005.04.242.

Epub 2005 Apr 4. Erratum in: J Clin Oncol. 2005 Sep 1;23(25):6281. Harousseau, Jean-Luc [corrected to Avet-Loiseau, Herve]. PMID: 15809451.

34. Palumbo A, Avet-Loiseau H, Oliva S, Lokhorst HM, Goldschmidt H, Rosinol L, Richardson P, Caltagirone S, Lahuerta JJ, Facon T, Bringhen S, Gay F, Attal M, Passera R, Spencer A, Offidani M, Kumar S, Musto P, Lonial S, Petrucci MT, Orlowski RZ, Zamagni E, Morgan G, Dimopoulos MA, Durie BG, Anderson KC, Sonneveld P, San Miguel J, Cavo M, Rajkumar SV, Moreau P. Revised international staging system for multiple myeloma: a report from international myeloma working group. J Clin Oncol. 2015;33(26):2863–9.
35. Kumar S, Rajkumar SV. The multiple myelomas—current concepts in cytogenetic classification and therapy. Nat Rev Clin Oncol. 2018;15:409–21.
36. Rajkumar SV, Kumar S. Multiple myeloma current treatment algorithms. Blood Cancer J. 2020;10:94.
37. Durie BGM, Hoering A, Abidi MH, Rajkumar SV, Epstein J, Kahanic SP, Thakuri M, Reu F, Reynolds CM, Sexton R, Orlowski RZ, Barlogie B, Dispenzieri A. Bortezomib with lenalidomide and dexamethasone versus lenalidomide and dexamethasone alone in patients with newly diagnosed myeloma without intent for immediate autologous stem-cell transplant (SWOG S0777): a randomised, open-label, phase 3 trial. Lancet. 2017;389(10068):519–27.
38. Attal M, Lauwers-Cances V, Hulin C, Leleu X, Caillot D, Escoffre M, Arnulf B, Macro M, Belhadj K, Garderet L, Roussel M, Payen C, Mathiot C, Fermand JP, Meuleman N, Rollet S, Maglio ME, Zeytoonjian AA, Weller EA, Munshi N, Anderson KC, Richardson PG, Facon T, Avet-Loiseau H, Harousseau JL, Moreau P, IFM 2009 Study. Lenalidomide, Bortezomib, and Dexamethasone with transplantation for myeloma. N Engl J Med. 2017;376(14):1311–20.
39. Attal M, et al. Autologous transplantation for multiple myeloma in the era of new drugs: a phase III study of the Intergroupe Francophone Du Myelome (IFM/DFCI 2009 Trial). Blood. 2015;126:391.
40. Reeder CB, Reece DE, Kukreti V, Chen C, Trudel S, Hentz J, Noble B, Pirooz NA, Spong JE, Piza JG, Zepeda VH, Mikhael JR, Leis JF, Bergsagel PL, Fonseca R, Stewart AK. Cyclophosphamide, bortezomib and dexamethasone induction for newly diagnosed multiple myeloma: high response rates in a phase II clinical trial. Leukemia. 2009;23(7):1337–41. https://doi.org/10.1038/leu.2009.26. Epub 2009 Feb 19. PMID: 19225538; PMCID: PMC2711213.
41. Voorhees PM, Kaufman JL, Laubach J, Sborov DW, Reeves B, Rodriguez C, Chari A, Silbermann R, Costa LJ, Anderson LD Jr, Nathwani N, Shah N, Efebera YA, Holstein SA, Costello C, Jakubowiak A, Wildes TM, Orlowski RZ, Shain KH, Cowan AJ, Murphy S, Lutska Y, Pei H, Ukropec J, Vermeulen J, de Boer C, Hoehn D, Lin TS, Richardson PG. Daratumumab, lenalidomide, bortezomib, and dexamethasone for transplant-eligible newly diagnosed multiple myeloma: the GRIFFIN trial. Blood. 2020;136(8):936–45.
42. https://clinicaltrials.gov/ct2/show/NCT04786028
43. Moreau P, Attal M, Hulin C, Arnulf B, Belhadj K, Benboubker L, Béné MC, Broijl A, Caillon H, Caillot D, Corre J, Delforge M, Dejoie T, Doyen C, Facon T, Sonntag C, Fontan J, Garderet L, Jie KS, Karlin L, Kuhnowski F, Lambert J, Leleu X, Lenain P, Macro M, Mathiot C, Orsini-Piocelle F, Perrot A, Stoppa AM, van de Donk NW, Wuilleme S, Zweegman S, Kolb B, Touzeau C, Roussel M, Tiab M, Marolleau JP, Meuleman N, Vekemans MC, Westerman M, Klein SK, Levin MD, Fermand JP, Escoffre-Barbe M, Eveillard JR, Garidi R, Ahmadi T, Zhuang S, Chiu C, Pei L, de Boer C, Smith E, Deraedt W, Kampfenkel T, Schecter J, Vermeulen J, Avet-Loiseau H, Sonneveld P. Bortezomib, thalidomide, and dexamethasone with or without daratumumab before and after autologous stem-cell transplantation for newly diagnosed multiple myeloma (CASSIOPEIA): a randomised, open-label, phase 3 study. Lancet. 2019;394(10192):29–38.
44. Laubach J, Garderet L, Mahindra A, et al. Management of relapsed multiple myeloma: recommendations of the international myeloma working group. Leukemia. 2016;30:1005–1017A.
45. Palumbo A, Chanan-Khan A, Weisel K, et al. Daratumumab, bortezomib, and dexamethasone for multiple myeloma. N Engl J Med. 2016;375:754–66.

46. Moreau P, Kumar SK, San Miguel J, Davies F, Zamagni E, Bahlis N, Ludwig H, Mikhael J, Terpos E, Schjesvold F, Martin T, Yong K, Durie BGM, Facon T, Jurczyszyn A, Sidana S, Raje N, van de Donk N, Lonial S, Cavo M, Kristinsson SY, Lentzsch S, Hajek R, Anderson KC, João C, Einsele H, Sonneveld P, Engelhardt M, Fonseca R, Vangsted A, Weisel K, Baz R, Hungria V, Berdeja JG, da Costa FL, Maiolino A, Waage A, Vesole DH, Ocio EM, Quach H, Driessen C, Bladé J, Leleu X, Riva E, Bergsagel PL, Hou J, Chng WJ, Mellqvist U-H, Dytfeld D, Harousseau J-L, Goldschmidt H, Laubach J, Munshi NC, Gay F, Beksac M, Costa LJ, Kaiser M, Hari P, Boccadoro M, Usmani SZ, Zweegman S, Holstein S, Sezer O, Harrison S, Nahi H, Cook G, Mateos M-V, Rajkumar SV, Dimopoulos MA, Richardson PG. Treatment of relapsed and refractory multiple myeloma: recommendations from the international myeloma working group. Lancet Oncol. 2021;22(3):e105–18.
47. Dimopoulos M, Quach H, Mateos MV, et al. Carfilzomib, dexamethasone, and daratumumab versus carfilzomib and dexamethasone for patients with relapsed or refractory multiple myeloma (CANDOR): results from a randomised, multicentre, open-label, phase 3 study. Lancet. 2020;396:186–97.
48. Moreau P, Dimopoulos MA, Mikhael J, Yong K, Capra M, Facon T, Hajek R, Špička I, Baker R, Kim K, Martinez G, Min CK, Pour L, Leleu X, Oriol A, Koh Y, Suzuki K, Risse ML, Asset G, Macé S, Martin T, IKEMA Study Group. Isatuximab, carfilzomib, and dexamethasone in relapsed multiple myeloma (IKEMA): a multicentre, open-label, randomised phase 3 trial. Lancet. 2021;397(10292):2361–71. https://doi.org/10.1016/S0140-6736(21)00592-4. Epub 2021 Jun 4.
49. Dimopoulos MA, Oriol A, Nahi H, et al. Daratumumab, lenalidomide, and dexamethasone for multiple myeloma. N Engl J Med. 2016;375:1319–31.
50. Miguel JS, Weisel K, Moreau P, et al. Pomalidomide plus low-dose dexamethasone versus high-dose dexamethasone alone for patients with relapsed and refractory multiple myeloma (MM-003): a randomised, open-label, phase 3 trial. Lancet Oncol. 2013;14:1055–66.
51. Attal M, Richardson PG, Rajkumar SV, et al. Isatuximab plus pomalidomide and low-dose dexamethasone versus pomalidomide and low-dose dexamethasone in patients with relapsed and refractory multiple myeloma (ICARIA-MM): a randomised, multicentre, open-label, phase 3 study. Lancet. 2019;394:2096–107.
52. Bergsagel DE. Total body irradiation for myelomatosis. Br Med J. 1971;2:325. https://doi.org/10.1136/bmj.2.5757.325-a.
53. Talamo G, Dimaio C, Abbi KK, et al. Current role of radiation therapy for multiple myeloma. Front Oncol. 2015;5:40. Published 2015 Feb 18. https://doi.org/10.3389/fonc.2015.00040.
54. Kumar S, Paiva B, Anderson KC, Durie B, Landgren O, Moreau P, Munshi N, Lonial S, Bladé J, Mateos MV, Dimopoulos M, Kastritis E, Boccadoro M, Orlowski R, Goldschmidt H, Spencer A, Hou J, Chng WJ, Usmani SZ, Zamagni E, Shimizu K, Jagannath S, Johnsen HE, Terpos E, Reiman A, Kyle RA, Sonneveld P, Richardson PG, McCarthy P, Ludwig H, Chen W, Cavo M, Harousseau JL, Lentzsch S, Hillengass J, Palumbo A, Orfao A, Rajkumar SV, Miguel JS, Avet-Loiseau H. International myeloma working group consensus criteria for response and minimal residual disease assessment in multiple myeloma. Lancet Oncol. 2016;17(8):e328–46. https://doi.org/10.1016/S1470-2045(16)30206-6.
55. LeBlanc R, Bergstrom DJ, Côté J, Kotb R, Louzada ML, Sutherland HJ. Management of myeloma manifestations and complications: the cornerstone of supportive care: recommendation of the Canadian Myeloma Research Group (formerly Myeloma Canada Research Network) consensus guideline consortium. Clin Lymphoma Myeloma Leuk. 2022;22(1):e41–56. https://doi.org/10.1016/j.clml.2021.07.028. S2152-2650(21)00311-6. Epub ahead of print. PMID: 34456159.

Chapter 12
Monoclonal Gammopathy of Undetermined Significance (MGUS) and Highlight on Monoclonal Gammopathy of Neurological Significance (MGNS)

Hadi Goubran, Vinita Sundaram, Julie Stakiw, and Mohamed Elemary

Abbreviations

CANOMAD	Chronic ataxic neuropathy with ophthalmoplegia, monoclonal gammopathy, cold agglutinins, and disialosyl ganglioside (anti-GD1b, anti-GT1b or anti-GQ1b) antibodies
CIDP	Chronic idiopathic demyelinating polyneuropathy
CRAB	Calcium, renal affection, anemia, and bone disease
DADS-M	Demyelinating symmetric neuropathy with monoclonal gammopathy
IMWG	International Myeloma Working Group
iSTOPMM	Iceland Screens, Treats or Prevents Multiple Myeloma
IVIG	Intravenous gamma globulins
KLoSHA	The Korean Longitudinal Study on Health and Aging
M protein	Monoclonal protein
MAG	Myelin-associated glycoprotein
MGNS	Monoclonal gammopathy of neurological significance

H. Goubran (✉) · J. Stakiw · M. Elemary
Saskatoon Cancer Centre and College of Medicine, University of Saskatchewan, Saskatoon, SK, Canada
e-mail: hadi.goubranmessih@saskcancer.ca; Julie.stakiw@saskcancer.ca; Mohamed.Elemary@saskcancer.ca

V. Sundaram
Saskatoon Cancer Centre, Saskatoon, SK, Canada
e-mail: Vinita.sundaram@saskcancer.ca

© The Author(s), under exclusive license to Springer Nature Switzerland AG 2022
G. Ragab et al. (eds.), *Paraproteinemia and Related Disorders*,
https://doi.org/10.1007/978-3-031-10131-1_12

MGRS	Monoclonal gammopathy of renal significance
MGUS	Monoclonal gammopathy of undetermined significance
MM	Multiple myeloma
PN	Peripheral neuritis
POEMS	Polyneuropathy, organomegaly, endocrinopathy, monoclonal protein, and skin changes syndrome
PROMISE	Predicting Progression of Developing Myeloma in a High-Risk Screened Population study in the United States
Py	Patient-year
sFLC	Serum free light chain
SPEP	Serum protein electrophoresis
WBLDCT	Whole-body low-dose CT scan

Introduction and Classification

Monoclonal gammopathy of undetermined significance (MGUS) is an incidental premalignant diagnosis that is characterized by the presence of a serum monoclonal protein less than 30 g/L noted on serum protein electrophoresis [SPEP], less than 10% plasma cells in the bone marrow and the absence of end-organ damage (defined by the acronym CRAB for hypercalcemia, renal insufficiency, anemia, or bone lesions) and lack of B-cell lymphoma or other diseases known to produce an M-protein [1, 2]. The term MGUS was coined in 1978, and the latest International myeloma working group (IMWG) classification of MGUS was updated in 2014 [3, 4].

A. Non-IgM monoclonal gammopathy of undetermined significance
• Serum monoclonal protein (non-IgM type) <30 g/L
• Clonal bone marrow plasma cells <10%
• Absence of end-organ damage such as CRAB
B. IgM monoclonal gammopathy of undetermined significance
• Serum IgM monoclonal protein <30 g/L
• Bone marrow lymphoplasmacytic infiltration <10%
• No evidence of anemia, constitutional symptoms, hyperviscosity, lymphadenopathy, hepatosplenomegaly, or other end-organ damage that can be attributed to the underlying lymphoproliferative malignancy
C. Light chain monoclonal gammopathy of undetermined significance
• Abnormal serum free light chain (sFLC) ratio (<0.26 or >1.65)
• Increased level of the appropriate involved light chain (increased κ FLC in patients with ratio >1.65 and increased λ FLC in patients with ratio <0.26). No immunoglobulin heavy chain expression on immunofixation
• Absence of end-organ damage such as CRAB or amyloidosis that can be attributed to the plasma cell proliferative disorder
• Clonal bone marrow plasma cells <10%
• Urinary monoclonal protein <500 mg/24 h

Despite the benign nature of MGUS, mounting data are associating MGUS with the development of organ dysfunction, specifically, the kidneys leading to monoclonal gammopathy of renal significance (MGRS) and the neurological system in the form of a monoclonal gammopathy of neurological significance (MGNS).

IMWG has delineated the risk factors for progression and management. A helpful risk stratification model created by Rajkumar et al. provides an absolute risk of progression at 20 years of 58% if all three risk factors are present, compared with 37% when two risk factors were present; 21% when one risk factor was present; and only 5% when none of the risk factors were present [5, 6].

MGUS-risk factors:

1.	Serum monoclonal protein level greater than or equal to 15 g/L (1.5 g/dL)
2.	Non-IgG MGUS
3.	Abnormal serum free light chain ratio

These risk factors and used to calculate the overall risk of progression of MGUS.

Low-risk MGUS	No risk factors
Low-intermediate risk MGUS	One risk factor
High-intermediate risk MGUS	Two risk factors
High-risk MGUS includes	All three factors

The significance of recognizing MGUS is essential due to the risk of progression to plasmacytic or lymphoproliferative malignancies at 1% per year in non-IgM MGUS, 1.5% in IgM MGUS, and 0.3% in light chain MGUS [7]. Furthermore, even though the prevalence of MGUS increased with advancing age, there is no evidence of an increase in the annual risk of progression to malignancy by age or the duration of MGUS [6].

Prevalence

A review of the literature shows that the prevalence rate of MGUS varies across the globe. The landmark study is a large population-based study in Olmsted County, MN, from January 1, 1995 to December 31, 2001, which obtained samples from 21,463 of the 28,038 residents above the age of 50 years [6]. MGUS was identified in 3.2% of this sample, and prevalence increased with an increase in age. This crude prevalence of MGUS was calculated in a predominantly white population. It showed a higher prevalence rate of MGUS in the general population than previous studies and showed a definite increase with advancing age. It also showed an increased prevalence in men as compared to women.

Racial/Ethnic Differences in Prevalence

A population-based study of 12,482 persons over the age of 50 years from the National Health and Nutritional Examination Survey revealed racial disparities in the prevalence of MGUS [8]. Previously documented increased incidence of Multiple Myeloma (MM) in Black Americans was attributed to the higher prevalence of MGUS [9]. The adjusted prevalence of MGUS was calculated as 3.7% for Black, 1.8% for Mexican, and 2.3% for White Americans. This study did show that the adjusted prevalence of MGUS varies depending on the geographical location in the United States. As expected, the prevalence increased with age for all racial groups, but there appeared to be an earlier age of onset for Black Americans. There is documentation of the increased prevalence of MGUS in various African populations [10–12].

The Japanese study on the Nagasaki population of 52,000 atomic bomb survivors, including 1000 diagnosed MGUS individuals, showed some exciting features. The effects of radiation did not increase the prevalence unless higher radiation exposure was before the age of 20 years [13]. An overall prevalence of 2.1% was lower than what had been observed in White and African populations.

A prospective epidemiological study on the Chinese population reported an overall prevalence of 2.73% [14]. This multicenter prospective study enrolled 1797 healthy subjects showed that the majority by different age groups was 1.19% in the age group of 41–50 years, 3.08% in those over 50 years, and 7.76% in the age group over 81 years [14]. Another more recent study on the Chinese population showed that the overall prevalence of MGUS was 1.11% (95% CI 1.02–1.18%) among participants aged ≥50 years and 2.57% (95% CI 2.22–2.98%) among those aged ≥70 years [15].

In a study of 3260 participants in Thailand, 1104 males (33.9%) and 2156 females (66.1%) were undertaken [16]. The median age was 57 years (range 50–93 years). The overall prevalence of MGUS was 2.3%, which is comparable to Japan.

The Korean Longitudinal Study on Health and Aging (KLoSHA) is a population-based prospective cohort comprised of individuals above the age of 65 years. The overall crude prevalence of MGUS was 3.1% [95% confidence interval (CI) = 1.8–4.4]. The age-adjusted and sex-adjusted prevalence rates in Korean elders aged 65 years or older were both estimated as 3.3% (95% CI = 2.0–4.6) [17]. It was unusual to find that IgA was the most common isotype of immunoglobulin (43%) in this study. However, the Korean myeloma registry reporting shows that IgG myeloma was diagnosed predominantly in their population [18].

In contrast to the slightly higher global prevalence, over 10 years, the Italian study analyzed the samples of patients of the Ospedale di Busto Arsizio, a district (provincial) general hospital. Furthermore, the serum protein electrophoresis used less sensitive methods of testing M protein on cellulose acetate membranes yielding a low prevalence rate of 0.3% [19].

One of the earliest studies done in southern Sweden on 70% of a population above 25 years reports a prevalence of MGUS of 0.9% [20]. A relatively lower prevalence rate could be due to the inclusion of younger age groups in the cohort.

Data from various studies using IMWG diagnostic criteria show approximately a twofold increase in prevalence in the black races compared to the white populations [21]. Chinese Japanese, Korean, and Thai studies have reported a less than white people prevalence rate. The Mexican ethnic group did show a prevalence, half of that seen in Caucasians [8, 10].

Therefore, there is considerable variability in MGUS prevalence data reported globally. The overall prevalence is influenced by the study design and sampling size and the demographic composition of the study cohorts. Data from the general population rather than inpatient clinics or hospitals are ideal for population-based screening studies. Epidemiological studies need to be population based to provide accurate prevalence rates, using defined criteria and standardized equipment.

Age and Sex

The global studies on the prevalence of MGUS show progressive increment in the prevalence rate with increased age. Kyle et al. published a large population-based study on residents of Olmsted County, Minnesota [6]. This study provided accurate epidemiological data for assessing the overall prevalence of MGUS. Serum samples obtained from 21,463 residents above 50 years were sent for serum electrophoresis with agarose gel and immunofixation. Due to the location, the demographic composition of the study cohort was predominantly White Americans.

In the age group 50–59, the total prevalence was 1.7, which increased to 3 in 60–69 years. In men above the age of 80 years, there was a fourfold increase to 8.3. After 85 years, there is a plateauing of the prevalence in men, a phenomenon observed in women only after the age of 90 years [6].

All the studies have shown the prevalence of MGUS increased in the male sex. On average, the prevalence of MGUS is 1.5 times higher in men than in women [21]. However, the rate in men is almost the same as that of women a decade older. The overall age-adjusted prevalence rate in men is 4% (95% CI, 3.5–4.4) while that of women in 2.7% (95% CI, 2.4–3.0) ($p < 0.001$) [6]. The fact that men are found to be 60% of patients with multiple myeloma (MM) in this community confirms these findings [22].

Immunoglobulins

Monoclonal proteins produced by the clonal plasma cells can produce immunoglobulins, heavy plus light chains, or light chains. The immunoglobulin type was IgG in 70% of the patients, IgA in 12%, and IgM in 15% [23].

IgD and IgE MGUS are relatively rare. However, biclonal gammopathy and triclonal gammopathy have also been reported. The light chain type was kappa in 61% and lambda in 39% [23].

Associations

The presence of monoclonal gammopathy is seen in proliferative lymphoplasmacytic clonal disorders and associated with various connective tissue disorders, neurological disease with peripheral sensorimotor neuropathies, motor neuron disease, myasthenia gravis, nemaline myopathy, ataxia telangiectasia, and POEMS (polyneuropathy, organomegaly, endocrinopathy, monoclonal protein, and skin changes) syndrome. Association with dermatological disease and endocrine disorders are numerous but may be coincidental [24]. In their study, Bida et al., 2009, obtained samples from 21,463 of the 28,038 enumerated residents in Olmsted County, Minnesota. They identified 605 cases of MGUS and 16,793 negative controls among 17,398 samples tested between 1975 and 2006, for a total of 422,663 person-years of observations. These diagnostic codes were analyzed to identify and confirm previously reported associations, adjusting for age, sex, and total person-year observation [24]. A significant association between MGUS and other disorders was noted in 14 (19%) of 75, including vertebral and hip fractures and osteoporosis. The authors had previously reported an increased frequency of osteoporosis and bone fractures in patients with MGUS, independent of progression to myeloma. In contrast, previously reported associations with certain infections or lupus were not reported [24].

Documentation of MGUS after renal, liver, heart, and autologous bone marrow transplantation may be attributed to immune suppression [25]. In addition, environmental factors may influence prevalence, such as exposure to toxins like asbestos, fertilizers, and pesticides [26]. Finally, a familial predisposition to MGUS is reported, with one study showing almost threefold increased risk of MGUS among first-degree relatives [27]. The presence of MGUS at a younger age has also been reported with Gaucher's disease [28].

Risk Stratification and Progression

The resources required to monitor MGUS in an increasingly aging population are substantial. Therefore, it is essential to follow evidence-supported algorithms of follow-up based on population prevalence and risk stratification with the risk factors, including the amount of M-protein, non-IgG MGUS, and abnormal free light chain ratios.

Risk Stratification

The risk stratification proposed by Rajkumar et al., 2005 is based on the number of risk factors present translating into a relative risk of progression [5]:

- No risk factors present: relative risk (1), Absolute risk of progression at 20 years (5%)
- Low/Intermediate (1 risk factor): relative risk (5.4), Absolute risk of progression at 20 years (21%)
- High/Intermediate (2 risk factors): relative risk (10.1), Absolute risk of progression at 20 years (37%)
- High: All three risk factors present: relative risk (20.8), Absolute risk of progression at 20 years (58%).

The resources required to monitor an increasingly aging population with a highly prevalent premalignant precursor are substantial. Therefore, evaluation of the impact on the health systems is essential. Outcomes of ongoing clinical trials, The Iceland Screens, Treats, or Prevents Multiple Myeloma (iSTOPMM) study, and the Predicting Progression of Developing myeloma in a High-Risk Screened Population (PROMISE) study in the United States should provide insight into the benefits and harms of screening for MGUS [29]. This knowledge should clarify whether the early detection of MGUS will affect the overall survival of MM and define strategies for high-risk populations.

The two primary biological subtypes are classified as IgM and non-IgM MGUS due to variations in the progression of the disease type. Progression in non-IgM results in MM, plasmacytomas, and amyloidosis. IgM MGUS is associated with a risk of progression to lymphoplasmacytic lymphoma or amyloidosis [13].

IgM MGUS

IgM MGUS typically arises from a CD20+ lymphoplasmacytic cell. The overall IgM MGUS prevalence from various studies is calculated at approximately 0.55% [30]. IgM MGUS is known to have better survival, and the vast majority progresses to lymphoplasmacytic lymphoma [31].

The overall risk of progression was approximately 1.5% per year. Therefore, investigations such as bone marrow studies and imaging were deferred when IgM was less than 1.5 g/L with no other abnormal indices [4].

Singh et al. observed that MGUS prevalence in Black Americans was almost double that of White patients at the Veterans Administration hospital [12]. IgM subtype was seen in 20% of the White Americans compared to 6.3% in Black.

Interestingly the study on Ghanese men revealed IgM prevalence was only 5.6% [10]. It was shown in these studies that the African populations do have a reduced progression to lymphoplasmacytic lymphoma.

Overall, IgM MGUS constitutes an increased proportion of MGUS in descendants of Western Europe [6]. However, it was not as high in the Swedish or Dutch populations [20, 32]. Moreover, Eastern European countries have reported a lower prevalence of IgM MGUS [33]. A similar lower IgM MGUS prevalence was observed in Japan, Spain and China [13, 34, 35].

Non-IgM MGUS

Non-IgM MGUS is considered a precursor to plasma cell malignancies. This group of immunoglobulin composes up to 85% of MGUS [4]. The category denotes IgG, IgA, IgD, and E, and as we have previously stated, the IgG is the most commonly diagnosed. The IgG and IgA subtype progress to MM and have shorter survival than the IgM MGUS [31, 36].

The IgD and IgE MGUS are documented but relatively rare [37, 38]. Biclonal gammopathy is seen in 3–6% of MGUS, while triclonal gammopathy is rare, and only 24 cases have been documented [35, 36].

Light Chain MGUS

Light chain MGUS has a prevalence of 0.8% of the predominantly Caucasian population [39]. The Olmsted County population over 50 years showed the age-standardized prevalence of light chain MGUS in men and women was 1.0% (95% CI, 0.8–1.2) and 0.6% (95% CI, 0.5–0.8), respectively [23, 25]. Of the total MGUS cases detected, light chain MGUS was seen in 19%. Renal impairment was present in 23% of light chain MGUS, which is confounding, as this elevates the serum free light chain kappa and lambda and may alter the kappa to lambda ratio. Overall, the light chain MGUS has a lower progression rate to MM, similar to low-risk MGUS with normal serum free light chain ratio.

Monoclonal Gammopathy of Renal Significance (MGRS)

In contrast to frank progression, monoclonal gammopathy of renal significance (MGRS) is a term that was first introduced by the International Kidney and Monoclonal Gammopathy Research Group (IKMG) in 2012 and may represent an association rather than progression [40]. It is an umbrella term that encompasses renal damage mediated directly or indirectly by monoclonal protein. It includes all B-cell/plasma cell clonal proliferative disorders not requiring immediate treatment of the clonal disease: MGUS, smoldering MM, smoldering Waldenström macroglobulinemia, low-grade chronic lymphatic leukemia, and low-grade non-Hodgkin lymphoma (marginal zone lymphoma, mantle cell lymphoma, and mucosa-associated lymphoid tissue lymphoma) [41]. MGRS has been estimated from previous observations at 10% of cases of MGUS, with a prevalence of 0.32% and 0.53% in people older than 50 years and 70 years, respectively [42, 43]. The topic of MGRS is discussed in Chap. 13.

Monoclonal Gammopathy of Neurological Significance (MGNS)

Despite the benign nature of MGUS, mounting data are associating MGUS with the development of organ dysfunction, specifically MGRS and affection of the neurological symptoms in the form of a monoclonal gammopathy of neurological significance (MGNS), which could be associated with substantial morbidity [44]. The association between MGUS and peripheral neuropathy (PN) was established in a population-based study in which the relative risk of PN was increased in individuals with MGUS, yet it may not be causal [24]. Monoclonal IgM paraproteinemia is more commonly associated with PN than IgG or IgA paraproteins which deposition can be difficult to distinguish from chronic idiopathic demyelinating polyneuropathy (CIDP) [45]. The diagnostic workup for a patient with PN and IgG/IgA MGUS should exclude other PN causes rather than prove the correlation. Such patients usually mimic the management of CIDP without paraproteinemia [46]. Therefore, MGNS refers to IgM-mediated PN.

MGNS is typically sensory rather than the motor and symmetrical in distribution and is length-dependent and slowly progressive. This clinical syndrome is known as distal acquired demyelinating symmetric neuropathy with monoclonal gammopathy (DADS-M), with half of the patients exhibiting an anti-myelin-associated glycoprotein (MAG) [44, 47]. Its progression is insidious in up to 50% of patients [47], reaching significant disability in10–15 years [48]. Rarely is it asymmetrical as in chronic ataxic neuropathy with ophthalmoplegia, monoclonal gammopathy, cold agglutinins, and disialosyl ganglioside (anti-GD1b, anti-GT1b, or anti-GQ1b) antibodies (CANOMAD). It is a rare condition characterized by asymmetrical PN, ataxia, ophthalmoplegia, and sometimes other cranial nerve involvement [49].

In addition to their routine lab work, these patients may need to be investigated by advanced imaging to assess the liver and spleen size and rule out any bone disease. Invasive testing with bone marrow, cerebrospinal fluid analysis, or nerve biopsies may also be needed in conjunction with electromyography and nerve conduction studies.

As the spectrum of MGNS is likely to keep expanding, more research is needed to understand and better define better its multiple clinical syndromes [44].

Overall, the treatment of MGNS represents a challenge as data on the treatment of MGNS is derived from few studies and case reports. Patients with DADS-M without anti-MAG antibodies seem to have lower response rates to immunomodulating therapies or plasma exchange than idiopathic CIDP, with combination chemoimmunotherapy being more effective than monotherapy in IgM-mediated PN [50]. In contrast, patients with CANOMAD may benefit from a combination of IVIG and rituximab [51]. Multicentric, prospective clinical trials exclusively focused on improving outcomes in patients with MGNS are therefore needed to address this evolving medical condition.

Comparison Between the Progression of Different Subclasses

When differentiating IgM MGUS from non-IgM MGUS and using paraproteinemia of >15 g/L and abnormal sFLC ratio as risk factors, the progression (at 20 years) was respectively [27]:

- No risk factors: 19 vs 07%
- One risk factor: 41 vs 20%
- Two risk factors: 55 vs 30%

In a study by Steiner et al. (2017), in 44/2935 (1.5%) patients, MGRS was diagnosed. In MGRS patients, significantly more progressions to MM were observed than in MGUS patients (18% vs. 3%; $P < 0.001$). MGRS patients showed a higher risk for progression with a median time to progression of 23 years for MGUS and 18.8 years for MGRS patients. The corresponding progression rate was 8.8 [7.2–10.7] per 1000 patient-years (py) for MGUS patients and 30.6 [15.3–61] for the MGRS group. Risk for progression within the first year after diagnosis was 1% [0.6–1.4] in the MGUS group and 10% [4–28] among MGRS patients.

Therefore, a significantly higher risk for progression to MM means MGRS patients should be monitored carefully and treated in a specialized center [43].

Progression of MGNS parallels the IgM-MGUS class.

Diagnosis

It is imperative to recognize that MGUS is a diagnosis of exclusion, with the primary diagnostic workup goal being to rule out other disorders.

The recent recommendations of the Myeloma Canada Research Network Consensus Guideline Consortium [52] proposed an initial assessment to confirm the diagnosis that includes:

Laboratory Assessment (Table 12.1 Illustrates the Routine Testing for all MGUS Patients)

Table 12.1 Laboratory tests needed for the assessment of patients with MGUS

• Complete blood count with white cell count
• Peripheral smear
• Serum calcium
• Albumin
• Creatinine clearance and/or serum creatinine
• Total serum protein and serum protein electrophoresis
• Immunofixation
• Serum free light chain assay
• 24 h total protein with urine protein electrophoresis and immune fixation
• Quantitative total immune globulin testing with IgA, IgM, IgG
• Hepatic and renal functions are assessed with additional tests done based on clinical presentation

Bone Marrow Examination

It should be offered to intermediate to high-risk patients with cytogenetic testing using FISH for t(4;14)(p16;q32), t(14;16)(q32;q23), del(17p13) be processed only if bone marrow plasma cells are more than 10%.

Imaging

Table 12.2 illustrates the imaging needed for patients with MGUS based on their risk stratifications [53, 54].

Table 12.2 Imaging investigations for patients with MGUS based on their type and risk factors

Low-risk MGUS	Consider skeletal survey by conventional radiology or whole-body low-dose CT (WBLDCT) scan or MRI or 18F FDG-PET/CT scan
Low and high intermediate High-risk MGUS	WBLDCT is the recommended tool Other tools offered if WBLDCT is unavailable [53, 54]
IgM-MGUS	Abdominal ultrasound and/or CT of the abdomen

Monitoring

Clinical assessment is needed in conjunction with laboratory testing and imaging to allow for proper monitoring of patients. Therefore, indefinite follow-up by a hematologist is not necessary. However, following initial investigations and follow-up, their family doctor could follow patients deemed stable by the hematologist [40].

Laboratory assessment should include general evaluations of hematologic, hepatic, and renal parameters to examine for features that are defining MM or conditions such as AL amyloidosis.

Low-risk MGUS (no risk factors present):

- Repeat CBC, calcium with albumin, SPEP, sFLC, and creatinine in 6 months.
  - If stable, repeat annually
- Bone marrow examination and skeletal survey are not required in the absence of symptoms.

Low-intermediate, high-intermediate, and high-risk MGUS; with >1 risk factor present:

- Repeat CBC, calcium with albumin, SPEP, sFLC, and creatinine in 6 months.
  - If stable, repeat annually
- Bone marrow examination, imaging, and more frequent monitoring may be clinically indicated based on suspicion of progression.

For all MGUS:

Periodic assessment of osteoporosis and related bone features to initiate timely and appropriate treatment as per clinical practice guidelines published by Osteoporosis Canada [55–57].

Conclusions

MGUS is an incidental premalignant condition identified in around 3% of the older population with an increased prevalence with age advancement. It is a diagnosis of exclusion, with the primary diagnostic protocol aims to rule out other disorders. The significance of recognizing MGUS is justifiable due to the risk of progression to plasmacytic or lymphoproliferative malignancies at 1% per year in non-IgM MGUS, 1.5% in IgM MGUS, and 0.3% in the light chain MGUS. It is also essential to be aware of the potential associations of MGUS with infections, immune and metabolic disorders. Establishing and adhering to an algorithm for monitoring is also needed to ensure that progression is diagnosed promptly.

Furthermore, it is crucial to identify patients with MGRS (Chap. 13), and those with MGNS as these entities will necessitate therapeutic interventions.

References

1. Rajkumar SV, Dimopoulos MA, Palumbo A, Blade J, Merlini G, Mateos MV, Kumar S, Hillengass J, Kastritis E, Richardson P, Landgren O, Paiva B, Dispenzieri A, Weiss B, LeLeu X, Zweegman S, Lonial S, Rosinol L, Zamagni E, Jagannath S, Sezer O, Kristinsson SY, Caers

J, Usmani SZ, Lahuerta JJ, Johnsen HE, Beksac M, Cavo M, Goldschmidt H, Terpos E, Kyle RA, Anderson KC, Durie BG, Miguel JF. International myeloma working group updated criteria for the diagnosis of multiple myeloma. Lancet Oncol. 2014;15(12):e538–48.
2. Kaseb H, Annamaraju P, Babiker HM. Monoclonal gammopathy of undetermined significance. [Updated 2020 Dec 14]. In: StatPearls [Internet]. Treasure Island: StatPearls Publishing; 2021.
3. Kyle RA. Monoclonal gammopathy of undetermined significance. Natural history in 241 cases. Am J Med. 1978;64(5):814–26. https://doi.org/10.1016/0002-9343(78)90522-3. PMID: 645746.
4. Kyle RA, Durie BG, Rajkumar SV, et al. Monoclonal gammopathy of undetermined significance (MGUS) and smoldering (asymptomatic) multiple myeloma: IMWG consensus perspectives risk factors for progression and guidelines for monitoring and management. Leukemia. 2010;24(6):1121–7. https://doi.org/10.1038/leu.2010.60.
5. Rajkumar SV, Kyle RA, Therneau TM, Melton LJ 3rd, Bradwell AR, Clark RJ, Larson DR, Plevak MF, Dispenzieri A, Katzmann JA. Serum free light chain ratio is an independent risk factor for progression in monoclonal gammopathy of undetermined significance. Blood. 2005;106(3):812–7. https://doi.org/10.1182/blood-2005-03-1038. Epub 2005 Apr 26. PMID: 15855274; PMCID: PMC1895159.
6. Kyle RA, Therneau TM, Rajkumar SV, Larson DR, Plevak MF, Offord JR, Dispenzieri A, Katzmann JA, Melton LJ 3rd. Prevalence of monoclonal gammopathy of undetermined significance. N Engl J Med. 2006;354(13):1362–9. https://doi.org/10.1056/NEJMoa054494. PMID: 16571879.
7. Kyle RA, Therneau TM, Rajkumar SV, et al. A long term study of prognosis of monoclonal gammopathy of undetermined significance. NEJM. 2002;346:564–9.
8. Landgren O, Graubard BI, Katzmann JA, et al. Racial disparities in the prevalence of monoclonal gammopathies: a population-based study of 12,482 persons from the National Health and Nutritional Examination Survey. Leukemia. 2014;28:1537–42.
9. Greenberg AJ, Vachon CM, Rajkumar SV. Disparities in the prevalence, pathogenesis and progression of monoclonal gammopathy of undetermined significance and multiple myeloma between blacks and whites. Leukemia. 2012;26(4):609–14. https://doi.org/10.1038/leu.2011.368.
10. Landgren O, Katzmann JA, Hsing AW, Pfeiffer RM, Kyle RA, Yeboah ED, Biritwum RB, Tettey Y, Adjei AA, Larson DR, Dispenzieri A, Melton LJ 3rd, Goldin LR, McMaster ML, Caporaso NE, Rajkumar SV. Prevalence of monoclonal gammopathy of undetermined significance among men in Ghana. Mayo Clin Proc. 2007;82(12):1468–73. https://doi.org/10.1016/S0025-6196(11)61089-6. PMID: 18053453.
11. Waxman AJ, Mink PJ, Devesa SS, et al. Racial disparities in incidence and outcome in multiple myeloma: a population-based study. Blood. 2010;116(25):5501–6. https://doi.org/10.1182/blood-2010-07-298760.
12. Singh J, Dudley AW Jr, Kulig KA. Increased incidence of monoclonal gammopathy of undetermined significance in blacks and its age-related differences with whites on the basis of a study of 397 men and one woman in a hospital setting. J Lab Clin Med. 1990;116:785–9.
13. Iwanaga M, Tagawa M, Tsukasaki K, Kamihira S, Tomonaga M. Prevalence of monoclonal gammopathy of undetermined significance: study of 52,802 persons in Nagasaki City, Japan. Mayo Clin Proc. 2007;82(12):1474–9. https://doi.org/10.1016/S0025-6196(11)61090-2. PMID: 18053454.
14. Ma L, Xu S, Qu J, et al. Monoclonal gammopathy of undetermined significance in Chinese population: a prospective epidemiological study. Hematol Oncol. 2019;37:75–9. https://doi.org/10.1002/hon.2548.
15. Han JH, Wang JN, Zhang YL, Cao XX, Zhou DB, Xu TD, Su W, Li J. Prevalence of monoclonal gammopathy of undetermined significance in a large population with annual medical check-ups in China. Blood Cancer J. 2020;10(3):34. https://doi.org/10.1038/s41408-020-0303-8. PMID: 32152278; PMCID: PMC7062721.
16. Watanaboonyongcharoen P, Nakorn TN, Rojnuckarin P, Lawasut P, Intragumtornchai T. Prevalence of monoclonal gammopathy of undetermined significance in Thailand. Int J Hematol. 2012;95(2):176–81. https://doi.org/10.1007/s12185-011-0995-4. Epub 2012 Jan 12. PMID: 22234527.

17. Park H-K, Lee K-R, Kim Y-J, Cho H-I, Eun Kim J, Woong Kim K, Jung Kim Y, Lee K-W, Hyun Kim J, Bang S-M, Lee J-S. Prevalence of monoclonal gammopathy of undetermined significance in an elderly urban Korean population. Am J Hematol. 2011;86:752–5. https://doi.org/10.1002/ajh.22095.
18. Kim SJ, Kim K, Kim BS, et al. Clinical features and survival outcomes in patients with multiple myeloma: analysis of web-based data from the Korean Myeloma Registry. Acta Haematol. 2009;122:200–10.
19. Malacrida V, De Francesco D, Banfi G, Porta FA, Riches PG. Laboratory investigation of monoclonal gammopathy during 10 years of screening in a general hospital. J Clin Pathol. 1987;40(7):793–7. https://doi.org/10.1136/jcp.40.7.793. PMID: 3114329; PMCID: PMC1141100.
20. Axelsson U, Bachmann R, Hällén J. Frequency of pathological proteins (M-components) om 6,995 sera from an adult population. Acta Med Scand. 1966;179(2):235–47. https://doi.org/10.1111/j.0954-6820.1966.tb05453.x. PMID: 4160039.
21. Wadhera RK, Rajkumar SV. Prevalence of monoclonal gammopathy of undetermined significance: a systematic review. Mayo Clin Proc. 2010;85(10):933–42. https://doi.org/10.4065/mcp.2010.0337. Epub 2010 Aug 16. PMID: 20713974; PMCID: PMC2947966.
22. Kyle RA, Gertz MA, Witzig TE, et al. Review of 1027 patients with newly diagnosed multiple myeloma. Mayo Clin Proc. 2003;78:21–33.
23. Kyle RA, Larson DR, Therneau TM, Dispenzieri A, Kumar S, Cerhan JR, Rajkumar SV. Long-term follow-up of monoclonal Gammopathy of undetermined significance. N Engl J Med. 2018;378(3):241–9. https://doi.org/10.1056/NEJMoa1709974. PMID: 29342381; PMCID: PMC5852672.
24. Bida JP, Kyle RA, Therneau TM, et al. Disease associations with monoclonal gammopathy of undetermined significance: a population-based study of 17,398 patients. Mayo Clin Proc. 2009;84(8):685–93. https://doi.org/10.1016/S0025-6196(11)60518-1.
25. Gagnon MF, Cardinal H, Emond JP, Latour M, Lemieux B. The evolution of monoclonal gammopathy of undetermined significance in kidney transplant recipients. Transplant Direct. 2019;5(10):e489. Published 2019 Sep 19. https://doi.org/10.1097/TXD.0000000000000937.
26. Landgren O, Kyle RA, Hoppin JA, Beane Freeman LE, Cerhan JR, Katzmann JA, Rajkumar SV, Alavanja MC. Pesticide exposure and risk of monoclonal gammopathy of undetermined significance in the Agricultural Health Study. Blood. 2009;113(25):6386–91. https://doi.org/10.1182/blood-2009-02-203471.
27. Clay-Gilmour AI, Kumar S, Rajkumar SV, Rishi A, Kyle RA, Katzmann JA, Murray DL, Norman AD, Greenberg AJ, Larson DR, O'Byrne MM, Slager SL, Vachon CM. Risk of MGUS in relatives of multiple myeloma cases by clinical and tumor characteristics. Leukemia. 2019;33(2):499–507. https://doi.org/10.1038/s41375-018-0246-2. Epub 2018 Sep 10. PMID: 30201985; PMCID: PMC6371786.
28. Weinreb NJ, Mistry PK, Rosenbloom BE, Dhodapkar MV. MGUS, lymphoplasmacytic malignancies, and Gaucher disease: the significance of the clinical association. Blood. 2018;131(22):2500–1.
29. ClinicalTrials.gov. Identifier NCT03689595. NCT03327597. https://clinicaltrials.gov/ct2/show/NCT03689595, https://clinicaltrials.gov/ct2/show/NCT03327597.
30. McMaster ML, Landgren O. Prevalence, clinical aspects, and natural history of IgM MGUS. Cytometry B Clin Cytom. 2010;78 Suppl 1(Suppl 1):S91–7. https://doi.org/10.1002/cyto.b.20550.
31. Kristinsson SY, Björkholm M, Andersson TM, et al. Patterns of survival and causes of death following a diagnosis of monoclonal gammopathy of undetermined significance: a population-based study. Haematologica. 2009;94(12):1714–20. https://doi.org/10.3324/haematol.2009.010066.
32. Ong F, Hermans J, Noordijk EM, Wijermans PW, Seelen PJ, de Kieviet W, Gerrits WB, Kluin PM, Kluin-Nelemans JC. A population-based registry on paraproteinaemia in the Netherlands. Comprehensive Cancer Centre West, Leiden, the Netherlands. Br J Haematol. 1997;99(4):914–20. https://doi.org/10.1046/j.1365-2141.1997.4943298.x. PMID: 9432042.

33. Vuckovic J, Ilic A, Knezevic N, Marinkovic M, Zemunik T, Dubravcic M. Prognosis in monoclonal gammopathy of undetermined significance. Br J Haematol. 1997;97(3):649–51. https://doi.org/10.1046/j.1365-2141.1997.1072923.x. PMID: 9207414.
34. Bergón E, Miravalles E. Retrospective study of monoclonal gammopathies detected in the clinical laboratory of a Spanish healthcare district: 14-year series. Clin Chem Lab Med. 2007;45(2):190–6. https://doi.org/10.1515/CCLM.2007.029. PMID: 17311507.
35. Lolin YI, Chow J, Wickham NW. Monoclonal gammopathy of unknown significance and malignant paraproteinemia in Hong Kong. Am J Clin Pathol. 1996;106:449–56.
36. Kyle RA, Rajkumar SV. Monoclonal gammopathy of undetermined significance. Br J Haematol. 2006;134(6):573–89. https://doi.org/10.1111/j.1365-2141.2006.06235.x. PMID: 16938117.
37. Bladé J, Kyle RA. IgD monoclonal gammopathy with long-term follow-up. Br J Haematol. 1994;88(2):395–6. https://doi.org/10.1111/j.1365-2141.1994.tb05037.x. PMID: 7803288.
38. Ayto RM, Lambert C, Lampert I, Salooja N. Monoclonal gammopathy of undetermined significance with an IgE paraprotein. Blood. 2007;110(11):4744. https://doi.org/10.1182/blood.V110.11.4744.4744.
39. Dispenzieri A, Katzmann JA, Kyle RA, Larson DR, Melton LJ 3rd, Colby CL, Therneau TM, Clark R, Kumar SK, Bradwell A, Fonseca R, Jelinek DF, Rajkumar SV. Prevalence and risk of progression of light-chain monoclonal gammopathy of undetermined significance: a retrospective population-based cohort study. Lancet (London, England). 2010;375(9727):1721–8. https://doi.org/10.1016/S0140-6736(10)60482-5.
40. Leung N, Bridoux F, Hutchison CA, Nasr SH, Cockwell P, Fermand JP, Dispenzieri A, Song KW, Kyle RA. International kidney and monoclonal gammopathy research group monoclonal gammopathy of renal significance: when MGUS is no longer undetermined or insignificance. Blood. 2012;120(22):4292–5. https://doi.org/10.1182/blood-2012-07-445304.
41. Leung N, Bridoux F, Batuman V, Chaidos A, Cockwell P, D'Agati VD, Dispenzieri A, Fervenza FC, Fermand JP, Gibbs S, Gillmore JD, Herrera GA, Jaccard A, Jevremovic D, Kastritis E, Kukreti V, Kyle RA, Lachmann HJ, Larsen CP, Ludwig H, Markowitz GS, Merlini G, Mollee P, Picken MM, Rajkumar VS, Royal V, Sanders PW, Sethi S, Venner CP, Voorhees PM, Wechalekar AD, Weiss BM, Nasr SH. The evaluation of monoclonal gammopathy of renal significance: a consensus report of the international kidney and monoclonal gammopathy research group. Nat Rev Nephrol. 2019;15(1):45–59. https://doi.org/10.1038/s41581-018-0077-4. Erratum in: Nat Rev Nephrol. 2019 Feb;15(2):121. PMID: 30510265; PMCID: PMC7136169.
42. Ciocchini M, Arbelbide J, Musso CG. Monoclonal gammopathy of renal significance (MGRS): the characteristics and significance of a new meta-entity. Int Urol Nephrol. 2017;49(12):2171–5. https://doi.org/10.1007/s11255-017-1594-y.
43. Steiner N, Göbel G, Suchecki P, Prokop W, Neuwirt H, Gunsilius E. Monoclonal gammopathy of renal significance (MGRS) increases the risk for progression to multiple myeloma: an observational study of 2935 MGUS patients. Oncotarget. 2017;9(2):2344–56. https://doi.org/10.18632/oncotarget.23412. eCollection 2018 Jan 5.
44. Castillo JJ, Callander NS, Baljevic M, Sborov DW, Kumar S. The evaluation and management of monoclonal gammopathy of renal significance and monoclonal gammopathy of neurological significance. Am J Hematol. 2021;96(7):846–53. https://doi.org/10.1002/ajh.26155.
45. Yeung KB, Thomas PK, King RH, et al. The clinical spectrum of peripheral neuropathies associated with benign monoclonal IgM, IgG and IgA paraproteinaemia. Comparative clinical, immunological and nerve biopsy findings. J Neurol. 1991;238(7):383–91.
46. Chaudhry HM, Mauermann ML, Rajkumar SV. Monoclonal gammopathy-associated peripheral neuropathy Latov N. Pathogenesis and therapy of neuropathies associated with monoclonal gammopathies. Ann Neurol. 1995;37(Suppl 1):S32-S42.hy: diagnosis and management. Mayo Clin Proc. 2017;92(5):838–50.
47. D'Sa S, Kersten MJ, Castillo JJ, et al. Investigation and management of IgM and Waldenstrom-associated peripheral neuropathies: recommendations from the IWWM-8 consensus panel. Br J Haematol. 2017;176(5):728–42.

48. Nobile-Orazio E, Meucci N, Baldini L, Di Troia A, Scarlato G. Long-term prognosis of neuropathy associated with anti-MAG IgM M-proteins and its relationship to immune therapies. Brain. 2000;123(Pt 4):710–7.
49. Willison HJ, O'Leary CP, Veitch J, et al. The clinical and laboratory features of chronic sensory ataxic neuropathy with anti-disialosyl IgM antibodies. Brain. 2001;124(Pt 10):1968–77.
50. Hospital MA, Viala K, Dragomir S, et al. Immunotherapy-based regimen in anti-MAG neuropathy: results in 45 patients. Haematologica. 2013;98(12):e155–7.
51. Loscher WN, Woertz A, Wallnofer M, Wanschitz JV, Luef G. Successful treatment of CANOMAD with IVIg and rituximab. J Neurol. 2013;260(4):1168–70.
52. Bergstrom DJ, Kotb R, Louzada ML, Sutherland HJ, Tavoularis S, Venner CP, Myeloma Canada Research Network Consensus Guideline Consortium. Consensus guidelines on the diagnosis of multiple myeloma and related disorders: recommendations of the Myeloma Canada Research Network Consensus Guideline Consortium. Clin Lymphoma Myeloma Leuk. 2020;20(7):e352–67. https://doi.org/10.1016/j.clml.2020.01.017. Epub 2020 Feb 4.
53. Go RS, Rajkumar SV. How I manage monoclonal gammopathy of undetermined significance. Blood. 2018;131:163–73.
54. Hillengass J, Usmani S, Rajkumar SV, et al. International myeloma working group consensus recommendations on imaging in monoclonal plasma cell disorders. Lancet Oncol. 2019;20:e302–12.
55. Van de Donk NW, Palumbo A, Johnsen HE, et al.; European Myeloma Network. The clinical relevance and management of monoclonal gammopathy of undetermined significance and related disorders: recommendations from the European Myeloma Network. Haematologica. 2014;99:984–996.
56. Berenson JR, Yellin O, Boccia RV, et al. Zoledronic acid markedly improves bone mineral density for patients with monoclonal gammopathy of undetermined significance and bone loss. Clin Cancer Res. 2008;14:6289–95.
57. Papaioannou A, Morin S, Cheung AM, et al.; Scientific Advisory Council of Osteoporosis Canada. 2010 clinical practice guidelines for the diagnosis and management of osteoporosis in Canada: summary. CMAJ. 2010;182:1864–1873.

Chapter 13
Monoclonal Gammopathy of Renal Significance: An Insight

James Barton, Waleed Sabry, and Hadi Goubran

Abbreviations

BM	Bone marrow
CBD	Cyclophosphamide, bortezomib, and dexamethasone
CG	Crystaloglobulin
CKD	Chronic kidney disease
Cryo GN	Cryoglobulinemic glomerulonephritis
CSH	Crystal storing histiocytosis
EM	Electron microscopy
FISH	Fluorescence in situ hybridization
FS	Fanconi syndrome
GFR	Glomerular filtration rate
GN	Glomerulonephritis
HDM	High dose melphalan
IF	Immunofluorescence
IKMG	International Kidney and Monoclonal Gammopathy Research Group
IMiD	Immunomodulatory drugs

J. Barton (✉)
Division of Nephrology, College of Medicine, University of Saskatchewan,
Saskatoon, SK, Canada
e-mail: james.barton@usask.ca

W. Sabry · H. Goubran
Saskatoon Cancer Centre and College of Medicine, University of Saskatchewan,
Saskatoon, SK, Canada
e-mail: Waleed.Sabry@saskcancer.ca; Hadi.goubranmessiha@saskcancer.ca

© The Author(s), under exclusive license to Springer Nature Switzerland AG 2022

G. Ragab et al. (eds.), *Paraproteinemia and Related Disorders*,
https://doi.org/10.1007/978-3-031-10131-1_13

IMWG	International Myeloma Working Group
LCPT	Light-chain proximal tubulopathy
LM	Light microscopy
mAB	Monoclonal antibody
MG	Monoclonal gammopathy
MGCS	Monoclonal gammopathy of clinical significance
MGRS	Monoclonal gammopathy of renal significance
MGUS	Monoclonal gammopathy of undetermined significance
MIDD	Monoclonal immunoglobulin deposition disease
MIg	Monoclonal immunoglobulin
MM	Multiple myeloma
MN	Membranous nephropathy
MP	Monoclonal protein
MPGN	Membranoproliferative GN
NS	Nephrotic syndrome
PGNMID	Proliferative glomerulonephritis and monoclonal immunoglobulin deposits
POEMS	Polyneuropathy, organomegaly, endocrinopathy, monoclonal protein, and skin changes syndrome
RAS	Renin angiotensin system
sFLCs	Serum free light chains
TMA	Thrombotic microangiopathy
WM	Waldenström macroglobulinemia

Introduction

Two categories of renal disorders are associated with monoclonal gammopathies [MG]. The first group occurs in the context of high tumor masses with the production of large amounts of monoclonal immunoglobulins, as in multiple myeloma (MM), resulting in the so-called myeloma cast nephropathy. The second group includes all renal disorders caused by a monoclonal immunoglobulin (MIg) secreted by a non-malignant or premalignant B-cell clone. Currently, it is referred to as a "monoclonal gammopathy of renal significance (MGRS)" [1].

Robert Kyle, in 1978, was the first to describe and classify monoclonal gammopathy of undetermined significance (MGUS). This premalignant condition (as described in Chap. 12) is present in patients who do not display any organ damage attributable to MIgs while presenting with a serum monoclonal immunoglobulin of less than 30 g/l and clonal bone marrow plasma cells of less than 10% [2].

Progression of MGUS to overt malignancy is signaled by the development of disease-specific features. Conversion to MM in patients with a plasma cell clone is indicated by the occurrence of one or more myeloma-defining events, including elevated calcium, renal impairment, anemia and bone disease (CRAB) [3]. In contrast, progression of a B-cell clone to Waldenström macroglobulinemia (WM) is characterized by anemia, thrombocytopenia, lymphadenopathy or organomegaly, blood hyperviscosity, neuropathy, cryoglobulinemia, and cold agglutinin disease [4].

The term MGRS was first introduced by the International Kidney and Monoclonal Gammopathy Research Group (IKMG) in 2012 [5]. It regrouped all renal disorders caused directly or indirectly by an MIg secreted by a non-malignant or premalignant B-cell clone and does not meet the criteria for overt MM or B-cell lymphoma [6]. It includes a broad spectrum of conditions that can only be determined by renal biopsy and encompasses old entities such as AL amyloidosis and the newly described lesions, proliferative glomerulonephritis with monoclonal Ig deposits, and C3 glomerulopathy with monoclonal gammopathy [5]. The IKMG redefined and revised the definition of MGRS and its related disorders in April 2017. MGRS became a broader term encompassing renal damage mediated directly or indirectly by monoclonal protein (MP). It, therefore, included all renal disorders associated with MIg in the context of plasma/B-cell-clonal proliferative disorders not requiring immediate treatment ranging from smouldering MM and smouldering WM to low-grade chronic lymphocytic leukemia and low-grade non-Hodgkin lymphomas (marginal zone lymphoma, mantle cell lymphoma, and mucosa-associated lymphoid tissue lymphoma) [7]. Due to its high morbidity, early recognition is crucial to improve outcomes [5].

Background

MGs refer to monoclonal immunoglobulin in the serum/urine as an immunoglobulin in its intact form or as free heavy or light chains. It is produced by an expanded clone of plasma cells or lymphoplasmacytic cells [7–9].

A small percentage of patients with renal impairment have MGUS at the initial presentation or detected later during their subsequent follow-up. A retrospective review of 5410 kidney biopsies showed that 2.5% had MIg deposition [10]. Typically, these patients with a small paraprotein in the serum and/or urine were labeled as having MGUS, as per the International Myeloma Working Group [IMWG] diagnostic criteria [2]. The pathophysiology of MGRS, described by IKMG, is direct through the deposition of an MIg in the renal tissue or indirect through complement activation mediating renal damage [7]. It results from the MIg unique physicochemical properties and does not relate to the tumor bulk per se [11].

This definition is, however, limited by the fact that patients with the renal-limited atypical hemolytic uremic syndrome (aHUS), thrombotic microangiopathy (TMA), MG and patients with C3 glomerulopathy (C3G) do not demonstrate MP deposition in the kidney, and some patients with MGRS lack an identifiable MP in serum [12, 13].

Epidemiology

Despite the increasing awareness of MGRS in recent years, there is still a gap between the actual incidence and the reported cases. The estimated prevalence of MGRS derived from previous observations is approximately 10% of cases of MGUS, with 0.32% and 0.53% in people older than 50 and 70 years, respectively [10, 14, 15]. As their renal function declines, patients with MGRS have worse renal survival than those without MGRS [16].

In 2020, Klomjit et al. identified patients with MG who had undergone a kidney biopsy from the medical records of the Mayo Clinic from 2013 to 2018. One hundred and sixty patients out of 6300 (2.5%) had undergone a diagnostic kidney biopsy. They reported that 64 out of 160 patients (40%) had an MGRS lesion. Light chain amyloidosis was the most common finding, accounting for nearly half of these lesions. Proteinuria ≥1.5 g/day, hematuria, and an elevated free light chain ratio increased the clinical likelihood of finding MGRS and the presence of such findings; a biopsy should be highly considered [17].

Another report from Latin America describes 27 patients from Chile, Argentina, Ecuador, and Uruguay. Half of the patients presented with a nephrotic syndrome and one-third required dialysis. When reviewing their pathology, proliferative glomerulonephritis with monoclonal immunoglobulin deposits was found in 33%, amyloidosis in 26% and monoclonal immunoglobulin deposition disease in 26%. IgG Kappa was the most identified MP in renal biopsies, and a paraprotein was detected in 67% of cases [18].

Few reports describe the clinical course and prognosis of MGUS patients on long-term immunosuppression following renal transplantation and the possible progression to MM or lymphoma.

Classification of MGRS

The spectrum of renal diseases in MGRS is vast. Its classification relies on the localization of renal lesions within the nephron, being either glomerular, tubular, or vascular, and the ultrastructural MIg deposits pattern [1]. Occasionally, no deposits can be identified, yet the changes seen are attributed to MIg [15]. Interestingly, the IKMG recommended referring to an MGRS-associated disease when the findings are confined to the kidney without an associated symptomatic tumor mass [7].

The type of renal lesion is governed by the MIg's innate structural and physicochemical characteristics rather than by the clone features that produced it [19].

Based on the findings of immunofluorescence studies, MGRS-associated lesions are initially separated by the presence or absence of MIg deposits in kidney biopsy samples. The ultrastructural characteristics of the deposits further subcategorize them into organized and non-organized. Organized deposits are further subdivided into fibrillary (which include the immunoglobulin-related amyloidosis and monoclonal fibrillary glomerulonephritis (GN)), microtubular (including immunotactoid GN and cryoglobulinemic GN type I and II) and inclusions or crystalline categories. In the absence of immunoglobulin deposits by electron microscopy, light-chain proximal tubulopathy (LCPT), crystal storing histiocytosis, and cryo crystaloglobulin GN are organized patterns. Monoclonal immunoglobulin deposition disease (MIDD), proliferative glomerulonephritis (PGNMID), and MIg deposits are identified as non-organized [7].

MP cannot be demonstrated in the kidney biopsy in certain thrombotic MGRS entities, supporting an indirect role for MP in their pathogenesis [20]. TMA associated with monoclonal gammopathy [13] and a miscellaneous group including C3 GN and polyneuropathy, organomegaly, endocrinopathy, monoclonal protein, and skin changes syndrome (POEMS) (Chap. 21) were provisionally added as subcategories to the non-immunoglobulin deposits, non-organized category of the classification scheme. It is postulated that the MIg act as an autoantibody to complement regulatory proteins, especially complement factor H, or as a stabilizer of C3 convertase resulting in a dysregulation of the alternative complement pathway with downstream complement activation and membrane attack complex formation damaging the kidney [21, 22] in C3 GN and TMA. Recent reports described an unusually high MG incidence in C3GN and TMA patients compared with the age-matched general population [21]. Vascular endothelial growth factors released by the clonal plasma cells in POEMS syndrome led to microangiopathic renal lesions. The classification relying on histological and ultrastructural findings is relevant from a pathology, diagnostic standpoint.

Renal parenchyma is broadly divided into three structural and functional compartments: glomerulus, tubulointerstitium, and vasculature. Monoclonal deposits in MGRS can, therefore, conceptually involve any or all of the compartments [10]. MGRS can also be classified based on the dominant site of monoclonal deposition [10, 15] (Fig. 13.1). This classification seems to be more pertinent from the clinical aspect. Both schemes, however, are commonly used together in clinical practice for better clinicopathological correlation [10].

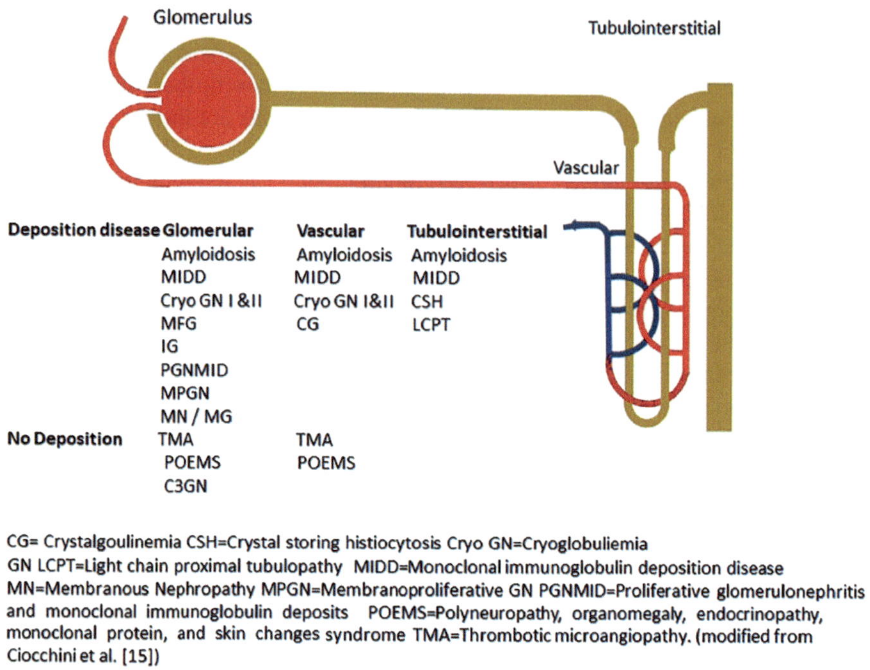

Fig. 13.1 Classification of MGRS based on the site of pathology and the presence or absence of deposits (Ciocchini et al. [15])

Clinical Presentation

MGRS presents with a broad clinical spectrum that ranges from proteinuria and hematuria to renal insufficiency and hypertension.

Clinically, the presentation depends on the dominant site of injury and is often slowly progressive. If the primary pathology targets the glomeruli, nephrotic syndrome (NS) is commonly noted as in amyloidosis and MIDD, whereas nephritic-nephrotic syndrome represents proliferative GN features. On the other hand, tubulointerstitial disorders usually present with tubular proteinuria, electrolyte abnormalities, with/without progressive renal insufficiency, metabolic acidosis, or Fanconi syndrome (FS) [20]. As expected, TMA presents with acute renal failure [6].

Progression

It was unclear if MGRS progresses more rapidly than non-IgM MGUS to a full MM with end-organ damage.

Steiner et al. (2017) identified 44 patients with MGRS from a cohort of 2935 patients with MGUS (1.5%). Significantly more progressions to MM were observed in the MGRS patient group than in the MGUS ones (18% vs. 3%; $P < 0.001$). MGRS' patients showed a higher risk and rate of progression with a rate of 30.6% and a median time to progression of 18.8 years for MGRS compared to only 8.8% and a median time to progression of 23 years for MGUS patients. Risk for advancement within the first year after diagnosis was ten times higher in the MGRS population. Therefore, a significantly higher risk for progression to MM means MGRS patients should be monitored carefully and treated in specialized centers [14].

From the renal perspective and with the decline of their renal functions, patients with MGRS have worse renal survival than those without MGRS [16].

Evaluation of Suspected MGRS

From a therapeutic and prognostic perspective, it is essential to distinguish MGRS-associated disorders from other acute or chronic kidney diseases (CKD) due to their different clinical characteristics and therapy [23, 24]. Furthermore, identifying any extrarenal involvement secondary to the MG is critical. The recognition of the presence of a POEMS syndrome would also be of crucial importance in the diagnostic workup.

A multidisciplinary approach is often needed to reach the proper diagnosis with nephrologists and hematologists, supported by heme and renal pathologists and, in some cases, cardiologists. The aim is to identify with certainty the clinicopathological evidence of MGRS-associated abnormalities from the renal perspective, identify B cell or plasma cell clonality from the hematological one, and document any extrarenal involvement that could alter the treatment strategy. Any discrepancy between MG and the MIg deposit in the renal biopsy specimen would argue against the diagnosis of MGRS [7].

Jain et al. (2019) suggested a four-step diagnostic approach in patients with MGRS after ruling out target-organ damage [10], which includes:

1. Renal biopsy for patients with MG associated with kidney disease, unexplained kidney disease and those with known risk factors for chronic kidney disease following an atypical clinical course. It is also recommended for patients with kidney disease and monoclonal gammopathy aged <50 years [7].

   Biopsy specimens should be processed for light microscopy (LM) and immunofluorescence (IF) using anti-IgG subclass fluorescence, and the demonstration of complement deposition (C3 with or without C1q) is also needed. Although the IKMG classification encourages but does not mandate the use of electron microscopy (EM), the information it provides can help identify non-organized deposits [7]. In some instances, one can obtain additional valuable information with protease immunofluorescence on kidney biopsy, renal amyloid typing by liquid chromatography or mass spectrometry.

Clinicians, however, will need to balance the risk of missing a diagnosis against those of the complications of the procedure. Biopsies from less-invasive sites (abdominal fat pad, gingival, or rectal) can successfully demonstrate amyloid deposits sparing the patients' risks of renal biopsy [25].

2. Identification of paraproteins in the serum and urine of patients suspected to have MGRS using serum protein electrophoresis demonstrating MG in the γ and/or α/β regions, immunoglobulin assay, and immunofixation and serum free light chains (sFLCs) assay. Serum/urine immunofixation electrophoresis is more sensitive than electrophoresis as it characterizes the type of MP [9]. The normal range for sFLCs ratio (k/λ ratio) is 0.26–1.65 in the context of normal renal functions. In contrast, the "renal range" of the sFLCs ratio has been defined as 0.37–3.17, with perturbations of these ratios pointing to monoclonality.
3. After establishing the presence of an MG and its correlation to the renal biopsy findings, the diagnostic approach should focus on the characterization of the underlying clonal population of cells based on the type of paraproteins. A plasma cell clone necessitates a confirmatory bone marrow (BM biopsy), whereas a lymphoplasmacytic clone necessitates a confirmatory biopsy from the BM or lymph nodes.

   Tissue specimens should be subjected to LM, immunostaining and flow cytometry, and the use of Congo red staining.

   A plasma cell clone is managed along with plasma cell disorders and MM. Flow cytometry or additional immunophenotyping help identify neoplastic plasma cells frequently showing aberrant loss of CD45 and CD19 and aberrant expression of CD56 and CD117; in addition to κ and λ light chains and CD38 helps identify small plasma cell clones. On the other hand, a B-cell/lymphoplasmacytic clone affects the therapeutic decision as it typically implies anti-CD20 antibodies in the treatment regimen. When the presence of B cells clones is suspected, identifying CD5 and CD20 bearing cells by immunophenotyping can separate small clones from polytypic cells. Immunohistochemistry might be helpful to the evaluation of focal atypical lymphoid infiltrates [7].

   Additionally, mutation testing may help identify the MYD88 L265P mutation found in over 90% of patients with lymphoplasmacytic lymphoma or Waldenström macroglobulinemia and only 40–60% of individuals with IgM MGUS [26–28]. Furthermore, FISH Cyclin D1, FISH with immunostaining for CD10, BCL2, and BCL6, can subclassify diffuse large cell lymphoma, and prognostic FISH panels for MM and chronic lymphocytic leukemia can also be helpful.
4. A full comprehensive assessment for any extrarenal involvement secondary to the MG is critical from a diagnostic, therapeutic, and prognostic perspective. For

example, cardiac involvement in AL amyloidosis confers a poor prognosis and necessitates urgent chemotherapy initiation to reduce the disease burden and reverse some patients' renal dysfunction [29]. Its multisystem involvement may also be a clue to the diagnosis [30]. Cryoglobulinemic GN Vasculitis is often associated with Raynaud's phenomenon, livedo reticularis, arthralgia, and peripheral neuropathy (Chap. 16) [31], whereas POEMS affects the sensory-motor system and leads to organomegaly, endocrinopathy, and skin affection (Chaps. 19 and 21) [32].

The careful ruling out of target organ damage associated with overt malignant paraproteinemias should precede this four-step approach to diagnose MGRS. Radiologic assessment using conventional radiology skeletal surveys and whole-body low-dose CT scans is often needed.

Treatment of MGRS

The ultimate aim of MGRS treatment is to preserve or improve organ function by targeting the MIg-producing plasma or B-cell clone. Although it is not an evidently malignant clone per se, current evidence strongly supports a clone-directed therapy strategy. The best results are possibly achieved when targeting the underlying MGUS clone induces the most profound hematologic response protecting the organ and preventing its damage [5, 33]. The isotype of the underlying clone in the BM (IgG, IgA, or LCs only versus IgM clone), the renal metabolism and potential renal and neurological toxicity of the therapeutic protocol will guide the treatment strategy [7].

Renal and Supportive Care

MGRS should be monitored and managed according to usual best practices, including, for example, thrombotic and infectious risk prevention in the case of nephrotic syndrome.

All patients with hypertension and/or proteinuria should be treated, preferably if renal functions allow with renin-angiotensin system inhibitors combined with salt restriction. Diuretics can be used with caution to treat hypertension or fluid retention [33]. Managing renal bone disease with a bisphosphonate is also suggested.

MGRS should not be considered a contraindication to renal transplantation, given the fact that the risk of patients dying from their clone is low. However, reducing the MIg by obtaining the best hematologic response is a critical issue in allograft survival [34].

Clone-Directed Therapy

In general, non-IgM clone-directed therapy is more in line with MM treatment with chemotherapy with or without a monoclonal antibody offered to induce a remission followed by autologous stem cell transplantation (ASCT) to be provided for eligible patients. IgM clones are addressed with the combination of monoclonal antibodies and specific chemotherapy.

MGRS with Plasma Cell Dyscrasia with IgG, IgA, or FLCs Only Clone

In the case of MGRS with an IgG, IgA, or FLC-only-producing plasma cell clone (non-IgM MGUS), therapy should be directed at eradicating the plasma cell clone with anti-myeloma agents while preserving kidney functions.

As in MM cases, patients with an IgG or an IgA clone should be stratified into transplant eligible (based on age and performance status) and non-eligible.

Transplant eligible patients would receive induction chemotherapy to reduce the tumor burden followed by stem cell collection and ASCT with melphalan as a conditioning agent before stem cell reinfusion. Interestingly, kidney disease is not a contraindication to ASCT and has no adverse effects on the quality of stem cell collection or their engraftment. ASCT is also possible in dialysis patients [35]. High rates of complete remission and very good partial response have been reported after treatment with bortezomib-based regimens and high dose melphalan (HDM) conditioned ASCT [36]. If the GFR is less than 40 mL/min, the melphalan dose should be reduced. Induction therapy prior to ASCT can be omitted in patients with a small clone, but is beneficial for patients with a poor performance status due to MGRS. The treatment-related mortality of ASCT is <1% [33].

The cornerstone induction therapy is a combination of proteasome inhibitors like bortezomib with dexamethasone. The agent has a non-renal metabolism and the most robust data in the treatment of MGRS. Bortezomib-containing regimens have demonstrated in MM patients a rapid reduction of tumor load and improved kidney functions [37]. Furthermore, the medication proved to be a highly effective drug in AL amyloidosis and seems to be the most effective agent in MIDD.

Immunomodulatory drugs (IMiD) such as thalidomide, lenalidomide, or pomalidomide are suitable alternatives in transplant non-eligible settings and relapsed cases. Lenalidomide, however, is secreted by the kidney, necessitating dose adjustment [38].

There are limited data on the use of daratumumab, an IgG1Κ human monoclonal antibody (mAb) that targets CD38 on the surface of cells in a variety of hematological malignancies, in patients with MGRS. The results of daratumumab-based therapy in 25 MGRS patients, 12 of whom were previously untreated, were recently published [39]. The hematologic response rate was 83% vs. 69% for previously untreated and treated, respectively. It was 91% vs. 64% when daratumumab was combined with conventional

MM treatments compared to daratumumab monotherapy. It seems, therefore, that daratumumab-based therapy is a new option for patients with MGRS [39].

In patients with MGRS and FLCs, AL (AH and ALH) amyloid deposits, a low-grade plasma cell clone, most often secreting γLC, are observed. The amyloid in AL is composed of monoclonal ALs, whereas it is composed of monoclonal AHs in AH, and ALH contains the entire immunoglobulin [34]. As the patients are often frail due to their cardiac involvement, treatment should be carefully adapted to achieve the best and most durable hematologic response. In patients with stage I and II cardiac diseases (based on New York Heart Association classification), a first-line treatment used to be based on melphalan and dexamethasone. In the last decade, bortezomib proved effective in those patients and increased hematologic and organ response rates [40, 41]. Selected eligible patients can benefit from ASCT. In patients with advanced CKD, cyclophosphamide may replace melphalan [34]. Based on small case series, the cyclophosphamide, bortezomib, and dexamethasone (CBD) regimen significantly reduces the early death rate in the poor prognosis patients with advanced heart disease [42].

In patients with rare MIDD, the therapeutic approach is based on consensus opinion as controlled studies are lacking. The IKMG recommended a bortezomib-based regimen followed by ASCT in eligible patients with low-grade renal disease. ASCT should only be offered to patients with advanced kidney disease if they are renal transplant eligible [34].

Observation alone is recommended in patients with type I cryoglobulinemia, with few systemic symptoms and a low-grade underlying plasma cell clonal proliferation. On the other hand, in patients with advanced disease and renal failure, bortezomib, cyclophosphamide, and/or thalidomide-based regimens should be used. In selected patients, HDM/ASCT may be considered [34] (Chap. 16).

In PGNMID with detectable MIg, monotypic glomerular deposits observed are the result of MIg deposition. Consequently, PGNMID invariably recurs after renal transplantation [43]. It seems, therefore, logical to follow patients with stage 1 and 2 CKD and mild proteinuria and consider CBD alone in non-eligible and CBD followed by HDM/ASCT in eligible patients with stage 1 and 2 and high-grade proteinuria and those with stage 3 and 4. In patients with stage 5 CKD who are candidates for renal transplantation, achieving a complete hematologic remission with chemotherapy and HDM/ASCT is a crucial goal. In contrast, in-patients ineligible for renal transplantation, the benefit of chemotherapy is highly questionable and conservative treatment should be recommended [34].

In patients with acquired FS—MGRS and crystal storing histiocytosis, steroids may be helpful. In contrast, for those with stages 1–3 CKD, chemotherapy should be considered to try to slow progression to ESRD. CBD or thalidomide-based regimens are the best options. Bendamustine may also be used. HDM/ASCT may be performed in selected nonresponding patients although the benefit of this strategy remains to be proven. Among patients with stages 4–5 CKD, only patients eligible for a renal allograft should be offered chemotherapy followed by HDM/ASCT.

In POEMS, where the etiology is related to growth factor production by the culprit clone, it is unknown if clonal-directed therapy can benefit. HDM/ASCT has shown long-term benefits with halting progressive neuropathy in some patients. On the other hand, in the novel, MGRS with isolated glomerular C3 deposits, autoantibody activity of the MIg against a complement alternative pathway regulatory protein is the central current hypothesis. Because the disease course is rapid, with a high risk of recurrence after renal transplantation, chemotherapy should be offered early [34].

MGRS with B-Cell Clone with IgM M-Paraprotein

IgM MGUS is less common, and there is little evidence supporting the choice of treatment in MGRS-related to IgM M-protein. Based on the limited studies in monoclonal gammopathy of neurological significance (MGNS) where the underlying BM clone is a CD20-expressing B-cell or lymphoplasmacytic one secreting IgM, clone-directed rituximab-based therapy would be the first choice of treatment [44].

Type II mixed cryoglobulins are composed of an MIg, usually an IgM k with a rheumatoid factor (RF) activity, associated with polyclonal immunoglobulin and reduced complement levels [34].

Most cases are associated with chronic hepatitis C virus infection. Other conditions include hepatitis B virus infection or autoimmune disorders implicating the presence of an underlying B-cell clone, most typically with less than 10% BM involvement. It progresses into overt lymphoid proliferation, usually a WM or a low-grade lymphoma, during follow-up [45]. Suppose the underlying etiology to the B clonal expansion is viral. In that case, antiviral therapy alone could be offered to stages 1 and 2 with mild proteinuria, whereas the approach of chemotherapy followed by HDM/ASCT, when applicable, should be provided to patients with advanced disease or those with end-stage renal disease eligible for allograft transplantation [34]. Preliminary reports suggest a beneficial effect of rituximab, including the effect in patients with or without a detectable B-cell clone [34, 46]. However, it seems reasonable to propose rituximab only to patients in whom an associated CD-20-positive B-cell clone can be demonstrated.

Rituximab can be combined with dexamethasone and cyclophosphamide or bendamustine with the last two medications necessitating dose adjustment in renal impairment [47, 48]. Figure 13.2 illustrates the algorithmic approach to diagnose and manage patients with MGRS.

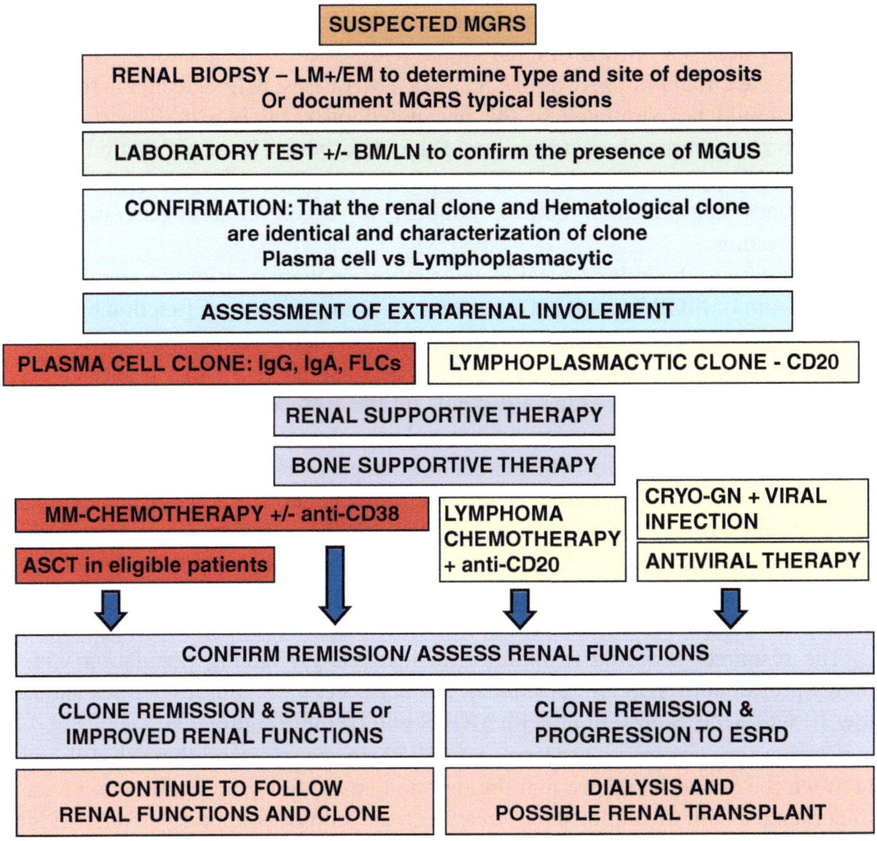

Fig. 13.2 Algorithmic approach for the confirmation of the diagnosis and the management of MGRS. *ASCT* Autologous stem cell transplantation, *BM* Bone marrow, *CRYO GN* Cryoglobulinemic glomerulonephritis, *EM* Electron microscopy, *ESRD* End-stage renal disease, *LM* Light microscopy, *LN* Lymph node, *MM* Multiple myeloma

Conclusions

Our understanding of the pathogenic property of MG and clonal expansions has grown significantly over the last few years. By their intrinsic physicochemical properties, MP can deposit in organs leading to their damage or induce a cascade of immune reactions resulting in the same effect. The umbrella term, monoclonal gammopathy of clinical significance (MGCS), has been coined to include various conditions attributed to these pathogenic proteins, including MGRS and MGNS. Many renal clinicopathological entities have been described in association with MGUS. MGRS was introduced to regroup all renal disorders caused by an MIg secreted by a non-malignant B-cell clone and does not meet the criteria for overt MM or B-cell proliferation.

The diagnosis of MGRS is established only by demonstrating monotypic immunoglobulin deposits on renal biopsy or showing evidence of pathology indirectly related to the circulating MIg as in C3 GN or TMA cases. MIg detected in the blood or BM should be correlated to the one noted on renal biopsy. The diagnostic approach rests on the characterization of the underlying clonal population of cells based on the type of paraproteins. Plasma cell dyscrasia with IgG, IgA, or FLCs-only clones can be identified in contrast to B-cell clones generating IgM M-paraproteins.

In addition to the kidney-specific and supportive therapy offered to patients, the ultimate aim of MGRS treatment is to preserve or improve organ function by targeting the organ-damaging plasma or B-cell clone producing the MIg. The best results are possibly achieved when targeting the underlying MGUS clone induces a deep hematologic response. Treatment depends on the isotype of the underlying clone, the renal metabolism and potential renal and neurological toxicity of therapy.

An approach similar to MM treatment strategies should be offered to patients with non-IgM MGRS, including ASCT in eligible patients. In contrast, chemotherapy combined with anti-CD20-based mAB should be provided to patients exhibiting a lymphoplasmacytic clone expressing B cells. More evidence-based data, however, are needed to solidify the treatment approaches and protocols.

MGRS is neither a contraindication to ASCT nor renal transplantation.

The resources required to monitor an increasingly ageing population with a highly prevalent MGUS are substantial. Furthermore, the resources to track and follow 10% of MGUS presenting with MGRS will be quite significant.

Despite the increasing awareness of MGRS in recent years, there is still a gap between the actual incidence and the reported cases. Early recognition is of great importance as timely administered treatment can stop or potentially reverse kidney disease. A multidisciplinary approach involving nephrologists, hematologists, and pathologists is often needed to establish the causative role of the M-protein in the pathogenesis of MGRS.

References

1. Javaugue V, Bouteau I, Sirac C, Quellard N, Diolez J, Colombo A, Desport E, Ecotière L, Goujon JM, Fermand JP, Touchard G, Jaccard A, Bridoux F. [Classification and therapeutic management of monoclonal gammopathies of renal significance]. Rev Med Interne. 2018;39(3):161–170. https://doi.org/10.1016/j.revmed.2017.03.012. Epub 2017 Apr 27. PMID: 28457684.
2. Kyle RA. Monoclonal gammopathy of undetermined significance. Natural history in 241 cases. Am J Med. 1978;64(5):814–26. https://doi.org/10.1016/0002-9343(78)90522-3.
3. Rajkumar SV, Dimopoulos MA, Palumbo A, Blade J, Merlini G, Mateos MV, Kumar S, Hillengass J, Kastritis E, Richardson P, Landgren O, Paiva B, Dispenzieri A, Weiss B, LeLeu X, Zweegman S, Lonial S, Rosinol L, Zamagni E, Jagannath S, Sezer O, Kristinsson SY, Caers J, Usmani SZ, Lahuerta JJ, Johnsen HE, Beksac M, Cavo M, Goldschmidt H, Terpos E, Kyle RA, Anderson KC, Durie BG, Miguel JF. International myeloma working group updated criteria for the diagnosis of multiple myeloma. Lancet Oncol. 2014;15(12):e538–48. https://doi.org/10.1016/S1470-2045(14)70442-5. Epub 2014 Oct 26. PMID: 25439696.

4. Dimopoulos MA, Gertz MA, Kastritis E, Garcia-Sanz R, Kimby EK, Leblond V, Fermand JP, Merlini G, Morel P, Morra E, Ocio EM, Owen R, Ghobrial IM, Seymour J, Kyle RA, Treon SP. Update on treatment recommendations from the fourth international workshop on Waldenstrom's macroglobulinemia. J Clin Oncol. 2009;27(1):120–6. https://doi.org/10.1200/JCO.2008.17.7865. Epub 2008 Dec 1. PMID: 19047284.
5. Leung N, Bridoux F, Hutchison CA, Nasr SH, Cockwell P, Fermand JP, Dispenzieri A, Song KW, Kyle RA. International kidney and monoclonal gammopathy research group monoclonal gammopathy of renal significance: when MGUS is no longer undetermined or insignificance. Blood. 2012;120(22):4292–5. https://doi.org/10.1182/blood-2012-07-445304.
6. Bridoux F, Leung N, Hutchison CA, Touchard G, Sethi S, Fermand JP, Picken MM, Herrera GA, Kastritis E, Merlini G, Roussel M, Fervenza FC, Dispenzieri A, Kyle RA, Nasr SH, International Kidney and Monoclonal Gammopathy Research Group. Diagnosis of monoclonal gammopathy of renal significance. Kidney Int. 2015;87(4):698–711. https://doi.org/10.1038/ki.2014.408. Epub 2015 Jan 21. PMID: 25607108.
7. Leung N, Bridoux F, Batuman V, Chaidos A, Cockwell P, D'Agati VD, Dispenzieri A, Fervenza FC, Fermand JP, Gibbs S, Gillmore JD, Herrera GA, Jaccard A, Jevremovic D, Kastritis E, Kukreti V, Kyle RA, Lachmann HJ, Larsen CP, Ludwig H, Markowitz GS, Merlini G, Mollee P, Picken MM, Rajkumar VS, Royal V, Sanders PW, Sethi S, Venner CP, Voorhees PM, Wechalekar AD, Weiss BM, Nasr SH. The evaluation of monoclonal gammopathy of renal significance: a consensus report of the international kidney and monoclonal gammopathy research group. Nat Rev Nephrol. 2019;15(1):45–59. https://doi.org/10.1038/s41581-018-0077-4. Erratum in: Nat Rev Nephrol. 2019 Feb;15(2):121. PMID: 30510265; PMCID: PMC7136169.
8. Hogan JJ, Weiss BM. Bridging the divide: an onco-nephrologic approach to the monoclonal gammopathies of renal significance. Clin J Am Soc Nephrol. 2016;11(9):1681–91. https://doi.org/10.2215/CJN.03160316.
9. Leung N, Barnidge DR, Hutchison CA. Laboratory testing in monoclonal gammopathy of renal significance (MGRS). Clin Chem Lab Med. 2016;54(6):929–37. https://doi.org/10.1515/cclm-2015-0994.
10. Jain A, Haynes R, Kothari J, Khera A, Soares M, Ramasamy K. Pathophysiology and management of monoclonal gammopathy of renal significance. Blood Adv. 2019;3(15):2409–23. https://doi.org/10.1182/bloodadvances.2019031914. PMID: 31409583; PMCID: PMC6693003.
11. Doshi M, Lahoti A, Danesh FR, Batuman V, Sanders PW, American Society of Nephrology Onco-Nephrology Forum. Paraprotein-related kidney disease: kidney injury from paraproteins-what determines the site of injury? Clin J Am Soc Nephrol. 2016;11(12):2288–94. https://doi.org/10.2215/CJN.02560316.
12. Chauvet S, Frémeaux-Bacchi V, Petitprez F, Karras A, Daniel L, Burtey S, Choukroun G, Delmas Y, Guerrot D, François A, Le Quintrec M, Javaugue V, Ribes D, Vrigneaud L, Arnulf B, Goujon JM, Ronco P, Touchard G, Bridoux F. Treatment of B-cell disorder improves renal outcome of patients with monoclonal gammopathy-associated C3 glomerulopathy. Blood. 2017;129(11):1437–47. https://doi.org/10.1182/blood-2016-08-737163. Epub 2017 Jan 9.
13. Ravindran A, Go RS, Fervenza FC, Sethi S. Thrombotic microangiopathy associated with monoclonal gammopathy. Kidney Int. 2017;91(3):691–8. https://doi.org/10.1016/j.kint.2016.09.045. Epub 2016 Dec 18.
14. Steiner N, Göbel G, Suchecki P, Prokop W, Neuwirt H, Gunsilius E. Monoclonal gammopathy of renal significance (MGRS) increases the risk for progression to multiple myeloma: an observational study of 2935 MGUS patients. Oncotarget. 2017;9(2):2344–56. https://doi.org/10.18632/oncotarget.23412. eCollection 2018 Jan 5.
15. Ciocchini M, Arbelbide J, Musso CG. Monoclonal gammopathy of renal significance (MGRS): the characteristics and significance of a new meta-entity. Int Urol Nephrol. 2017;49(12):2171–5. https://doi.org/10.1007/s11255-017-1594-y.
16. Shaik M, Al-Janadi A. Long term survival of monoclonal gammopathy of renal significance (MGRS): an analysis of Nhanes III. Blood. 2014;124:4849.
17. Klomjit N, Leung N, Fervenza F, Sethi S, Zand L. Rate and predictors of finding monoclonal gammopathy of renal significance (MGRS) lesions on kidney biopsy in patients with

monoclonal gammopathy. J Am Soc Nephrol. 2020;31(10):2400–11. https://doi.org/10.1681/ASN.2020010054. Epub 2020 Aug 3. PMID: 32747354.
18. Peña C, Schutz NP, Riva E, Valjalo R, Majlis A, López-Vidal H, Lois V, Zamora D, Ochoa P, Shanley C, Gonzalez JT, Fantl D, Correa G, Ramirez J, Mur P, Silva G, Verri V, Rojas C, Escobar K, Glavic G, Méndez GP, Grupo de estudio latinoamericano de mieloma múltiple (GELAMM). Epidemiological and clinical characteristics and outcome of monoclonal gammopathy of renal significance-related lesions in Latin America. Nephrology (Carlton). 2020;25(6):442–9. https://doi.org/10.1111/nep.13685. Epub 2019 Dec 19. PMID: 31825549.
19. Solomon A, Weiss DT, Kattine AA. Nephrotoxic potential of Bence Jones proteins. N Engl J Med. 1991;324:1845–51.
20. Sethi S, Rajkumar SV, D'Agati VD. The complexity and heterogeneity of monoclonal immunoglobulin-associated renal diseases. J Am Soc Nephrol. 2018;29(7):1810–23.
21. Ciocchini M, Musso CG. Which should be the correct treatment for monoclonal gammopathy of renal significance with complement alternative pathway dysregulation (C3 glomerulopathy and atypical hemolytic uremic syndrome): clone-directed or anticomplement therapy? Int Urol Nephrol. 2018;50(7):1365–6.
22. Lin M, Haas M. Paraprotein-associated thrombotic microangiopathy: expanding the spectrum of renal disease related to plasma cell dyscrasias. Kidney Int. 2017;91(3):532–4.
23. Chauvet S, Bridoux F, Ecotière L, Javaugue V, Sirac C, Arnulf B, Thierry A, Quellard N, Milin S, Bender S, Goujon JM, Jaccard A, Fermand JP, Touchard G. Kidney diseases associated with monoclonal immunoglobulin M-secreting B-cell lymphoproliferative disorders: a case series of 35 patients. Am J Kidney Dis. 2015;66(5):756–67. https://doi.org/10.1053/j.ajkd.2015.03.035. Epub 2015 May 16. PMID: 25987261.
24. Paueksakon P, Revelo MP, Horn RG, Shappell S, Fogo AB. Monoclonal gammopathy: significance and possible causality in renal disease. Am J Kidney Dis. 2003;42:87–95.
25. Merlini G, Wechalekar AD, Palladini G. Systemic light chain amyloidosis: an update for treating physicians. Blood. 2013;121(26):5124–30.
26. Kumar S, et al. International myeloma working group consensus criteria for response and minimal residual disease assessment in multiple myeloma. Lancet Oncol. 2019;17:e328–46.
27. Treon SP, et al. MYD88 L265P somatic mutation in Waldenström's macroglobulinemia. N Engl J Med. 2012;367:826–33.
28. Shanafelt TD, Ghia P, Lanasa MC, Landgren O, Rawstron AC. Monoclonal B cell; lymphocytosis (MBL): biology, natural history and clinical management. Leukemia. 2010;24:512–20.
29. Sayed RH, Wechalekar AD, Gilbertson JA, et al. Natural history and outcome of light chain deposition disease. Blood. 2015;126(26):2805–10.
30. Wechalekar AD, Gillmore JD, Hawkins PN. Systemic amyloidosis. Lancet. 2016;387 (10038):2641–54.
31. Sidana S, Rajkumar SV, Dispenzieri A, et al. Clinical presentation and outcomes of patients with type 1 monoclonal cryoglobulinemia. Am J Hematol. 2017;92(7):668–73.
32. Dispenzieri A. POEMS syndrome: 2017 update on diagnosis, risk stratification, and management. Am J Hematol. 2017;92(8):814–29.
33. Amaador K, Peeters H, Minnema MC, Nguyen TQ, Dendooven A, Vos JMI, Croockewit AJ, van de Donk NWCJ, Jacobs JFM, Wetzels JFM, Sprangers B, Abrahams AC. Monoclonal gammopathy of renal significance (MGRS) histopathologic classification, diagnostic workup, and therapeutic options. Neth J Med. 2019;77(7):243–54. PMID: 31582582.
34. Fermand JP, Bridoux F, Kyle RA, Kastritis E, Weiss BM, Cook MA, Drayson MT, Dispenzieri A, Leung N, International Kidney and Monoclonal Gammopathy Research Group. How I treat monoclonal gammopathy of renal significance (MGRS). Blood. 2013;122(22):3583–90. https://doi.org/10.1182/blood-2013-05-495929. Epub 2013 Oct 9. PMID: 24108460.
35. Yadav P, Cook M, Cockwell P. Current trends of renal impairment in multiple myeloma. Kidney Dis (Basel). 2016;1(4):241–57.

36. Cohen C, Royer B, Javaugue V, et al. Bortezomib produces high hematological response rates with prolonged renal survival in monoclonal immunoglobulin deposition disease. Kidney Int. 2015;88(5):1135–43.
37. Breitkreutz I, Heiss C, Perne A, et al. Bortezomib improves outcome after SCT in multiple myeloma patients with end-stage renal failure. Bone Marrow Transplant. 2014;49(11):1371–5.
38. Kintzel PE, Dorr RT. Anticancer drug renal toxicity and elimination: dosing guidelines for altered renal function. Cancer Treat Rev. 1995;21(1):33–64.
39. Kastritis E, Theodorakakou F, Roussou M, Psimenou E, Gakiopoulou C, Marinaki S, Gatou A, Fotiou D, Migkou M, Kanellias N, Eleutherakis-Papaiakovou E, Malandrakis P, Dialoupi I, Ntanasis-Stathopoulos I, Kostopoulos IV, Terpos E, Gavriatopoulou M, Dimopoulos MA. Daratumumab-based therapy for patients with monoclonal gammopathy of renal significance. Br J Haematol. 2021;193(1):113–8. https://doi.org/10.1111/bjh.17052. Epub 2020 Aug 23. PMID: 32829529.
40. Dubrey SW, Reece DE, Sanchorawala V, Hegenbart U, Merlini G, Palladini G, Fermand JP, Vescio RA, Bladé J, Heffner LT, Hassoun H, Liu X, Enny C, Ramaswami P, Elsayed Y, Van De Velde H, Mortimer S, Cakana A, Comenzo RL, Velcade Can2007 Study Group. Bortezomib in a phase 1 trial for patients with relapsed AL amyloidosis: cardiac responses and overall effects. QJM. 2011;104(11):957–70. https://doi.org/10.1093/qjmed/hcr105. Epub 2011 Jul 13. PMID: 21752867.
41. Kastritis E, Wechalekar AD, Dimopoulos MA, et al. Bortezomib with or without dexamethasone in primary systemic (light chain) amyloidosis. J Clin Oncol. 2010;28(6):1031–7.
42. Venner CP, Lane T, Foard D, et al. Cyclophosphamide, bortezomib, and dexamethasone therapy in AL amyloidosis is associated with high clonal response rates and prolonged progression-free survival. Blood. 2012;119(19):4387–90.
43. Nasr SH, Satoskar A, Markowitz GS, et al. Proliferative glomerulonephritis with monoclonal IgG deposits. J Am Soc Nephrol. 2009;20(9):2055–64.
44. Bergstrom DJ, Kotb R, Louzada ML, Sutherland HJ, Tavoularis S, Venner CP, Myeloma Canada Research Network Consensus Guideline Consortium. Consensus guidelines on the diagnosis of multiple myeloma and related disorders: recommendations of the myeloma canada research network consensus guideline consortium. Clin Lymphoma Myeloma Leuk. 2020;20(7):e352–67. https://doi.org/10.1016/j.clml.2020.01.017. Epub 2020 Feb 4.
45. Ferri C, Greco F, Longombardo G, et al. Association between hepatitis C virus and mixed Cryoglobulinemia. Clin Exp Rheumatol. 1991;9(6):621–4.
46. Dammacco F, Tucci FA, Lauletta G, et al. Pegylated interferon-alpha, ribavirin, and rituximab combined therapy of hepatitis C virus related mixed cryoglobulinemia: a long-term study. Blood. 2010;116(3):343–53.
47. Haubitz M, Bohnenstengel F, Brunkhorst R, Schwab M, Hofmann U, Busse D. Cyclophosphamide pharmacokinetics and dose requirements in patients with renal insufficiency. Kidney Int. 2002;61(4):1495–501.
48. Nordstrom BL, Knopf KB, Teltsch DY, Engle R, Beygi H, Sterchele JA. The safety of bendamustine in patients with chronic lymphocytic leukemia or non-Hodgkin lymphoma and concomitant renal impairment: a retrospective electronic medical record database analysis. Leuk Lymphoma. 2014;55(6):1266–73.

Chapter 14
Waldenström Macroglobulinemia

Mervat Mattar and Ali Bazerbachi

Abbreviations

alloHCT	Allogeneic hematopoietic cell transplant
anti-GM1	Anti-ganglioside M1
anti-MAG	Anti-myelin-associated globulin antibody
ARID1A	AT-rich interactive domain-containing protein 1A
ASO-PCR	Allele-Specific Polymerase Chain testing
BDR	Bendamustine, Dexamethasone, Rituximab
BR	Bendamustine, Rituximab
BTKi	Bruton tyrosine kinase inhibitors
CANOMAD	Chronic Ataxic Neuropathy Opthalmoplegia, IgM paraprotein, cold agglutinins, and disialosyl antibodies
CD	Cluster of differentiation
CXC4	Chemokine receptor type 4
CXCR4WT	Chemokine receptor type 4 wild-type gene
DRC	Dexamethasone, Rituximab, Cyclophosphamide
IG	Immunoglobulin
MGUS	Monoclonal gammopathies of undetermined significance
MLL2	Myeloid/lymphoid or mixed-lineage leukemia
MRR	Major response rate

M. Mattar (✉)
Clinical Hematology Unit, Kasr Alaini Faculty of Medicine, Cairo University, Cairo, Egypt

A. Bazerbachi
Department of Internal Medicine, American University of Beirut Medical Center, Beirut, Lebanon
e-mail: bazarbac@aub.edu.lb

© The Author(s), under exclusive license to Springer Nature Switzerland AG 2022

G. Ragab et al. (eds.), *Paraproteinemia and Related Disorders*,
https://doi.org/10.1007/978-3-031-10131-1_14

mSMARTt	Mayo Stratification of Macroglobulinemia and Risk-Adapted Therapy
MYD88L265*P*	Myeloid differentiation primary response gene mutation
MYD88^{WT}	Myeloid differentiation primary response gene wild-type
ORR	Overall response rate
PD-1	Programmed cell death protein 1
PFS	Progression-free survival
PI3Ki	Phosphatidylinositol 3-Kinase Inhibitor
R	Rituximab
VelR	Bortezomib-Rituximab
WM	Waldenström macroglobulinemia

Epidemiology

According to the American Surveillance, Epidemiology, and End Results Database, approximately 1000–1500 new WM cases are diagnosed every year in the United States with only 5% of African descent. At diagnosis, the median age is 63 years for blacks and 73 for whites with male/female ratio 1.6:1 [1, 2]. In the United Kingdom, the annual incidence of the disease is 10.3 per million [3]. A Japanese study reported a median age of 65 among 66 cases with a predominance of males (78.02%) [4].

WM is a chronic disease in most patients. The median survival has varied in studies, from 5 years to nearly 11 years [5].

Etiology

WM etiology is unknown. However, like in multiple myeloma (MM), a syndrome of IgM monoclonal gammopathy of undetermined significance (MGUS) may precede WM. Genetic predisposition has been noted with a positive family history of either WM or other lymphoproliferative disorders [6, 7].

The B-cell anti-apoptotic MYD88 L265P somatic mutation, where leucine is replaced by proline at position 265, is found in white blood cells in approximately 90% of WM cases. This causes overactivity of the altered MYD88 protein, stimulating the signaling molecules that activate nuclear factor-kappa-B [8].

Using sensitive Allele-Specific Oligonucleotide Polymerase Chain Reaction (ASO-PCR), it was found that MYD88 L265 was expressed in 93-97% of patients with WM and was identifiied in sorted malignant B cells and plasma cells [6, 7, 9]. Non-L265P MYD88 mutations were only present in 1–2% in WM [10].

Structural alterations on chromosome 3p can increase the allele burden of mutated MYD88 [11].

CXCR4 mutations are present in up to 40% of patients with WM, mostly co-expressing MYD88 mutations [12]. Cases with mutated CXCR4 experience less adenopathy, and those with nonsense CXCR4 mutations have increased bone marrow disease, higher serum IgM levels, and/or symptomatic hyperviscosity at presentation [13]. Inhibition of MYD88 causes apoptosis in both wild-type and mutated CXCR4-expressing WM cells, indicating a more critical role for mutated MYD88 survival signaling in WM [14].

Less common somatic genetic changes include variants in ARID1A, with increased disease burden, and variants in MLL2 [6].

Hepatitis C, hepatitis G, and human herpesvirus 8 have all been implicated, but no concrete data exists to link them to the disease [15].

Pathophysiology

Secretion of the IgM paraprotein by monoclonal B lymphoplasmacytic cells causes hyperviscosity. Serum viscosity is greater than water due to its protein content. Immunoglobulins are relatively large but also linear, unlike most serum proteins that are spherical in shape. When immunoglobulins pass through the serum, they spin around their longitudinal axis, increasing serum viscous drag, and therefore viscosity. IgM is pentameric and very large in size (970 kDa). Normal serum viscosity is 1.5–1.7 cP relative to water, and serum viscosity can increase with IgM levels of 3 g/dL or higher [16, 17].

Thus, paraprotein physical, chemical, and immunologic properties may cause hyperviscosity syndrome with coagulation abnormalities, including acquired Von Willebrand disease, types 1 and 2 cryoglobulinemia, cold agglutinin disease and anemia. Another consequence is the development of AL or AA amyloidosis.

Sensorimotor peripheral neuropathy may occur with the anti-myelin activity of IgM paraprotein. Tissue deposition of amorphous IgM in the skin, gastrointestinal tract, kidneys, and other organs is also seen. Besides IgM secretion, B-cell monoclonal lymphoplasmacytic cells also invade the bone marrow, spleen, and lymph nodes with rare extranodal involvement. This may contribute to cytopenias, mainly anemia and, to a lesser extent, thrombocytopenia. IgM paraprotein may also have rheumatoid factor and lupus anticoagulant activity [15].

Clinical Presentation

History

WM may be asymptomatic noted incidentally on a laboratory result. General symptoms such as weakness in 66% of cases, anorexia in 25%, weight loss in 17%, fever in 15%, and Raynaud phenomenon in 11% of cases may occur. Peripheral neuropathy was seen in 24% of cases. Central nervous system disturbances with disturbed consciousness and other neurologic deficits may either be due to infiltration, neuropathy, or hyperviscosity. The latter syndrome: manifests by bleeding diathesis, tinnitus, hearing loss, visual blurring, dizziness, or headache. Malabsorption or gastrointestinal bleeding may occur. Organomegaly causing abdominal swelling can also be noticed by the patient [18].

Physical Examination

The physical findings result from malignant B-cell infiltration, paraprotein increase with antigen-antibody reactions causing hyperviscosity, and derangement of the hemostatic system by the paraprotein, all of which contribute to the clinical manifestations [18], including hepatomegaly in 20%, splenomegaly in 19%, and lymphadenopathy in 15% of cases. Bleeding diathesis may occur with purpuric eruptions in 9% of cases and other hemorrhagic manifestations in 7% of cases.

Neurological deficits may manifest with slowly progressive neuropathy, distal symmetrical neuropathy, or chronic ataxic neuropathy (Miller-Fisher syndrome), a variant of Guillain-Barré syndrome which has been described with WM. [15] POEMS syndrome (polyneuropathy, organomegaly, endocrinopathy, M protein, and skin changes) (Chaps. 19 and 21) and Bing-Neel syndrome which involves infiltration of the central nervous system with neurological deficit have also been reported [18].

Ophthalmologic manifestations were detected in 19 out of 99 patients including flame-shaped hemorrhages, venous sausaging, papilledema, macular detachments, or central retinal vein occlusion in 16 patients; paraproteinemic keratopathy in 2; and a single case of CANOMAD syndrome (Chronic Ataxic Neuropathy Ophthalmoplegia, IgM paraprotein, Cold Agglutinins Disialosyl antibodies) [19].

Skin manifestations include purpura, bullous, nodular or papular skin lesions, chronic urticaria or Raynaud phenomenon. Vasculitic lesions, Livedo reticularis, or acrocyanosis may also be noted [18] (See Figs. 14.1, 14.2, and 14.3).

Other rare manifestations include pulmonary nodules or masses, parenchymal infiltrates, pleural effusion, periorbital masses, or osseous lesions. Congestive heart failure may ensue and may be amyloidosis related [18].

Complications

Complications of WM include diarrhea and malabsorption with gastrointestinal involvement, renal disease, amyloidosis of the heart, kidney, liver, lungs, and joints. Bleeding manifestations develop secondary to platelet dysfunction as well as coagulation factors and fibrinogen abnormalities due to interaction with plasma IgM

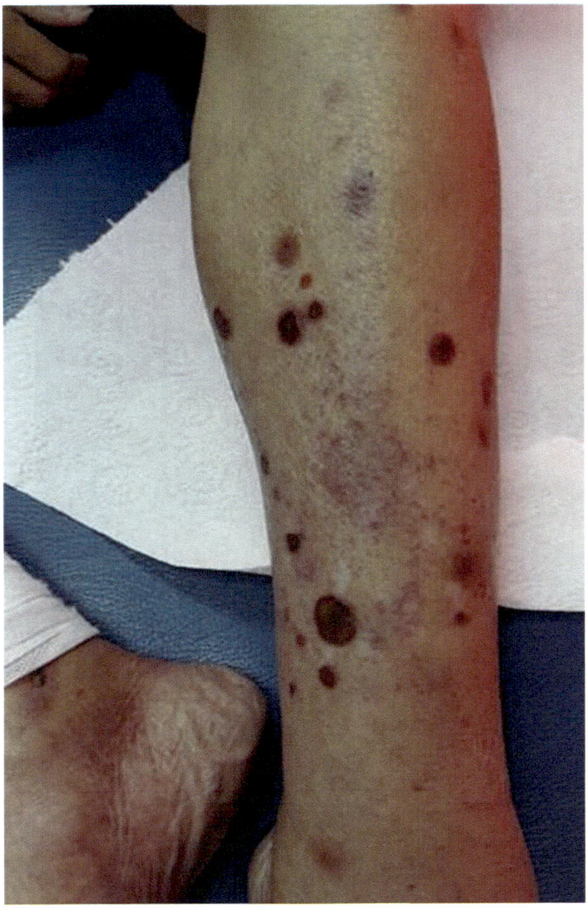

Fig. 14.1 A 50-year-old male, case of WM presenting with anemic manifestations, abdominal discomfort, and swelling with progressive weight loss. Legs showed vasculitic skin ulcers

and B-cell dysfunction which also lead to increased incidence of infections. Increased incidence of lymphomas, myelodysplasia, and leukemias is also seen [15].

Diagnosis

Diagnosis of WM includes history, physical exam, essential and other complimentary investigations [20–22]. Family history for WM and other B-cell lymphoproliferative disorders is important. Physical examination and a review of systems with funduscopic examination are all mandatory.

Laboratory investigations include complete blood count for possible findings of plasmacytoid lymphocytes, normocytic normochromic anemia, rouleaux formation,

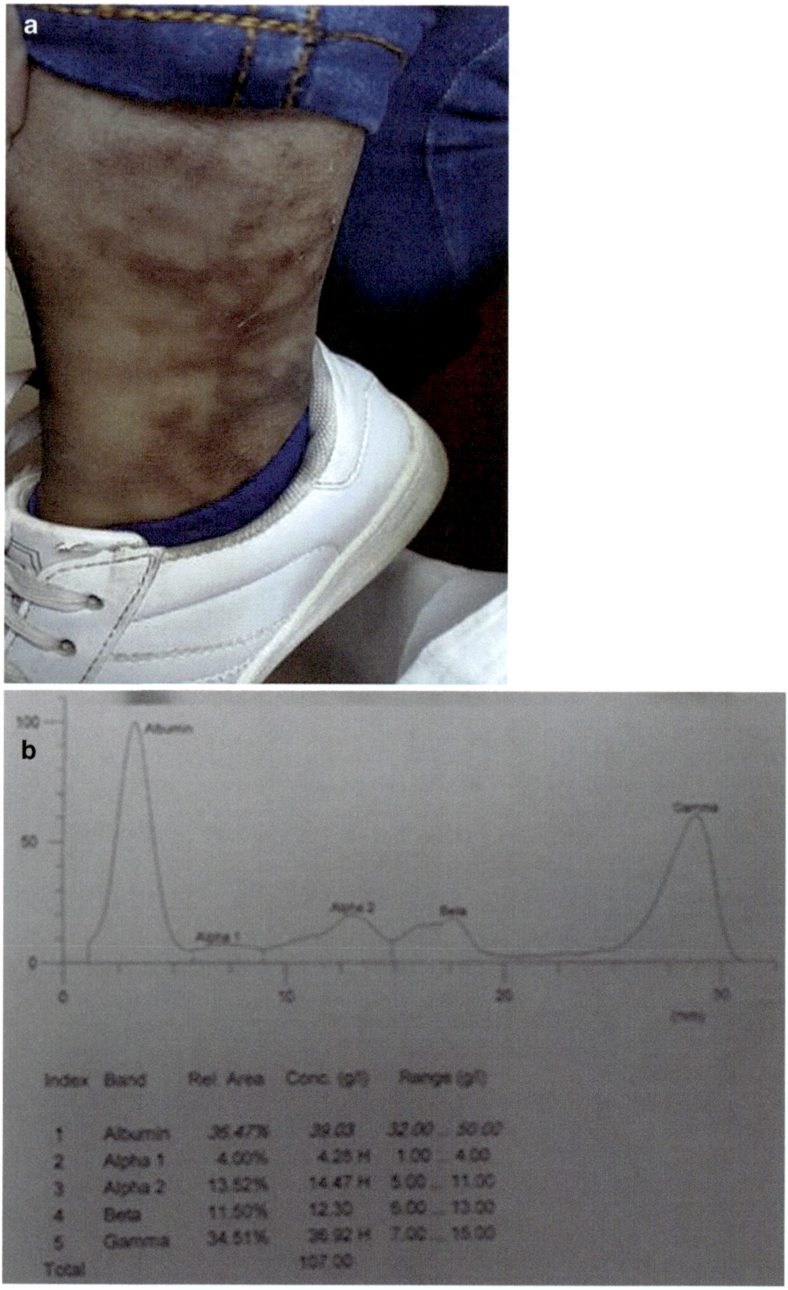

Fig. 14.2 WM with monoclonal band on plasma protein electrophoresis (**a**), IgM level of 4100 mg/dL, and serum viscosity of 4.1 cP. Reticulated skin lesions of livedo reticularis of the extremities were noted (**b**). Patient received multiple plasmapheresis sessions followed by Bendamustine/Dexamethasone/Rituximab. (**c**) shows plasma protein electrophoresis response following therapy

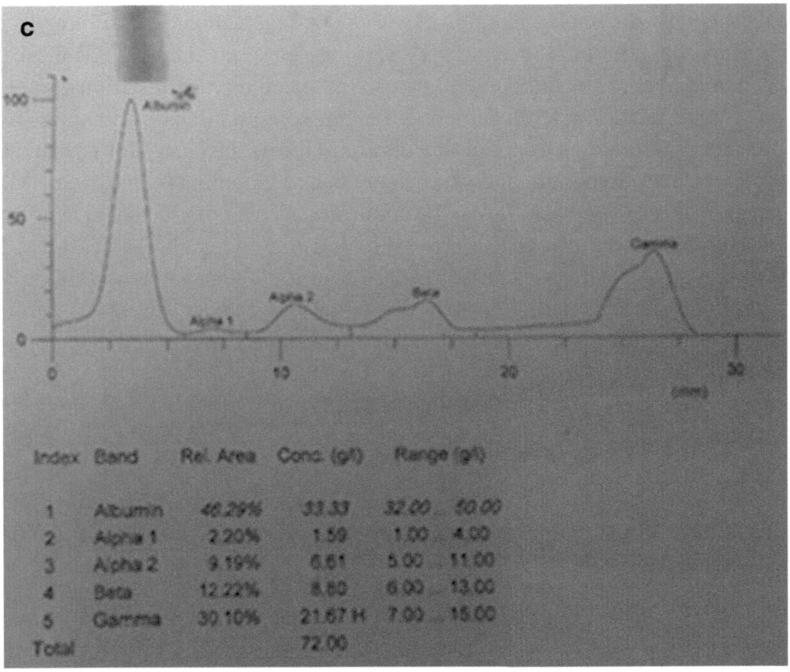

Fig. 14.2 (continued)

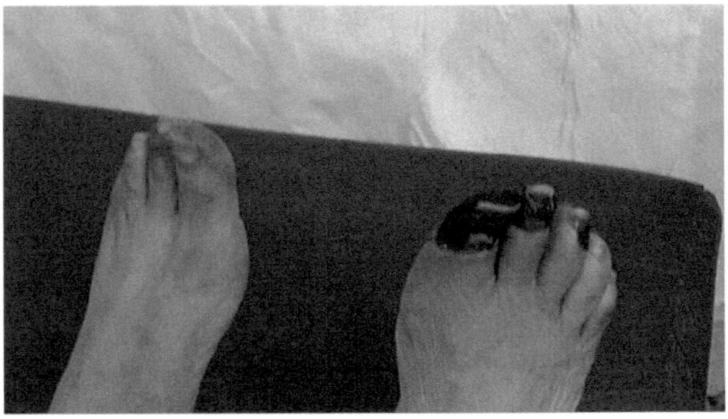

Fig. 14.3 Right foot of a 60-year-old male presenting splenomegaly and acrocyanosis with bluish gangrenous toes seen more on the right foot. WM was diagnosed with IgM level of 3800 mg/dL. IgM was estimated under warm conditions as cryoglobulins were also detected

neutropenia in some patients, and thrombocytopenia. Serum and urine electrophoresis with immunofixation and quantitative serum immunoglobulin levels (IgA, IgG, IgM) establish monoclonality. IgM heavy chain and type of light chain assay (usually Kappa subtype) are also required. IgM estimation should be repeated in warm conditions if cryoglobulinemia is detected.

Complications and risk of WM can be assessed by serum Beta-2-microglobulin level, 24-h urinary protein quantification. Cryoglobulin estimation, direct antiglobulin test for warm and cold antibodies, cold agglutinin titer and serum viscosity are needed especially if symptomatic. IgM level >4000 mg/dL mandates serum viscosity testing. Hepatitis B and C as well as HIV serology are needed to exclude these virological causes of cryoglobulinemia. In cases with bleeding manifestations, screening for coagulation factors and von Willebrand factor is required. N-terminal pro-b-type natriuretic peptide, cardiac troponins are also required as surrogates for possible amyloidosis. An electromyogram, anti-myelin-associated globulin antibody (anti-MAG), anti-ganglioside M1 (anti-GM1) may be abnormal in cases of associated neuropathy.

Bone marrow aspiration and biopsy showing intertrabecular monoclonal lymphoplasmacytic infiltrate is observed in >10% in a nodular, interstitial/nodular, or polymorphous pattern with possible detection of Dutcher bodies (perinuclear deposits of IgM). Congo red stain is done if amyloidosis is suspected with confirmatory fat pad aspirate.

Bone marrow immunohistochemistry and flow cytometry tests will show expression of surface IgM, CD19, CD20, CD22 (dim), CD25, and CD27 and negative expression of CD5, CD10, CD23, and CD103. Cytogenetic and molecular studies for establishment of (*MYD88L265P*) and (CXC4) gene mutations may be done.

Radiological investigations include computed tomography to detect organomegaly and lymphadenopathy. PET-CT may be helpful for follow-up of therapy [20–22].

Differential Diagnosis

Differential diagnosis includes [23]:

1. IgM monoclonal gammopathy of undetermined significance (MGUS) with high IgM but <3 g/dL and <10% bone marrow infiltration.
2. Smouldering WM (sWM) an asymptomatic type with a high IgM level >3 g/dL and bone marrow lymphocytoplasmic infiltration >10% .
3. Type 2 cryoglobulins, cold agglutinin hemolytic anemia, neuropathy, and amyloidosis may be associated with raised serum IgM with or without bone marrow lymphoplasmacytic infiltration. Lymphadenopathy or organomegaly, however, are uncommon.
4. Overt MM will be associated with bone or renal problems, usually IgG or IgA gammopathy type with >10% plasma bone marrow infiltration and no MYD88 mutation.
5. Chronic lymphocytic leukemia is characteristically associated with lymphadenopathy and/or splenomegaly. Peripheral and marrow lymphocytosis is evident. Immunophenotyping shows CD5, CD23 positivity. Auto-immune features may be present.
6. Mantle cell lymphoma shows a peculiar monomorphous small- to medium-sized lymphocyte appearance with irregular nuclei. The cells are usually CD5-positive, CD23 negative, with t(11,14) (q13,q32) and cyclin D1.
7. Marginal zone lymphoma involves lymph node or extra nodal site infiltration. Bone marrow usually shows a nodular non-paratrabecular lymphoplasmacytic pattern. MYD 88 mutation may be positive in 5–10% of cases.

Prognosis

The median survival for younger patients exceeds 10 years. For elderly patients, the median survival is shorter, but a significant proportion will die due to causes unrelated to the underlying WM [24]. Many prognostic scores have been devised trying to adapt treatment decisions in order to attain a survival benefit balanced to drug toxicity. Comparison of different prognostic scores is depicted in Table 14.1.

Table 14.1 Prognostic scoring for WM (Adapted from [24–32])

Southwest Oncology Group Prognostic Score [24]	Revised International Prognostic Score System for WM [25]	Mayo Clinic Prognostic Score [26]	Independent predictors of progression [27–32]
Stage A Low Rrisk Beta2 microglobulin <3 mg/dL and Hb >12 g/dL 5-year overall survival 87% Stage B Medium risk Beta2 microglobulin <3 mg/dL + Hb < 12 G/dL 5-year survival 63% Stage C Medium risk Beta2 microglobulin > 3 mg/dL and IgM <40 g/L 5-year survival 53% Stage D High risk Beta 2 microglobulin >3 mg/dL and IgM >40 g/L 5-year survival 21%	Risk factors • Age: • ≤65 years, 0 points • 66–75 years, 1 point • ≥76 years, 2 points • Beta2-microglobulin > 4 mg/L: 1 point • LDH >250 IU/L (upper limit of normal < 225 IU/L): 1 point • Serum albumin <3.5 g/dL: 1 point Risk Score 0 points very low risk (10-year OS = 84%) • 1 point low risk (10-year OS = 59%) • 2 points intermediate risk (10-year OS = 37%) • 3 points high risk (10 year OS = 19%) • 4–5 points very high risk (10-year OS = 9%)	Age >65 years organomegaly No risk factors 10 year OS = 57% Any risk factor 10 year OS = 16% > 1 risk factor 10 year OS = 5%	• IgM ≥ 4500 mg/dL • Bone marrow, lymphoplasmacytic infiltration ≥70% Diffuse infiltration rather than nodular infiltration • Beta2-microglobulin ≥4.0 mg/dL • Serum albumin ≤3.5 g/day Mutational status Wild-type MYD88 + additional mutations, MYD88 mutation + Wild type CXCR4 Better response to Ibrutinib Soluble PD-1 ligands

CXCR4wt CXC4:chemokine receptor type 4 wild-type, *IgM*: Immunoglobulin M, *LDH*: lactic acid dehydrogenase, *MYD88*: Myeloid differentiation primary response gene mutation, *Os*: overall survival, *PD-1*: Programmed cell death protein 1, *WM*: Waldenström macroglobulinemia

When to Treat WM?

The most common indications for treatment are represented by peripheral cytopenias due to bone marrow infiltration (mostly anemia with hemoglobin <10 g/dL or platelet count<100,000/cm), constitutional symptoms, bulky lymphadenopathies or splenomegaly, symptoms and signs due to the paraprotein (mainly hyperviscosity, peripheral neuropathy, symptomatic cryoglobulinemia, amyloidosis, and cold agglutinin disease), nephropathy or amyloidosis [20, 33].

Watchful waiting in asymptomatic cases is advised with monitoring without intervention every 3 months for clinical evaluation and laboratory studies including serum immunoglobulin levels [21]. Yearly funduscopic examination is recommended in all WM patients with serum IgM levels ≥3000 mg/dL [34].

How to Treat WM?

Treatment of Hyperviscosity

Hyperviscosity syndrome usually occurs when serum viscosity is 4.4 cP or above with IgM of >4000 mg/dL, being a clinical emergency. Immediate management is the removal of IgM by daily 3–4 L of total plasma exchange sessions with replacement by albumin. A single plasma exchange reduces viscosity by 20–30% [35] as approximately 75% of IgM is intravascular [36]. Blood warmers should be considered during apheresis if cryoglobulins are present [37]. Avoidance of blood and plasma transfusion is advised so as not to further increase viscosity. Daily sessions are repeated until normal serum viscosity is reached and symptoms are better. This should be followed by definitive therapy.

Definitive First-Line Therapy

Combinations of rituximab with either an alkylator, nucleoside analogs, or proteasome inhibitor-based, or Bruton tyrosine kinase (BTK) inhibitor-based therapy are the most commonly used frontline therapies [23].

Primary therapy with Dexamethasone/Rituximab/Cyclophosphamide (DRC) yielded an overall response rate (ORR) of 83% with 3-year progression-free survival (PFS) of 45%, and a median time to next treatment of 51 months [29]. Retreatment with a rituximab-based regimen achieved the second response rate of 82%. Transformation to diffuse large B-cell lymphoma occurred in 10% and myelodysplasia in 3% [29]. The 8-year and estimated 10-year overall survival (OS) were 64% and 53%, respectively [30]. This regimen may be recommended in patients with low disease burden [31].

Bendamustine-Rituximab combination was found to be comparable to Dexa/Rituximab/Cyclophosphamide with similar reductions in IgM, and activity independent of *MYD88*^{L265P} status [32] but with better median time to best response (6.1 vs. 11 months, respectively) [33]. Bendamustine-Rituximab therapy is well tolerated and has durable responses in relapsed/refractory cases [34, 35].

Maintenance rituximab had a higher major response rate (MRR) (97 vs. 68%) with superior PFS and OS [36]. However, a 2-year rituximab maintenance was not of better benefit post Bendamustine-Rituximab [37].

The combination of bortezomib, dexamethasone, and rituximab (VelDR) showed an ORR (Overall Response Rate) of 96%, MRR of 83%, and CR of 22%, respectively [38]. Peripheral neuropathy was the most common adverse event. Novel less neurotoxic proteasome inhibitors have also been tried including Carfilizomib (in non-cardiac patients) [39] and oral Ixazomib [40] and Oprozomib [41].

Single-agent rituximab has been advised by mSMART (Mayo Stratification of Macroglobulinemia and Risk-Adapted Therapy) in cases of Hb < 11 g/dL, Platelets <120,00/cmm, hemolysis, or cryoglobulinemia [42].

Plasmapheresis may still be needed if a paradoxical increase in monoclonal protein levels occurs after starting rituximab therapy, the so-called rituximab flare [43]. Initial rituximab therapy is associated with an increase in serum IgM concentrations in 30–70% of patients. Peak IgM was observed at a mean of 4 weeks, ranging from 1 to 8 weeks, from the start of rituximab use and may persist for up to 4 months. Thus, the use of rituximab is recommended only when the serum IgM level is <4000 mg/dL [44, 45].

Ibrutinib is an oral irreversible inhibitor of Bruton kinase which gives the best responses observed in cases with *MYD88*^{L265P} and *CXCR4*^{WT} mutations [46, 47]. It may be used to treat Bing-Neel syndrome, as it can cross the blood–brain barrier [48]. Oral ibrutinib was tried in Rituximab-resistant cases. ORR and MRR were achieved in 90% and 71%, respectively. Response rates were similar in individuals with MYD88^{L265P} and MYD88^{WT}. Median PFS was not reached at the median follow-up (18.1 months), and OS was 97% at 18 months [49] with positive impact on quality of life. Hematologic, gastrointestinal, and infectious side effects along with cardiac arrhythmias are possible side effects. An ibrutinib-rituximab combination [50], second- and third-generation Bruton kinase inhibitors Acalabrutinib [51] and Zanubrutinib [52] were also tried.

Venetoclax, an oral BCL2 inhibitor, at a maximum dose of 800 mg daily, demonstrated an ORR and major response rates of 87% and 80%, respectively [53]. The median time to response was 1.9 months, but a slower response was noted in 16 patients (52%) previously treated by BTK inhibitors. No tumor lysis syndrome or IgM flares were observed, and cytopenias and diarrhea were the most common adverse events.

Idelalisib, a (Phosphatidylinositol 3-Kinase Inhibitor PI3Ki) was tried in combination with obinutuzumab (anti-CD20 antibody) in patients with Relapsed/Refractory WM [54] with an ORR of 90% after a median follow-up of 18.3 months. It is noteworthy that 96% of the patients had *MYD88* mutation. Hepatotoxicity of

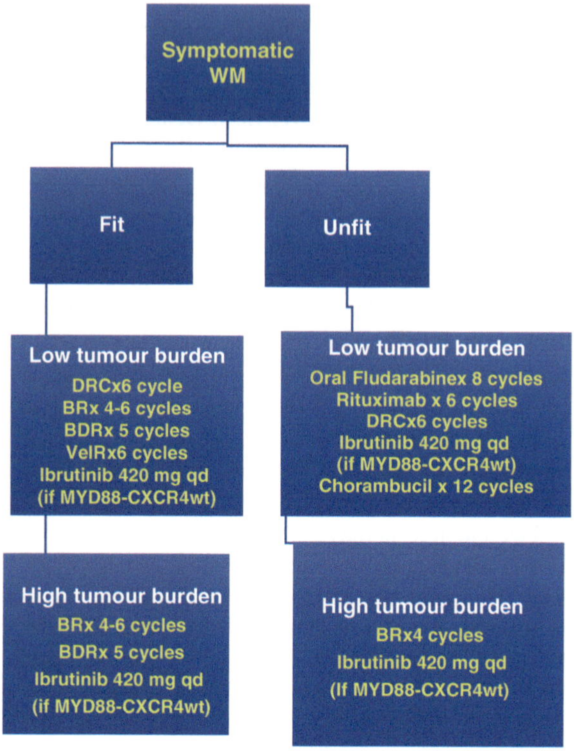

Fig. 14.4 First-line treatment of symptomatic WM (Adapted from [60]). *BDR* Bendamustine/dexamethasone/rituximab, *BR* Bendamustine/rituximab, *CXCR4wt* CXC4:chemokine receptor type 4 wild-type, *DRC* Dexamethasone/rituximab/cyclophosphamide, *MYD88* Myeloid differentiation primary response gene mutation, *VelR* Bortezomib/rituximab, *WM* Waldenström macroglobulinemia

Idelalisib was lower with use of other PI3K inhibitors, such as duvelisib and umbralisib (TGR- 1202), which are still being evaluated in WM [55, 56].

Ulocuplumab is a fully human IgG4 monoclonal antibody which inhibits the binding of *CXCR4* to *CXCL12*, resulting in decreased WM cell proliferation [57]. It is being combined with ibrutinib in a phase 1/2 clinical trial for symptomatic patients who have *CXCR4*^{MUT} [58]. Mavorixafor is an oral small molecule the non-competitive antagonist of chemokine receptor *CXCR4* small molecule, currently under trial [59]. Figure 14.4 demonstrates first-line treatment algorithm.

Role of Stem Cell Transplant in WM

Autologous and allogeneic hematopoietic cell transplants (alloHCT) are less commonly used to treat patients with WM. This may be used for long-term disease control and prevention of hyperviscosity syndrome. After alloHCT, 46% of 144 cases achieve progression-free survival 5 years, with a relapse rate of 24% [59].

Response Criteria

The term complete response indicates full disappearance of symptoms and signs including non-detection of lymphadenopathy and organomegaly. Laboratory investigations should demonstrate normal serum and urine immunofixation on two separate occasions, 6 weeks apart, normal serum IgM level, and no lymphocytic infiltration of bone marrow. Very good partial response denotes complete disappearance of symptoms, signs, lymphadenopathy, organomegaly, and at least 90% reduction in serum IgM. Partial response with at least 50% reduction in adenopathy and organomegaly, with no new signs or symptoms of active disease and 50–90% reduction in serum monoclonal IgM is less promising. Cases with minor response may suffer new symptoms or signs of active disease with only 25–50% reduction in serum monoclonal IgM. Major response includes complete response, very good partial response or partial response [61].

Worse cases are those with progressive disease with worsening of anemia, thrombocytopenia, or leukopenia, and more adenopathy or organomegaly or increase in symptoms attributed to WM with two measurements showing at least 25% increase in serum monoclonal IgM. Stable disease neither meets the criteria for minor response nor progressive disease [61].

Treatment of Relapsed WM

Treatment depends on the duration of the first response. Early relapses require introduction of new agents while late relapses may benefit from the same first-line regimens (see Fig. 14.5).

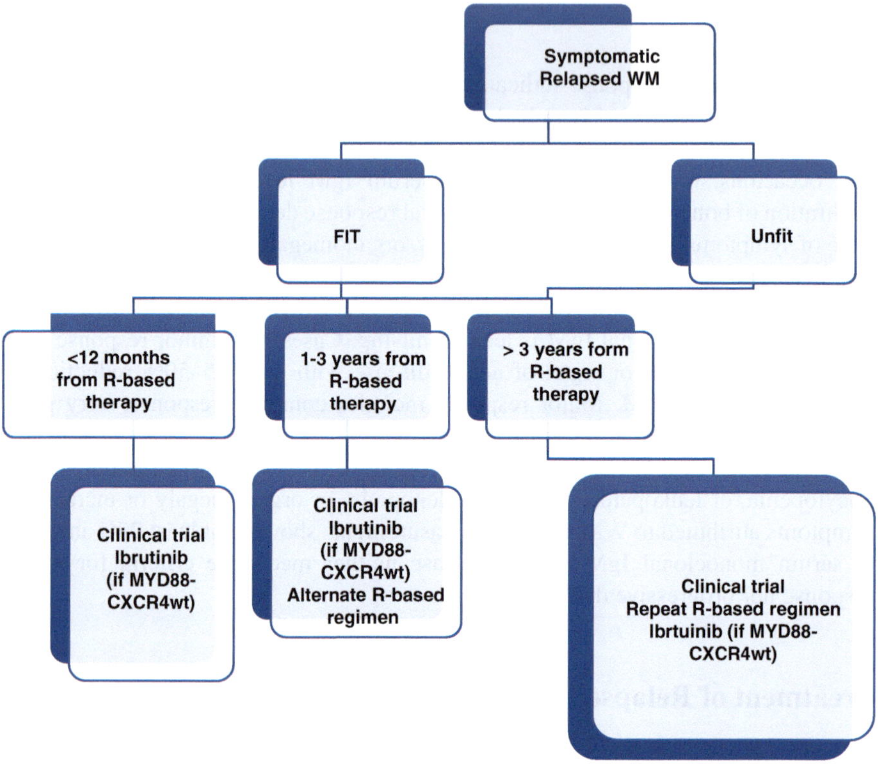

Fig. 14.5 Treatment of relapsed WM (Adapted from [60]). *CXCR4wt* CXC4:Chemokine receptor type 4 wild-type, *MYD88* Myeloid differentiation primary response gene mutation, *R* Rituximab, *WM* Waldenström macroglobulinemia

Conclusion

WM is a clonal B-cell lymphoproliferative disorder with many clinical aspects. Overactivity of the altered MYD88 protein, stimulating the signaling molecules that activate nuclear factor-kappa-B can be detected in 93–97% of cases. Physical findings include hepatomegaly, splenomegaly, lymphadenopathy, purpura, ocular, and neurological as well as skin manifestations along with hyperviscosity syndrome.

Treatment includes plasmapheresis for hyperviscosity together with combination chemo/immunotherapy. Stem cell transplant is less commonly used in WM.

References

1. Yun S, Johnson AC, Okolo ON, Arnold SJ, McBride A, et al. Waldenström macroglobulinemia: review of pathogenesis and management. Clin Lymphoma Myeloma Leuk. 2017;17(5):252–62.
2. Sekhar J, Sanfilippo K, Zhang Q, Trinkaus K, Vij R, Morgensztern D. Waldenström macroglobulinemia: a surveillance, epidemiology, and end results database review from 1988 to 2005. Leuk Lymphoma. 2012;53(8):1625–6.
3. Wang H, Chen Y, Li F, Delasalle K, Wang J, Alexanian R, et al. Temporal and geographic variations of Waldenstrom macroglobulinemia incidence: a large population-based study. Cancer. 2011;118:3793.
4. Zou H, Yang H, Liao Z-X. Serum markers in the differential diagnosis of Waldenstrom macroglobulinemia and other IgM monoclonal gammopathies. J Clin Lab Anal. 2019;33:e22827. https://doi.org/10.1002/jcla.22827.
5. Morel P, Duhamel A, Gobbi P, Dimopoulos MA, Dhodapkar MV, et al. International prognostic scoring system for Waldenstrom macroglobulinemia. Blood. 2009;113:4163–70.
6. Xu L, Hunter ZR, Yang G, Zhou Y, Cao Y, et al. MYD88 L265P in Waldenströ̈m macroglobulinemia, immunoglobulin M monoclonal gammopathy, and other B-cell lymphoproliferative disorders using conventional and quantitative allele-specific polymerase chain reaction. Blood. 2011;21:2051–20583.
7. Gustine J, Meid K, Xu L, Hunter Z, Castillo J, Treon SP. To select or not to select? The role of B-cell selection in determining the MYD88 mutation status in Waldenstrom macroglobulinemia. Br J Haematol. 2017;176:822–4.
8. Treon SP, Xu L, Hunter Z. MYD88 mutations and response to ibrutinib in Waldenstrom's macroglobulinemia. N Engl J Med. 2015;373:584–6.
9. Varettoni M, Arcaini L, Zibellini S, Boveri E, Rattotti S, et al. Prevalence and clinical significance of the MYD88(L265P) somatic mutation in Waldenstrom's macroglobulinemia and related lymphoid neoplasms. Blood. 2013;121:2522–8.
10. Varettoni M, Zibellini S, Defrancesco I, Ferretti V, Rizzo E, et al. Pattern of somatic mutations in patients with Waldenstrom macroglobulinemia or IgM monoclonal gammopathy of undetermined significance. Haematologica. 2017;102:2077–85.
11. Hunter ZR, Xu L, Yang G, Zhou Y, Liu X, et al. The genomic landscape of Waldenstrom macroglobulinemia is characterized by highly recurring MYD88 and WHIM-likeCXCR4 mutations, and small somatic deletions associated with B-cell lymphomagenesis. Blood. 2014;123:1637–46.
12. Treon SP, Xu L, Guerrera ML, Jimenez C. Genomic landscape of Waldenstrom macroglobulinemia and its impact on treatment strategies. J Clin Oncol. 2020;38:1198–208.
13. Treon SP, Cao Y, Xu L, Yang G, Liu X, Hunter Z. Somatic mutations in MYD88 and CXCR4 are determinants of clinical presentation and overall survival in Waldenstrom macroglobulinemia. Blood. 2014;123:2791–6.
14. Cao Y, Hunter ZR, Liu X, Xu L, Yang G, et al. CXCR4 WHIM-like frameshift and nonsense mutations promote ibrutinib resistance but do not supplant MYD88(L265P)-directed survival signaling in Waldenstrom macroglobulinaemia cells. Br J Haematol. 2015;168:701–7.
15. Seiter K Waldenstrom macroglobulinemia: on Medscape.com; Besa, EC ed Updated: Feb 1, 2021.
16. Kwaan HC, Bongu A. The hyperviscosity syndromes. Semin Thromb Hemost. 1999;25:199–208. https://doi.org/10.1055/s-2007-994921.
17. Gustine JN, Meid K, Dubeau T, Hunter ZR, Xu L, Yang G, et al. Serum IgM level as predictor of symptomatic hyperviscosity in patients with Waldenstrom macroglobulinaemia. Br J Haematol. 2017;177:717–25. https://doi.org/10.1111/bjh.14743.
18. Merlini G, Baldini L, Broglia C, Comelli M, Goldaniga M, et al. Prognostic factors in symptomatic Waldenstrom's macroglobulinemia. Semin Oncol. 2003;30(2):211–5.

19. Dammacco R, Lisch W, Kivelä TT, et al. The spectrum of ocular manifestations in patients with Waldenström's macroglobulinemia. J Ocular Immunol Inflamm. 2021. https://doi.org/10.1080/09273948.2021.1933068.
20. Tedeschi A, Conticello C, Rizzi R, Benevolo G, Varettoni M. Diagnostic framing of IgM monoclonal gammopathy: focus on Waldenström macroglobulinemia. Hematol Oncol. 2019;37:117–28. https://doi.org/10.1002/hon.2539.
21. Gertz MA. Waldenström macroglobulinemia: 2019 update on diagnosis, risk stratification, and management. Am J Hematol. 2019;94(2):266–76. https://doi.org/10.1002/ajh.25292.
22. Castillo J, Treon SP. Management of Waldenstrom macroglobulinemia in 2020. Hematology Am Soc Hematol Educ Program. 2020;2020(1):372–9.
23. Christopher N, Grimont CN, Almeida N, Gertz MA. Current and emerging treatments for Waldenström macroglobulinemia. Acta Haematol. 2021;144:146–57. https://doi.org/10.1159/000509286.
24. Dhodapkar MV, Jacobson JL, Gertz MA, Rivkin SE, Roodman GD, et al. Prognostic factors and response to fludarabine therapy in patients with Waldenstrom macroglobulinemia: results of United States intergroup trial (Southwest Oncology Group S9003). Blood. 2001;98:41–8.
25. Kastritis E, Morel P, Duhamel A, Gavriatopoulou M, Kyrtsonis MC, et al. A revised international prognostic score system for Waldenström's macroglobulinemia. Leukemia. 2019;33(11):2654–61.
26. Ghobrial IM, Fonseca R, Gertz MA, Plevak MF, Larson DR, et al. Prognostic model for disease-specific and overall mortality in newly diagnosed symptomatic patients with Waldenstrom macroglobulinaemia. Br J Haematol. 2006;133:158–64.
27. Bustoros M, Sklavenitis-Pistofidis R, Kapoor P, Liu C-H, Kastritis E, et al. Progression risk stratification of asymptomatic Waldenström macroglobulinemia. J Clin Oncol. 2019;37(16):1403–11.
28. Advani P, Paulus A, Ailawadhi S. Updates in prognostication and treatment of Waldenström's macroglobulinemia. Hematol Oncol Stem Cell Ther. 2019;12(4):179–88.
29. Treon SP, Gustine J, Xu L, Manning RJ, Tsakmaklis N, et al. MYD88 wild type Waldenstrom macroglobulinaemia: differential diagnosis, risk of histological transformation, and overall survival. Br J Haematol. 2018;180:374–80.
30. Hunter ZR, Xu L, Tsakmaklis N, Demos MG, Kofedis A, et al. Insights into the genomic landscape of MYD88 wild-type Waldenstrom macroglobulinemia. Blood Adv. 2018;2:2937–46.
31. Treon SP, Tripsas CK, Meid K, Warren D, Varma G, et al. Ibrutinib in previously treated Waldenstrom's macroglobulinemia. N Engl J Med. 2015;372:1430–40.
32. Jalali S, Price-Troska T, Paludo J, Villasboas J, Kim HJ, et al. Soluble PD-1 ligands regulate T-cell function in Waldenstrom macroglobulinemia. Blood Adv. 2018;2(15):1985–97.
33. Dimopoulos MA, Kastritis E. How I treat Waldenstro¨m macroglobulinemia. Blood. 2019; 134(23):2022–35.
34. Gustine JN, Meid K, Dubeau T, Hunter ZH, Xu L, et al. Serum IgM level as predictor of symptomatic hyperviscosity in patients with Waldenstrom macroglobulinaemia. Br J Haematol. 2017;177(5):717–25.
35. Ballestri M, Ferrari F, Magistroni R, Mariano M, Ceccherelli GB, et al. Plasma exchange in acute and chronic hyperviscosity syndrome: a rheological approach and guidelines study. Ann Ist Super Sanita. 2007;43:171–5.
36. Kaplan A. A practical guide to therapeutic plasma exchange. Malden: Blackwell Science; 1999.
37. Stone MJ. Waldenstrom's macroglobulinemia: hyperviscosity syndrome and cryoglobulinemia. Clin Lymphoma Myeloma. 2009;9(1):97–9.
38. Treon SP, Ioakimidis L, Soumerai JD, Patterson CJ, Sheehy P, et al. Primary therapy of Waldenström macroglobulinemia with bortezomib, dexamethasone, and rituximab: WMCTG clinical trial 05-180. J Clin Oncol. 2009;27(23):3830–5.
39. Chaudhry M, Steiner R, Claussen C, Patel K, Lee H, et al. Carfilzomib-based combination regimens are highly effective frontline therapies for multiple myeloma and Waldenström's macroglobulinemia. Leuk Lymphoma. 2019;60(4):964–70.

40. Shirley M. Ixazomib: first global approval. Drugs. 2016;76(3):405–11.
41. Ghobrial IM, Vij R, Siegel D, Badros A, Kaufman J, Raje N, et al. A phase Ib/II study of oprozomib in patients with advanced multiple myeloma and Waldenström macroglobulinemia. Clin Cancer Res. 2019;25(16):4907–16.
42. Castillo JJ, Advani RH, Branagan AR, Buske C, Dimopoulos MA, et al. Consensus treatment recommendations from the tenth international workshop for Waldenström macroglobulinaemia. Lancet Haematol. 2020;7(11):e827–37.
43. Ansell SM, Kyle RA, Reeder CB, Fonseca R, Mikhael JR, Morice WG, et al. Diagnosis and management of Waldenstrom macroglobulinemia: Mayo stratification of macroglobulinemia and risk-adapted therapy (mSMART) guidelines. Mayo Clin Proc. 2010;85:824–33.
44. Dimopoulos MA, Zervas C, Zomas A, Kiamouris C, Viniou NA, Grigoraki V, et al. Treatment of Waldenstrom's macroglobulinemia with rituximab. J Clin Oncol. 2002;20:2327–33. https://doi.org/10.1200/JCO.2002.09.039.
45. Treon SP, Branagan AR, Hunter Z, Santos D, Tournhilac O, Anderson KC. Paradoxical increases in serum IgM and viscosity levels following rituximab in Waldenstrom's macroglobulinemia. Ann Oncol. 2004;15:1481–3. https://doi.org/10.1093/annonc/mdh403.
46. Cao Y, Hunter ZR, Liu X, Xu L, Yang G, Chen J, et al. The WHIM-like CXCR4(S338X) somatic mutation activates AKT and ERK, and promotes resistance to ibrutinib and other agents used in the treatment of Waldenstrom's macroglobulinemia. Leukemia. 2015;29(1):169–76.
47. Treon SP, Tripsas CK, Meid K, Warren D, Varma G, Green R, et al. Ibrutinib in previously treated Waldenström's macroglobulinemia. N Engl J Med. 2015;372(15):1430–40.
48. Hartsell L, Janes A, Larck C, Park S, Arnall JR. Ibrutinib for the treatment of Bing-Neel syndrome, a complication of Waldenström macroglobulinemia: patient case report. J Oncol Pharm Pract. 2019;25(6):1534–9.
49. Dimopoulos MA, Trotman J, Tedeschi A, Matous JV, Macdonald D, Tam C, et al.; iNNOVATE Study Group and the European Consortium for Waldenström's Macroglobulinemia. Ibrutinib for patients with rituximab-refractory Waldenström's macroglobulinaemia (iNNOVATE): an open-label substudy of an international, multicentre, phase 3 trial. Lancet Oncol. 2017;18(2):241–250.
50. Dimopoulos MA, Tedeschi A, Trotman J, García-Sanz R, Macdonald D, Leblond V, et al.; iNNOVATE Study Group and the European Consortium for Waldenström's Macroglobulinemia. Phase 3 trial of Ibrutinib plus rituximab in Waldenström's macroglobulinemia. N Engl J Med. 2018;378(25):2399–2410.
51. Owen RG, McCarthy H, Rule S, D'Sa S, Thomas SK, Tournilhac O, et al. Acalabrutinib monotherapy in patients with Waldenström macroglobulinemia: a single-arm, multicentre, phase 2 study. Lancet Haematol. 2020;7(2):e112–21.
52. Tam CS, Trotman J, Opat S, Burger JA, Cull G, et al. Phase 1 study of the selective BTK inhibitor zanubrutinib in B-cell malignancies and safety and efficacy evaluation in CLL. Blood. 2019;134(11):851–9.
53. Castillo JJ, Gustine J, Meid K, Dubeau T, Keezer A, Allan JN, et al. Multicenter prospective phase II study of Venetoclax in patients with previously treated Waldenstrom macroglobulinemia. Blood. 2018;132(Suppl 1):132.
54. Tomowiak C, Desseaux K, Poulain S, Herbaux C, Perrot A, Mahe B, et al. Open label non-randomized phase II study exploring "chemo-free" treatment association with Idelalisib plus Obinutuzumab in patients with relapsed/refractory (R/R) Waldenstrom's macroglobulinemia (MW), a filo trial: results of the intermediary analysis of the induction phase. Blood. 2019;134
55. Flinn IW, O'Brien S, Kahl B, Patel M, Oki Y, Foss FF, et al. Duvelisib, a novel oral dual inhibitor of PI3K-δ,γ, is clinically active in advanced hematologic malignancies. Blood. 2018;131(8):877–87.
56. NIH. Study to assess the efficacy and safety of Umbralisib in patients with non-follicular indolent non-Hodgkin's lymphoma. https://clinicaltrials.gov/ct2/show/study/NCT03364231.
57. Kuhne MR, Mulvey T, Belanger B, Chen S, Pan C, Chong C, et al. BMS-936564/MDX-1338: a fully human anti-CXCR4 antibody in- duces apoptosis in vitro and shows antitumor activity in vivo in hematologic malignancies. Clin Cancer Res. 2013;19(2):357–66.

58. A study of Ulocuplumab and Ibrutinib in symptomatic patients with mutated CXCR4 Waldenstrom's macroglobulinemia. 2020. https://clinicaltrials.gov/ct2/show/record/NCT03225716.
59. Cornell RF, Bachanova V, D'Souza A, Woo-Ahn K, Martens M, Huang J, et al. Allogeneic transplantation for relapsed Waldenstrom macroglobulinemia and lymphoplasmacytic lymphoma. Biol Blood Marrow Transplant. 2017;23:60–6. https://doi.org/10.1016/j.bbmt.2016.10.010.
60. Kastritis, E, Leblond V, Dimopoulos MA, Kimby E, Staber P, Kersten MJ, et al, on behalf of the ESMO Guidelines Committee. Clinical practice guidelines—Waldenstrom's macroglobulinaemia. Ann Oncol. 2018;29(Suppl 4):iv41–iv50.
61. Oza A, Rajkumar SV. Waldenstrom macroglobulinemia: prognosis management. Blood Cancer J. 2015;5:e296. https://doi.org/10.1038/bcj.2015.28. www.nature.com/bcj.

Chapter 15
IgG4-Related Disease Overview: Pathology, Clinical Picture, and Treatment

Emanuel Della-Torre, Yoh Zen, and John H. Stone

Introduction

IgG4-related disease (IgG4-RD) is a fibro-inflammatory disorder characterized by mass-forming lesions with a relapsing-remitting course that can lead to organ failure if left untreated [1]. IgG4-RD derives its name from elevated concentrations of serum IgG4 detected in most patients and the accumulation of IgG4 secreting plasma cells in affected tissues [1]. In healthy individuals, IgG4 is the least abundant of all IgG subclasses. In contrast, among some patients with IgG4-RD, the serum concentration rises to 30–40 times the upper limit of normal. A clear association between IgG4 antibodies and organ damage has not been established; however, the characteristic IgG4 paraproteinemia is now generally regarded as an epiphenomenon of the ongoing inflammatory response rather than a driver of disease pathogenesis [2].

First described in 2001 in the setting of type I autoimmune pancreatitis (AIP), IgG4-RD is now known to affect virtually any anatomical area [3]. The systemic nature of IgG4-RD was recognized in 2003 when conditions regarded as unrelated entities for decades—such as type I autoimmune pancreatitis (AIP), sclerosing

E. Della-Torre (✉)
Unit of Immunology, Rheumatology, Allergy, and Rare Diseases (UnIRAR), San Raffaele Hospital, Milan, Italy
e-mail: dellatorre.emanuel@hsr.it

Y. Zen
Institute of Liver Studies, King's College Hospital and King's College London, London, UK
e-mail: yoh.1.zen@kcl.ac.uk

J. H. Stone
Division of Rheumatology, Allergy, and Immunology, Massachusetts General Hospital, Boston, MA, USA
e-mail: jhstone@mgh.harvard.edu

© The Author(s), under exclusive license to Springer Nature Switzerland AG 2022

G. Ragab et al. (eds.), *Paraproteinemia and Related Disorders*,
https://doi.org/10.1007/978-3-031-10131-1_15

cholangitis, retroperitoneal fibrosis, hypertrophic pachymeningitis, Mikulicz's disease, and Riedel's thyroiditis—were shown not only to occur simultaneously in a proportion of patients but to have common histological findings across the organs involved [4–8]. IgG4-RD mainly affects middle age to elderly individuals, with a male to female ratio that ranges from 1.6:1 for head and neck manifestations to 4:1 for other sites of organ involvement [9]. The global incidence and prevalence of IgG4-RD remain largely under-studied. According to a national epidemiological survey, the incidence of AIP in Japan in 2016 was 3.1 cases per 100,000 individuals, but pancreatic involvement represents only one of more than a dozen organs potentially affected by IgG4-RD. Indeed, among 8000 patients with IgG4-RD referred to Japanese hospitals in a survey from 2009, 5190 did not exhibit pancreatic involvement, underscoring our poor appraisal of disease epidemiology in its multiple manifestations [10–12]. Nevertheless, awareness of IgG4-RD has rapidly increased across medical specialties in the last 10 years, and a number of international collaborative studies now provide clinicians with landmark guideline documents for implementing disease recognition and patient management, including the 2012 Consensus statement on the pathology of IgG4-RD and the 2015 International guidance statement of the management and treatment of IgG4-RD [13, 14]. More recently, the tissues indicate that IgG4-RD is likely sustained by an antigen-driven immune response but the nature of these antigen/s as well as the reason for disease targeting of particular organs remain unclear [15–19]. Indeed, a variety of self-antigens have been identified including galectin-3, annexin-A11, laminin-511, and prohibitin, suggesting that a breach of immunological tolerance might initiate the disease [20–23]. Similarly, although a Genome Wide Association Study on Japanese patients identified HLA-DRB1 and FC-gamma receptor IIb regions as susceptibility loci, there are currently no genetic risk factors clearly associated with disease pathogenesis [24].

The first "inflammatory" phase of IgG4-RD is characterized by antigen-experienced B and T lymphocytes that accumulate at disease sites, engage in mutual activating antigen-driven interactions, and secrete pro-fibrotic molecules such as interleukin (IL)-1β, IL-6, interferon (IFN)-γ, transforming growth factor (TGF)-β, platelet-derived growth factor (PDGF)-B, and lysyl oxidase homolog 2 (LOXL2) [25]. These populations of activated lymphocytes include circulating plasmablasts, T effector memory (TEM) cytotoxic T lymphocytes (CTLs), and CD45RA+ TEM (TEMRA) CTLs [26]. Both plasmablasts and effector memory T cells express the signaling lymphocytic activation molecule F7 (SLAMF7), a surface protein that has been implicated in cell–cell interaction and chronic lymphocyte activation [26].

Although TEM and TEMRA CTLs involvement in tissue fibrosis has not been proven, plasmablasts/plasma cells from patients with IgG4-RD have been shown to prompt fibroblast activation and collagen production in vitro, thus partially explaining the improvement of fibrotic lesions with B-cell depletion [25]. Other T cell subsets presumably involved in the "inflammatory" phase of IgG4-RD are CD4 follicular T-helper (Tfh) cells, T-regulatory cells, and Th2 cells [27–32]. Circulating Tfh1 and Tfh2 cells expressing programmed cell death protein 1 (PD1+) are expanded in patients with IgG4-RD. They also correlate with disease activity, plasmablasts numbers, serum levels of IgG4 and IL-4 [27–32].

PD1+ Tfh2 cells drive IgG4 class-switch in vitro, enhance proliferation of IgG4-committed B cells, and facilitate the differentiation of naive B cells into plasmablasts/plasma cells, resulting in increased IgG4 secretion [27–33]. Activated IL-4 and IL-21-expressing Tfh cells are also found in tertiary lymphoid structures of IgG4-RD affected tissues and likely contribute to germinal center formation [27–33]. On the other hand, the contribution of T-regulatory cells and Th2 cells to disease pathogenesis is controversial. Several lines of indirect evidence based on IL-5, IL-10, and IL-13 expression in disease lesions, in fact, suggest activation of Th2 and regulatory immune reactions, but other studies have failed to demonstrate a significant expansion of Th2 and T-regulatory cells in IgG4-RD [27–33].

The role of innate immunity in the pathogenesis of IgG4-RD has not been studied widely to date although innate immune cells appear implicated in the transition from the "inflammatory" to the "fibrotic" phase of the disease. In particular, M2 macrophages have been shown to accumulate in IgG4-RD lesions and to express pro-fibrotic cytokines such as TGF-β and CCL18, possibly upon engagement of MerTK receptor by plasmablasts and CTLs [34].

In this pathological scenario, the role of IgG4 antibodies remains controversial. Compared to other immunoglobulin subclasses, in fact, IgG4 antibodies are known to participate in the resolution of tissue inflammation because of intrinsic anti-inflammatory properties (Fig. 15.1) [2]. These properties are mainly due to structural changes occurring at disulfide bridges connecting the two heavy chains of the IgG4 molecule ("hinge region"). Specifically, as opposite to IgG1, IgG2, and IgG3, the hinge region of IgG4 presents a proline instead of a serine amino

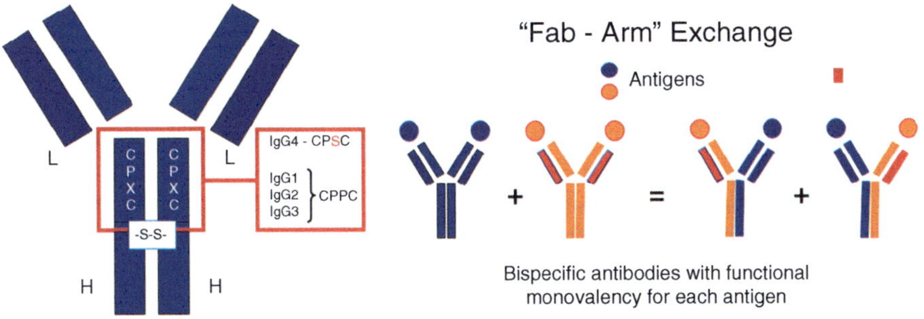

	IgG1	IgG2	IgG3	IgG4
Biological target	Protein	Carbohydrate	Protein	Protein
Functional form	Monomeric, bivalent	Dimeric, bivalent or tetravalent	Monomeric, bivalent	Bispecific, monovalent for each antigen
Serum levels (mg/dl)	5 - 11	1.5 - 6	0.2 - 1	0.08 - 1.4
Proportion of total IgG (%)	43 - 75	16 - 48	1.7 - 7	0.8 - 11.7
Complement fixation	+++	+	+++	-
Binding to FC gamma receptors				
FC gamma RI	++	+	+++	+
FC gamma RII	++	+	+++	-
FC gamma RIII	++	+	++	-

Fig. 15.1 Molecular basis of the "Fab-arm" exchange and physiopathological properties of IgG4 antibodies

acid residue at position 228 (P288S) leading to a greater stereometric flexibility compared to other IgG subclasses [35]. This flexibility allows additional disulfide bridges to form within the same heavy chain ("intra-chain" disulfide bonds) instead of connecting the two heavy chains ("inter-chain" disulfide bonds). Under reducing conditions, the two heavy chains of the IgG4 antibody can dissociate and recombine randomly with other heavy chains from different nearby IgG4 hemi-molecules in a process termed "Fab-arm exchange" [35]. The new antibody resulting from the combination of two hemi-molecules (namely, paired heavy and light chains from two IgG4 molecules) are bispecific because they can cross-link two different antigens instead of two antigens of the same kind. As a consequence, IgG4 is not able to form large immune complexes, to activate the classic complement pathway, or to bind activating Fc receptors on immune cells. The relevance of these properties to IgG4-RD pathogenesis is presently unknown. On the one hand, in fact, there is a diffused tendency to consider the aberrant IgG4 production occurring in IgG4-RD as an epiphenomenon of underlying pathological Th2 and T-regulatory responses. However, the evidence of immune-mediated diseases caused by auto-reactive IgG4 such as pemphigus and anti-MuSK myasthenia gravis does not completely rule out the possibility that IgG4-RD might also be sustained by IgG4 autoantibodies [36].

The increase in serum IgG4 in IgG4-RD might, therefore, represent a counter-regulatory response in which serum IgG4 concentrations rise in an attempt to dampen the ongoing inflammation. On the other hand, IgG1 and IgG4 purified from IgG4-RD patients (specifically patients with IgG4-related autoimmune pancreatitis) and administered subcutaneously to neonatal Balb/c mice have been shown to recapitulate pancreatic and salivary gland disease in recipient mice, suggesting a possible direct contribution of IgG4 antibodies to tissue damage [37]. Moreover, monoclonal IgG4 antibodies targeting ovalbumin-expressing pancreatic cells have also been shown to induce pancreatic inflammation in mice only when injected with ovalbumin-specific CTLs and not when injected alone, further supporting a possible synergistic effect in causing tissue damage [37]. Overall, the precise pathophysiological role of the IgG4 molecule remains debated, but the many clinical and epidemiological correlations between serum IgG4 elevation and disease activity warrant additional investigation.

Clinical Picture

Presentation

IgG4-RD is typically an indolent disease [38]. Fevers are rarely to ever present in IgG4-RD except in case of infectious complications such as ascending cholangitis [39, 40]. It is frequently possible to determine that patients have had the disease unrecognized for many months or even years before the diagnosis is established. Organ involvement often occurs in—or is recognized in—a "metachronous" fashion, i.e., one organ is recognized initially to be abnormal followed months later by the identification of an abnormality in another organ, followed perhaps by yet another organ somewhat later. Eventually, this pattern triggers a thorough evaluation leading to a diagnosis. Because of growing awareness of the disease, the interval between first recognized abnormality and clinical diagnosis has likely grown shorter, but long latency periods are still common. The very nature of the disease, which culminates in major organ damage but usually only slowly, is an important reason for this.

Although fevers and rapidly progressive disease do not typify IgG4-RD, weight loss—on the order of 5–15 kg—is common. When present, it is often a clue to exocrine pancreatic insufficiency.

Organs Affected

IgG4-RD has the capability of affecting essentially any organ but has particular predilections for the following, listed from approximately the most common to least common: pancreas (often accompanied by intra- and extra-pancreatic bile duct disease); the lacrimal and major salivary glands; the orbits (extraocular muscles, retrobulbar masses); the retroperitoneum (with aortic or peri-aortic disease); the kidneys; the lungs; the pachymeninges; and the thyroid gland. Riedel's thyroiditis is in fact IgG4-RD of the thyroid. In the 2019 Classification Criteria developed by the American College of Rheumatology and the European League Against Rheumatism, these organs are considered "typical" IgG4-RD organs. In order to be classified as having IgG4-RD, a patient must have at least one of these organs affected.

Approximately 40% of patients present with clinically evident disease in a single organ, but presentations involving five or six organs are not uncommon. Even patients with multi-organ involvement can remain remarkably asymptomatic for long periods of time despite substantial disease burden within individual organs.

Damage

The ability of the disease to persist undetected for lengthy periods leads to irreversible organ injury that can occur even before the patient is aware of being ill. The pancreas is perhaps the organ injured most commonly. Substantial weight loss in a patient with IgG4-RD usually implicates an injury to the exocrine pancreas, impairing the patient's ability to produce digestive enzymes and therefore to absorb nutrients. Such patients often have low serum amylase or lipase concentrations, reflective of "burned-out" autoimmune pancreatitis. The diagnosis of exocrine pancreatic insufficiency can be confirmed by the finding of low concentrations of elastase in stool. Management requires dietary supplementation with pancreatic replacement enzymes. Endocrine pancreatic insufficiency in IgG4-RD leads to diabetes mellitus.

Disease Subsets

Two large subtypes of disease are clear on a clinical basis. These subtypes have been termed the proliferative subtype and the fibrotic subtype. The glandular and epithelial tissues are primarily affected in patients with the proliferative subtype. Lymphadenopathy, dacryoadenitis, sialadenitis, autoimmune pancreatitis, IgG4-related sclerosing cholangitis, lung disease, tubulointerstitial nephritis, paranasal sinusitis, and hypophysitis are common manifestations of this subtypes. In terms of laboratory assessments, the proliferative subtype typically demonstrates high serum concentrations of IgG4, IgG1 and IgE, hypocomplementemia, and peripheral eosinophilia. Multi-organ involvement is usually found in the proliferative IgG4-RD subset, and atopy is also a frequent disease accompaniment.

The fibrotic subtype, in contrast, tends to affect extra-glandular sites and may be concentrated more on a specific body region than a discrete organ per se. Retroperitoneal fibrosis, sclerosing mesenteritis, and fibrosing mediastinitis are the best examples of the fibrotic subtype, but Riedel's thyroiditis and pachymeningitis also often fit the overall profile of a patient in the fibrotic subtype. Compared with the proliferative subtype, those in the fibrotic subtype have fewer organs affected and a lower degree of serological activity.

A latent class analysis of data from the study from which the American College of Rheumatology and European League Against Rheumatism Classification Criteria for IgG4-related disease were derived identified four phenotypic groups [39]. These groups included: (1) pancreatic-hepato-biliary disease (31%); (2) retroperitoneal fibrosis with or without aortitis (24%); (3) head and neck-limited disease (24%); and (4) a classic Mikulicz syndrome with systemic involvement (22%) (Fig. 15.2). These phenotypic subgroups fit well into the proliferative/fibrotic subtype paradigm outlined above.

Pathology

Tissue enlargement due to a massive inflammatory infiltrate and fibrosis is a typical morphological alteration of IgG4-RD. Solid organs (e.g., pancreas, salivary glands) exhibit global swelling or localized mass lesions, while ductal organs (e.g., bile duct, aorta) transform to a pipe stem-like appearance with diffuse wall thickening [41]. Retroperitoneal or mediastinal manifestations present with either a well circumscribed nodule or ill-defined infiltrative lesion. Morphological transformations

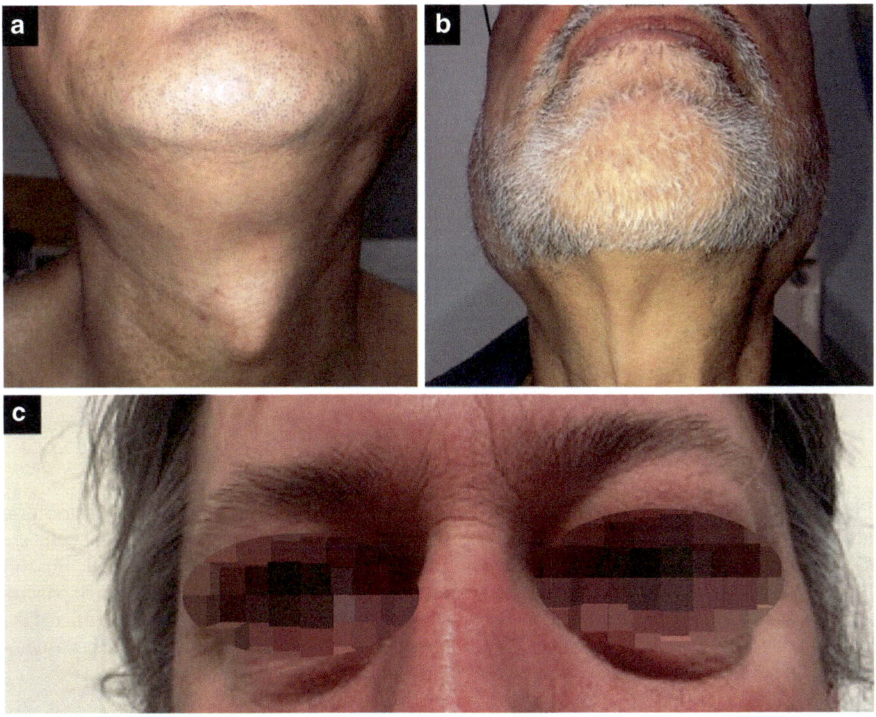

Fig. 15.2 Common physical examination manifestations of IgG4-RD. (**a**) Bilateral submandibular gland enlargement. (**b**) Bilateral parotid gland enlargement. (**c**) Periorbital swelling associated with inflammation of the extraocular muscles

in the respiratory system are most diverse, potentially mimicking a primary nodular neoplasm, central airway disease, and diffuse interstitial pneumonia [42, 43].

All organ manifestations of IgG4-RD share basic histological changes, and three characteristic findings are dense lymphoplasmacytic infiltration, storiform fibrosis, and obliterative phlebitis [13]. Affected tissue is diffusely infiltrated by mature small lymphocytes and plasma cells (Fig. 15.3a). Co-existence of B lymphocytes with variable degrees of maturation (e.g., plasmablasts, immunoblasts) exhibits a polymorphic microscopic appearance, a finding useful for the differential diagnosis from lymphoid malignancies with a monomorphic cellular infiltrate. Formation of lymphoid follicles with germinal centers can occur, being more commonly observed in case of salivary or lacrimal glands involvement [44]. IgG4 immunostaining often reveals IgG4+ B lymphocytes within germinal centers (Fig. 15.3b), indicating that IgG4 class switch occurs in those tertiary lymphoid structures or regional lymph nodes.

Fibrosis is another essential histological element of IgG4-RD. In particular, collagen fibers are arranged in an irregularly whorled pattern, somewhat resembling the spokes of a cartwheel or the net of a straw mat, and this spatial organization is typically referred to as storiform fibrosis (Fig. 15.3a). Immunostaining for alpha

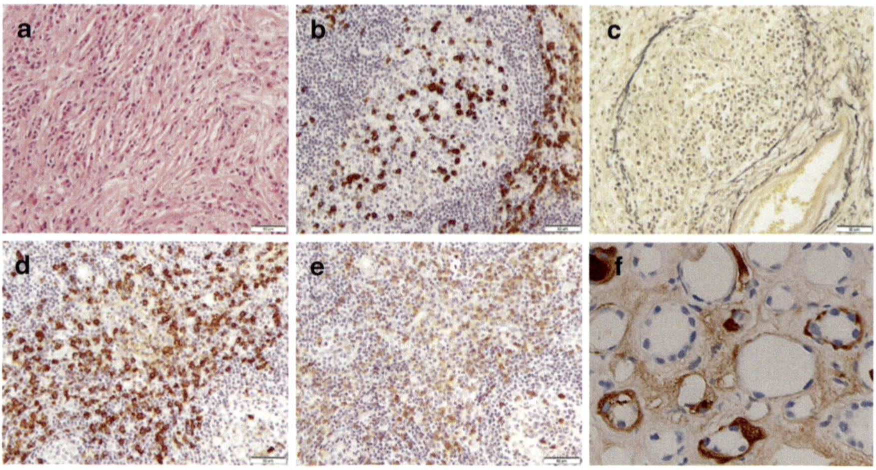

Fig. 15.3 Histopathology of IgG4-RD. (**a**) Diffuse lymphoplasmacytic infiltration with storiform fibrosis is observed in a case of IgG4-related sclerosing cholangitis. (**b**) Many IgG4+ cells are identified in a germinal center of the lymphoid follicle developed in IgG4-related sialadenitis. (**c**) Elastica van Gieson staining highlights obliterative phlebitis in IgG4-related autoimmune pancreatitis. (**d** and **e**) Immunostaining demonstrates many IgG4+ (**d**) and IgG+ plasma cells (**e**), and the ratio of IgG4/IgG+ cells is greater than 70% (at the same field; a case of IgG4-related dacryoadenitis). (**f**) Deposits around the tubular basement are positive for IgG4 immunostaining

smooth muscle actin shows only a small number of active myofibroblasts [45], while CD168 immunostaining uncovers abundant M2-type macrophages in fibrotic areas [46], indicating that storiform fibrosis is not a simple fibrotic process, but a macrophage-rich stromal response. This may explain why IgG4-RD responds well to corticosteroids despite its fibrotic appearance.

Obliterative phlebitis is characterized by vascular channels partially or completely obliterated by the sclerosing inflammatory process [13]. Unlike non-specific fibrous obliteration of veins, which are seen in many other chronic inflammatory conditions, obliterative phlebitis contains many lymphocytes and plasma cells inside the obliterated vascular channel. A small fibrous nodule next to the patent artery is a microscopic guidepost for identifying obliterative phlebitis. Elastica staining often unexpectedly uncovers the completely obliterated veins on tissue sections (Fig. 15.3c), and this is particularly useful for biopsy specimens. It is usually a microscopic finding, but obliteration of the large veins (e.g., portal vein) adjacent to the affected organs can show similar obliterative changes and may be mistaken for malignant vascular involvement on imaging [47].

A less specific microscopic finding of IgG4-RD is eosinophilic infiltration. Eosinophilic infiltrate is typically moderate although extreme examples mimicking eosinophilic pancreatitis, cholecystitis, or pneumonitis have been reported [48]. Obliterative arteritis can also be seen in lung manifestations [13]. This finding needs to be distinguished from necrotizing vasculitis by the absence of fibrinoid necrosis.

Microscopic findings against the diagnosis of IgG4-RD include discrete granulomas, necrosis, and abscess [13]. Neutrophilic infiltration is also not expected in IgG4-RD except for lung manifestation [13]. Of note is that xanthogranulomatous organ injuries often present with a mass-like lesion and are potentially accompanied by many IgG4+ plasma cells, but the presence of abundant foamy macrophages basically excludes the possibility of IgG4-RD.

Immunostaining is an essential part of the histological diagnosis of IgG4-RD, requiring a careful assessment in three aspects: the number, ratio, and distribution of IgG4+ plasma cells. A recommendation is to count three high-power fields (hpf) with the highest number of IgG4+ plasma cells and calculate the average number of IgG4+ plasma cells within these fields. IgG+ plasma cells at the same three fields should be counted for the purpose of calculating the IgG4/IgG+ cell ratio [13]. The number of IgG4+ cells is at least >10 and typically >50 cells/hpf (Fig. 15.3d). Likewise, IgG4/IgG+ cell ratio is at least >40% and typically 70% in this condition (Fig. 15.3e). The diagnosis of IgG4-RD requires to meet both criteria, and an isolated increase in either the number or ratio does not suggest the diagnosis. Diffuse distribution of IgG4+ plasma cells also needs to be confirmed. Focal aggregation of IgG4+ plasma cells is not typical for IgG4-RD, even if it meets the number and ratio criteria. The diffuse distribution of IgG4+ plasma cells was not emphasized before, but its importance has been increasingly recognized for avoiding the over-diagnosis of IgG4-RD [49].

Bone marrow involvement in IgG4-RD is uncommon with only a handful of cases reported until now [50, 51]. The bone marrow abnormality is typically suspected by PDG-PET, which demonstrates partial or diffuse avidity in the bone marrow [51]. In a French study, only one of 21 cases had FDG avidity in the bone marrow [50]. A typical microscopic finding is a mild to moderate increase in polyclonal IgG4+ plasma cells (>10 cells/hpf; IgG4/IgG ratio >40%) [51, 52]. Although fibrosis and obliterative phlebitis are usually absent, a single case showed diffuse storiform fibrosis [53]. A differential diagnosis is IgG4-type plasma cell myeloma, which accounts for 4% of IgG-type myeloma [54]. No pathological association between IgG4-RD and IgG4-type plasma cell myeloma has been confirmed.

Approximately 5–10% of patients with IgG4-related kidney disease have membranous glomerulonephropathy (MGN) [55, 56]. IgG4-related MGN is characterized by IgG4-dominant subepithelial deposits [57]. That finding is similar to primary MGN but different from other secondary forms of MGN, which are associated with deposits that predominantly stain for IgG1, IgG2, or IgG3. However, unlike in the majority of cases of primary MGN, antibodies to PLA2R do not colocalize with the immune deposits in IgG4-related MGN [57]. IgG4-related tubulointerstitial nephritis can also show deposition of immune complexes along the tubular basement membrane, either on immunofluorescence studies or on electron microscopy, and immunoreactivity to IgG4 can be observed (Fig. 15.3f) [55, 56]. These microscopic findings are unique to IgG4-related kidney disease and may explain the common association with hypocomplementemia.

Histological findings of long-standing IgG4-RD are poorly understood. Based on our experience, two manifestations supposed to persist for a long time before clinical presentation such as IgG4-related retroperitoneal fibrosis and periaortitis are typically more fibrotic and pathological findings become less specific. In particular, the degree of lymphoplasmacytic infiltration decreases, and infiltration of IgG4+ plasma cells may be patchy. Obliterated veins are observed, but they are not associated with inflammation; therefore, it is not conclusive for obliterative phlebitis. A diagnostic clue for long-standing IgG4-RD is recognition of storiform fibrosis, which tends to persist at least focally even at the chronic phase.

The 2012 Consensus Statement of IgG4-RD Pathology proposed a diagnostic approach, in which a combination of three morphological findings (diffuse lymphoplasmacytic infiltration, obliterative phlebitis, and storiform fibrosis) and immunohistochemical results (the number and ratio of IgG4+ cells) were considered [13]. The document also provided required numbers of IgG4+ plasma cells for the diagnosis of individual organ manifestations (e.g., >100 cells/hpf for sialadenitis; >50 cells/hpf for pancreatitis). A minimum criterion of IgG4/IgG+ plasma cell ratio was 40% [13]. The 2019 ACR/EULAR Classification Criteria endorse a similar approach based on both morphological and immunohistochemical findings. Namely, diffuse lymphoplasmacytic infiltration with storiform fibrosis gives a higher score than lymphoplasmacytic infiltration with obliterative phlebitis [39, 58]. Two thresholds are then set for either the total number (10–50 or >50 cells/hpf) or the ratio (40–70 or >70%) of IgG4+ plasma cells [57]. Scores of immunohistochemical domain are calculated based on the combination of the number and ratio of IgG4+ plasma cells, and the highest score of 16 is given when both >50 cells/hpf and >70% are met [59].

Pathological differential diagnoses span from reactive to neoplastic conditions. Histological mimickers potentially accompanied by many IgG4+ plasma cells include granulomatosis with polyangiitis, multicentric Castleman disease (Chap. 21), Rosai-Dorfman disease, and inflammatory myofibroblastic tumor. Unlike IgG4-RD, granulomatosis with polyangiitis typically shows necrosis and/or granulomatous reaction [49]. Serological tests for ANCA also assist in the differential diagnosis. Multicentric Castleman disease often has extensive infiltration of IgG4+ plasma cells (>50 cells/hpf in 86% of cases), and the ratio of IgG4/IgG+ plasma cells can also increase over 40% in one third of cases [60]. However, storiform fibrosis, obliterative phlebitis and eosinophilic infiltration are uncommon in multicentric Castleman disease [60]. Unlike IgG4-RD, in which plasmacytic infiltration is associated with intervening lymphocytes, sheet-like plasmacytosis is characteristic for multicentric Castleman disease. The histological identification of abnormal large macrophages immunoreactive to S100 is crucial for the diagnosis of Rosai-Dorfman disease, but those cells are easily missed particularly if suspicion is low [61]. The neoplastic nature of inflammatory myofibroblastic tumor is usually suspected by sheets of atypical spindle cells, but the diagnosis by biopsies from an inflamed, hypocellular area requires immunohistochemistry or sequencing analysis of ALK, ROS1 and other tumor-related genes [62, 63].

Diagnostic Considerations

Definitive diagnosis of IgG4-RD requires rigorous clinical-pathological correlation because clinical assessments, laboratory evaluations, and imaging studies are often insufficient to distinguish neoplastic, inflammatory, and infectious mimickers. Serological findings in patients with IgG4-RD are largely non-specific. Erythrocyte sedimentation rate can be elevated to a moderate degree. C-reactive protein is usually normal except in some clinical manifestations (such as retroperitoneal and aortic involvement) where slight increase can be observed [64, 65]. Marked elevation of acute phase reactants should raise the concern of infectious or inflammatory conditions that closely mimic IgG4-RD such as ANCA-associated vasculitis and multicentric Castleman disease [64]. Peripheral blood eosinophilia and increased serum IgE occur in almost 30% of patients [64]. Some have low-titer antinuclear antibodies and/or positive rheumatoid factor [64].

Serum IgG4 elevation occurs in 55–97% of cases, especially in Asian patients, and correlates with the number of organs involved and the risk of relapse [1]. An increase in serum IgG4 has, however, poor specificity for diagnostic purposes because, similarly to the finding of IgG4+ plasma cells within tissue, it can be commonly observed in a broad spectrum of neoplastic, infectious, and autoimmune diseases [64]. In particular, a meta-analysis of nine case-control studies including 1235 IgG4-RD patients and 5696 controls, found that a cut-off value of serum IgG4 ranging from 1.35 to 1.44 g/L bears a pooled sensitivity of 87.2% (95% Confidence Interval, CI: 85.2–89.0%) and a specificity of 82.6% (95% CI: 81.6–83.6%) [66]. In addition, serum IgG4 measurement is not free from analytical errors. Most laboratories worldwide, in fact, perform IgG4 quantitation by either turbidimetry or nephelometry, with the former methodology giving spuriously normal IgG4 values in case of antigen excess "prozone phenomenon" [67]. Finally, serum IgG4 concentration does not correlate with indirect measures of fibrosis, and uncommonly returns to normal with treatment-induced remission making it an imperfect biomarker for tracking disease activity [68]. Other IgG subclasses—namely IgG1, IgG2, and IgG3—are frequently elevated, although generally not to the extent of IgG4, and may be responsible for the complement consumption observed in nearly a quarter of patients with active IgG4-RD [1]. In these patients, baseline urinalysis with evaluation of the urinary sediment is warranted because decreased serum C3 and C4 concentrations might indicate subclinical or overt renal involvement [69]. Disease-specific autoantibodies such as, ANCA, SSA/Ro or SSB/La, double-stranded DNA, RNP, and Sm, are not observed in IgG4-RD and should orient diagnosis towards mimicking autoimmune conditions [66]. Radiological findings are also largely non-specific in most affected organs. IgG4-related AIP with diffuse involvement is the sole exception because computed tomography and magnetic resonance imaging classically show a diffusely enlarged "sausage-shaped" pancreas with a surrounding halo of edematous tissue (Fig. 15.4) [70].

Because of the shortcomings of serological and radiological findings, histological examination according to available guidelines documents remains the mainstay

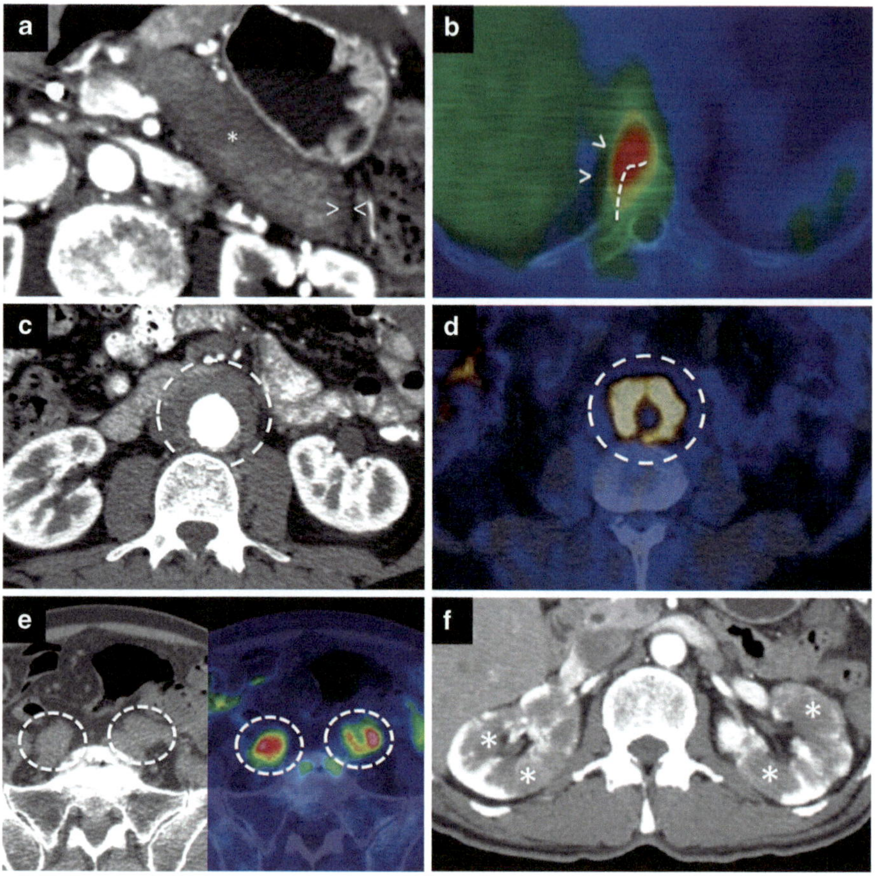

Fig. 15.4 Radiological findings suggestive of IgG4-RD included in the "ACR/EULAR Classification Criteria": (**a**) diffuse "sausage-like" pancreatic enlargement (asterisk) with surrounding "halo sign" (arrowheads); (**b**) paravertebral band-like soft tissue (arrowheads and dashed line); (**c**, **d**) circumferential tissue around the infrarenal aorta (dashed circle) or (**e**) iliac arteries (dashed circles); (**f**) bilateral renal cortex low-density areas (asterisks)

for definitive diagnosis and should be performed whenever possible. Indeed, depending on the availability of tissue specimen and on a combination of clinical and serological features, IgG4-RD can be diagnosed as "definitive," "probable," or "possible" according to the "2011 Comprehensive diagnostic criteria for IgG4-RD," with a "definitive" diagnosis formulated only in the presence of pathological confirmation [71]. Yet, obtaining optimal biopsies for histological studies might be challenging in many scenarios such as in case of retroperitoneal, biliary, or meningeal involvement. To overcome these major diagnostic challenges and to capture the majority of patients with homogeneous manifestations of IgG4-RD, experts from the ACR and EULAR developed the 2019 "ACR/EULAR Classification Criteria for IgG4-Related Disease" [39, 58]. Specifically, the "ACR/EULAR Classification

Criteria for IgG4-Related Disease" are based on a three-step classification process, consisting of a main entry criterion, a set of exclusion criteria, and a set of weighted inclusion criteria. According to this process, involvement of at least one of 11 possible organs in a manner consistent with IgG4-RD (entry criteria) is required to enter the classification algorithm. Exclusion criteria are then applied and the presence of any of these criteria eliminates the patient from further IgG4-RD classification. Finally, a set of inclusion criteria addressing clinical, serological, radiological, and pathological findings is weighted, and a patient is classified if a cumulative score of ≥20 points is obtained [39, 58]. This classification algorithm showed excellent accuracy in distinguishing IgG4-RD from multiple mimickers, including malignant disorders, granulomatous conditions, small and large vessel vasculitis with a specificity of 97.8% and a sensitivity of 82.0% [39, 58]. In particular, the clinical and/or radiological manifestations that received the highest weight for IgG4-RD classification among the inclusion criteria were: (1) involvement of two or more sets of salivary and lacrimal glands (14 points); (2) paravertebral band-like soft tissue in the thorax (10 points); (3) diffuse pancreatic enlargement with capsule-like rim and biliary tree involvement (19 points); (4) bilateral renal cortex low-density areas (10 points); and (5) circumferential/anterolateral soft tissue around the infra-renal aorta (8 points) (Fig. 15.4). Of note, in a retrospective single center cohort analysis, 39/40 (97.5%) patients with definite IgG4-RD according to the Comprehensive Criteria were also classified as having IgG4-RD according to the Classification Criteria, further underscoring the encouraging performance of this novel algorithm [72]. It is, therefore, plausible that the 2019 ACR/EULAR Classification Criteria will be soon adopted worldwide not only for classifying patients with IgG4-RD but also as a useful framework for guiding disease diagnosis. The Criteria, however, were not meant for diagnostic purposes but rather to identify homogeneous groups of subjects for clinical trials, research, and observational studies. Clinicians should, therefore, be aware of the many cases of IgG4-RD that would not fulfill entry criteria or achieve classification due to atypical manifestation, low-to-no elevation of serum IgG4, or because they are less likely to be biopsied. These clinical scenarios, especially if presenting as isolated organ involvement, might include unusual sites of infiltration such as the hypophysis, the pericardium, and the thymus, as well as more frequent manifestations such as focal AIP, retroperitoneal fibrosis, inflammatory aortitis, and hypertrophic pachymeningitis.

Treatment

Essentially all patients with active, symptomatic IgG4-RD should be treated. A subset of patients,—for example, those with autoimmune pancreatitis, sclerosing cholangitis, tubulointerstitial nephritis, and certain other organ manifestations—may require treatment urgently, but such decisions need to be made on a case-by-case basis. Watchful waiting is appropriate in a minority of patients, for example, those with asymptomatic lymphadenopathy or mild submandibular gland enlargement [73].

The cornerstone of treatment for IgG4-RD remains glucocorticoids. Conventional disease-modifying anti-rheumatic drugs (DMARDs) are also employed widely as glucocorticoid-sparing agents, albeit the evidence that any DMARD works well for that purpose is slim. Advancing understanding of the pathophysiology of IgG4-RD has led increasingly to the development of targeted treatment approaches. A variety of approaches have been designed to target B cells, and several of these are the subject of ongoing clinical trials.

Glucocorticoids

Glucocorticoids are the cornerstone of treatment for most patients with IgG4-related disease [73–75]. So reliable is this treatment response that the failure of glucocorticoids to bring significant clinical benefit constitutes an exclusion criterion in the ACR/EULAR Classification Criteria [39, 58]. Unfortunately, glucocorticoids are accompanied by substantial potential for treatment-related toxicity. The fact that many patients with IgG4-RD are middle-aged to elderly and frequently have comorbidities such as diabetes, obesity, osteoporosis, and hypertension poses in aggregate a major contraindication to prolonged glucocorticoid therapy. Moreover, IgG4-RD often has a substantial impact on the pancreas, and this further complicates glucocorticoid treatment in this disease.

A prospective, multicenter trial in Japan that described the adverse events observed during glucocorticoid treatment in patients with IgG4-related disease reported glucose intolerance in 41% of patients, dyslipidemia in 26%, and major infections in 18%, despite a maintenance dose of only 5–10 mg/day in most patients [76]. Careful monitoring for glucocorticoid toxicity and proactive interventions to limit such toxicity, particularly by reducing treatment duration and using effective glucocorticoid-sparing agents when available, are critical concepts in management. Treatment strategies vary across countries but at many centers the overall goal of induction therapy with glucocorticoids is to discontinue glucocorticoids within 3–4 months [14]. There has been a strong tendency in Asian countries, however, to rely upon longer glucocorticoid courses.

An international consensus guidance document concurred that prednisone at a dosage of 30–40 mg/day is appropriate for initial treatment [14]. A randomized trial in China evaluated the effect of a high-dose prednisone regimen (0.8–1.0 mg/kg/day) compared to a medium-dose regimen (0.5–0.6 mg/kg/day) [77]. Patients with more organ involvement and a higher IgG4-related disease responder index [78] score were more likely to relapse on the medium-dose regimen. In practice, the initial dosage of glucocorticoids varies widely. Some authors have reported the use of higher doses in patients with severe complications (pancreatic, pulmonary, renal, and retroperitoneal involvement) but lower doses in elderly patients or those with comorbidities. One reasonable approach is to maintain the starting dose of prednisone for 2–4 weeks and to taper the prednisone by 5 mg/day every 1–2 weeks until discontinuation.

Sustained remissions are unlikely to be induced without glucocorticoid courses lengthy enough to cause substantial toxicity in patients who have multi-organ disease and extremely high serum IgG4 concentrations at baseline. In such patients, early consideration should be given to a glucocorticoid-sparing agent.

Conventional DMARDs

Azathioprine, mycophenolate mofetil, methotrexate, leflunomide, and cyclophosphamide are commonly used worldwide in combination with glucocorticoids in patients with IgG4-related disease [14]. Despite the frequency with which they are used, however, there exists scant evidence that these agents add significantly to the efficacy of glucocorticoids. Most of the data on these drugs in IgG4-RD derive from retrospective analyses of case series in which glucocorticoids were used simultaneously, making it difficult to differentiate how much of the positive treatment effect was due to the "steroid-sparing agent" and how much was due to the persisting impact of glucocorticoids.

Biologic Agents

The current pathophysiologic understanding of IgG4-RD has identified certain targeted treatment approaches, some of which are now under study in clinical trials. Several of the approaches center around the interactions reported between cells of the B lymphocyte lineage and CD4+ T cells, particularly CD4 + CTLs that express SLAMF7.

The elevated concentrations of IgG4 seen in most patients with IgG4-RD provided evidence for a role of humoral immunity and inspiration for the use of rituximab in treatment. B cell depletion, which is highly effective in IgG4-RD, likely operates through several mechanisms. First, B cell depletion interrupts antigen presentation to CD4 + CTLs; indeed, the concentration of CD4 + CTLs in the peripheral blood and in tissue declines following targeted B cell depletion [26, 79, 80]. B cell depletion also decreases tissue fibrosis [68] and reduces cytokine production by B cells. It remains unclear whether the reduction of serum IgG4 concentrations is beneficial in IgG4-RD, but in theory this may be helpful in patients prone to developing immune complexes because of extremely high serum IgG4 concentrations.

B-Cell-Depleting Strategies

Rituximab, a chimeric monoclonal antibody directed against CD20 (a B-cell antigen) showed evidence of substantial efficacy in a trial of 30 patients with IgG4-related disease [81]. Seventy-seven percent of the patients achieved the primary outcome of remission at 6 months. Forty percent remained in complete remission at 12 months even though rituximab was not re-dosed. Rituximab has not been studied in randomized, double-blind trials, however, and this treatment strategy does have potential limitations. In a multicenter nationwide study from France assessing long-term safety and efficacy of rituximab over 2 years [82], only 52% of patients achieved glucocorticoid withdrawal and 40% of the patients experienced disease relapses. Serious infections and hypogammaglobulinemia were observed in approximately 15% of patients.

The efficacy evident for rituximab led directly to a trial of inebilizumab, a randomized double-blind, placebo-controlled study. Inebilizumab is a humanized monoclonal antibody directed against CD19, an antigen expressed even more broadly in the B lymphocyte lineage than CD20. Investigators in this trial plan to enroll 160 patients at 80 sites across the world [83].

Non-Depleting B-Cell Strategies

Other treatment strategies directed against B cells also appear promising [84]. A phase 2 trial of XmAb5871, a monoclonal antibody directed against both Fc-gammaRIIb and CD19, elicited positive treatment responses in 12 of 15 patients, with disease control obtained in the absence of glucocorticoid use in most subjects [85].

Approaches Targeting T Lymphocytes

Abatacept (anti-CTLA4-Ig), which interferes with T cell co-stimulation, was reportedly effective in one anecdotal report [86]. A phase 2 trial of abatacept that included ten patients, however, was less encouraging, with good treatment responses observed in only five of the ten patients [87].

SLAMF7 is a highly appealing drug target because it is present on both CD4 + CTLs and B cells. Depletion of activated cells that bear this surface molecule on would therefore directly address the interaction between CD4 + CTLs and the antigen-presenting B lineage cells that is felt to be fundamental to IgG4-related disease. A phase 2/3 trial with the anti-SLAM7 monoclonal antibody elotuzumab, a drug approved for the treatment of refractory multiple myeloma, was approved to begin enrollment in late 2021 [88].

Conclusions

IgG4-RD was recognized as a unified disease entity only in 2003 and awareness of this novel fibro-inflammatory condition has rapidly increased worldwide. IgG4-RD is characterized by the development of tumor-like masses and fibro-inflammatory strictures, and by the accumulation of IgG4-expressing B cells, T cells, and macrophages enmeshed in fibrotic material within lesions. Involvement of the pancreatobiliary tract, retroperitoneum/aorta, head and neck, and salivary glands are the most frequently observed disease phenotypes, differing in epidemiological features, serological findings, and prognostic outcomes. The optimal management of patients with IgG4-RD has to be grounded in careful clinical-pathological correlation and should take into account all of the potential presentations of this diverse condition. Continued follow-up is crucial, as the cumulative effects of indolent disease or repeated flares can lead to severe organ damage over time.

IgG4-RD is highly responsive to glucocorticoids but can lead to end-stage organ failure and even death if unrecognized. Prolonged courses of corticosteroids are often needed to maintain remission because the disease relapses in most patients. Flares are currently managed with repeated courses of glucocorticoids and with the introduction of immunomodulators or B-cell-depleting agents to maintain disease remission. Targeted therapeutic strategies are eagerly awaited as prolonged exposure to glucocorticoid therapy and immunosuppressive treatments can also expose patients to long-term toxicity. In this regard, substantial advancements have been made in understanding the pathophysiology of IgG4-RD, unveiling therapeutic targets that will offer valuable alternatives in the years ahead.

Yet, many other areas of uncertainty and questions remain to be addressed while welcoming novel therapeutic opportunities. First, it is important to understand whether emerging treatment options can replace corticosteroid therapy or whether they should only be used as steroid-sparing agents. Second, the right timing of treatment administration represents a relevant matter of discussion as some therapies might be more effective than others in inducing and/or maintaining disease remission as well as in targeting established tissue fibrosis. Third, as IgG4-RD is largely considered a life-long disorder that can relapse many years after original diagnosis and therapy, treatment duration represents a still unanswered question. Choosing the best therapy for the individual patient, based on the stage of presentation (inflammatory phase or more fibrotic), clinical disease phenotype (isolated pancreatic involvement versus multi-systemic disease), urgency of presentation (jaundice with biliary stricture, sight-threatening orbital mass, or generalized lymphadenopathy) and established predictors of relapse (serum IgG4 level, multi-organ disease) will represent, therefore, the most important goal for the future. Finally, we currently ignore whether clinical phenotypes of IgG4-RD also differ in pathophysiologic mechanisms and, thus, whether specific agents should be preferred over others. In this sense, the identification of distinct and replicable disease phenotypes as well as the recently released ACR/EULAR classification criteria will represent an invaluable platform for designing high quality clinical and research studies to address most of these fundamental questions.

Looking ahead, the field of IgG4-RD is evolving towards a more personalized approach based on multidisciplinary evaluations and tailored therapeutic strategies. The emergence of a variety of targeted treatments is fostering this process but proper validation of their safety and efficacy in randomized clinical trials will be required to offer patients the best available therapeutic option.

References

1. Lanzillotta M, Mancuso G, Della-Torre E. Advances in the diagnosis and management of IgG4 related disease. BMJ. 2020;369:m1067. https://doi.org/10.1136/bmj.m1067.
2. Mahajan VS, Mattoo H, Deshpande V, Pillai SS, Stone JH. IgG4-related disease. Annu Rev Pathol. 2014;9:315–47.
3. Hamano H, Kawa S, Horiuchi A, et al. High serum IgG4 concentrations in patients with sclerosing pancreatitis. N Engl J Med. 2001;344:732–8.
4. Kuttner H. Über entzündliche tumoren der submaxillar-speicheldrüse. Beitr Klin Chir. 1896;15:815–34.
5. Mikulicz J. Über eine eigenartige symmetrische erkränkung der thränen—und mundspeicheldrüsen. In: Billroth T, editor. Beiträge zur Chir Festschrift Gewidmet Stuttgart Ger Ferdinand Enke. 1892. pp. 610–630.
6. Ormond JK. Bilateral ureteral obstruction due to envelopment and compression by an inflammatory retroperitoneal process. J Urol. 1948;59:1072–9.
7. Zinkraf E. A case of exocrine and endocrine pancreatic insufficiency following sclerosing pancreatitis complicating an unusual pancreatic deformity. Frankf Z Pathol. 1951;62:13–21.
8. Riedel B. Die chronische zur Bildung eisenharter Tumoren fuhrende Entzündung der Schildrüse. Verhandlung der Dtsch Gesellschaft für Chir. 1896;25:101.
9. Della-Torre E, Lanzillotta M, Doglioni C. Immunology of IgG4-related disease. Clin Exp Immunol. 2015;181:191–206.
10. Kanno A, Nishimori I, Masamune A, et al.; the Research Committee on Intractable Diseases of Pancreas. Nationwide epidemiological survey of autoimmune pancreatitis in Japan. Pancreas. 2012;41:835–839.
11. Masamune A, Kikuta K, Hamada S, et al. Nationwide epidemiological survey of autoimmune pancreatitis in Japan in 2016. J Gastroenterol. 2019;55:462. https://doi.org/10.1007/s00535-019-01658-7.
12. Uchida K, Masamune A, Shimosegawa T, Okazaki K. Prevalence of IgG4-related disease in Japan based on Nationwide survey in 2009. Int J Rheumatol. 2012;2012:358371.
13. Deshpande V, Zen Y, Chan JK, Yi EE, Sato Y, Yoshino T, et al. Consensus statement on the pathology of IgG4-related disease. Mod Pathol. 2012;25:1181–92.
14. Khosroshahi A, Wallace ZS, Crowe JL, et al. International consensus guidance statement on the management and treatment of IgG4-related disease. Arthritis Rheumatol. 2015;67:1688–99.
15. Della-Torre E, Bozzalla-Cassione E, Sciorati C, et al. A CD8α− subset of CD4+SLAMF7+ cytotoxic T cells is expanded in patients with IgG4-related disease and decreases following glucocorticoid treatment. Arthritis Rheumatol. 2018;70:1133–43.

16. Mattoo H, Mahajan VS, Della-Torre E, et al. De novo oligoclonal expansions of circulating plasmablasts in active and relapsing IgG4-related disease. J Allergy Clin Immunol. 2014;134:679–87.
17. Maehara T, Mattoo H, Ohta M, et al. Lesional CD4+ IFN-γ+ cytotoxic T lymphocytes in IgG4-related dacryoadenitis and sialoadenitis. Ann Rheum Dis. 2017;76:377–85.
18. Perugino C, Kaneko N, Kers J, et al. Clonal expansion of a specific subset of cytotoxic CD4+T cells and tissue apoptosis in patients with IgG4-related disease [abstract]. Arthritis Rheumatol. 2019;71(suppl 10).
19. Perugino C, Kaneko N, Maehara T, et al. CD8+ cytotoxic T lymphocytes are clonally-expanded in IgG4-related disease and home to affected tissues [abstract]. Arthritis Rheumatol. 2019;71(suppl 10).
20. Perugino CA, AlSalem SB, Mattoo H, et al. Identification of galectin-3 as an autoantigen in patients with IgG4-related disease. J Allergy Clin Immunol. 2019;143:736–45.e6.
21. Hubers LM, Vos H, Schuurman AR, et al. Annexin A11 is targeted by IgG4 and IgG1 autoantibodies in IgG4-related disease. Gut. 2018;67:728–35.
22. Shiokawa M, Kodama Y, Sekiguchi K, et al. Laminin 511 is a target antigen in autoimmune pancreatitis. Sci Transl Med. 2018;10(453):eaaq0997.
23. Du H, Shi L, Chen P, et al. Prohibitin is involved in patients with IgG4 related disease. PLoS One. 2015;10:e0125331.
24. Terao C, Ota M, Iwasaki T, et al. IgG4-related disease in the Japanese population: a genome-wide association study. Lancet Rheumatol. 2019;1:e14–22. https://doi.org/10.1016/S2665-9913(19)30006-2.
25. Della-Torre E, Rigamonti E, Perugino C, et al. B lymphocytes directly contribute to tissue fibrosis in patients with IgG4-related disease. J Allergy Clin Immunol. 2019;145:968. https://doi.org/10.1016/j.jaci.2019.07.004.
26. Mattoo H, Mahajan VS, Maehara T, et al. Clonal expansion of CD4(+) cytotoxic T lymphocytes in patients with IgG4-related disease. J Allergy Clin Immunol. 2016;138:825–38.
27. Akiyama M, Suzuki K, Yamaoka K, et al. Number of circulating follicular helper 2 T cells correlates with IgG4 and Interleukin-4 levels and plasmablast numbers in IgG4-related disease. Arthritis Rheumatol. 2015;67:2476–81.
28. Grados A, Ebbo M, Piperoglou C, et al. T cell polarization toward TH2/TFH2 and TH17/TFH17 in patients with IgG4-related disease. Front Immunol. 2017;8:235.
29. Cargill T, Makuch M, Sadler R, et al. Activated T-follicular helper 2 cells are associated with disease activity in IgG4-related Sclerosing cholangitis and pancreatitis. Clin Transl Gastroenterol. 2019;10:e00020.
30. Akiyama M, Yasuoka H, Yamaoka K, et al. Enhanced IgG4 production by follicular helper 2 T cells and the involvement of follicular helper 1 T cells in the pathogenesis of IgG4-related disease. Arthritis Res Ther. 2016;18:167.
31. Chen Y, Lin W, Yang H, et al. Aberrant expansion and function of follicular helper T cell subsets in IgG4-related disease. Arthritis Rheumatol. 2018;70:1853–65.
32. Zen Y, Fujii T, Harada K, et al. Th2 and regulatory immune reactions are increased in immunoglobin G4-related sclerosing pancreatitis and cholangitis. Hepatology. 2007;45:1538–46.
33. Tanaka A, Moriyama M, Nakashima H, et al. Th2 and regulatory immune reactions contribute to IgG4 production and the initiation of Mikulicz disease. Arthritis Rheum. 2012;64:254–63.
34. Furukawa S, Moriyama M, Miyake K, et al. Interleukin-33 produced by M2 macrophages and other immune cells contributes to Th2 immune reaction of IgG4-related disease. Sci Rep. 2017;7:42413.
35. van der Neut KM, Schuurman J, Losen M, Bleeker WK, Martinez-Martinez P, Vermeulen E, et al. Anti-inflammatory activity of human IgG4 antibodies by dynamic Fab arm exchange. Science. 2007;317:1554–7.
36. Koneczny I. A new classification system for IgG4 autoantibodies. Front Immunol. 2018;9:97.
37. Sasaki T, Yajima T, Shimaoka T, et al. Synergistic effect of IgG4 antibody and CTLs causes tissue inflammation in IgG4-related disease. Int Immunol. 2020;32(3):163–74. https://doi.org/10.1093/intimm/dxz073.
38. Zhang W, Stone JH. Management of IgG4-related disease. Lancet Rheumatol. 2019;1:e55–65.

39. Wallace ZS, Naden RP, Chari S, et al. The 2019 American College of Rheumatology/European League Against Rheumatism Classification criteria for IgG4-related disease. Arthritis Rheumatol. 2020;72:7–19.
40. Wallace ZS, Zhang Y, Perugino CA, Naden R, Choi HK, Stone JH. Clinical phenotypes of IgG4-related disease: an analysis of two international cross-sectional cohorts. Ann Rheum Dis. 2019;78:406–12.
41. Kamisawa T, Zen Y, Pillai S, Stone JH. IgG4-related disease. Lancet. 2015;385:1460–71.
42. Zen Y, Inoue D, Kitao A, Onodera M, Abo H, Miyayama S, Gabata T, Matsui O, Nakanuma Y. IgG4-related lung and pleural disease: a clinicopathologic study of 21 cases. Am J Surg Pathol. 2009;33:1886–93.
43. Inoue D, Zen Y, Abo H, Gabata T, Demachi H, Kobayashi T, Yoshikawa J, Miyayama S, Yasui M, Nakanuma Y, Matsui O. Immunoglobulin G4-related lung disease: CT findings with pathologic correlations. Radiology. 2009;251:260–70.
44. Zen Y, Nakanuma Y. IgG4-related disease: a cross-sectional study of 114 cases. Am J Surg Pathol. 2010;34:1812–9.
45. Zen Y, Fujii T, Sato Y, Masuda S, Nakanuma Y. Pathological classification of hepatic inflammatory pseudotumor with respect to IgG4-related disease. Mod Pathol. 2007;20:884–94.
46. Zen Y, Britton D, Mitra V, Pike I, Heaton N, Quaglia A. A global proteomic study identifies distinct pathological features of IgG4-related and primary sclerosing cholangitis. Histopathology. 2015;68:796–809.
47. Ishikawa T, Itoh A, Kawashima H, Ohno E, Itoh Y, Nakamura Y, Hiramatsu T, Miyahara R, Ohmiya N, Haruta J, Goto H, Hirooka Y. Peripancreatic vascular involvements of autoimmune pancreatitis. J Gastroenterol Hepatol. 2012;27:1790–5.
48. Abraham SC, Leach S, Yeo CJ, Cameron JL, Murakata LA, Boitnott JK, Albores-Saavedra J, Hruban RH. Eosinophilic pancreatitis and increased eosinophils in the pancreas. Am J Surg Pathol. 2003;27:334–42.
49. Zen Y, Kawakami H, Kim JH. IgG4-related sclerosing cholangitis: all we need to know. J Gastroenterol. 2016;51:295–312.
50. Ebbo M, Grados A, Guedj E, Gobert D, Colavolpe C, Zaidan M, Masseau A, Bernard F, Berthelot JM, Morel N, Lifermann F, Palat S, Haroche J, Mariette X, Godeau B, Bernit E, Costedoat-Chalumeau N, Papo T, Hamidou M, Harlé JR, Schleinitz N. Usefulness of 2-[18F]-fluoro-2-deoxy-D-glucose-positron emission tomography/computed tomography for staging and evaluation of treatment response in IgG4-related disease: a retrospective multicenter study. Arthritis Care Res (Hoboken). 2014;66:86–96.
51. Ichiki A, Hashimoto N, Ueda T, Hiraiwa S, Tajiri T, Nakamura N, Ando K, Yokoyama K. IgG4-related disease with bone marrow involvement. Intern Med. 2016;55:2295–9.
52. Kamisawa T, Funata N, Hayashi Y, Eishi Y, Koike M, Tsuruta K, Okamoto A, Egawa N, Nakajima H. A new clinicopathological entity of IgG4-related autoimmune disease. J Gastroenterol. 2003;38:982–4.
53. van den Elshout-den UD, Spoto CPE, de Boer M, Leiner T, Leavis HL, Leguit RJ. First report of IgG4 related disease primary presenting as vertebral bone marrow lesions. Front Immunol. 2019;10:1910.
54. Geyer JT, Niesvizky R, Jayabalan DS, Mathew S, Subramaniyam S, Geyer AI, Orazi A, Ely SA. IgG4 plasma cell myeloma: new insights into the pathogenesis of IgG4-related disease. Mod Pathol. 2014;27:375–81.
55. Raissian Y, Nasr SH, Larsen CP, Colvin RB, Smyrk TC, Takahashi N, Bhalodia A, Sohani AR, Zhang L, Chari S, Sethi S, Fidler ME, Cornell LD. Diagnosis of IgG4-related tubulointerstitial nephritis. J Am Soc Nephrol. 2011;22:1343–52.
56. Saeki T, Nishi S, Imai N, Ito T, Yamazaki H, Kawano M, et al. Clinicopathological characteristics of patients with IgG4-related tubulointerstitial nephritis. Kidney Int. 2010;78:1016–23.

57. Alexander MP, Larsen CP, Gibson IW, Nasr SH, Sethi S, Fidler ME, Raissian Y, Takahashi N, Chari S, Smyrk TC, Cornell LD. Membranous glomerulonephritis is a manifestation of IgG4-related disease. Kidney Int. 2013;83:455–62.
58. Wallace ZS, Naden RP, Chari S, et al. The 2019 American College of Rheumatology/European League against Rheumatism classification criteria for IgG4-related disease. Ann Rheum Dis. 2020;79:77–87.
59. Chang SY, Keogh KA, Lewis JE, Ryu JH, Cornell LD, Garrity JA, et al. IgG4-positive plasma cells in granulomatosis with polyangiitis (Wegener's): a clinicopathologic and immunohistochemical study on 43 granulomatosis with polyangiitis and 20 control cases. Hum Pathol. 2013;44:2432–7.
60. Otani K, Inoue D, Fujikura K, Komori T, Abe-Suzuki S, Tajiri T, Itoh T, Zen Y. Idiopathic multicentric Castleman's disease: a clinicopathologic study in comparison with IgG4-related disease. Oncotarget. 2018;9(6):6691–706.
61. Tracht J, Reid MD, Xue Y, Madrigal E, Sarmiento JM, Kooby D, Alese OB, Krasinskas AM. Rosai-Dorfman disease of the pancreas shows significant histologic overlap with IgG4-related disease. Am J Surg Pathol. 2019;43:1536–46.
62. Yamamoto H, Yamaguchi H, Aishima S, Oda Y, Kohashi K, Oshiro Y, et al. Inflammatory myofibroblastic tumor versus IgG4-related sclerosing disease and inflammatory pseudotumor: a comparative clinicopathologic study. Am J Surg Pathol. 2009;33:1330–40.
63. Taylor MS, Chougule A, MacLeay AR, Kurzawa P, Chebib I, Le L, Deshpande V. Morphologic overlap between inflammatory myofibroblastic tumor and IgG4-related disease: lessons from next-generation sequencing. Am J Surg Pathol. 2019;43:314–24.
64. Della-Torre E, Stone JH. "How I manage" IgG4-related disease. J Clin Immunol. 2016;36:754–63.
65. Carruthers MN, Khosroshahi A, Augustin T, Deshpande V, Stone JH. The diagnostic utility of serum IgG4 concentrations in IgG4-related disease. Ann Rheum Dis. 2015;74:14–8.
66. Hao M, Liu M, Fan G, Yang X, Li J. Diagnostic value of serum IgG4 for igg4-related disease: a PRISMA-compliant systematic review and meta-analysis. Medicine (Baltimore). 2016;95:e3785.
67. Khosroshahi A, Cheryk LA, Carruthers MN, Edwards JA, Bloch DB, Stone JH. Brief report: spuriously low serum IgG4 concentrations caused by the prozone phenomenon in patients with IgG4-related disease. Arthritis Rheumatol. 2014;66:213–7.
68. Della-Torre E, Feeney E, Deshpande V, et al. B-cell depletion attenuates serological biomarkers of fibrosis and myofibroblast activation in IgG4-related disease. Ann Rheum Dis. 2014;74:2236–43.
69. Wallace ZS, Deshpande V, Mattoo H, et al. IgG4-related disease: clinical and laboratory features in one hundred twenty-five patients. Arthritis Rheumatol. 2015;67:2466–75.
70. Lopes Vendrami C, Shin JS, Hammond NA, Kothari K, Mittal PK, Miller FH. Differentiation of focal autoimmune pancreatitis from pancreatic ductal adenocarcinoma. Abdom Radiol. 2019;45:1371. https://doi.org/10.1007/s00261-019-02210-0.
71. Umehara H, Okazaki K, Masaki Y, et al. Comprehensive diagnostic criteria for IgG4-related disease (IgG4-RD), 2011. Mod Rheumatol. 2012;22:21–30.
72. Yoo BW, Song JJ, Park YB, Lee SW. 2019 American College of Rheumatology/European League Against Rheumatism classification criteria for IgG4-related disease by Wallace et al. Ann Rheum Dis. 2020;79(1):77–87. https://doi.org/10.1136/annrheumdis-2020-217086.
73. Kubota K, Iida H, Fujisawa T, et al. Clinical factors predictive of spontaneous remission or relapse in cases of autoimmune pancreatitis. Gastrointest Endosc. 2007;66:1142–51.
74. Brito-Zeron P, Kostov B, Bosch X, Acar-Denizli N, Ramos-Casals M, Stone JH. Therapeutic approach to IgG4-related disease: a systematic review. Medicine (Baltimore). 2016;95:e4002.
75. Hart PA, Kamisawa T, Brugge WR, et al. Long-term outcomes of autoimmune pancreatitis: a multicentre, international analysis. Gut. 2013;62:1771–6.

76. Masaki Y, Matsui S, Saeki T, et al. A multicenter phase II prospective clinical trial of glucocorticoid for patients with untreated IgG4-related disease. Mod Rheumatol. 2017;27:849–54.
77. Wu Q, Chang J, Chen H, et al. Efficacy between high and medium doses of glucocorticoid therapy in remission induction of IgG4-related diseases: a preliminary randomized controlled trial. Int J Rheum Dis. 2017;20:639–46.
78. Wallace ZS, Khosroshahi A, Carruthers MD, et al. An international multispecialty validation study of the IgG4-related disease responder index. Arthritis Care Res. 2018;70:1671–8.
79. Khosroshahi A, Bloch DB, Deshpande V, Stone JH. Rituximab therapy leads to rapid decline of serum IgG4 levels and prompt clinical improvement in IgG4-related systemic disease. Arthritis Rheum. 2010;62:1755–62.
80. Khosroshahi A, Carruthers MD, Deshpande V, Leb L, Reed JI, Stone JH. Cutaneous immunoglobulin G4-related systemic disease. AJM. 2011;124:e7.
81. Carruthers MN, Topazian MD, Khosroshahi A, et al. Rituximab for IgG4-related disease: a prospective, open-label trial. Ann Rheum Dis. 2015;74:1171–7.
82. Ebbo M, Grados A, Samson M, et al. Long-term efficacy and safety of rituximab in IgG4-related disease: data from a French nationwide study of thirty-three patients. PLoS One. 2017;12:e0183844.
83. clinicaltrials.gov: NCT04540497.
84. Stone JH, Wallace ZS, Perugino CA, et al. Final results of an open label phase 2 study of a reversible B cell inhibitor, XmAb5871,in IgG4-related disease. Arthritis Rheumatol. 2017;9:A169.
85. clinicialtrials.gov: NCT0272547.
86. Yamamoto M, Takahashi H, Takano K, et al. Efficacy of abatacept for IgG4-related disease over 8 months. Ann Rheum Dis. 2016;75:1576–8.
87. Matza MA, Perugino CA, Harvey L, Wallace ZS, Liu H, Pillai S, Stone JH. Abatacept for the treatment of IgG4-related disease (abstract). American College of Rheumatology. 2020.
88. clinicaltrials.gov: NCT04918147.

Chapter 16
Type I Cryoglobulinemia

Adrien Mirouse, David Saadoun, and Patrice Cacoub

Abbreviations

CNS	Central nervous system
IV	Intravenous
MGCS	Monoclonal gammopathy of clinical significance
PAS	Periodic acid–Schiff

Introduction

Cryoglobulins are immunoglobulins that precipitate when serum is incubated at temperatures lower than 37 °C. The existence of circulating cryoglobulins (cryoglobulinemia) is not always related to the presence of symptomatology. Cryoglobulinemia are usually classified according to Brouet et al. classification [1]. Type I cryoglobulinemia corresponds to a monoclonal immunoglobulin. In the first description, the monoclonal component corresponded to a monoclonal IgM, IgG, or a monoclonal light chain and monoclonal IgM was the most frequent. Type I cryoglobulins account for 10–25% of total cryoglobulinemias [2]. Type II and III

A. Mirouse · D. Saadoun · P. Cacoub (✉)
Department of Internal Medicine and Clinical Immunology, AP-HP, Groupe Hospitalier Pitié-Salpêtrière, Centre national de références Maladies Autoimmunes et systémiques rares, Centre national de références Maladies Autoinflammatoires rares et Amylose inflammatoire, Paris, France

Sorbonne Université, Paris, France

INSERM, UMR S 959, Immunology-Immunopathology- Immunotherapy (I3), Paris, France
e-mail: adrien.mirouse@aphp.fr; david.saadoun@aphp.fr; patrice.cacoub@aphp.fr

© The Author(s), under exclusive license to Springer Nature Switzerland AG 2022
G. Ragab et al. (eds.), *Paraproteinemia and Related Disorders*,
https://doi.org/10.1007/978-3-031-10131-1_16

cryoglobulinemias (Chap. 17) correspond to either a monoclonal immunoglobulin with polyclonal immunoglobulin or polyclonal immunoglobulin, respectively. The distinction of these subtypes is meaningful because underlying diseases vary according to each subtype. Moreover, physiopathological mechanisms and manifestations of type I cryoglobulinemia differ substantially from those of type II and III cryoglobulinemias.

Pathophysiology

Cryoglobulin cold-induced precipitation depends upon concentration, hydrophobicity, size and surface charge, as well as the solution temperature, pH, and ionic strength [3]. Cryoprecipitation is thought to be favored in small vessels because of higher cryoglobulin concentration with increased steric overload. Type I cryoglobulin, especially when made of monoclonal IgM with pentamer structure, may obstruct small vessels' lumen [4]. Steric and intrinsic properties of cryoglobulin may explain why some subtypes of immunoglobulin like IgG1 and IgG3 are more frequently diagnosed in type I cryoglobulinemia [5].

Besides cryoglobulin itself, other serum components like fibronectin influence the ability to precipitate [6]. Another study reported that cryoprecipitation is a property not only of immune complexes themselves but also of a group of large normal serum proteins [7]. Non-immunoglobulin cryoproteins were found to precipitate when exposed to cold, in association with immunoglobulin. In inflammatory diseases, the concentrations of some of these proteins may increase to the point where intermolecular attractive forces become prominent, particularly in the cold. However, cryoprecipitation upon cold exposure does not explain why tissues that are distant from the site of exposure to cold (like kidney) may be affected. Alterations of ion concentration like chloride and calcium in the renal interstitium may influence cryoglobulin structure and aggregation [3, 8].

Type I cryoglobulinemia should be considered, in the majority of cases, as a micro-thrombotic disease, with absence or minor signs of vasculitis. Cryoprecipitation explains ischemic manifestation and small vessels occlusion. Complement consumption which may be a diagnostic feature of cryoglobulinemic vasculitis is less frequently found in type I as compared to mixed cryoglobulinemia [9].

Epidemiology

The prevalence and incidence of cryoglobulinemia are unknown, in particular because of the heterogeneity in the cause, clinical presentation, and geographical distribution of the disease. The prevalence of clinically significant cryoglobulinemia has been estimated as approximately 1:100,000 individuals [10]. The real prevalence of cryoglobulinemia is probably higher, due to asymptomatic cryoglobulinemia.

Manifestations

Cryoglobulin-related symptoms cover a large scope of manifestations (Fig. 16.1). Of note, the presence of a cryoglobulin in the serum may be found in healthy individuals. As type I cryoglobulinemia is monoclonal, it is reflecting the presence of a B-lineage clone, but it also can be asymptomatic. Type I cryoglobulinemia may be asymptomatic in 13–25% patients and diagnosed during the work-up for a monoclonal gammopathy or a lymphoid neoplasm [5, 11, 12]. Type II and III cryoglobulinemia manifestations are linked to a medium/small vessels vasculitis. It can involve every organ, but typical manifestations are purpura, neuropathy, and kidney

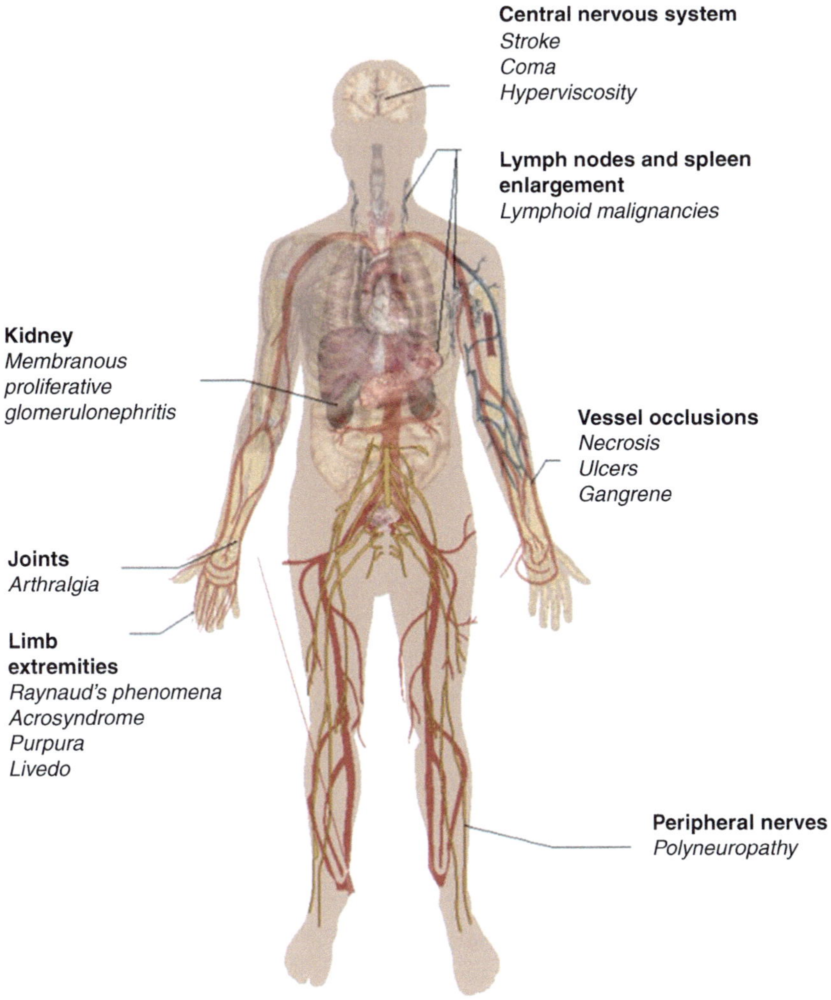

Fig. 16.1 Type I cryoglobulinemia manifestations

disease. In type I cryoglobulinemia, clinical manifestations may be directly linked to vascular occlusion, favored by cold-induced precipitation and less frequently by immune complex vasculitis. When compared to other types of cryoglobulinemia, patients with type I cryoglobulinemia exhibit more severe cutaneous involvement, and a lower frequency of glomerulonephritis [13].

For the purpose of this review, we analyzed the main characteristics of patients with type I cryoglobulinemia published in four recent series [13] (Table 16.1).

Skin Manifestations

Cold-induced manifestations in type I cryoglobulinemia include Raynaud's phenomena or other forms of acrosyndrome, livedo, and necrosis of extremities (fingers, nose, ears) or limb ischemia (Fig. 16.2) [1]. Rarely, ischemic manifestations and vasculitis may coexist in patients with type I cryoglobulinemia. Skin biopsy is consistent with thrombotic vasculopathy. In a retrospective study of 102 patients,

Table 16.1 Characteristics of patients with type I cryoglobulinemia

Characteristics	Type I cryoglobulinemia [5, 11–13] $n = 266$	Non-infectious mixed cryoglobulinemia [10] $n = 242$
Gender, man	**51%** (135/266)	**33%** (79/242)
Skin manifestations		
Purpura	**45%** (119/266)	**75%** (182/242)
Ulcers/gangrene	**35%** (94/266)	**16%** (39/242)
Raynaud's phenomena	**17%** (45/266)	
Livedo	**16%** (37/230)	
Acrocyanosis	**10%** (24/230)	**26%** (64/242)
Cold-induced urticaria	**6%** (13/230)	
Neurological		
Peripheral neuropathy	**33%** (87/266)	**52%** (125/242)
Sensory	**22%** (59/266)	**21%** (50/242)
Mixed	**8%** (22/266)	**31%** (75/242)
Motor	**1%** (2/266)	
CNS symptoms	**4%** (9/230)	**2%** (5/242)
Renal	**21%** (57/266)	**35%** (84/242)
Arthralgia	**15%** (39/266)	**30%** (72/242)
Asymptomatic	**13%** (29/230)	
Underlying disease		
Hematological malignancy	**97%** (258/266)	**22%** (52/242)
MGCS	**40%** (106/266)	
Lymphoma	**39%** (103/266)	
Myeloma	**18%** (49/266)	
None	**3%** (8/266)	

CNS central nervous system, *MGCS* monoclonal gammopathy of clinical significance

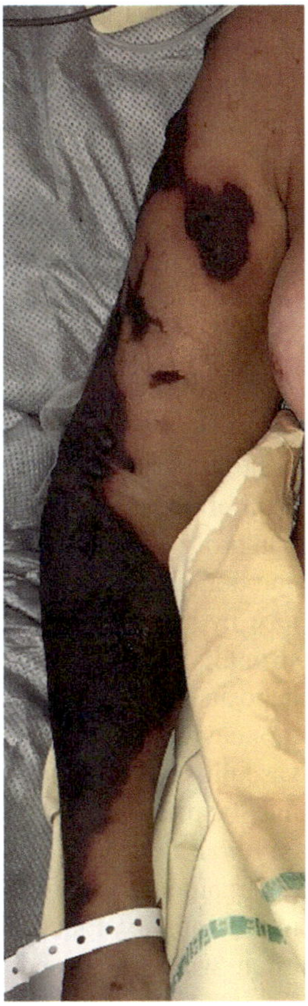

Fig. 16.2 Type I cryoglobulinemia with limb ischemia

63% of patients had skin manifestations, with purpura being most common (67%), followed by ulcers or gangrene in 55% of patients, livedo reticularis in 28% of patients with cutaneous findings, and 2% experienced cold-induced urticaria [11]. One quarter of patients reported vasomotor symptoms with 88% experiencing Raynaud's phenomenon and 20% acrocyanosis. Cryoglobulin lesions may involve nasal and oral mucosa [14].

Neurological Involvement

Peripheral nerve involvement consists in sensitory and/or motor neuropathy. Polyneuropathy and mononeuritis have been reported. Sensory neuropathy is the most frequent peripheral nerve involvement reported in patients with type I cryoglobulinemia [11, 13]. The pathogenesis of neuropathy may be due to three mechanisms, including immunologically mediated demyelination, microcirculation occlusion by cryoglobulin, and vasa nervorum vasculitis. When performed, nerve biopsy may reveal vasculitis but also ischemic lesions. Reported lesions include distal neuropathy due to *vasa nervorum* microcirculation occlusion caused by intravascular deposits of cryoglobulins associated with necrotizing vasculitis [15]. Central nervous system involvement is rarely described, consisting in ischemic stroke [5].

Kidney Involvement

The kidney is the most frequently involved organ in 20–30% of patients with type I cryoglobulinemia. Its presentation is consistent with nephrotic syndrome with arterial hypertension, proteinuria, hematuria, and acute kidney injury. Urine analysis usually shows hematuria. Kidney biopsy is consistent with a type I membranous proliferative glomerulonephritis. Examination with light microscopy reveals mesangial proliferation, inflammatory cells infiltration with neutrophils and macrophages, and double contour with silver staining. It may show diffuse and global endocapillary hyper-cellularity. Eosinophilic refractile intracapillary "cryo-plugs" that are strongly periodic acid–Schiff (PAS) positive is due to the IgM component of these deposits (Fig. 16.3). The acute phase has frequent neutrophils, with increased monocyte/macrophages. Arterioles and small arteries may show leukocytoclastic vasculitis. Cryoglobulin thrombi may obliterate small capillaries' lumen. Crescents may be present. Immunofluorescence staining shows mesangial and irregular capillary wall deposits. There is prominent IgM, C3, C4, and light chain deposits with lesser amounts of IgG or C1q. In type I cryoglobulin, cryo-plugs staining confirms monoclonality. Electron microscopy shows mesangial and subendothelial deposits, often with interposed cells and double contours due to new glomerular basal

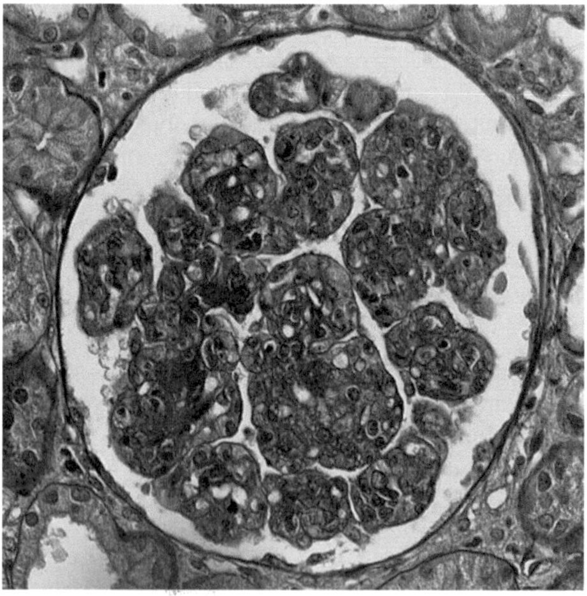

Fig. 16.3 Type I cryoglobulinemia kidney histology. Type I glomerunonephritis shows variable intracapillary hypercellularity, mostly due to mononuclear cells with intracapillary PAS + pseudothrombi, and glomerular basement membrane duplication. PAS stain

membrane formation beneath subendothelial deposits. Intracapillary deposits, extensive foot process effacement, and endocapillary hypercellularity also occur. Monoclonal cryoglobulin deposits may be microtubular and highly organized [16]. It has been suggested that the cryoprecipitation in kidney capillaries was the trigger of glomerulonephritis [17].

Rheumatologic and Systemic Symptoms

Among patients with type I cryoglobulinemia, 10–20% report inflammatory arthralgia [13]. Arthritis is less frequent. X-ray evaluation is usually normal. Patients may present with systemic symptoms like fever >38 °C, asthenia, and weight loss, due to the monoclonal immunoglobulin or the underlying hematological malignancy [5].

Hyperviscosity Syndrome

Hyperviscosity syndrome is a life-threatening complication. The classic triad of hyperviscosity reported by Waldenström includes mucosal bleeding, visual, and neurological abnormalities (Chap. 15) [18]. The most serious ophthalmic manifestation of hyperviscosity is bilateral central retinal vein occlusion. Headaches, nonspecific light-headedness, and hearing loss may appear. Funduscopic examination is a key exam because abnormalities are well correlated with abnormal plasma viscosity [19]. Funduscopic examination may reveal retinal vein dilation, tortuosity, and voluminous central hemorrhages. Viscosity is the highest in small venules and induces a venule wall tearing if there is not adequate underlying tissue support. Therefore, bleeding is seen where the veins are exposed on the surface with no superimposed epithelial tissue. This most commonly occurs in the lining of the nose, the gum, the retina, the lumen of the gastrointestinal tract, and the surface of the brain. Type I cryoglobulinemia is a well-described cause of hyperviscosity as the gelling phenomenon–which is highly temperature dependent—that occurs in the peripheral circulation rapidly raises the serum viscosity. In Waldenström disease, the mean monoclonal protein concentration is 41 g/L. In IgG myeloma with hyperviscosity, the mean monoclonal protein concentration is 64 g/L. [20]

Cryoglobulin Diagnosis

Cryoglobulin Identification

One of the diagnostic difficulties to the diagnosis of cryoglobulin is linked to the need to respect a well-defined procedure, including the need to keep samples warm at 37 °C [21]. There is no internationally accepted standard for the diagnostic methods of cryoglobulinemia. A survey of 137 laboratories on detection, analysis, and reporting of cryoglobulinemia demonstrated that only 36% of laboratories used procedures to ensure that the temperature did not drop below 37 °C [22]. There was wide variability in the time allowed for cryoprecipitation with 30% of laboratories allowing precipitation for less than 3 days. Cryoprecipitate was not immunotyped by 20% of laboratories. A non-respect of sampling and analysis exposes to the risk of false-negative results. A cryoglobulinemia research requires a sample of 10–20 mL in a 37 °C warmed tube. Samples are to be quickly transported to the laboratory and placed at 37 °C until coagulation. After centrifugation, sample is place at 4 °C. A result is negative if no cryoprecipitate is seen after 5–7 days. Cryoprecipitate concentration is variable from 0.01 g/L to more than 50 g/L and it is usually considered as positive above 0.05 g/L.

Indirect Diagnosis

Despite repetitive searches, type I cryoglobulinemia isolation may be difficult. In these cases, some indirect elements, in addition to clinical symptoms may help to diagnose cryoglobulinemia. Typical histologic findings are sufficient to diagnose cryoglobulinemia. Serum electrophoresis and immunofixation may detect a monoclonal immunoglobulin in patients' sera, reflecting B-cell lineage clonal proliferation. Complement consumption (i.e., low C4 level) and rheumatoid factor activity may be present in type I cryoglobulinemia although less frequently than in type II and III cryoglobulinemia [13]. The presence of type I cryoglobulinemia may disrupt routine laboratory exams and induce pseudo-thrombosis, pseudo-leukocytosis, pseudo-macrocytosis, and false positivity in sedimentation rate elevation.

Underlying Disease

As type I cryoglobulinemia corresponds to a monoclonal gammopathy, it is always associated with a B-cell lineage clonal disorder, especially multiple myeloma, monoclonal gammopathy of clinical significance (MGCS), and lymphoproliferative disorders (see Chaps. 12 and 21). Therefore, the initial diagnostic evaluation includes serum protein electrophoresis, whole-body imaging, CT-scan or PET-scan, bone marrow evaluation with aspiration and/or biopsy. Hematological malignancy is diagnosed in about 60% of cases of type I cryoglobulinemia including non-Hodgkin lymphoma (20%), multiple myeloma (19%), Waldenström disease (16%), and chronic lymphoid leukemia (2%). In other cases, the diagnosis of MGCS is made [13].

Treatment and Prognosis

Treatment of type I cryoglobulinemia depends on the underlying cause, i.e., MGCS or hemopathy (Fig. 16.4). Indications to treat are linked to the underlying malignancy in case of high tumor mass or associated manifestations such as cryoglobulinemia-related symptoms. In case of MGCS, treatment depends on the severity of cryoglobulinemia manifestations. In case of uncomplicated Raynaud's phenomena, or even when skin necrosis of extremities is present, avoidance of cold-exposition may be sufficient. In other cases with more severe cryoglobulin-related symptoms, treatment of monoclonal gammopathy is based on multiple myeloma regimen. Depending on the type of monoclonal immunoglobulin, we can define a better selection among the drugs used in myeloma. In case of MGCS with monoclonal IgG or IgA, treatment regimens include bortezomib, immunomodulators like pomalidomide or revlimid and dexamethasone. Monoclonal antibodies targeting plasma cells like anti-CD38 daratumumab are currently assessed. In case of MGCS with monoclonal IgM, treatment is based on rituximab in association with alkylating drugs, proteasome inhibitors or Bruton tyrosine kinase inhibitors. In case of

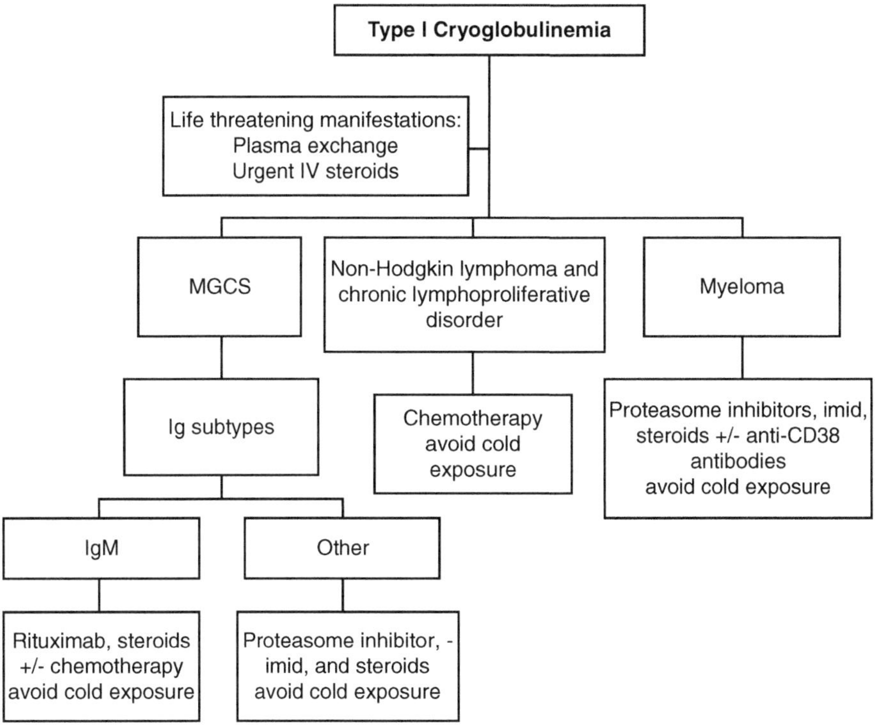

Fig. 16.4 Treatment strategy of patients with symptomatic type I cryoglobulinemia

identified hematological malignancy, treatment is decided jointly with a hematologist and is based on current recommendations.

In addition, in case of severe or life-threatening manifestations like extensive necrosis, acute kidney injury, or hyperviscosity syndrome plasma exchanges may be useful in association with high-dose steroids and chemotherapy to quickly remove the monoclonal immunoglobulin. Besides initial life-threatening manifestations, prognosis is linked to the underlying malignancy [5, 11–13].

Conclusion

Type I cryoglobulinemia is a rare but potentially life-threatening condition. It is always associated with a B-cell clonal proliferation. Treatment should be adapted the type and severity of cryoglobulin-related symptoms, and the type of underlying B-cell lymphoproliferative disorder.

References

1. Brouet JC, Clauvel JP, Danon F, Klein M, Seligmann M. Biologic and clinical significance of cryoglobulins. A report of 86 cases. Am J Med. 1974;57:775–88.
2. Tedeschi A, Baratè C, Minola E, Morra E. Cryoglobulinemia. Blood Rev. 2007;21:183–200.
3. Qi M, Steiger G, Schifferli JA. A calcium-dependent cryoglobulin IgM kappa/polyclonal IgG. J Immunol. 1992;149:2345–51.
4. Hiramoto E, et al. The IgM pentamer is an asymmetric pentagon with an open groove that binds the AIM protein. Sci Adv. 2018;4:eaau1199.
5. Harel S, et al. Clinico-biological characteristics and treatment of type I monoclonal cryoglobulinaemia: a study of 64 cases. Br J Haematol. 2015;168:671–8.
6. Strevey J, et al. The role of fibronectin in the cryoprecipitation of monoclonal cryoglobulins. Clin Exp Immunol. 1984;55:340–6.
7. Hardin JA. Cryoprecipitogogue from normal serum: mechanism for cryoprecipitation of immune complexes. Proc Natl Acad Sci U S A. 1981;78:4562–5.
8. Di Stasio E, et al. Cl− regulates cryoglobulin structure: a new hypothesis for the physiopathological mechanism of temperature non-dependent cryoprecipitation. Clin Chem Lab Med. 2004;42:614–20.
9. Vita SD, et al. Preliminary classification criteria for the cryoglobulinaemic vasculitis. Ann Rheum Dis. 2011;70:1183–90.
10. Terrier B, et al. Management of noninfectious mixed cryoglobulinemia vasculitis: data from 242 cases included in the CryoVas survey. Blood. 2012;119:5996–6004.
11. Sidana S, et al. Clinical presentation and outcomes of patients with type 1 monoclonal cryoglobulinemia. Am J Hematol. 2017;92:668–73.
12. Néel A, et al. Long-term outcome of monoclonal (type 1) cryoglobulinemia. Am J Hematol. 2014;89:156–61.
13. Terrier B, et al. The spectrum of type I cryoglobulinemia vasculitis: new insights based on 64 cases. Medicine (Baltimore). 2013;92:61–8.
14. Cohen SJ, Pittelkow MR, Su WP. Cutaneous manifestations of cryoglobulinemia: clinical and histopathologic study of seventy-two patients. J Am Acad Dermatol. 1991;25:21–7.

15. Garcia-Bragado F, Fernandez JM, Navarro C, Villar M, Bonaventura I. Peripheral neuropathy in essential mixed cryoglobulinemia. Arch Neurol. 1988;45:1210–4.
16. Fogo AB, Lusco MA, Najafian B, Alpers CE. AJKD atlas of renal pathology: cryoglobulinemic glomerulonephritis. Am J Kidney Dis. 2016;67:e5–7.
17. Reininger L, et al. Cryoglobulinemia induced by a murine IgG3 rheumatoid factor: skin vasculitis and glomerulonephritis arise from distinct pathogenic mechanisms. Proc Natl Acad Sci U S A. 1990;87:10038–42.
18. Waldenstrom J. Incipient myelomatosis or 'essential' hyperglobnlinemia with fibrinogenopenia—a new syndrome? Acta Med Scand. 1944;117:216–47.
19. Dumas G, Gabarre P, Bigé N, Maury E. Hyperviscosity syndrome. Intensive Care Med. 2018;44:1151–2.
20. Gertz MA. Acute hyperviscosity: syndromes and management. Blood. 2018;132:1379–85.
21. Sargur R, White P, Egner W. Cryoglobulin evaluation: best practice? 2010. https://journals.sagepub.com/doi/10.1258/acb.2009.009180?url_ver=Z39.88-2003&rfr_id=ori%3Arid%3Acrossref.org&rfr_dat=cr_pub++0pubmed&.
22. Vermeersch P, et al. A critical appraisal of current practice in the detection, analysis, and reporting of cryoglobulins. Clin Chem. 2008;54:39–43.

Chapter 17
Paraproteinemias Associated with Autoimmune Diseases

Luca Quartuccio, Elena Treppo, and Salvatore De Vita

Abbreviations

AA	Systemic inflammatory-associated (AA) amyloidosis
AS	Ankylosing spondylitis
BD	Bechet's disease
FLCs	Free light chains
GCA	Giant cell arteritis
GPA	Granulomatosis with polyangiitis
HR	Hazard ratio
MGUS	Monoclonal gammopathy of undetermined significance
mIg	Monoclonal immunoglobulins
MM	Multiple myeloma
PMR	Polymyalgia rheumatica
PsA	Psoriatic arthritis
PSO	Psoriasis
pSS	Primary Sjögren's syndrome
RA	Rheumatoid arthritis
RTX	Rituximab
SAA	Serum amyloid A
SIRs	Standardized incidence ratios
SLE	Systemic lupus erythematosus
SMM	Smoldering multiple myeloma

L. Quartuccio (✉) · E. Treppo · S. De Vita
Rheumatology Clinic, Department of Medicine, University of Udine, Udine, Italy
e-mail: luca.quartuccio@uniud.it; salvatore.devita@uniud.it

© The Author(s), under exclusive license to Springer Nature Switzerland AG 2022

G. Ragab et al. (eds.), *Paraproteinemia and Related Disorders*,
https://doi.org/10.1007/978-3-031-10131-1_17

SSc	Systemic sclerosis
TAK	Takayasu's arteritis

Introduction

A paraprotein is a monoclonal immunoglobulin or immunoglobulin light chain, arising from the clonal proliferation of B cell lineage, usually plasma cells or B-lymphocytes [1]. Paraproteins can be detected in the blood or urine and are characterized by a homogenous electrophoretic migration and the expression of a single light chain type, either kappa or lambda [1]. In this chapter, we focus on paraproteinemia associated with systemic autoimmune diseases.

The presence of paraproteinemia should be tested in patients with suspected clinical findings (Table 17.1). To increase the ability to detect a paraprotein, it is necessary to screen both blood and urine. To identify Bence-Jones protein, it is required to perform both serum protein electrophoresis and urinary protein electrophoresis. To detect free light chains, it is useful to perform serum-free chain analysis.

When monoclonal paraproteinemia is detected, the main issue is to distinguish between monoclonal gammopathy of uncertain significance (MGUS), smoldering multiple myeloma (SMM), and multiple myeloma (MM) (Table 17.2). MGUS is a

Table 17.1 Symptoms and clinical findings to suspect paraproteinemia

Symptoms	Persistent back pain
	Paresthesias
	Recurrent bacterial infections
Clinical findings	Lytic bone lesions
	Unexplained impaired renal function
	Normochromic normocytic anemia
	Pancytopenia
	Hypercalcemia
	Hyperviscosity syndrome
	Nephrotic syndrome
	Unexplained peripheral neuropathy

Table 17.2 Diagnostic criteria for monoclonal gammopathy of uncertain significance (MGUS), smoldering multiple myeloma (SMM), and multiple myeloma (MM)

	MGUS	SMM	MM
Paraprotein in serum	<30 g/L	>30 g/L	Presence in serum and/or urine
Clonal plasma cells in bone marrow	<10%	>10%	Presence
Myeloma-related organ impairment[a]	Absent	Absent	Presence

[a]Increased calcium levels, renal insufficiency, anemia, bone lesions, symptomatic hyperviscosity syndrome, amyloidosis, recurrent bacterial infections

CD19+, CD45−, and CD56+ plasma cell disorder, having a 1% average annual progression rate to MM [2]. MGUS maintains low proliferation rates and can evolve into MM or Waldenström's macroglobulinemia or AL amyloidosis or lymphoma [2]. Its association with autoimmune diseases has been suggested, arising from persistent antigenic stimulation and cytogenetic abnormalities due to chronic, persistent, pro-inflammatory microenvironment [2].

Monoclonal Gammopathy and Autoimmune Diseases

Several systematic reviews [3, 4] investigated autoimmune diseases and subsequently the risk of MGUS, SMM, and MM. Autoimmune conditions are markers of immune dysregulation, which may manifest with the development of plasma cell disorder [3]. Monoclonal gammopathy could be also associated with measures of disease activity including longer disease duration and higher sedimentation rate [5].

In 2016, a Swedish study [6] identified 12,140 MGUS patients (during the period 1987–2012) and 769,991 patients with any autoimmune diseases (during the period 1964–2012). Combining these data with a Swedish nationwide family registry, the authors provided familial risk for MGUS in patients whose first-degree relatives had any autoimmune diseases. Standardized incidence ratios (SIRs) were calculated as the ratio of observed to the expected number of cases. As expected, the mean age at diagnosis of MGUS was 70 years, and men slightly outnumbered (51%) women. For autoimmune diseases, the mean age was 39 years and women outnumbered (56%) men. Overall, 332 familial cases were found with SIR for MGUS of 1.63. The highest male SIR for MGUS was 9.18 when a family member was diagnosed with rheumatic fever. For women, the highest MGUS association of 6.18 was with granulomatosis with polyangiitis (GPA). SIRs were found to increase with 10 associations, the highest SIRs were observed in case of family history for rheumatic fever (6.04), polymyositis/dermatomyositis (5.66), and dermatitis herpetiformis (5.21). Association with rheumatoid arthritis (RA) and psoriasis (PSO), which are common autoimmune diseases, were 1.49 and 1.56, respectively. Table 17.3 shows the details of this study.

Notably, the overall risk for MGUS among any autoimmune diseases was 1.63, suggesting a strong impact of autoimmune stimulation on MGUS.

In reverse, authors [6] provided the risk for autoimmune disease in patients whose first-degree relatives had MGUS. Overall, 1893 familial cases were detected and the overall SIR was 1.10 (higher for men [1.13] than women [1.08]). For men, the highest risk was for Takayasu's arteritis (TA) (11.75), followed by Guillain-Barre syndrome, myasthenia gravis, polymyositis/dermatomyositis, and GPA in this order. For women, the risks for RA (1.24) and sarcoidosis (1.69) were found. Table 17.4 shows the details.

An earlier study [7] in 2012 examined the risks of MM (SIR) and survival in MM (hazard ratio, HR) systematically in patients who had been hospitalized for any of 33 autoimmune diseases covering the total Swedish population. For MM after any autoimmune diseases, the SIR was increased to 1.12 (95% CI 1.02–1.23),

Table 17.3 SIR for MGUS with a family history of autoimmune disease (1964–2012). (Modified by Hemminki K et al., Leukemia (2016) 1742–1792)

An autoimmune disorder in a family member	Men SIR (95% CI)	Women SIR (95% CI)	All SIR (95% CI)
Amyotrophic lateral sclerosis	2.13 (0.55–5.50)	2.78 (0.88–6.53)	***2.44 (1.11–4.66)***
Dermatitis herpetiformis	5.00 (0.47–18.40)	5.44 (0.51–20.01)	**5.21 (1.36–13.48)**
Giant cell arteritis	**2.88 (1.14–5.96)**	0.82 (0.08–3.02)	1.85 (0.84–3.52)
Multiple sclerosis	**2.50 (1.07–4.94)**	0.63 (0.06–2.30)	1.56 (0.74–2.88)
Pemphigoid	1.79 (0.17–6.59)	**4.49 (1.42–10.56)**	**3.14 (1.24–6.51)**
Polymyalgia rheumatica	1.69 (0.90–2.90)	**2.45 (1.45–3.89)**	**2.06 (1.40–2.93)**
Polymyositis/dermatomyositis	**7.07 (1.33–20.91)**	4.36 (0.41–16.05)	**5.66 (1.79–13.32)**
Psoriasis	**1.88 (1.26–2.70)**	1.23 (0.74–1.93)	**1.56 (1.15–2.07)**
Rheumatic fever	**9.18 (3.30–20.11)**	2.98 (0.28–10.95)	**6.04 (2.58–11.95)**
Rheumatoid arthritis	**1.53 (1.04–2.17)**	1.46 (0.98–2.10)	**1.49 (1.14–1.92)**
Sarcoidosis	**2.87 (1.30–5.48)**	1.61 (0.51–3.78)	**2.24 (1.22–3.77)**
Sjögren's syndrome	1.34 (0.13–4.91)	**3.50 (1.10–8.23)**	2.39 (0.95–4.95)
Ulcerative colitis	1.41 (0.67–2.60)	**1.95 (1.07–3.29)**	**1.68 (1.08–2.51)**
Granulomatosis with polyangiitis	–	**6.18 (1.16–18.28)**	3.24 (0.61–9.60)
All	**1.61 (1.37–1.87)**	**1.65 (1.41–1.92)**	**1.63 (1.46–1.81)**

SIR standardized incidence ratio, *CI* confidence interval

Table 17.4 SIR for autoimmune disease with a family history of MGUS (1987–2012). (Modified by Hemminki K et al., Leukemia (2016) 1742–1792)

Autoimmune disorder	Men SIR (95% CI)	Women SIR (95% CI)	All SIR (95% CI)
Guillain-Barre syndrome	**2.53 (1.38–4.25)**	0.88 (0.17–2.59)	**1.90 (1.10–3.04)**
Myasthenia gravis	**2.60 (1.11–5.16)**	0.77 (0.15–2.29)	1.58 (0.79–2.84)
Polymyositis/ dermatomyositis	**2.67 (1.06–5.54)**	0.89 (0.17–2.63)	1.67 (0.79–3.08)
Takayasu's arteritis	**11.75 (1.11–43.22)**	3.06 (0.29–11.26)	**4.86 (1.26–12.56)**
Granulomatosis with polyangiitis	**2.20 (1.00–4.19)**	0.93 (0.18–2.77)	1.64 (0.84–2.88)
All	**1.13 (1.06–1.22)**	**1.08 (1.02–1.15)**	**1.10 (1.05–1.15)**

SIR standardized incidence ratio, *CI* confidence interval

while the HR was 0.92 (95% CI 0.81–1.04) (not significant). SIRs were significantly increased after ankylosing spondylitis (AS) [2.02 (95% CI 1.15–3.28)] and systemic sclerosis (SSc) [2.63 (95% CI 1.58–4.11). No SIR was significantly decreased. Only the HR after rheumatic fever [5.27 (95% CI 2.37–11.75)] was significantly increased.

The data were analyzed also according to the age at MM diagnosis. The overall risk of MM was increased only for autoimmune diseases diagnosed before the age 60 (SIR 1.45). The risk of MM (SIRs) before age 60 years was increased in AS (3.31), chronic rheumatic heart disease (2.79), and systemic lupus erythematosus (SLE) (5.19). The HRs in young patients were increased after Graves/hyperthyroidism (2.48), rheumatic fever (21.17), and SSc (5.51). In MM patients diagnosed at age ≥60, only the risk for systemic sclerosis was increased (2.59). HRs were increased after polymyositis/dermatomyositis (5.40) and rheumatic fever (4.60).

To summarize, this study [7] showed an increase in MM SIR after two autoimmune diseases (AS and SSc) and HR after rheumatic fever.

The first comprehensive systematic review of the literature to investigate autoimmune conditions and MGUS and MM was performed in 2014 [4]. Overall, an elevated risk of both MGUS and MM in the presence of any autoimmune disease was found. However, the only condition with an elevated risk of both MGUS and MM was pernicious anemia. Vitamin B12 deficiency has been associated with several malignancies and has also been shown to disrupt normal homeostasis of methyl group metabolism as a result of abnormal DNA methylation and synthesis causing megaloblastic anemia, which is common in patients with MM. Autoimmune hemolytic anemia (AIHA) was also associated with MM and serum monoclonal gammopathy was a significant predictor for the appearance of lymphoproliferative disorders [4, 8]. PSO was found to be negatively associated with MM [4], and MM is infrequent in patients with psoriatic arthritis (PsA) [9]. These results could also depend on medication bias. In fact, another study [10] reported the development of monoclonal gammopathy among 8 out 300 patients with PSO or PsA who were treated with anti-TNF-alpha agents. Treatment with anti-TNF-alpha agents may be a marker of more active disease, thus the presence of MGUS may reflect the level of immune dysregulation [9].

RA was not demonstrate a significantly increased risk for MM, whereas a significant excess risk was observed for MGUS [4, 11].

In a large population-based, study Lindqvist EK et al. [11] included almost 20,000 MM patients, >5000 MGUS patients, and nearly 100,000 matched controls. The authors found that a personal history of several specific immune-related conditions was associated with an increased risk of MM and MGUS. Interestingly, they also found that a family history of an autoimmune disease increased the risk of MGUS, and not MM. This implies that immune-related conditions or their treatment are of importance in the pathogenesis of MGUS and possibly MM.

A personal history of all inflammatory conditions (OR = 1.4; 95% CI, 1.2–1.5), and autoimmune diseases (OR = 2.1; 95% CI, 1.9–2.4) was associated with a significantly increased risk of MGUS. A family history of autoimmune disease was associated with a significantly increased risk of MGUS (OR = 1.1; 95% CI, 1.00–1.2), but not MM. A personal history of polymyalgia rheumatica (PMR) and GCA was associated with an increased risk of both MM (OR = 7.8 and 1.“ for GCA and PMR, respectively) and MGUS (OR = 11.3 and 2.9 for GCA and PMR, respectively) [11]. PMR and GCA have been associated with lymphoplasmacytic lymphoma and Waldenström macroglobulinemia [12]. In addition, a family history of these disorders was associated with an increased risk of MGUS. The underlying mechanisms for these findings are not clear but may involve shared susceptibility or an effect of chronic immune stimulation.

Primary Sjögren's syndrome (pSS) is typically considered as a crossroad disease between autoimmunity and lymphoproliferation [13–15]. PSS presents with sicca symptomatology and its histological hallmark is focal lymphocytic infiltration of exocrine glands. PSS can extend to systemic involvement and may be complicated by lymphoma. Its analytical features are typically cytopenias, hypergammaglobulinemia, positivity of antinuclear antibodies, anti-Ro/SSA, and, less frequently, cryoglobulins as well as hypocomplementemia. A meta-analysis [16] showed that 21% of pSS had serum monoclonal immunoglobulins (mIg). Clinically, pSS patients with monoclonal gammopathy had a higher prevalence of parotid enlargement (38% vs 20%, $p = 0.021$), vasculitis (21% vs 6%, $p = 0.003$) and neurological involvement (42% vs 23%, $p = 0.016$) compared with those without monoclonal gammopathy [17]. Patients with monoclonal gammopathy had higher mean values of circulating gamma globulins (23.4% vs 20.6%, $p = 0.026$), erythrocyte sedimentation rate (56.6 vs 37.6 mm/h, $p = 0.003$) [17]. Furthermore, a higher prevalence of rheumatoid factor, low C3 and C4 levels, and cryoglobulins are detected in patients with monoclonal gammopathy. The predominant isotype in pSS is IgGk [16–18]. The isotype of mIg has less prognostic significance in pSS than MGUS. In MGUS, in fact, studies support an association between IgM isotype and B cell lymphoma, and between IgG isotype and MM (Chap. 12). This is less evident in pSS with mIg, nevertheless, pSS with monoclonal gammopathy has a poor prognosis. The clinical significance of circulating mIgs in pSS has been scarcely studied [17]. Interestingly, persistent rather than transient cryoglobulins were associated with type II rather than type III cryoglobulins, and they were associated with a more active disease (i.e., vasculitis) or lymphoma [19].

Bechet's disease (BD) straddles the interphase between autoinflammatory and autoimmune diseases. Few cases of BD and MGUS have been documented. Recent observations sustained the role of epigenetics in the pathogenesis of BD. The genetics and environmental factors influence also MGUS predisposition. Thus, it is supposed that BD and MGUS might be linked by similar pathogenetic mechanisms [2].

In conclusion, systemic autoimmune diseases are examples of non-hematologic diseases which often present with monoclonal gammopathy. Monoclonal gammopathy is observed in patients with several rheumatic disorders, with IgG being the most frequent type of M protein. The presence of monoclonal gammopathy seems to be associated with higher disease activity of the underlying autoimmune process [20]. Although the development of MM was considered unusual as reported in the literature, there are more patients with MM than with lymphoma [20]. The risk for MM has been reportedly higher in AS and SSc patients [7]. To facilitate an early diagnosis and timely intervention, we recommend the inclusion of monoclonal gammopathy screening in immunocompromised and rheumatic diseases patients especially when they exhibit a phenotype with high ESR, albumin/globulin inversion, rheumatoid factor positivity, hypergammaglobulinemia, hypocomplementemia, or renal injury of unknown reasons [3, 20].

Amyloidosis and Autoimmune Diseases

Systemic inflammatory-associated (AA) amyloidosis is also known as secondary amyloidosis. It is a long-recognized complication of chronic inflammatory diseases. The organ damage is caused by extracellular deposition of the soluble acute-phase reactant serum amyloid A (SAA) protein as insoluble amyloid fibrils. A sustained high concentration of SAA produced by the liver during a chronic inflammatory state is the prerequisite for developing AA amyloidosis [21, 22].

The diagnosis of AA amyloid was classified as proven, possible, or problematic [23]. Proven diagnosis: amyloid deposits had to be characterized histochemically by positive staining with Congo red, which also showed typical anomalous colors under polarized light, or the amyloid deposits had to be characterized by electron microscopy. Possible diagnosis: amyloid deposits had to be characterized histochemically by positive staining with any of the usual amyloid stains, including immunohistochemistry and there could not be evidence of non-AA amyloid. Problematic diagnosis: no report on any results of one of the usual amyloid stains, or in case there is evidence of a non-AA type of amyloid.

Among autoimmune diseases, strong disease associations were established in mixed connective tissue disease, SLE, and RA [21]. Where PMR was often followed by GCA, the combination was more strongly associated with AA amyloidosis than with PMR alone [21]. Table 17.5 shows the grade of association between inflammatory diseases and AA amyloidosis.

The production of SAA is regulated not only by cytokines such as interleukin-1, interleukin-6, and tumor necrosis factor, but also by glucocorticoids and

Table 17.5 Grades of associations between inflammatory diseases and AA amyloidosis

	Strong association	Unclear association	Unlikely association	Weak association
Rheumatic diseases	Rheumatoid arthritis	Rheumatic heart disease	Reactive arthritis	Adult-onset Still's disease
	Psoriatic arthritis	Myositis/antisynthetase syndrome	SAPHO syndrome	
	Seronegative spondyloarthropathy	Systemic sclerosis	Primary Sjögren's syndrome	
	Juvenile idiopathic arthritis			
	Gout			
	Systemic lupus erythematosus			
	Mixed connective tissue disease			
Vasculitis	Giant cell arteritis		ANCA-associated vasculitis	
	Polymyalgia rheumatica		Inflammatory aneurysm	
	Takayasu's arteritis			
	Bechet's disease			
Skin and subcutaneous tissue		Psoriasis		
Other			IgG4-related disease	Retroperitoneal fibrosis
			Schnitzler's syndrome	

SAPHO synovitis, acne, pustulosis, hyperostosis, and osteitis, *ANCA* anti-neutrophil cytoplasmic antibody

lipopolysaccharide [24]. The liver is the main site of SAA production, but monocyte-derived macrophages also can produce SAA [25]. Although chronically elevated SAA serum levels are a prerequisite, they are not sufficient alone to develop AA amyloidosis. Even in longstanding and severe inflammatory rheumatic diseases no more than 10–30% of the patients develop amyloidosis [26, 27]. The question that arises is whether there are protective factors in these patients with chronic inflammation who do not develop amyloidosis or facilitating factors other than elevated SAA in patients who do develop amyloidosis. Fibril-derived amyloid-enhancing factor appeared to be such a facilitating factor in animal studies and AA amyloidosis appeared to be transmissible by oral ingestion of food containing AA-amyloid in a mouse model. These observations suggest that exposure to exogenous substances with fibril-derived amyloid-enhancing factor activity might facilitate the development of AA amyloidosis in susceptible patients [28]. The SAA1 genotype is another factor probably influencing amyloidogenesis [29]. Knowing the underlying disease of AA amyloidosis provides an opportunity to look for targeted therapy. The normalization of SAA serum levels by adequate underlying disease control determines the prognosis of AA amyloidosis (Chaps. 7 and 8).

Serum Immunoglobulin-Free Light Chain Levels and Their Significance in Autoimmune Diseases

Breaking of the immunological tolerance towards one or more self-antigens is the cornerstone of an autoimmune disease. Subsequently, B cell activation may result in an increased secretion of immunoglobulin-free light chains (FLCs). Immunoglobulins have a tetrameric structure composed of two heavy and two light chains linked by non-covalent forces and disulfide bonds [30]. The serum concentration of FLCs is dependent on the balance between FLC production (from plasma cells and their progenitors) and FLC renal clearance [31]. The concentration of polyclonal FLCs reflects the inflammatory status in inflammatory disorders [32].

Over the years, different studies have been performed on serum and urinary FLCs of patients with SLE, demonstrating an intriguing association between the concentration of FLCs and overall SLE activity. Their authors [33, 34] suggested that measurement of urinary FLC levels in patients with SLE could be used to identify or monitor in vivo polyclonal B cell activation and predict disease relapses. Many other studies [35, 36] have confirmed that patients with SLE have high serum levels of FLCs even in comparison with healthy subjects. FLC concentrations changed based on therapies by determining the concentration of serum IgG, IgA, IgM, and serum FLCs before or after rituximab (RTX) treatment: in particular, it has been observed that κ and λ FLC concentrations decreased significantly after RTX therapy, while total IgG, IgA, and IgM levels decreased though remaining in a normal range [35]. That study confirmed a strong correlation between κ FLC levels and C3 consumption, which is characteristic of active SLE, proving that this correlation is preserved even after B cell depletion. Moreover, serum FLCs correlated with anti-dsDNA antibody titers and total serum IgG and IgA, confirming the strong relationship between plasma cell productivity and SLE disease activity [36].

In RA, patients have significantly higher mean concentrations of total, κ, and λ FLCs as compared to healthy subjects [31]. FLC levels markedly increased along with the Disease Activity Score 28, supporting a potential relationship between B cell activation and overall disease activity in RA [37]. High concentrations of FLCs in the synovial fluid from inflamed joints were also found [38]. Thus, it was noted a positive correlation between serum FLC amounts and disease activity. Interestingly, the treatment with Abatacept can reduce signs of polyclonal B cell activation, inducing a trend towards normalization of serum levels of different classes of Ig and FLCs, reducing titers of anti-citrullinated protein antibodies and rheumatoid factor, and also decreasing circulating post-switch memory B cells [39]. Changes in FLCs were also noted after treatment with RTX, and the effect of treatment on FLC concentrations distinguished clinical responders from non-responders [38]. These studies indicated that FLCs could be used as early prognostic biomarkers to monitor treatment response in patients with RA. As a side note, some authors [40] also observed that serum levels of FLCs might predict higher mortality in patients with RA.

Increased FLC levels were associated with extraglandular involvement in pSS. Serum levels of FLCs were higher in patients with pSS displaying systemic features than in those with only glandular involvement. High levels of FLCs with normal FLC ratio were more often detected in patients with concomitant monoclonal gammopathy of undetermined significance compared to patients with only pSS [37]. Moreover, other biological markers of B cell activation have been reported to be correlated with FLCs in patients with pSS, such as anti-SSA and anti-SSB autoantibodies, rheumatoid factor, serum levels of IgA, IgG, and IgM, serum B cell-activating factor, and serum β2-microglobulin [37, 41]. The correlation between FLC levels with the ESSDAI (EULAR Sjögren's Syndrome Disease Activity Index) showed that the κ chain was significantly and more strongly correlated than the λ chain [42, 43]. Therefore, increased disease activity of pSS is not only associated with increased polyclonal B cell activity, but remarkably also with the preferential increase of the κ chain clone [41, 44].

Only two studies investigated the role of FLCs in SSc [45, 46]. Serum κ chains and κ/λ ratio were significantly higher when compared with healthy subjects, while serum λ chains were similar. A correlation between FLCs and Interleukin-6, C-reactive protein, erythrocyte sedimentation rate, and the Rodnan skin score was found, showing also an independent association with lung disease and overall disease severity.

The role of FLCs in the management of autoimmune disorders is resumed in Fig. 17.1.

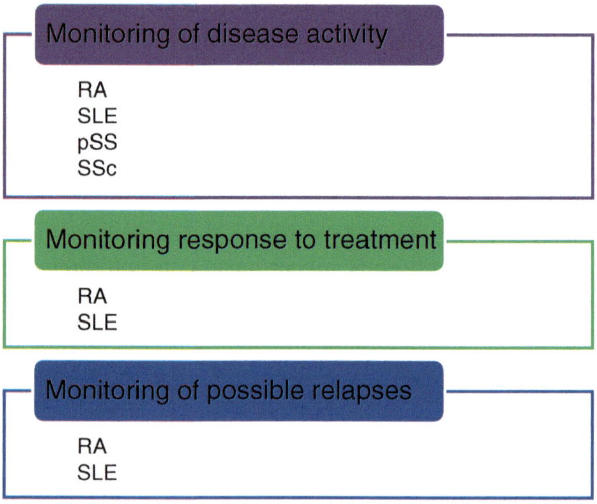

Fig. 17.1 Role of FLCs in systemic autoimmune diseases. (Modified by Napodano C et al., Autoimmunity Reviews. 2019). *RA* rheumatoid arthritis, *SLE* systemic lupus erythematosus, *pSS* primary Sjögren's syndrome, *SSc* systemic sclerosis

Conclusions

Paraproteinemias are heterogeneous disorders and can also be secondary to a wide range of clinical conditions, including systemic autoimmune diseases. The connection between paraproteinemias and autoimmune diseases is supported by inflammatory microenvironment and epigenetic contribution, which may promote the development of aberrant plasma cell clones leading to monoclonal gammopathy. Increased FLC levels correlates with disease activity and there is increasing interest in studying the potential use of FLC assessment as a biomarker of response to treatment. A well-known complication of chronic inflammatory diseases is AA amyloidosis, caused by increased SAA serum levels. An adequate control of the underlying inflammatory disease can influence the prognosis of AA amyloidosis.

In summary, immune dysregulation represents the link between paraproteinemias and autoimmune diseases and further investigations will provide a better understanding of pathogenesis and clinical role of paraproteinemias in the context of an autoimmune milieu.

References

1. Frank L-A, Rabin N. Paraproteinaemia. Br J Hosp Med. 2015;76:C82–5. https://doi.org/10.12968/hmed.2015.76.6.C82.
2. Chikanza I, Akpenyi O. Association of monoclonal gammopathy of undetermined significance with Behcet's disease: a review of shared common disease pathogenetic mechanisms. Mediterr J Rheumatol. 2018;29:80–5. https://doi.org/10.31138/mjr.29.2.80.
3. Castaneda-Avila MA, Ulbricht CM, Epstein MM. Risk factors for monoclonal gammopathy of undetermined significance: a systematic review. Ann Hematol. 2021;100:855–63. https://doi.org/10.1007/s00277-021-04400-7.
4. McShane CM, Murray LJ, Landgren O, O'Rorke MA, Korde N, Kunzmann AT, Ismail MR, Anderson LA. Prior autoimmune disease and risk of monoclonal gammopathy of undetermined significance and multiple myeloma: a systematic review. Cancer Epidemiol Biomark Prev. 2014;23:332–42. https://doi.org/10.1158/1055-9965.EPI-13-0695.
5. Ali YM, Urowitz MB, Ibanez D, Gladman DD. Monoclonal gammopathy in systemic lupus erythematosus. Lupus. 2007;16:426–9. https://doi.org/10.1177/0961203307079045.
6. Hemminki K, Försti A, Sundquist K, Sundquist J, Li X. Familial associations of monoclonal gammopathy of unknown significance with autoimmune diseases. Leukemia. 2016;30:1766–9. https://doi.org/10.1038/leu.2016.43.
7. Hemminki K, Liu X, Försti A, Ji J, Sundquist J, Sundquist K. Effect of autoimmune diseases on incidence and survival in subsequent multiple myeloma. J Hematol Oncol. 2012;5:59. https://doi.org/10.1186/1756-8722-5-59.
8. Sallah S, Wan JY, Hanrahan LR. Future development of lymphoproliferative disorders in patients with autoimmune hemolytic anemia. Clin Cancer Res. 2001;7:791–4.
9. Eder L, Thavaneswaran A, Pereira D, Sussman G, Gladman DD. Prevalence of monoclonal gammopathy among patients with psoriatic arthritis. J Rheumatol. 2012;39:564–7. https://doi.org/10.3899/jrheum.111054.
10. Prignano F, Pescitelli L, Ricceri F, Ermini A, Lotti T. Development of MGUS in psoriatic patients: a possible undiagnosed event during anti-TNF-α-treatment. J Eur Acad Dermatol Venereol. 2012;26:1444–8. https://doi.org/10.1111/j.1468-3083.2011.04216.x.

11. Lindqvist EK, Goldin LR, Landgren O, Blimark C, Mellqvist U-H, Turesson I, Wahlin A, Björkholm M, Kristinsson SY. Personal and family history of immune-related conditions increase the risk of plasma cell disorders: a population-based study. Blood. 2011;118:6284–91. https://doi.org/10.1182/blood-2011-04-347559.
12. Kristinsson SY, Koshiol J, Björkholm M, Goldin LR, McMaster ML, Turesson I, Landgren O. Immune-related and inflammatory conditions and risk of lymphoplasmacytic lymphoma or Waldenstrom macroglobulinemia. J Natl Cancer Inst. 2010;102:557–67. https://doi.org/10.1093/jnci/djq043.
13. Quartuccio L, Baldini C, Priori R, Bartoloni E, Carubbi F, Alunno A, Gandolfo S, Colafrancesco S, Giacomelli R, Gerli R, et al. Cryoglobulinemia in Sjögren syndrome: a disease subset that links higher systemic disease activity, autoimmunity, and local B cell proliferation in mucosa-associated lymphoid tissue. J Rheumatol. 2017;44:1179–83. https://doi.org/10.3899/jrheum.161465.
14. Argyropoulou OD, Pezoulas V, Chatzis L, Critselis E, Gandolfo S, Ferro F, Quartuccio L, Donati V, Treppo E, Bassoli CR, et al. Cryoglobulinemic vasculitis in primary Sjögren's syndrome: clinical presentation, association with lymphoma and comparison with hepatitis C-related disease. Semin Arthritis Rheum. 2020;50:846–53. https://doi.org/10.1016/j.semarthrit.2020.07.013.
15. Gandolfo S, Fabro C, Kapsogeorgou E, Colafrancesco S, Ferro F, Bartoloni E, Quartuccio L, Goules A, Priori R, Alunno A, et al. Validation of thymic stromal lymphopoietin as a biomarker of primary Sjögren's syndrome and related Lymphoproliferation: results in independent cohorts. Clin Exp Rheumatol. 2020;38(Suppl 126):189–94.
16. Brito-Zerón P, Ramos-Casals M, Nardi N, Cervera R, Yagüe J, Ingelmo M, Font J. Circulating monoclonal immunoglobulins in Sjögren syndrome: prevalence and clinical significance in 237 patients. Medicine (Baltimore). 2005;84:90–7. https://doi.org/10.1097/01.md.0000157398.37679.47.
17. Brito-Zerón P, Retamozo S, Gandía M, Akasbi M, Pérez-De-Lis M, Diaz-Lagares C, Bosch X, Bové A, Pérez-Alvarez R, Soto-Cárdenas M-J, et al. Monoclonal gammopathy related to Sjögren syndrome: a key marker of disease prognosis and outcomes. J Autoimmun. 2012;39:43–8. https://doi.org/10.1016/j.jaut.2012.01.010.
18. Varettoni M, Corso A, Cocito F, Mangiacavalli S, Pascutto C, Zappasodi P, Pica G, Lazzarino M. Changing pattern of presentation in monoclonal gammopathy of undetermined significance: a single-center experience with 1400 patients. Medicine (Baltimore). 2010;89:211–6. https://doi.org/10.1097/MD.0b013e3181e763be.
19. Quartuccio L, Corazza L, Gandolfo S, Vita SD. AB0586 persistent rather than fluctuating serum cryoglobulins are associated with cryoglobulinemic vasculitis in primary Sjögren's syndrome, and related to the risk of lymphoma. Ann Rheum Dis. 2015;74:1096. https://doi.org/10.1136/annrheumdis-2015-eular.3095.
20. Yang Y, Chen L, Jia Y, Liu Y, Wen L, Liang Y, An Y, Chen S, Su Y, Li Z. Monoclonal gammopathy in rheumatic diseases. Clin Rheumatol. 2018;37:1751–62. https://doi.org/10.1007/s10067-018-4064-8.
21. Brunger AF, Nienhuis HLA, Bijzet J, Hazenberg BPC. Causes of AA amyloidosis: a systematic review. Amyloid. 2020;27:1–12. https://doi.org/10.1080/13506129.2019.1693359.
22. Obici L, Merlini G. AA amyloidosis: basic knowledge, unmet needs and future treatments. Swiss Med Wkly. 2012;142:w13580. https://doi.org/10.4414/smw.2012.13580.
23. Benson MD, Buxbaum JN, Eisenberg DS, Merlini G, Saraiva MJM, Sekijima Y, Sipe JD, Westermark P. Amyloid nomenclature 2018: recommendations by the International Society of Amyloidosis (ISA) nomenclature committee. Amyloid. 2018;25:215–9. https://doi.org/10.1080/13506129.2018.1549825.
24. De Buck M, Gouwy M, Wang JM, Van Snick J, Proost P, Struyf S, Van Damme J. The cytokine-serum amyloid A-chemokine network. Cytokine Growth Factor Rev. 2016;30:55–69. https://doi.org/10.1016/j.cytogfr.2015.12.010.

25. Jumeau C, Awad F, Assrawi E, Cobret L, Duquesnoy P, Giurgea I, Valeyre D, Grateau G, Amselem S, Bernaudin J-F, et al. Expression of SAA1, SAA2 and SAA4 genes in human primary monocytes and monocyte-derived macrophages. PLoS One. 2019;14:e0217005. https://doi.org/10.1371/journal.pone.0217005.
26. Dhillon V, Woo P, Isenberg D. Amyloidosis in the rheumatic diseases. Ann Rheum Dis. 1989;48:696–701. https://doi.org/10.1136/ard.48.8.696.
27. Obici L, Raimondi S, Lavatelli F, Bellotti V, Merlini G. Susceptibility to AA amyloidosis in rheumatic diseases: a critical overview. Arthritis Rheum. 2009;61:1435–40. https://doi.org/10.1002/art.24735.
28. Solomon A, Richey T, Murphy CL, Weiss DT, Wall JS, Westermark GT, Westermark P. Amyloidogenic potential of foie gras. Proc Natl Acad Sci U S A. 2007;104:10998–1001. https://doi.org/10.1073/pnas.0700848104.
29. Westermark GT, Fändrich M, Westermark P. AA amyloidosis: pathogenesis and targeted therapy. Annu Rev Pathol. 2015;10:321–44. https://doi.org/10.1146/annurev-pathol-020712-163913.
30. Janeway Jr C, Travers P, Walport M, Shlomchik MJ. Immunobiology, 5th ed. Garland Science; 2001. isbn:978-0-8153-3642-6.
31. Napodano C, Pocino K, Rigante D, Stefanile A, Gulli F, Marino M, Basile V, Rapaccini GL, Basile U. Free light chains and autoimmunity. Autoimmun Rev. 2019;18:484–92. https://doi.org/10.1016/j.autrev.2019.03.003.
32. Bettacchioli E, Le Gaffric C, Mazeas M, Borghi MO, Frostegard J, Barturen G, Makowska Z, Babei S, Lesche R, PRECISESADS Clinical Consortium, et al. An elevated polyclonal free light chain level reflects a strong interferon signature in patients with systemic autoimmune diseases. J Transl Autoimmun. 2021;4:100090. https://doi.org/10.1016/j.jtauto.2021.100090.
33. Hopper JE, Sequeira W, Martellotto J, Papagiannes E, Perna L, Skosey JL. Clinical relapse in systemic lupus erythematosus: correlation with antecedent elevation of urinary free light-chain immunoglobulin. J Clin Immunol. 1989;9:338–50. https://doi.org/10.1007/BF00918666.
34. Epstein WV, Tan M. Increase of L-chain proteins in the sera of patients with systemic lupus erythematosus and the synovial fluids of patients with peripheral rheumatoid arthritis. Arthritis Rheum. 1966;9:713–9. https://doi.org/10.1002/art.1780090508.
35. Chiche L, Cournac JM, Mancini J, Bardin N, Thomas G, Jean R, Schleinitz N, Kaplanski G, Durand JM, Boucraut J, et al. Normalization of serum-free light chains in patients with systemic lupus erythematosus upon rituximab treatment and correlation with biological disease activity. Clin Rheumatol. 2011;30:685–9. https://doi.org/10.1007/s10067-010-1674-1.
36. Draborg AH, Lydolph MC, Westergaard M, Olesen Larsen S, Nielsen CT, Duus K, Jacobsen S, Houen G. Correction: elevated concentrations of serum immunoglobulin free light chains in systemic lupus erythematosus patients in relation to disease activity, inflammatory status, B cell activity and Epstein-Barr virus antibodies. PLoS One. 2016;11:e0148151. https://doi.org/10.1371/journal.pone.0148151.
37. Gottenberg J-E, Aucouturier F, Goetz J, Sordet C, Jahn I, Busson M, Cayuela J-M, Sibilia J, Mariette X. Serum immunoglobulin free light chain assessment in rheumatoid arthritis and primary Sjogren's syndrome. Ann Rheum Dis. 2007;66:23–7. https://doi.org/10.1136/ard.2006.052159.
38. Kormelink TG, Tekstra J, Thurlings RM, Boumans MHJ, Vos K, Tak PP, Bijlsma JWJ, Lafeber FPJG, Redegeld FA, van Roon JAG. Decrease in immunoglobulin free light chains in patients with rheumatoid arthritis upon rituximab (anti-CD20) treatment correlates with decrease in disease activity. Ann Rheum Dis. 2010;69:2137–44. https://doi.org/10.1136/ard.2009.126441.
39. Scarsi M, Paolini L, Ricotta D, Pedrini A, Piantoni S, Caimi L, Tincani A, Airò P. Abatacept reduces levels of switched memory B cells, autoantibodies, and immunoglobulins in patients with rheumatoid arthritis. J Rheumatol. 2014;41:666–72. https://doi.org/10.3899/jrheum.130905.
40. Deng X, Crowson CS, Rajkumar SV, Dispenzieri A, Larson DR, Therneau TM, Matteson EL, Kyle RA, Katzmann JA, Gabriel SE, et al. Elevation of serum immunoglobulin free light

chains during the preclinical period of rheumatoid arthritis. J Rheumatol. 2015;42:181–7. https://doi.org/10.3899/jrheum.140543.

41. Gottenberg J-E, Busson M, Cohen-Solal J, Lavie F, Abbed K, Kimberly RP, Sibilia J, Mariette X. Correlation of serum B lymphocyte stimulator and Beta2 microglobulin with autoantibody secretion and systemic involvement in primary Sjogren's syndrome. Ann Rheum Dis. 2005;64:1050–5. https://doi.org/10.1136/ard.2004.030643.
42. Verstappen GM, Moerman RV, van Nimwegen JF, van Ginkel MS, Bijzet J, Mossel E, Vissink A, Hazenberg BPC, Arends S, Kroese FGM, et al. Serum immunoglobulin free light chains are sensitive biomarkers for monitoring disease activity and treatment response in primary Sjögren's syndrome. Rheumatology (Oxford). 2018;57:1812–21. https://doi.org/10.1093/rheumatology/key180.
43. Seror R, Ravaud P, Bowman SJ, Baron G, Tzioufas A, Theander E, Gottenberg J-E, Bootsma H, Mariette X, Vitali C, et al. EULAR Sjogren's syndrome disease activity index: development of a consensus systemic disease activity index for primary Sjogren's syndrome. Ann Rheum Dis. 2010;69:1103–9. https://doi.org/10.1136/ard.2009.110619.
44. Nocturne G, Seror R, Fogel O, Belkhir R, Boudaoud S, Saraux A, Larroche C, Le Guern V, Gottenberg JE, Mariette X. CXCL13 and CCL11 serum levels and lymphoma and disease activity in primary Sjögren's syndrome. Arthritis Rheumatol. 2015;67:3226–33. https://doi.org/10.1002/art.39315.
45. Bosello S, De Luca G, Tolusso B, Lama G, Angelucci C, Sica G, Ferraccioli G. B cells in systemic sclerosis: a possible target for therapy. Autoimmun Rev. 2011;10:624–30. https://doi.org/10.1016/j.autrev.2011.04.013.
46. Lanteri A, Sobanski V, Langlois C, Lefèvre G, Hauspie C, Sanges S, Lambert M, Morell-Dubois S, Hatron P-Y, Hachulla E, et al. Serum free light chains of immunoglobulins as biomarkers for systemic sclerosis characteristics, activity and severity. Autoimmun Rev. 2014;13:974–80. https://doi.org/10.1016/j.autrev.2014.07.003.

Chapter 18
Infections and Paraproteinemia

Alessandro Visentin, Matilde Rocchi, Anna Giulia Salvadori, Paola Del Bravo, and Elda Righi

Abbreviations

AMS	Antimicrobial Stewardship
CMV	Cytomegalovirus
EBV	Epstein–Barr Virus
HBV	Hepatitis B Virus
HCV	Hepatitis C Virus
HIV	Human Immunodeficiency Virus
HPV	Human Papilloma Virus
HSCT	Hematopoietic Stem-Cell Transplantation
HSV	Herpes Simplex Virus
HZ	Herpes Zoster
IMiDs	Immunomodulatory Drugs
IPA	Invasive Pulmonary Aspergillosis
MGUS	Monoclonal Gammopathy of Undetermined Significance
MM	Multiple Myeloma
PIs	Proteasome Inhibitors
SLE	Systemic Lupus Erythematosus
TMP-SMX	Trimethoprim-Sulfamethoxazole
VZV	Varicella–Zoster Virus
WM	Waldenström's Macroglobulinemia

A. Visentin · M. Rocchi · A. G. Salvadori · P. Del Bravo · E. Righi (✉)
Infectious Diseases Division, Verona University Hospital, Verona, Italy
e-mail: alessandro.visentin@studenti.univr.it; matilde.rocchi@studenti.univr.it; paola.delbravo@aovr.veneto.it; elda.righi@univr.it

© The Author(s), under exclusive license to Springer Nature Switzerland AG 2022
G. Ragab et al. (eds.), *Paraproteinemia and Related Disorders*,
https://doi.org/10.1007/978-3-031-10131-1_18

Introduction

Paraproteinemia is a condition that is common to a wide spectrum of different rheumatological and hematological entities, ranging from monoclonal gammopathy of undetermined significance (MGUS) to amyloidosis and cryoglobulinemia [1]. Clinical manifestations, pathophysiology, and prevalence are extremely variable, the severity and prognosis of each condition being different. In this setting, infections represent threatening complication, as the individual's responses are compromised in multifaceted ways [2, 3], but also potential triggers [3, 4]. Various reports and population studies focus on both a direct oncogenic role of the infectious agent [3] and on the role of chronic inflammation in promoting abnormal cell proliferation [3, 4]. However, while some infections have been recognized as directly promoting paraproteinemia, evidence is controversial for many others.

A crucial element favoring infections as a consequence of paraproteinemia is the immune impairment following the altered expression of humoral immunity proteins. T-cell defects may also coexist, along with mucositis, comorbidities, use of vascular catheters, and other risk factors for infections that are common to immunocompromised patients requiring hospitalization [2, 3]. Due to the main nature of the immunosuppression, involving the expression of B cells, various reports have underlined that the impaired antibody production, particularly in multiple myeloma (MM), MGUS and Waldenström's macroglobulinemia (WM), is one of the key factors responsible for an increased risk of infectious complications [4]. Neutropenia and lymphocytopenia, linked to both disease progression and to selected chemotherapy regimens, also increase the infectious risk in these patient populations, including the potential for invasive mycoses and viral reactivation [5–7]. Other factors contributing to an overall increased risk for infectious complications include the placement of vascular catheters and impaired mucosal integrity, the former being a prerequisite for and the latter a consequence of chemotherapy. Moreover, impaired respiratory function and secretion clearance may occur in response to disease progression and organ impairment, including bone damage and palliative treatment [8, 9].

Paraproteinemia also tends to have higher prevalence in aging populations (e.g., from 60 years of age). Elderly patients with rheumatological or hematological disease are particularly vulnerable in developing infections. Higher morbidity and at least three-fold higher mortality rates have been reported compared to younger patients [10]. This unfavorable impact on patients' outcome, however, is likely to be multifactorial, and caused by age-related immune dysfunction, decreased physiologic reserve, frailty, geriatric syndromes, cognitive dysfunction, and even social isolation [11, 12].

Moreover, preventive measures such as vaccinations may have suboptimal efficacy and fail to guarantee an adequate response in this frail, immunocompromised population [13, 14]. Higher doses, or adjuvant use, or multiple vaccine administrations are often necessary to ensure normal levels of antibodies against common threats such as encapsulated bacteria, respiratory viruses, and VZV reactivation [15–17]. Finally, novel drugs have been introduced for the treatment of paraproteinemia, and also the use of biologics has become common in rheumatological diseases, in certain instances reducing the rates of infectious complications but also creating new scenarios for infections.

Here we present the most common infectious causes as well as complications associated with paraproteinemia and the main cornerstones for the management of this patient population [18].

Potential Infectious Triggers of Paraproteinemia

Infections have long been hypothesized to be potential triggers of various conditions, including cancer [19]. In paraproteinemia, infections are thought to act either as direct carcinogens, as exemplified by oncogenic viruses, or playing an indirect role in the pathogenesis as chronic inflammation promoters, which is consequently responsible for cell proliferation [4]. These findings embrace many different pathogen–disease associations, as exemplified in Table 18.1, but the available evidence is often controversial.

Bacterial Triggers of Paraproteinemia

Reports of paraproteinemia associated with bacterial infections are numerous [3, 19, 52]. In the setting of MM and MGUS, a higher percentage of IgG targeting *Helicobacter pylori* have been observed compared to normal sera [20], even though the clinical meaning of this finding remains controversial. As for WM, a large population study including 2470 affected patients showed that bacterial infections such as pneumonia, sinusitis, pyelonephritis, and sepsis were associated with a 30% increased risk of developing the condition [24]. Infections caused by Gram-positive bacteria, especially *Staphylococcus aureus*, as well as *Mycobacterium tuberculosis* have been reported in patients affected by IgG4-related disease [27, 28]. Previous studies also supported the role of *H. pylori* infection in triggering the disease, but a recent cohort study published by Culver et al. including 5 cases and 52 controls does not support this evidence, and the role of *H. pylori* infection remains debated [53]. Various bacterial infections including *S. aureus, Streptococcus pneumoniae, Salmonella* spp., *Escherichia coli,* and *M. tuberculosis* have been considered as potential triggers in SLE [30, 31], but solid data are still lacking. In the context of cryoglobulinemia, a plethora of bacterial infections have been associated with the disease, including brucellosis, leprosy, Lyme disease, *Rickettsial infections*, and syphilis [32]. Prior to effective therapy most cases of AA amyloidosis secondary to infections were secondary to *M. tuberculosis* infection [32–34]. Even in recent

Table 18.1 Potential infectious triggers of paraproteinemia

Disease	Bacteria	Virus	Fungi	Parasites	Reference
MM	*H. pylori*	HIV, HCV, EBV, HPV	–	–	[3, 20–23]
MGUS	*H. pylori*	HIV, HCV, EBV, HPV	–	–	[3, 20, 22, 23]
WM	Various infections (pneumonia, sinusitis, pyelonephritis, sepsis)	HCV, HIV, HBV, influenza, VZV	–	–	[19, 24–26]
IgG4-related disease	*S. aureus*, *M. tuberculosis*	–	–	–	[27–29]
SLE	*S. aureus*, *S. pneumoniae*, *E. coli*, *Salmonella*, *M. tuberculosis*	EBV, HIV, HCV	–	–	[30, 31]
Cryoglobulinemia	*Brucella*, *M. leprae*, Borreliosis, Rickettsiosis, *T. pallidum*	HCV, HIV, HBV, CMV, Parvovirus B19, Rubella	Coccidioides spp.	Echinococcosis, Leishmaniasis, Malaria, Schistosomiasis, Toxoplasmosis, Trypanosomiasis	[23, 32]
AA Amyloidosis	*M. tuberculosis, non-tuberculous mycobacteria, M. leprae, T. pallidum, T. whipplei, C. burnetii, Brucella* Various infections (osteomyelitis, chronic pyelonephritis, untreated abscesses, prosthetic infection, endocarditis)	HCV, HIV, HBV	Aspergillus spp., Coccidioides spp., Actinomycosis, Mucormycosis	Schistosomiasis, Echinococcosis, Giardiasis, Leishmaniasis, Malaria, Filariasis	[32–51]

MM multiple myeloma, *MGUS* monoclonal gammopathy of undetermined significance, *WM* Waldenström's Macroglobulinemia, *SLE* systemic lupus erythematosus times, tuberculosis remains a potential cause of AA amyloidosis in endemic countries [35] and complicates up to 5% of the diagnosed cases [36]. Exceptionally, cases of amyloidosis secondary to non-tuberculous mycobacteria and lepromatous leprosy have been described [37–40]. Other infections known as potential sources of secondary amyloidosis include syphilis prior to effective antimicrobial treatment [41, 42], *Tropheryma whipplei* [43], and anecdotal cases of brucellosis and Q fever [44, 45] as well as focal chronic infections such as osteomyelitis, chronic pyelonephritis, untreated abscess, prosthetic infections, or endocarditis [52]. A recent narrative review including articles up to 2019 showed a decrease from 50 to less than 20% after the 2000s in the frequency of AA amyloidosis secondary to infections; however, the percentage remains high, including the involvement of infections in low resource countries [52]. These data advocate for better management, control, and screening of infections requiring prolonged treatment.

Viral Triggers of Paraproteinemia

Viral infections have been reported as potential causative agents in many conditions associated with paraproteinemia [3, 19, 52]. For instance, prior to the development of the highly active antiretroviral therapy (HAART), the incidence of MGUS in HIV-infected patients was thought to be significantly higher, ranging from 4 to 26% [22, 23]. Viruses such as Epstein–Barr Virus (EBV), hepatitis C (HCV), and human papilloma virus (HPV), as well as *H. pylori* have been considered as potentially playing an indirect role in the pathogenesis of MGUS and MM as chronic inflammation promoters [3], which consequently can lead to cell proliferation [4]. A population-based study found a significant association between HCV infection and MM [21], whereas a retrospective study conducted at the US Veterans Affairs healthcare facilities from 1997 to 2004 reported that patients with chronic HCV had a three-time higher risk for WM compared to non-HCV-infected patients [25]. In a population study, Kristinsson et al. demonstrated an increased excess risk of developing WM not only in the setting of bacterial infections, but also for infections caused by influenza and herpes zoster (HZ) [24]. Other studies found an increased risk of WM following HZ infection [19, 26]. EBV has been recognized as a potential trigger also in SLE, either alone or in combination with HIV and HCV [29]. Though the mechanism behind it is not yet clearly understood, it is thought that EBV works via structural molecular mimicry with common SLE antigens and functional molecular mimicry with critical immune-regulatory components [22, 54]. Solid evidence is available for the pathogenetic role of HCV in the development of type II and III cryoglobulinemia [23]. In up to 45–65% of HCV-infected individuals, detectable levels of circulating paraproteins have been observed with or without clinical manifestations [32]. Other infections associated with cryoglobulinemia include HIV, HBV, CMV, parvovirus B19, and rubella [32], which potentially share the pathogenetic mechanism of B-cell hyperactivation and/or proliferation with subsequent selective expansion of cryoglobulin-producing B-cell clones. More robust evidence is also available for HIV infection and amyloidosis, which is responsible for up to 10% cases of kidney diseases in this subset of patients [46], whereas confounders make it difficult to ascertain the role of HCV. HBV chronic infection has also been shown to be associated with the development of AA amyloidosis, even though not as frequently as HIV infection [47, 52]. All in all, the presence of confounders makes it difficult to ascertain the role of chronic HCV in the setting of AA amyloidosis.

Fungal and Parasitic Triggers of Paraproteinemia

Chronic inflammation during fungal or parasitic infection can also predispose to the development of paraproteinemia, even though the evidence in this field is rather scarce [32, 52]. Data on fungi mostly involve aspergillus chronic infection as a potential trigger for amyloidosis [48]. However, it is unknown whether the condition is primarily sustained by the pathogen itself or by bronchiectasis. Seldom, association of coccidioidomycosis, actinomycosis, and mucormycosis with amyloidosis have been reported [49–51]. Similarly, evidence of paraproteinemia in chronic parasitic infections is rare and mostly limited to AA amyloidosis [52]. In fact, schistosomiasis, echinococcosis, giardiasis, leishmaniasis, malaria, and filariasis have all been linked to secondary amyloidosis [52], even though the evidence is mainly anecdotal. This is also true for cryoglobulinemia, which has been associated with chronic fungal (e.g., coccidiomycosis) and parasitic diseases (e.g., echinococcosis, leishmaniasis, malaria, schistosomiasis, toxoplasmosis, trypanosomiasis) [32].

Multiple Myeloma

MM is characterized by a defect of B cells, manifested by hypogammaglobulinemia, that is known to increase the risk of infections caused by encapsulated bacteria such as *S. pneumoniae* and *Haemophilus influenzae* [55]. Lymphocytopenia and neutropenia may be associated and derived from bone marrow infiltration, contributing to the risk of severe infections. Moreover, cytokines released by MM cells promote an imbalance in the TH1/TH2 ratio, resulting in a defective TH1 response. An overall increased risk of infection is also caused by MM-related multisystem involvement, resulting from iron overload and bone damage, and patients' older age [56]. Immunosuppressive treatments can also increase the risk for infection development.

As summarized in Table 18.2, numerous factors contribute to increased infection risk in patients with myeloma.

Table 18.2 Multifactorial risk factors for increased risk of infections in patients with MM

Risk type	Characteristics
Immunological	Impaired antibody production (decreased polyclonal Ig of 75%) Neutropenia Lymphopenia CD4/CD8 imbalance Defect of granulocyte adhesiveness Impaired leukocyte migration
Treatment related	IV catheters High-dose steroid use Chemotherapy-related mucositis
Others	Comorbidities (renal impairment) Impaired ventilation and secretions clearance Older age

Infections Associated with MM

In MM, the rate of infection is increased compared to the general population, with bacterial and viral infections predominating due to the plasma cellular dysfunction typical of the disease. MM has been associated with a 10-time greater risk of infection compared to WM. A study performed in Sweden between 2004 and 2007 including 9253 MM patients and 34,931 matched controls without hematologic malignancy showed that patients with MM had a seven-fold higher risk of infection compared with controls [57]. Specifically, the risk was 11-fold greater during the first year following diagnosis. Infections represented a major threat in this population, representing the underlying cause of death in 22% of patients at one-year follow-up. The most frequent infections reported in MM included pneumonia, bacteremia, cellulitis, pyelonephritis, osteomyelitis, and meningitis. The overall risk for viral infections was ten-fold higher for this group compared to matched controls with an 18-fold higher risk during the first year. Influenza and HZ virus were the most frequent viral infections detected [57]. While infections may occur at any stage, the incidence, etiology, and clinical syndromes or presentation vary according to different types of treatment and disease phases of MM. The first year following diagnosis, however, appears consistently as the most threatening for myeloma patients across studies. Blade et al. reported an overall incidence of severe infections between 0.8 and 2.22 per patient-year, ranging from 0.49 per patient-year during plateau phases and increasing to 1.9 during active disease [58]. Timing from treatment initiation shorter than 2 months, renal failure, and relapsed or refractory disease were additional risk factors for severe infections [59, 60]. Augustson et al. enrolled 3107 newly diagnosed patients in the UK from 1980 to 2002 analyzing risk factors for early mortality. Death within 60 days occurred in 10% of patients with 45% of deaths that were attributable to infection [61]. High tumor burden, poor performance status, and high comorbidity scores were common factors aggravating the infectious risk and should be taken into consideration while planning patients' follow-up and infectious risk assessment. Elevated baseline serum lactic dehydrogenase, a marker of tumor burden, was reported as an independent risk factor for infection occurring in the first year following disease diagnosis in transplant ineligible patients (incidence rate ratio 2.43, 95% CI 1.39–4.26). Smoking was also reported as a risk factor for infection (IRR 2.11, 95% CI 1.12–3.98), while receipt of more than 6 cycles of therapy appeared protective (IRR 0.49, 95% CI 0.28–0.88) [62].

Treatment-Associated Infections in Multiple Myeloma

From a therapeutic point of view, the use of novel agents in MM has increased the potential for patients' survival and may also have an impact on the occurrence of infections although the studies are still scarce and do not clearly compare the rates of infection among different treatment arms [63]. A report evaluating the predictors of early mortality (within 1 year from diagnosis) among 542 MM patients receiving novel agents identified age-adjusted Charlson comorbidity score ≥4, low body mass index (<20 kg/m^2), thrombocytopenia, and renal failure as independently associated to unfavorable outcomes. Additional factors associated with early mortality due to infection included hyperglycemia, lymphocytopenia, and low serum values of immunoglobulins [64]. As MM progresses, host defenses become severely impaired, with profound T-cell immunodeficiency, hypogammaglobulinemia, and neutropenia leading to a broadening of the spectrum of pathogens responsible for infections, including bacteria, fungi, viruses, mycobacteria, and parasites. While invasive fungal infections and CMV disease are uncommon early during MM treatment, in the advanced phases of the disease the risk for opportunistic infections increases due to the effect of cumulative immunosuppression [65, 66].

Invasive pulmonary aspergillosis (IPA) may also occur as a consequence of patients' use of high doses of steroids and in case of concomitant neutropenia. Similar to other immunocompromised patients, the clinical manifestations of infections may be mild or atypical, and imaging may not be suggestive of IPA [67]. Typical signs of IPA such as macronodules with the halo sign, well-circumscribed infiltrates, air crescent, or cavities may be replaced by small centrilobular micronodules, ground-glass opacities, tree-in-bud infiltrates, and focal bronchiectasis [68]. Most cases of CMV infections remain asymptomatic in MM patients. Routine CMV DNA testing in asymptomatic patients is not indicated in MM unless autologous HCT is performed. Reactivation and burden of CMV infection among patients receiving specific treatments, however, remains limited to few reports [69]. Gram-positive bacteria represent the most frequent causative pathogens following MM diagnosis, accounting for over 50% of causes of infections. *S. pneumoniae* and *S. aureus*, in particular, are frequently isolated and pneumonia represents a frequent cause of death in patients with MM. Among Gram-negative bacteria, *E. coli*, *H. influenzae*, *Neisseria* species, and enteric organisms are the leading pathogens [70]. With the introduction of bortezomib, HSV has also become a frequent cause of infection in the first months of treatment, along with other viruses such as

Enterovirus. Regimens that are known to increase the risk of severe infections include "traditional" chemotherapy, steroid use, and more recent regimens such as immunomodulatory drugs (IMiDs) and proteasome inhibitors (PIs). IMiDs like lenalidomide and pomalidomide may cause neutropenia. Among PIs, bortezomib is associated with VZ reactivation due to impairment of T-cell function [71]. A longitudinal study including 199 patients and 771 episodes of infection between 2008- and 2012 showed that, among chemotherapy regimens, intensive combination systemic chemotherapy (HR = 1.86) and specifically high-dose melphalan (HR = 2.07), IV cyclophosphamide (HR = 1.96), and cumulative doses of corticosteroids (HR = 3.06 at highest dose) were independently associated with increased risk of infection overall ($P < 0.05$). Conversely, IMiDs, PIs, and other clinical factors were not associated with infectious risk [72]. Renal failure, in particular, has been identified as a key risk factor in patients receiving chemotherapy, and is associated with a risk of death of 30% in the first 2 months of treatment [61].

Clinical Management of Infections in Multiple Myeloma

Clinical management of MM patients with infections include a timely diagnosis and a correct antimicrobial treatment according to patients' disease phase, risk factors, and potential pathogens involved. Fever should be considered of infectious origin unless proven otherwise and carefully investigated, also considering that the most frequent sites of infections are the respiratory tract, skin and soft tissues, and the urinary tract. Blood cultures should be prioritized in case of fever or if there is a high suspicion for sepsis [72]. The type of pathogens that can be isolated generally depends on the local epidemiology and on the patient's history, comorbidities, exposures, previous infections, or bacterial colonization. Patient's overall net state of immunosuppression should always be considered and related to the stage of the disease and its treatment phase (e.g., induction or consolidation, maintenance or salvage, relapse or refractory disease), the type of treatment, and the extent and intensity of prior therapies [73]. Local epidemiology should be also taken into account, as an increase in resistant bacteria, especially Gram-negative Enterobacterales (e.g., *Klebsiella pneumoniae* and *Pseudomonas aeruginosa*) with resistance to beta-lactams (e.g., extended-spectrum-beta-lactamases producing Enterobacterales) or to last resort antibiotic, such as carbapenems, has been registered worldwide and causes increased morbidity and mortality in immunocompromised hosts [74, 75].

According to the clinical scenario, for example, in case of advanced disease or heavily immunosuppressed patients (e.g., patients receiving blood stem cell transplantation) opportunistic infections such as CMV disease and invasive fungal should also be considered. Invasive aspergillosis can be investigated through pulmonary imaging and serum or bronchoalveolar lavage (BAL) *Aspergillus* galactomannan antigen testing. The role of 1,3-beta-D-glucan in this setting is yet to be determined but may be relevant to rule out *Pneumocystis jirovecii* pneumonia especially in patients receiving high-dose steroids [68, 76, 77]. A pre-emptive or prophylactic approach in the management of infection during this period should be targeted and based on thorough assessments and, when necessary, invasive diagnostics, taking into consideration the most frequent sites of infection and pathogens involved [61]. In case of suspicion for opportunistic pathogens and considering that immunocompromised patients may present with atypical or fewer symptoms compared to immunocompetent patients, high-resolution computerized tomography (CT) scans should be preferred to chest X-rays, and BAL may be performed along with nasopharyngeal swab for respiratory viruses (e.g., influenza, parainfluenza, respiratory syncytial virus, adenovirus, human metapneumovirus) if respiratory infections are suspected. Among these, *S. pneumoniae* may be fatal if not adequately treated. The presence of abdominal symptoms and/or diarrhea should prompt the collection of stool samples for *C. difficile* testing and cultures and PCR for enteric pathogens, including microscopic testing for parasites also according to the geographic area. Persistent fever of undetermined etiology despite a comprehensive workup may require further imaging such as fluorodeoxyglucose (FDG)-positron emission tomography (FDG PET-CT) to identify potential infectious foci [78, 79]. Reactivation of HBV may be clinically silent, manifesting as an increase in HBV-DNA and serum aminotransferase levels, but patients may also present with nausea and vomiting, which can progress to fulminant hepatic failure and death. Reactivation of HBV can also lead to an interruption of anti-MM therapy, with a potentially negative impact on the underlying disease [80]. Empiric antimicrobial therapy may be necessary in case of suspected sepsis, during neutropenic fever episodes, and should be performed according to the local epidemiology and national and international recommendations. Empiric antibiotic therapy is also essential during episodes of neutropenic fever [81]. To optimize diagnostics through a correct use of microbiological cultures to control for the potential emergence of resistance following the use of broad-spectrum antibiotics, preserving the efficacy of antibiotic therapy, antimicrobial stewardship measures (AMS) should be put in place when managing patients with MM. Recent reports advocate the use of AMS in hematological and rheumatological settings, including diagnostics stewardship principles (e.g., prompt availability of microbiological results and implementation of rapid techniques for identification of antibiotic susceptibility profiles) and antimicrobial principles to optimize therapy (e.g., use of antibiotics according to local patterns of resistance, consideration for de-escalation or treatment discontinuation as soon as possible to avoid prolonged treatment) [81].

Chemoprophylaxis and Vaccination in Patients with Multiple Myeloma

Despite improvements in the treatment of MM and the advent of novel drugs, a significant proportion of patients still face unfavorable outcomes especially within the first months following diagnosis and/or the beginning of chemotherapy. Infections remain the leading cause of death early after MM diagnosis. Antibiotic and/or antiviral prophylaxis and vaccinations have been proposed to reduce the infective burden in MM. A multicenter, double-blinded, phase 3 RCT conducted from 2012 to 2016 enrolled 489 patients receiving levofloxacin prophylaxis vs. 488 receiving placebo, showing higher mortality or first febrile episodes in the placebo vs. treatment arm (27% vs. 19%, HR 0.66, 95% CI 0.51–0.86; $p = 0.0018$) within the first 12 weeks of trial treatment [82]. Other prophylaxes that may be considered during chemotherapy include acyclovir for HSV prophylaxis and cotrimoxazole for *P. jirovecii* prophylaxis, especially among patients receiving steroids, although recommendations on duration or risk factors are unclear in favoring prophylaxis in non-transplanted immunocompromised patients and the risk assessment for opportunistic infections is usually performed on an individual basis [83]. Antibacterial prophylaxis is usually continued in patients who fail to respond to 3–4 cycles of induction chemotherapy until the disease is under control, while in responders it is not recommended [84]. A few RCTs have evaluated the effect of antibacterial prophylaxis in newly diagnosed MM patients. A trial compared trimethoprim-sulfamethoxazole (TMP-SMX) 160/800 mg every 12 h daily for 2 months with no prophylaxis in 54 MM patients. Bacterial infections occurred in 2 of 28 patients (7%) in the TMP-SMX group versus 11 of 26 patients (42%) in the control group ($P = 0.04$), with rates of 0.29 episodes per patient-year for TMP-SMX recipients and 2.43 per patient-year for controls [84]. Another prospective randomized trial that included 212 patients compared ciprofloxacin (500 mg orally twice daily) to either TMP-SMX (160/800 mg twice daily) given for 2 months or no prophylaxis. Differences between groups were not statistically significant, with rates of severe infections observed in 12.5% of ciprofloxacin recipients, 6.8% of TMP-SMX recipients, and 15.9% of placebo recipients [85]. In this trial, antibiotic prophylaxis did not decrease the incidence of serious infection (≥grade 3 and/or hospitalization) or any infection <2 months of treatment or infection upon completion of 2 months of therapy (nor at any time during the subsequent 2 years) or the response to therapy or to overall survival. Specific prophylaxis may be considered according to the type of chemotherapy received. Patients receiving a proteasome inhibitor (bortezomib, carfilzomib, ixazomib) or patients receiving antimyeloma regimens containing elotuzumab, isatuximab, or daratumumab are at high risk for VZV and HSV infections, therefore antiviral prophylaxis with acyclovir or valacyclovir may be considered before starting treatment. It has been suggested that antiviral prophylaxis be continued until 6 weeks after discontinuation of proteasome inhibitors [83]. Furthermore, testing for HBV surface antigen (HBsAg) and HBV core antibody (anti-HBc) as well as circulating HBV DNA is recommended. If a moderate to high risk for HBV reactivation is detected, patients should receive antiviral prophylaxis prior to commencing anti-MM therapy.

Data regarding the clinical effectiveness of vaccines in MM patients are limited. Patients who are not treated with HSCT have low probability of restoring long-term immunity and may present with reduced responses to vaccination also caused by hypogammaglobulinemia or the production of ineffective antibodies. While live attenuated vaccines are generally contraindicated, inactivated vaccines are safe and recommended especially for pneumococcal disease, influenza and reactivation of VZV due to the increased risks of invasive disease cased by these pathogens in this patient population [86].

MGUS

MGUS is a cell dyscrasia occurring in 3–7% in those aged >50 years [87, 88], characterized by the production of a monoclonal paraprotein detectable in the serum. The condition can further progress to MM, WM, amyloid light-chain amyloidosis or other lymphoproliferative diseases in 1% of patients per year [89]. MGUS itself is associated with a wide range of complications, either with a causal relationship to paraprotein production or related to paraprotein deposition in tissues: these include renal impairment, bone involvement, thrombosis, neuropathy, skin disorders, and increased rates of infection [3, 20, 90]. More specifically, infections play multiple roles in plasma cell dyscrasias like MGUS and MM, as mentioned before. There is an increasing body of evidence supporting the role of microorganisms not only in immunomodulation and disease progression, as gut microbiota is thought to contribute to the development of MM [91], but also as regulator of response and toxicity of immune-based therapies in MM [10, 92]. While the role of infectious agents as promoters in paraproteinemia is still under investigation, the presence of infective complications in MGUS patients is well known and, similar to MM, may be attributable to multiple mechanisms. Hypogammaglobulinemia due to suppression of normal plasma cells plays a central role [87, 93–96]. Karlsson et al. compared humoral immunity in patients with MM, WM, and MGUS with age-matched controls and found that the MGUS group displayed low antibody levels to a number of pathogens, notably staphylococcal antigens, *Moraxella* spp., VZV, and fungal antigens [97]. Hypogammaglobulinemia was present in up to 92% of MM patients, as opposed 56% of the MGUS patients, even though later studies displayed hypogammaglobulinemia levels of 25–28% in this population [20, 87]. Apparently, levels of expression of M protein also play a role; MGUS patients with M protein concentrations over 2.5 g/dL at diagnosis were found to display higher risks of infections compared to those with concentrations less than 0.5 g/dL, but compared to controls, the risk of infections was still significantly increased among MGUS patients irrespective of M protein concentrations. This was similar for IgG, IgA, and IgM MGUS isotypes [98]. Another issue related to the immunological alteration of MGUS patients is the lower absolute numbers of both CD4+ and CD8+ cells [99], which might impair host response mechanisms.

Further considerations on immune dysregulation must take into account the fact that MGUS patients, as an increasingly aging population, have a high incidence of underlying diseases, such as autoimmune disorders and non-hematological malignancies, that may contribute additionally to the increased susceptibility to infections [90, 98, 100–102]. Moreover, even though MGUS is often an incidental diagnosis and there is no known role for chemotherapy in the management of this condition, some protein-related complications such as monoclonal gammopathy of renal significance (MGRS) and MGUS-associated peripheral neuropathies warrant appropriate therapy [90, 103, 104], inevitably leading to further immune impairment. Overall, MGUS patients appear as a heterogeneous group with a variable degree of immunosuppression. Notable examples of infections in MGUS patients include a study of Gregersen et al. published in 1998, where an association between MGUS and risk of bacteremia was found with a standardized incidence ratio (SIR) of 2.2 [98]. Another study based on US screening data published in 2009 found a higher risk of upper respiratory bacterial infection, spontaneous bacterial peritonitis, and mycobacterium infection in patients with MGUS compared with controls [11]. Reports on association with selected inflammatory disease or infections are also available, such as pyoderma gangrenosum [12] and sterile abscess [105]. More recently, the population study performed in Sweden in 2012 by Kristinsson et al. [94] found that MGUS patients had a 2.1-fold increased risk of developing any infection, and that the risk was very similar at 10-year follow-up. When assessing individual bacterial infections, osteomyelitis, bacteremia, and meningitis presented a hazard risk (HR) above 3%. As for viral infections, associated risk was 2.7 and 2.8 times higher for influenza and VZV reactivation, respectively. In a case series of 25 renal-transplanted patients with MGUS, an increased frequency of EBV reactivation was noted [106] associated with higher viral loads. Currently, studies on infection prevention in this group of paraproteinemia are lacking, as indications are typically designed for patients with MM [107]. Ultimately, MGUS patients have a lower life expectancy when compared to the general population [93, 96, 98], with a median survival of 8.1 years vs 11.8 years in a large cohort study [11], and this mortality excess is due not only to malignant transformation, but mostly to a combination of non-hematologic cancers, infections, and organ dysfunction typical of the disease [90].

Waldenström's Macroglobulinemia

WM is a rare chronic lymphoproliferative malignancy with a reported annual incidence rate of 3–4 cases per million people [108, 109]. It is often preceded by MGUS, a precursor condition with a transformation rate of 1–2% per year [110]. There are several conditions considered at augmented risk of WM, including personal or family history of autoimmune diseases (Sjögren syndrome, autoimmune hemolytic anemia) and infective disorders, as well as other B-cell disorders [111, 112]. Clinical manifestations include anemia, constitutional symptoms, and IgM paraprotein-attributable symptoms such as Bing–Neel syndrome, peripheral neuropathy, hyperviscosity, and infectious complications [113]. Infections are common in WM, particularly those of the respiratory tract. A population-based study found that WM patients have a 3.4-fold (95% CI 3.1–3.6) elevated risk of developing any infection than controls, with 3.2 and 6.0 higher risk for bacterial and viral infections, respectively [19]. The infectious risk is considered to be higher due to hypogammaglobulinemia [97], a condition common to MGUS, WM and MM, and augmented by immunosuppressive therapy needed to control progression and complications. Nevertheless, one group found no cases of *P. jirovecii* pneumonia among WM patients treated with ibrutinib, even though prophylaxis rate was low [114]. Guidelines currently recommend anti-pneumocystis and antiviral prophylaxis, especially targeted at HSV and VZV, in patients requiring intensive or prolonged immunosuppressive treatment, including treatment with BTKi and bortezomib, respectively [115]. Antimicrobial prophylaxis based on local epidemiology should also be considered for patients with hypogammaglobulinemia who develop recurrent bacterial infections, whereas patients with secondary recurrent infection despite antimicrobial prophylaxis should be considered for immunoglobulin replacement [115, 116]. Similar to MM, patients diagnosed with WM should be tested for previous viral hepatitis infection to avoid viral reactivation [117]. Infection prevention with vaccination is also warranted, including seasonal influenza vaccine. Furthermore, all patients with WM should be offered pneumococcal vaccination [118]. Live vaccines are not recommended and, for patients eligible for VZV vaccine, the non-live vaccine should be used [115, 116].

IgG4-Related Disease

IgG4-related disease is a rare fibro-inflammatory multiorgan condition, commonly characterized by polyclonal lymphoplasmacytic infiltrate with IgG4+ plasma cells, storiform fibrosis, and obliterative phlebitis [119, 120]. The pathogenetic mechanism for IgG4-related disease development is poorly understood. Studies found that Th2 cytokines like IL-4, IL-5, IL-10, and IL-13, which activate B-cell IgE production and eosinophil recruitment, are at increased production in some organ dysfunction in IgG4-related disease [121, 122]. Evidence of genetic susceptibility prominently focuses on pancreatitis presentation [123, 124] and is generally scarce. Reactive eosinophilia is also present in 40% of the patients, usually alongside asthma and atopy [125]; IgE is also markedly increased, whereas IgA and IgM levels are normal or moderately elevated. All patients with symptomatic disease require some degree of immunosuppressive therapy, including short-term glucocorticoids use or monoclonal antibodies such as rituximab for disease relapse [126–128]. Therefore, infectious complications also arise in response to treatment [128, 129], as shown by Campochiaro et al. reporting upper respiratory tract infections and urinary tract infections in 6 out of 14 patients receiving rituximab [128]. Another study conducted in France found rates of severe infection up to 12.1/100 patient-days in patients who received rituximab [129]. Overall, many patients followed an indolent course and responded well to treatment, but a significant proportion showed morbid or fatal complications such as periaortitis, pachymeningitis, and severe infections. Further studies to stratify infectious risk in this group are needed, and careful monitoring for severe infection development during immunosuppressive treatment is warranted.

Systemic Lupus Erythematosus

Although not classified among paraproteinemias but potentially associated with transient occurrence of paraproteinemia is systemic lupus erythematosus (SLE), an inflammatory and multi-systemic autoimmune disorder which may affect every organ and tissue. SLE is characterized by an uncontrolled auto-reactivity of B and T cells; this condition causes the production of autoantibodies that act against self-tissues [130]. The clinical manifestations and the pattern of organ involvement are widely heterogenous, reflecting the complex mosaic of disrupted molecular pathways converging into the SLE clinical phenotype. Morbidity and mortality in SLE are not only caused by the disease itself but are also due to treatment-associated complications such as coronary artery disease and increased infection risk as a consequence of corticosteroids [130].

Factors associated with increased risk of infections include high disease activity, specific immune dysregulation, drug-induced immune deficiency, and organ failure with irreversible damage. Furthermore, immunosuppressive agents may make patients more susceptible to opportunistic infections [131]. Distinguishing between infections and flares of SLE can be challenging, as infections may mimic them, leading to delays in diagnosis and appropriate management [131]. Specific biomarkers allowing for an accurate differential diagnosis in this disease are lacking, as serum markers may be nonspecific (e.g., C reactive protein) or may be relevant only for certain infections (e.g., beta-D-glucan for fungal infections). Procalcitonin may increase the accuracy of detection of severe bacterial infections in SLE; however, false-positive results are possible, and its measurement should not replace an accurate workup to establish the real need for antibiotic use [132]. Research is needed to determine specific immune dysregulation underlying the increased susceptibility to specific infections, predictors of infection in SLE such as genetic markers, and biomarkers that discriminate between disease activity and active infections. Bacterial infections are the most frequent infections in SLE, followed by viral and fungal infections. Among risk factors for infection in SLE are the impaired cellular and humoral immune functions, disease activity, prednisone doses above 7.5–10 mg/day, and high doses of methylprednisolone or cyclophosphamide [30, 133]. A recent review has investigated in vivo and human models analyzing specific bacterial species associated with SLE, and the potential roles of certain common bacterial infections in promoting lupus progression [30]. A total of 8 studies performed over a 20-year period (1999–2020) encompassing over 100,000 patients showed rates of infections between 18 and 72% [134–141]. A large variety of infectious sites and pathogens were reported, including opportunistic pathogens or bacteria that are typical of the hospital setting (Table 18.3). Increased age, leukopenia, and prednisone treatment were identified among risk factors for infection [30].

Despite increased awareness and improved management, infections remain a major source of morbidity, mortality, hospitalization, and death in patients with

Table 18.3 Most frequently reported sites of infections and related pathogens in patients with SLE

Site of infection	Meningitis, meningoencephalitis	[134–137]
	Endocarditis	[134]
	Hepatitis	[134]
	Respiratory	[134–141]
	Bacteremia	[134–137, 139]
	Peritonitis	[137]
	Urinary tract infection	[137–141]
	Abdominal	[136–138, 141]
	Skin and soft tissue	[137, 141]
Pathogens	Staphylococci	[136–139]
	Klebsiella spp.	[134, 136, 140]
	Pseudomonas spp.	[134, 136, 140]
	Acinetobacter spp.	[136, 140]
	Enterococcus spp.	[136]
	E. coli	[136, 137, 139, 140]
	Salmonella spp.	[136, 137]
	Nocardia spp.	[136]
	Mycobacterium tuberculosis	[137]
	Neisseria meningitidis	[137]
	Campylobacter spp.	[137]
	Legionella pneumophila	[137]
	Serratia spp.	[137]

SLE. Infections range from opportunistic to common bacterial and viral infections with typical or atypical presentations. Infections are common, particularly from encapsulated bacteria [142]. Pneumonia due to *S. pneumoniae* has been documented in these patients and is associated with increased mortality [133]. A retrospective study performed during 2011–2014 analyzing 443 patients with various autoimmune rheumatic diseases showed that 24/70 (34%) patients with suspected CMV infection had positive CMV-Ag, particularly in SLE (59%). At the time of CMV infection, SLE patients had moderate to severe disease activity and main CMV sites involved were the lungs (46%) and the gastrointestinal tract (27%). Mortality rates reported in the study were high reaching 46% and were associated with higher doses of daily oral corticosteroids ($p = 0.07$) and lower number of lymphocytes ($p = 0.06$). As increased CMV disease severity has been associated with SLE, CMV monitoring in patients with symptoms or laboratory tests suggestive for CMV disease should be performed [143]. Immunization in SLE is recommended due to an increase in vaccine-preventable disease in this patient population. In addition to routine immunization schedules, pneumococcal and seasonal influenza vaccination should be considered as key immunizations. Also, measures must be evaluated appropriately to prevent infections and their complications in SLE [131].

Cryoglobulinemia

Cryoglobulinemia is a condition that may be associated with various diseases such as infections, autoimmune disorders, and malignancies [32]. As previously mentioned, cryoglobulins are detected in the serum of patients suffering from chronic infection and/or inflammation including viral infections, particularly HCV and less frequently HIV [23, 32]. The French cohort study of Bonnet et al. and the multicenter HISPAMEC registry, mostly incorporating patients from Southern Europe, North America, and Japan, found the condition in 40–65% of those with HCV infection and HCV/HIV coinfection, whereas prevalence was 15–20% in case of HIV infection. The treatment of mixed cryoglobulinemia (defined as cryoglobulins in the serum that contain more than one immunoglobulin component) is performed using immunosuppressants such as corticosteroids. Considering both immunosuppressive therapy and the comorbidities that are often associated with the underlying condition, it is usually recommended to start an antibiotic prophylaxis against opportunistic infection such as *P. jirovecii* especially among patients receiving high-dose prednisone. Patients should also receive age-appropriate immunizations before the initiation of immunosuppression [144, 145].

Amyloidosis

Amyloidosis is defined as the extracellular tissue deposition of subunits of various proteins, which usually circulate as normal constituents of plasma. The clinical manifestations of amyloid deposits depend on their type, location, and amount [146]. There are more than 30 different types of amyloidosis, both systemic and localized. The principal forms of amyloid subunit proteins include immunoglobulin light chain (AL) amyloid, transthyretin (ATTR) amyloid, and secondary (AA) amyloidosis [147]. AA amyloidosis is described as an occurring complication of chronic diseases associated with ongoing or recurring inflammation, including infections [52, 148]. Risk factors for developing infections in patients with amyloidosis include hyposplenism, hypogammaglobulinemia, treatment-related neutropenia, melphalan-induced mucositis, and nosocomial infections related to prolonged hospital stay [149]. AL amyloidosis has a poor long-term prognosis when detected at an advanced stage, with a median survival between 4 and 6 months. Infections are one of the major causes of death, alongside cardiac, renal, or hepatic failure [150]. Taimur et al. analyzed 493 patients with AL amyloidosis undergoing treatment with high dose melphalan and autologous SCT between 1994 and 2009. Microbiologically documented infections occurred in 24% of patients with mortality within 100 days of SCT reported in 21%, showing a three-fold relative risk of treatment-related mortality (3.42, 95% CI 2.02–5.79). Infections were caused by Gram-positive bacteria in 51%, anaerobic bacteria in 16%, Gram-negative bacteria in 13%, and fungi in 9%

of cases. Serum creatinine >2 mg/dL was associated with increased risk of post-SCT infection (38% vs. 21%, $P = 0.0007$, OR 2.27). Infection did not appear associated with age, gender, cardiac involvement, steroid therapy, melphalan dose, or multiorgan involvement [149]. Among other treatments, bortezomib therapy may be associated with an increased risk of HZ [151]. Clinical trials have also shown that patients receiving daratumumab have an increased risk of infections such as pneumonia, upper respiratory tract infections, and bacteremia. Such infections lead to significant morbidity and mortality although these results may be related to the frailty of the population treated [152, 153].

Discussion and Conclusions

Paraproteinemia accounts for several diseases with complex presentations and multiple immune defects. Infections have sometimes been considered as triggers for paraproteinemia or may arise as a consequence of immunosuppression linked to the underlying disease or to the associated chemotherapy. The types and timing of infections remain poorly studied especially in rare paraproteinemias, and several studies appear to focus on infections as a predisposing cause for autoimmune or hematological diseases rather than infections as a consequence of paraproteinemia. For MM, severe infections mainly occur early after diagnosis, or during initial chemotherapy. Various factors including age, prolonged hospitalization, organ failure, and disease stage may impact on the type and severity of infections. Bacteria (compared to viruses, parasites, or fungi) are more commonly isolated in patients with paraproteinemia, including both community-acquired (e.g., *E. coli*, *S. pneumoniae*) and hospital-acquired (e.g., *P. aeruginosa*, *K. pneumoniae*, *S. aureus*) bacteria. Viral infections include mainly herpesvirus reactivation. Fungal infections are less common although candidemia because of prolonged hospitalization and invasive aspergillosis may occur and are characterized by high mortality rates.

Some key points to consider in the management of infections in paraproteinemia are reported in Fig. 18.1.

Some of these points apply to the wider population of immunocompromised patients, including performance of molecular tests or rapid diagnostics to obtain etiological diagnosis and to target antimicrobial treatment. Empiric antibiotic therapy is currently deeply affected by antimicrobial resistance [75]. Infections due to multidrug-resistant pathogens, especially Gram-negative bacteria such ESBL-producing or carbapenemase-producing *K. pneumoniae* or *P. aeruginosa* are responsible for high mortality rates and may leave few effective antimicrobial options [74, 75]. Furthermore, although novel compounds have become available for multidrug-resistant bacteria, they have high costs, their efficacy have been mainly tested in vitro, and they may develop resistance as well. Factors such as clinical severity, underlying comorbidities, prolonged hospitalization or antibiotic

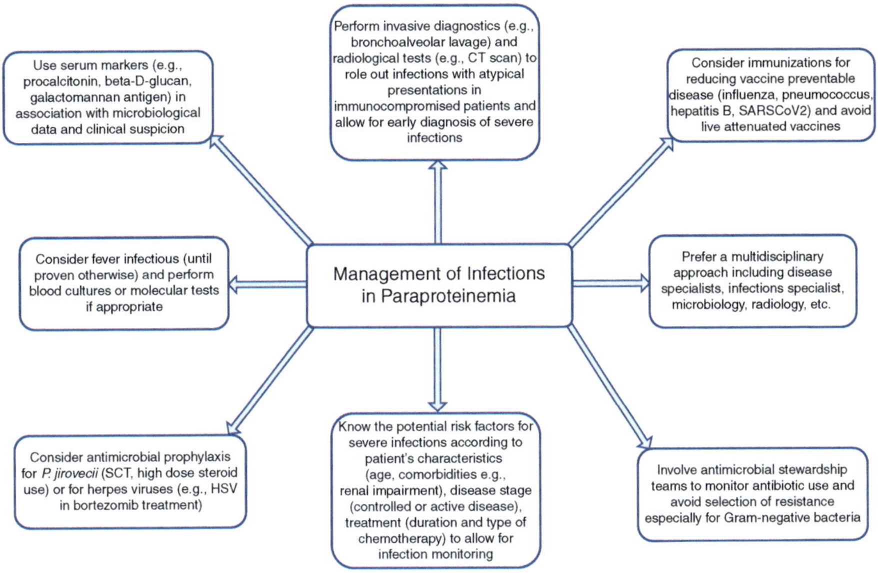

Fig. 18.1 Key elements for the management of infections in paraproteinemia

use, and previous history of colonization or infections due to multidrug-resistant bacteria represent key points in approaching an immunocompromised patient with signs of infection and may warrant for increased antibiotic resistance [74, 75]. Antimicrobial stewardship principles should be put in place while managing patients with severe or recurrent infections to spare last resort antibiotics, such as carbapenems, and reduce the ecological impact preserving treatment efficacy. A de-escalation therapy with initial use of wide-spectrum antimicrobials (e.g., carbapenems with or without an aminoglycoside and/or a glycopeptide) followed by clinical and microbiological reassessment after 72 h of treatment may represent a good option in severe infections or in febrile neutropenia if a resistant pathogen is suspected [74, 75]. Epidemiological surveillance through performance of prevalence studies is paramount in centers managing immunocompromised patients [67, 74, 75].

Finally, prevention remains one of the best strategies to reduce the infection burden in immunocompromised hosts. Clear guidelines on antibiotic prophylaxis in immunocompromised patients other than HSC and solid organ transplant are lacking, although some clinical trials support the use of cotrimoxazole in patients receiving high-dose steroids. Antiviral prophylaxis should also be considered in patients receiving selected chemotherapy who are at risk for herpesvirus infections or hepatitis B infections. Immunizations should be performed prior to chemotherapy and live attenuated vaccinations should be avoided, while vaccinations against pneumococcal disease, influenza virus, and, most recently, SARS-CoV-2 are recommended [45, 86].

References

1. Cook L, Macdonald DHC. Management of paraproteinaemia. Postgrad Med J. 2007;83(978):217–23. https://doi.org/10.1136/pgmj.2006.054627.
2. Nakamura K, Smyth MJ, Martinet L. Cancer immunoediting and immune dysregulation in multiple myeloma. Blood. 2020;136(24):2731–40. https://doi.org/10.1182/blood.2020006540.
3. Caro J, Braunstein M, Williams L, et al. Inflammation and infection in plasma cell disorders: how pathogens shape the fate of patients. Leukemia. 2022;36(3):613–24. https://doi.org/10.1038/s41375-021-01506-9.
4. Karlsson J, Andréasson B, Kondori N, et al. Comparative study of immune status to infectious agents in elderly patients with multiple myeloma, Waldenstrom's macroglobulinemia, and monoclonal gammopathy of undetermined significance. Clin Vaccine Immunol. 2011;18(6):969–77. https://doi.org/10.1128/CVI.00021-11.
5. Pal R, Monaghan SA, Hassett AC, et al. Immunomodulatory derivatives induce PU.1 downregulation, myeloid maturation arrest, and neutropenia. Blood. 2010;115(3):605–14. https://doi.org/10.1182/blood-2009-05-221077.
6. Teh BW, Harrison SJ, Worth LJ, Thursky KA, Slavin MA. Infection risk with immunomodulatory and proteasome inhibitor–based therapies across treatment phases for multiple myeloma: a systematic review and meta-analysis. Eur J Cancer. 2016;67:21–37. https://doi.org/10.1016/j.ejca.2016.07.025.
7. Teh BW, Harrison SJ, Pellegrini M, Thursky KA, Worth LJ, Slavin MA. Changing treatment paradigms for patients with plasma cell myeloma: impact upon immune determinants of infection. Blood Rev. 2014;28(2):75–86. https://doi.org/10.1016/j.blre.2014.01.004.
8. Mermel LA, Allon M, Bouza E, et al. Clinical practice guidelines for the diagnosis and management of intravascular catheter-related infection: 2009 update by the Infectious Diseases Society of America. Clin Infect Dis. 2009;49(1):1–45. https://doi.org/10.1086/599376.
9. Teh BW, Harrison SJ, Slavin MA, Worth LJ. Epidemiology of bloodstream infections in patients with myeloma receiving current era therapy. Eur J Haematol. 2017;98(2):149–53. https://doi.org/10.1111/ejh.12813.
10. Yoshikawa TT. Epidemiology and unique aspects of aging and infectious diseases. Clin Infect Dis. 2000;30(6):931–3. https://doi.org/10.1086/313792.
11. Nucci M, Anaissie E. Infections in patients with multiple myeloma in the era of high-dose therapy and novel agents. Clin Infect Dis. 2009;49(8):1211–25. https://doi.org/10.1086/605664.
12. Solana R, Tarazona R, Gayoso I, Lesur O, Dupuis G, Fulop T. Innate immunosenescence: effect of aging on cells and receptors of the innate immune system in humans. Semin Immunol. 2012;24(5):331–41. https://doi.org/10.1016/j.smim.2012.04.008.
13. Montecino-Rodriguez E, Berent-Maoz B, Dorshkind K. Causes, consequences, and reversal of immune system aging. J Clin Invest. 2013;123(3):958–65. https://doi.org/10.1172/JCI64096.
14. Pratt G, Goodyear O, Moss P. Immunodeficiency and immunotherapy in multiple myeloma. Br J Haematol. 2007;138(5):563–79. https://doi.org/10.1111/j.1365-2141.2007.06705.x.
15. Stadtmauer EA, Vogl DT, Luning Prak E, et al. Transfer of influenza vaccine–primed costimulated autologous T cells after stem cell transplantation for multiple myeloma leads to reconstitution of influenza immunity: results of a randomized clinical trial. Blood. 2011;117(1):63–71. https://doi.org/10.1182/blood-2010-07-296822.
16. Hahn M, Schnitzler P, Schweiger B, et al. Efficacy of single versus boost vaccination against influenza virus in patients with multiple myeloma. Haematologica. 2015;100(7):e285–8. https://doi.org/10.3324/haematol.2014.116772.
17. Branagan AR, Duffy E, Albrecht RA, et al. Clinical and serologic responses after a two-dose series of high-dose influenza vaccine in plasma cell disorders: a prospective, single-arm trial. Clin Lymphoma Myeloma Leuk. 2017;17(5):296–304.e2. https://doi.org/10.1016/j.clml.2017.02.025.

18. Quartuccio L, Zabotti A, Del Zotto S, Zanier L, De Vita S, Valent F. Risk of serious infection among patients receiving biologics for chronic inflammatory diseases: usefulness of administrative data. J Adv Res. 2019;15:87–93. https://doi.org/10.1016/j.jare.2018.09.003.
19. McShane CM, Murray LJ, Engels EA, Anderson LA. Community-acquired infections associated with increased risk of lymphoplasmacytic lymphoma/Waldenström macroglobulinaemia. Br J Haematol. 2014;164(5):653–8. https://doi.org/10.1111/bjh.12671.
20. Bosseboeuf A, Feron D, Tallet A, et al. Monoclonal IgG in MGUS and multiple myeloma targets infectious pathogens. JCI Insight. 2017;2(19):e95367. https://doi.org/10.1172/jci.insight.95367.
21. Duberg AS, Nordström M, Törner A, et al. Non-Hodgkin's lymphoma and other non-hepatic malignancies in Swedish patients with hepatitis C virus infection. Hepatology. 2005;41(3):652–9. https://doi.org/10.1002/hep.20608.
22. Perl A, Fernandez D, Telarico T, Phillips PE. Endogenous retroviral pathogenesis in lupus. Curr Opin Rheumatol. 2010;22(5):483–92. https://doi.org/10.1097/BOR.0b013e32833c6297.
23. Ramos-Casals M, Muñoz S, Medina F, et al. Systemic autoimmune diseases in patients with hepatitis C virus infection: characterization of 1020 cases (the HISPAMEC registry). J Rheumatol. 2009;36(7):1442–8. https://doi.org/10.3899/jrheum.080874.
24. Kristinsson SY, Koshiol J, Bjorkholm M, et al. Immune-related and inflammatory conditions and risk of lymphoplasmacytic lymphoma or Waldenstrom macroglobulinemia. J Natl Cancer Inst. 2010;102(8):557–67. https://doi.org/10.1093/jnci/djq043.
25. Giordano TP, Henderson L, Landgren O, et al. Risk of non-Hodgkin lymphoma and lymphoproliferative precursor diseases in US veterans with hepatitis C virus. JAMA. 2007;297(18):2010–7. https://doi.org/10.1001/jama.297.18.2010.
26. Koshiol J, Gridley G, Engels EA, McMaster ML, Landgren O. Chronic immune stimulation and subsequent Waldenström macroglobulinemia. Arch Intern Med. 2008;168(17):1903. https://doi.org/10.1001/archinternmed.2008.4.
27. Siddiquee Z, Zane NA, Smith RN, Stone JR. Dense IgG4 plasma cell infiltrates associated with chronic infectious aortitis: implications for the diagnosis of IgG4-related disease. Cardiovasc Pathol. 2012;21(6):470–5. https://doi.org/10.1016/j.carpath.2012.02.001.
28. Kawano M, Yamada K, Kakuchi Y, et al. A case of immunoglobulin G4-related chronic sclerosing sialadenitis and dacryoadenitis associated with tuberculosis. Mod Rheumatol. 2009;19(1):87–90. https://doi.org/10.3109/s10165-008-0127-z.
29. Lu F, Martin KA, Soldan SS, et al. Defective Epstein-Barr virus genomes and atypical viral gene expression in B-cell lines derived from multiple myeloma patients. J Virol. 2021;95(13):e0008821. https://doi.org/10.1128/JVI.00088-21.
30. Battaglia M, Garrett-Sinha LA. Bacterial infections in lupus: roles in promoting immune activation and in pathogenesis of the disease. J Transl Autoimmun. 2021;4:100078. https://doi.org/10.1016/j.jtauto.2020.100078.
31. Via CS, Handwerger BS. B-cell and T-cell function in systemic lupus erythematosus. Curr Opin Rheumatol. 1993;5(5):570–4. https://doi.org/10.1097/00002281-199305050-00004.
32. Bonnet F, Pineau JJ, Taupin JL, et al. Prevalence of cryoglobulinemia and serological markers of autoimmunity in human immunodeficiency virus infected individuals: a cross-sectional study of 97 patients. J Rheumatol. 2003;30(9):2005–10.
33. Rizvi SN, Gulati PD, Vaishnava H. Letter: tuberculosis and renal amyloidosis. Br Med J. 1974;4(5945):657. https://doi.org/10.1136/bmj.4.5945.657-a.
34. Chugh KS, Datta BN, Singhal PC, Jain SK, Sakhuja V, Dash SC. Pattern of renal amyloidosis in Indian patients. Postgrad Med J. 1981;57(663):31–5. https://doi.org/10.1136/pgmj.57.663.31.
35. Mengistu M. Incidence of renal amyloidosis in adult Ethiopian tuberculosis patients. East Afr Med J. 1983;60(11):773–7.
36. Erk O, Turfanda T, Uysal V. Frequency of renal amyloidosis secondary to tuberculosis. Nephron. 1995;71(3):367. https://doi.org/10.1159/000188751.

37. Tsuji K, Arai H, Furusu A, et al. A case of membranoproliferative glomerulonephritis and AA amyloidosis complicated with pulmonary nontuberculous mycobacterial infection. CEN Case Rep. 2015;4(1):24–30. https://doi.org/10.1007/s13730-014-0134-1.
38. Aharon A, Langevitz P, Maran R, Blank-Porat D, Shtrasburg S, Livneh A. Reactive amyloidosis in a patient with Mycobacterium simiae pulmonary infection. Respir Med. 1998;92(1):123–4. https://doi.org/10.1016/s0954-6111(98)90044-0.
39. Nakayama EE, Ura S, Fleury RN, Soares V. Renal lesions in leprosy: a retrospective study of 199 autopsies. Am J Kidney Dis. 2001;38(1):26–30. https://doi.org/10.1053/ajkd.2001.25177.
40. Amyloidosis and leprosy. Lancet. 1975;2(7935):589.
41. Secondary amyloidosis. Ann Intern Med. 1949;31(1):105. https://doi.org/10.7326/0003-4819-31-1-105
42. Nakagawa S, Suzue K. Amyloidosis in Japan. Pathobiology. 1964;27(5):850–4. https://doi.org/10.1159/000161539.
43. Sander S. Whipple's disease associated with amyloidosis. Acta Pathol Microbiol Scand. 1964;61:530–6. https://doi.org/10.1111/apm.1964.61.4.530.
44. Vanderbeke L, Peetermans WE, Saegeman V, De Munter P. Q fever: a contemporary case series from a Belgian hospital. Acta Clin Belg. 2016;71(5):290–6. https://doi.org/10.1080/17843286.2016.1165397.
45. Kollabathula A, Vishwajeet V, Gupta K, et al. Chronic brucellosis with hepatic brucelloma and AA amyloidosis in a patient with autosomal dominant polycystic kidney disease. Autops Case Rep. 2020;10(1):e2019128. https://doi.org/10.4322/acr.2019.128.
46. Lejmi H, Jen KY, Olson JL, James SH, Sam R. Characteristics of AA amyloidosis patients in San Francisco. Nephrology (Carlton). 2016;21(4):308–13. https://doi.org/10.1111/nep.12616.
47. Girnius S, Dember L, Doros G, Skinner M. The changing face of AA amyloidosis: a single center experience. Amyloid. 2011;18(sup1):226–8. https://doi.org/10.3109/13506129.2011.574354085.
48. Muthu V, Sehgal IS, Dhooria S, Bal A, Agarwal R. Allergic bronchopulmonary aspergillosis presenting as nephrotic syndrome due to secondary amyloidosis: case report and systematic review of the literature. Lung India. 2018;35(4):332–5. https://doi.org/10.4103/lungindia.lungindia_180_17.
49. Brownstein MH, Helwig EB. Secondary systemic amyloidosis: analysis of underlying disorders. South Med J. 1971;64(4):491–6. https://doi.org/10.1097/00007611-197104000-00024.
50. Symmers WS. Letter: amyloidosis complicating actinomycosis. BMJ. 1973;4(5889):423–4. https://doi.org/10.1136/bmj.4.5889.423-b.
51. Berns JS, Rapalino O, Fenves AZ, El Khoury JB, Klepeis VE, Anahtar MN. Case 11-2020: a 37-year-old man with facial droop, dysarthria, and kidney failure. Cabot RC, Rosenberg ES, Pierce VM, et al., eds. N Engl J Med. 2020;382(15):1457–66. https://doi.org/10.1056/NEJMcpc1916252.
52. Deshayes S, Aouba A, Grateau G, Georgin-Lavialle S. Infections and AA amyloidosis: an overview. Int J Clin Pract. 2021;75(6):e13966. https://doi.org/10.1111/ijcp.13966.
53. Culver EL, Smit WL, Evans C, et al. No evidence to support a role for Helicobacter pylori infection and plasminogen binding protein in autoimmune pancreatitis and IgG4-related disease in a UK cohort. Pancreatology. 2017;17(3):395–402. https://doi.org/10.1016/j.pan.2017.04.002.
54. Sekigawa I, Kaneko H, Hishikawa T, et al. HIV infection and SLE: their pathogenic relationship. Clin Exp Rheumatol. 1998;16(2):175–80.
55. Backhaus E, Berg S, Andersson R, et al. Epidemiology of invasive pneumococcal infections: manifestations, incidence and case fatality rate correlated to age, gender and risk factors. BMC Infect Dis. 2016;16(1):367. https://doi.org/10.1186/s12879-016-1648-2.
56. Miceli MH, Dong L, Grazziutti ML, et al. Iron overload is a major risk factor for severe infection after autologous stem cell transplantation: a study of 367 myeloma patients. Bone Marrow Transplant. 2006;37(9):857–64. https://doi.org/10.1038/sj.bmt.1705340.

57. Blimark C, Holmberg E, Mellqvist UH, et al. Multiple myeloma and infections: a population-based study on 9253 multiple myeloma patients. Haematologica. 2015;100(1):107–13. https://doi.org/10.3324/haematol.2014.107714.
58. Bladé J, San Miguel JF, Fontanillas M, et al. Increased conventional chemotherapy does not improve survival in multiple myeloma: long-term results of two PETHEMA trials including 914 patients. Hematol J. 2001;2(4):272–8. https://doi.org/10.1038/sj.thj.6200115.
59. Hargreaves RM, Lea JR, Griffiths H, et al. Immunological factors and risk of infection in plateau phase myeloma. J Clin Pathol. 1995;48(3):260–6. https://doi.org/10.1136/jcp.48.3.260.
60. Snowdon L, Gibson J, Joshua DE. Frequency of infection in plateau-phase multiple myeloma. Lancet. 1994;344(8917):262. https://doi.org/10.1016/S0140-6736(94)93028-7.
61. Augustson BM, Begum G, Dunn JA, et al. Early mortality after diagnosis of multiple myeloma: analysis of patients entered onto the United Kingdom Medical Research Council trials between 1980 and 2002—Medical Research Council Adult Leukaemia Working Party. JCO. 2005;23(36):9219–26. https://doi.org/10.1200/JCO.2005.03.2086.
62. Djebbari F, Panitsas F, Eyre TA, et al. Infection-related morbidity in a large study of transplant non-eligible newly diagnosed myeloma patients treated with UK standard of care. Haematologica. 2020;105(9):e474–9. https://doi.org/10.3324/haematol.2019.240762.
63. Moreau P, Touzeau C. Multiple myeloma: from front-line to relapsed therapies. Am Soc Clin Oncol Educ Book. 2015;35:e504–11. https://doi.org/10.14694/EdBook_AM.2015.35.e504.
64. Korean Multiple Myeloma Working Party (KMMWP), Jung SH, Cho MS, et al. Risk factors associated with early mortality in patients with multiple myeloma who were treated upfront with a novel agents containing regimen. BMC Cancer. 2016;16(1):613. https://doi.org/10.1186/s12885-016-2645-y.
65. Lortholary O, Ascioglu S, Moreau P, et al. Invasive aspergillosis as an opportunistic infection in Nonallografted patients with multiple myeloma: a European Organization for Research and Treatment of Cancer. Clin Infect Dis. 2000;30(1):41–6. https://doi.org/10.1086/313592.
66. Teh BW, Teng JC, Urbancic K, et al. Invasive fungal infections in patients with multiple myeloma: a multi-center study in the era of novel myeloma therapies. Haematologica. 2015;100(1):e28–31. https://doi.org/10.3324/haematol.2014.114025.
67. Bassetti M, Righi E. Overview of fungal infections—the Italian experience. Semin Respir Crit Care Med. 2015;36(5):796–806. https://doi.org/10.1055/s-0035-1562890.
68. Nucci M, Nouér SA, Grazziutti M, Kumar NS, Barlogie B, Anaissie E. Probable invasive aspergillosis without prespecified radiologic findings: proposal for inclusion of a new category of aspergillosis and implications for studying novel therapies. Clin Infect Dis. 2010;51(11):1273–80. https://doi.org/10.1086/657065.
69. Frerichs KA, Bosman PWC, Nijhof IS, Zweegman S, van de Donk NWCJ. Cytomegalovirus reactivation in a patient with extensively pretreated multiple myeloma during daratumumab treatment. Clin Lymphoma Myeloma Leuk. 2019;19(1):e9–e11. https://doi.org/10.1016/j.clml.2018.10.002.
70. Savage DG. Biphasic pattern of bacterial infection in multiple myeloma. Ann Intern Med. 1982;96(1):47. https://doi.org/10.7326/0003-4819-96-1-47.
71. Balmaceda N, Aziz M, Chandrasekar VT, et al. Infection risks in multiple myeloma: a systematic review and meta-analysis of randomized trials from 2015 to 2019. BMC Cancer. 2021;21(1):730. https://doi.org/10.1186/s12885-021-08451-x.
72. Teh BW, Harrison SJ, Worth LJ, Spelman T, Thursky KA, Slavin MA. Risks, severity and timing of infections in patients with multiple myeloma: a longitudinal cohort study in the era of immunomodulatory drug therapy. Br J Haematol. 2015;171(1):100–8. https://doi.org/10.1111/bjh.13532.
73. Schütt P, Brandhorst D, Stellberg W, et al. Immune parameters in multiple myeloma patients: influence of treatment and correlation with opportunistic infections. Leuk Lymphoma. 2006;47(8):1570–82. https://doi.org/10.1080/10428190500472503.

74. Righi E, Peri AM, Harris PNA, et al. Global prevalence of carbapenem resistance in neutropenic patients and association with mortality and carbapenem use: systematic review and meta-analysis. J Antimicrob Chemother. 2017;72(3):668–77. https://doi.org/10.1093/jac/dkw459.
75. Bassetti M, Righi E. Multidrug-resistant bacteria: what is the threat? Hematology. 2013;2013(1):428–32. https://doi.org/10.1182/asheducation-2013.1.428.
76. Kim JH, Goulston C, Sanders S, et al. Cytomegalovirus reactivation following autologous peripheral blood stem cell transplantation for multiple myeloma in the era of novel chemotherapeutics and tandem transplantation. Biol Blood Marrow Transplant. 2012;18(11):1753–8. https://doi.org/10.1016/j.bbmt.2012.06.008.
77. Karageorgopoulos DE, Qu JM, Korbila IP, Zhu YG, Vasileiou VA, Falagas ME. Accuracy of β -D-glucan for the diagnosis of Pneumocystis jirovecii pneumonia: a meta-analysis. Clin Microbiol Infect. 2013;19(1):39–49. https://doi.org/10.1111/j.1469-0691.2011.03760.x.
78. Miceli MH, Jones Jackson LB, Walker RC, Talamo G, Barlogie B, Anaissie EJ. Diagnosis of infection of implantable central venous catheters by [18F]fluorodeoxyglucose positron emission tomography. Nucl Med Commun. 2004;25(8):813–8. https://doi.org/10.1097/01.mnm.0000130247.37315.66.
79. Mahfouz T, Miceli MH, Saghafifar F, Stroud S, Jones-Jackson L, Walker R. 18 F-Fluorodeoxyglucose positron emission tomography contributes to the diagnosis and management of infections in patients with multiple myeloma: a study of 165 infectious episodes. JCO. 2005;23(31):7857–63.
80. Tsukune Y, Sasaki M, Odajima T, et al. Incidence and clinical background of hepatitis B virus reactivation in multiple myeloma in novel agents' era. Ann Hematol. 2016;95(9):1465–72. https://doi.org/10.1007/s00277-016-2742-7.
81. Bassetti M, Righi E, Akova M. Gram-negative infections. In: Cornely OA, Hoenigl M, editors. Infection management in hematology. Hematologic malignancies. Springer International Publishing; 2021. p. 161–179. https://doi.org/10.1007/978-3-030-57317-1_12.
82. Drayson MT, Bowcock S, Planche T, et al. Levofloxacin prophylaxis in patients with newly diagnosed myeloma (TEAMM): a multicentre, double-blind, placebo-controlled, randomised, phase 3 trial. Lancet Oncol. 2019;20(12):1760–72. https://doi.org/10.1016/S1470-2045(19)30506-6.
83. Terpos E, Kleber M, Engelhardt M, et al. European myeloma network guidelines for the management of multiple myeloma-related complications. Haematologica. 2015;100(10):1254–66. https://doi.org/10.3324/haematol.2014.117176.
84. Oken MM, Pomeroy C, Weisdorf D, Bennett JM. Prophylactic antibiotics for the prevention of early infection in multiple myeloma. Am J Med. 1996;100(6):624–8. https://doi.org/10.1016/S0002-9343(95)00043-7.
85. On behalf of the University of Rochester Cancer Center and the Eastern Cooperative Oncology Group, Vesole DH, Oken MM, et al. Oral antibiotic prophylaxis of early infection in multiple myeloma: a URCC/ECOG randomized phase III study. Leukemia. 2012;26(12):2517–20. https://doi.org/10.1038/leu.2012.124.
86. Righi E, Gallo T, Azzini AM, et al. A review of vaccinations in adult patients with secondary immunodeficiency. Infect Dis Ther. 2021;10(2):637–61. https://doi.org/10.1007/s40121-021-00404-y.
87. Atkin C, Reddy-Kolanu V, Drayson MT, Sapey E, Richter AG. The prevalence and significance of monoclonal gammopathy of undetermined significance in acute medical admissions. Br J Haematol. 2020;189(6):1127–35. https://doi.org/10.1111/bjh.16487.
88. On behalf of the International Myeloma Working Group, Kyle RA, Durie BGM, et al. Monoclonal gammopathy of undetermined significance (MGUS) and smoldering (asymptomatic) multiple myeloma: IMWG consensus perspectives risk factors for progression and guidelines for monitoring and management. Leukemia. 2010;24(6):1121–7. https://doi.org/10.1038/leu.2010.60.
89. van de Donk NWCJ, Palumbo A, Johnsen HE, et al. The clinical relevance and management of monoclonal gammopathy of undetermined significance and related disorders: recommen-

dations from the European Myeloma Network. Haematologica. 2014;99(6):984–96. https://doi.org/10.3324/haematol.2013.100552.
90. Garrett WS. Cancer and the microbiota. Science. 2015;348(6230):80–6. https://doi.org/10.1126/science.aaa4972.
91. Kristinsson SY, Bjorkholm M, Andersson TML, et al. Patterns of survival and causes of death following a diagnosis of monoclonal gammopathy of undetermined significance: a population-based study. Haematologica. 2009;94(12):1714–20. https://doi.org/10.3324/haematol.2009.010066.
92. La Torre G. Influenza and pneumococcal vaccination in hematological malignancies: a systematic review of efficacy, effectiveness and safety. Mediterr J Hematol Infect Dis. 2016;8:e2016044. https://doi.org/10.4084/mjhid.2016.044.
93. Gregersen H, Ibsen JS, Mellemkjœr L, Dahlerup JF, Olsen JH, Sørensen HT. Mortality and causes of death in patients with monoclonal gammopathy of undetermined significance: mortality in MGUS. Br J Haematol. 2001;112(2):353–7. https://doi.org/10.1046/j.1365-2141.2001.02533.x.
94. Kristinsson SY, Tang M, Pfeiffer RM, et al. Monoclonal gammopathy of undetermined significance and risk of infections: a population-based study. Haematologica. 2012;97(6):854–8. https://doi.org/10.3324/haematol.2011.054015.
95. Anderson LA, Pfeiffer R, Warren JL, et al. Hematopoietic malignancies associated with viral and alcoholic hepatitis. Cancer Epidemiol Biomark Prev. 2008;17(11):3069–75. https://doi.org/10.1158/1055-9965.EPI-08-0408.
96. Kyle RA, Therneau TM, Rajkumar SV, et al. Prevalence of monoclonal gammopathy of undetermined significance. N Engl J Med. 2006;354(13):1362–9. https://doi.org/10.1056/NEJMoa054494.
97. Leung N, Bridoux F, Hutchison CA, et al. Monoclonal gammopathy of renal significance: when MGUS is no longer undetermined or insignificant. Blood. 2012;120(22):4292–5. https://doi.org/10.1182/blood-2012-07-445304.
98. Gregersen H, Madsen KM, Sørensen HT, Schønheyder HC, Ibsen JS, Dahlerup JF. The risk of bacteremia in patients with monoclonal gammopathy of undetermined significance. Eur J Haematol. 2009;61(2):140–4. https://doi.org/10.1111/j.1600-0609.1998.tb01075.x.
99. Briault S, Courtois-Capella M, Duarte F, Aucouturier P, Preud'Homme JL. Isotypy of serum monoclonal immunoglobulins in human immunodeficiency virus-infected adults. Clin Exp Immunol. 1988;74(2):182–4.
100. Antoine Pepeljugoski C, Morgan G, Braunstein M. Analysis of intestinal microbiome in multiple myeloma reveals progressive dysbiosis compared to MGUS and healthy individuals. Blood. 2019;134(Supplement_1):3076. https://doi.org/10.1182/blood-2019-130643.
101. Kyle RA, Therneau TM, Rajkumar SV, et al. A long-term study of prognosis in monoclonal gammopathy of undetermined significance. N Engl J Med. 2002;346(8):564–9. https://doi.org/10.1056/NEJMoa01133202.
102. Cesana C, Klersy C, Barbarano L, et al. Prognostic factors for malignant transformation in monoclonal gammopathy of undetermined significance and smoldering multiple myeloma. JCO. 2002;20(6):1625–34. https://doi.org/10.1200/JCO.2002.20.6.1625.
103. Pérez-Persona E, Vidriales MB, Mateo G, et al. New criteria to identify risk of progression in monoclonal gammopathy of uncertain significance and smoldering multiple myeloma based on multiparameter flow cytometry analysis of bone marrow plasma cells. Blood. 2007;110(7):2586–92. https://doi.org/10.1182/blood-2007-05-088443.
104. Isaksson E, Björkholm M, Holm G, et al. Blood clonal B-cell excess in patients with monoclonal gammopathy of undetermined significance (MGUS): association with malignant transformation. Br J Haematol. 1996;92(1):71–6. https://doi.org/10.1046/j.1365-2141.1996.294826.x.
105. Fermand JP, Bridoux F, Kyle RA, et al. How I treat monoclonal gammopathy of renal significance (MGRS). Blood. 2013;122(22):3583–90. https://doi.org/10.1182/blood-2013-05-495929.

106. Glavey SV, Leung N. Monoclonal gammopathy: the good, the bad and the ugly. Blood Rev. 2016;30(3):223–31. https://doi.org/10.1016/j.blre.2015.12.001.
107. Bida JP, Kyle RA, Therneau TM, et al. Disease associations with monoclonal gammopathy of undetermined significance: a population-based study of 17,398 patients. Mayo Clin Proc. 2009;84(8):685–93. https://doi.org/10.1016/S0025-6196(11)60518-1.
108. Babel N, Schwarzmann F, Pruss A, Volk HD, Reinke P. Monoclonal gammopathy of undetermined significance (MGUS) is associated with an increased frequency of Epstein-Barr virus (EBV) latently infected B lymphocytes in long-term renal transplant patients. Transplant Proc. 2004;36(9):2679–82. https://doi.org/10.1016/j.transproceed.2004.09.046.
109. Aoki H, Takishita M, Kosaka M, Saito S. Frequent somatic mutations in D and/or JH segments of Ig gene in Waldenström's macroglobulinemia and chronic lymphocytic leukemia (CLL) with Richter's syndrome but not in common CLL. Blood. 1995;85(7):1913–9.
110. Weltgesundheitsorganisation. In: Swerdlow SH, Campo E, Harris NL, et al., editors. WHO classification of tumours of haematopoietic and lymphoid tissues. Revised 4th ed. International Agency for Research on Cancer; 2017.
111. Kristinsson SY, Björkholm M, Goldin LR, McMaster ML, Turesson I, Landgren O. Risk of lymphoproliferative disorders among first-degree relatives of lymphoplasmacytic lymphoma/ Waldenström macroglobulinemia patients: a population-based study in Sweden. Blood. 2008;112(8):3052–6. https://doi.org/10.1182/blood-2008-06-162768.
112. Treon SP, Hunter ZR, Aggarwal A, et al. Characterization of familial Waldenström's macroglobulinemia. Ann Oncol. 2006;17(3):488–94. https://doi.org/10.1093/annonc/mdj111.
113. Owen RG. Developing diagnostic criteria in Waldenstrom's macroglobulinemia. Semin Oncol. 2003;30(2):196–200. https://doi.org/10.1053/sonc.2003.50069.
114. Cheng MP, Kusztos AE, Gustine JN, et al. Low risk of *Pneumocystis jirovecii* pneumonia and invasive aspergillosis in patients with Waldenström macroglobulinaemia on ibrutinib. Br J Haematol. 2019;185(4):788–90. https://doi.org/10.1111/bjh.15627.
115. Pratt G, El-Sharkawi D, Kothari J, et al. Guidelines on the diagnosis and management of Waldenström macroglobulinaemia—A *British Society for Haematology* guideline. Br J Haematol. 2022;197(2):171–87. https://doi.org/10.1111/bjh.18036.
116. Schuh AH, Parry-Jones N, Appleby N, et al. Guideline for the treatment of chronic lymphocytic leukaemia: a British Society for Haematology guideline. Br J Haematol. 2018;182(3):344–59. https://doi.org/10.1111/bjh.15460.
117. Lampertico P, Agarwal K, Berg T, et al. EASL 2017 clinical practice guidelines on the management of hepatitis B virus infection. J Hepatol. 2017;67(2):370–98. https://doi.org/10.1016/j.jhep.2017.03.021.
118. Durot E, Kanagaratnam L, Zanwar S, et al. A prognostic index predicting survival in transformed Waldenström macroglobulinemia. Haematologica. 2021;106(11):2940–6. https://doi.org/10.3324/haematol.2020.262899.
119. Kamisawa T, Okamoto A. IgG4-related sclerosing disease. WJG. 2008;14(25):3948. https://doi.org/10.3748/wjg.14.3948.
120. Wallace ZS, Naden RP, Chari S, et al. The 2019 American College of Rheumatology/ European League Against Rheumatism Classification criteria for IgG4-related disease. Arthritis Rheumatol. 2020;72(1):7–19. https://doi.org/10.1002/art.41120.
121. Aalberse RC, Schuurman J. IgG4 breaking the rules. Immunology. 2002;105(1):9–19. https://doi.org/10.1046/j.0019-2805.2001.01341.x.
122. Zen Y, Fujii T, Harada K, et al. Th2 and regulatory immune reactions are increased in immunoglobin G4-related sclerosing pancreatitis and cholangitis. Hepatology. 2007;45(6): 1538–46. https://doi.org/10.1002/hep.21697.
123. Kawa S, Ota M, Yoshizawa K, et al. HLA DRB1*0405-DQB1*0401 haplotype is associated with autoimmune pancreatitis in the Japanese population. Gastroenterology. 2002;122(5):1264–9. https://doi.org/10.1053/gast.2002.33022.
124. Ota M, Katsuyama Y, Hamano H, et al. Two critical genes (HLA-DRB1 and ABCF1) in the HLA region are associated with the susceptibility to autoimmune pancreatitis. Immunogenetics. 2006;59(1):45–52. https://doi.org/10.1007/s00251-006-0178-2.

125. Della Torre E, Mattoo H, Mahajan VS, Carruthers M, Pillai S, Stone JH. Prevalence of atopy, eosinophilia, and IgE elevation in IgG4-related disease. Allergy. 2014;69(2):269–72. https://doi.org/10.1111/all.12320.
126. Khosroshahi A, Wallace ZS, Crowe JL, et al. International consensus guidance statement on the management and treatment of IgG4-related disease: international consensus statement on IgG4-RD management. Arthritis Rheumatol. 2015;67(7):1688–99. https://doi.org/10.1002/art.39132.
127. Okazaki K, Chari ST, Frulloni L, et al. International consensus for the treatment of autoimmune pancreatitis. Pancreatology. 2017;17(1):1–6. https://doi.org/10.1016/j.pan.2016.12.003.
128. Campochiaro C, Della-Torre E, Lanzillotta M, et al. Long-term efficacy of maintenance therapy with rituximab for IgG4-related disease. Eur J Intern Med. 2020;74:92–8. https://doi.org/10.1016/j.ejim.2019.12.029.
129. Ebbo M, Grados A, Samson M, et al. Long-term efficacy and safety of rituximab in IgG4-related disease: data from a French nationwide study of thirty-three patients. PLoS One. 2017;12(9):e0183844. https://doi.org/10.1371/journal.pone.0183844.
130. Fava A, Petri M. Systemic lupus erythematosus: diagnosis and clinical management. J Autoimmun. 2019;96:1–13. https://doi.org/10.1016/j.jaut.2018.11.001.
131. Singh BK, Singh S. Systemic lupus erythematosus and infections. Reumatismo. 2020;72(3):154–69. https://doi.org/10.4081/reumatismo.2020.1303.
132. Buhaescu I, Yood RA, Izzedine H. Serum procalcitonin in systemic autoimmune diseases—where are we now? Semin Arthritis Rheum. 2010;40(2):176–83. https://doi.org/10.1016/j.semarthrit.2009.10.004.
133. Danza A, Ruiz-Irastorza G. Infection risk in systemic lupus erythematosus patients: susceptibility factors and preventive strategies. Lupus. 2013;22(12):1286–94. https://doi.org/10.1177/0961203313493032.
134. Cervera R, Khamashta MA, Font J, et al. Morbidity and mortality in systemic lupus erythematosus during a 5-year period: a multicenter prospective study of 1,000 patients. Medicine. 1999;78(3):167–75. https://doi.org/10.1097/00005792-199905000-00003.
135. Kang K, Kwok SK, Ju J, et al. The causes of death in Korean patients with systemic lupus erythematosus over 11 years. Lupus. 2011;20(9):989–97. https://doi.org/10.1177/0961203311402245.
136. Jacobsen S, Petersen J, Ullman S, Junker P. Mortality and causes of death of 513 Danish patients with systemic lupus erythematosus. Scand J Rheumatol. 1999;28(2):75–80.
137. Fei Y, Shi X, Gan F, et al. Death causes and pathogens analysis of systemic lupus erythematosus during the past 26 years. Clin Rheumatol. 2014;33(1):57–63. https://doi.org/10.1007/s10067-013-2383-3.
138. Tsai PH, Jang SS, Liou LB. Septicaemia is associated with increased disease activity and mortality in systemic lupus erythematosus: a retrospective analysis from Taiwan. Lupus. 2020;29(2):191–8. https://doi.org/10.1177/0961203319899162.
139. Bharath G, Kumar P, Makkar N, et al. Mortality in systemic lupus erythematosus at a teaching hospital in India: a 5-year retrospective study. J Fam Med Prim Care. 2019;8(7):2511. https://doi.org/10.4103/jfmpc.jfmpc_362_19.
140. Oud L. Epidemiology and outcomes of sepsis among hospitalizations with systemic lupus erythematosus admitted to the ICU: a population-based cohort study. J Intensive Care. 2020;8(1):3. https://doi.org/10.1186/s40560-019-0424-y.
141. Ruiz-Irastorza G, Olivares N, Ruiz-Arruza I, Martinez-Berriotxoa A, Egurbide MV, Aguirre C. Predictors of major infections in systemic lupus erythematosus. Arthritis Res Ther. 2009;11(4):R109. https://doi.org/10.1186/ar2764.
142. Ross SC, Densen P. Complement deficiency states and infection: epidemiology, pathogenesis and consequences of neisserial and other infections in an immune deficiency. Medicine (Baltimore). 1984;63(5):243–73.
143. Santos RP, dos Reis-Neto ET, Pinheiro MM. Incidence of cytomegalovirus antigenemia in patients with autoimmune rheumatic diseases: a 3-year retrospective study. Adv Rheumatol. 2019;59(1):18. https://doi.org/10.1186/s42358-019-0061-0.

144. Ognibene FP, Shelhamer JH, Hoffman GS, et al. Pneumocystis carinii pneumonia: a major complication of immunosuppressive therapy in patients with Wegener's granulomatosis. Am J Respir Crit Care Med. 1995;151(3 Pt 1):795–9. https://doi.org/10.1164/ajrccm/151.3_Pt_1.795.
145. Suryaprasad A, Stone JH. When is it safe to stop *Pneumocystis jiroveci* pneumonia prophylaxis? Insights from three cases complicating autoimmune diseases. Arthritis Rheum. 2008;59(7):1034–9. https://doi.org/10.1002/art.23822.
146. Ke PC, Zhou R, Serpell LC, et al. Half a century of amyloids: past, present and future. Chem Soc Rev. 2020;49(15):5473–509. https://doi.org/10.1039/C9CS00199A.
147. Benson MD, Buxbaum JN, Eisenberg DS, et al. Amyloid nomenclature 2020: update and recommendations by the International Society of Amyloidosis (ISA) nomenclature committee. Amyloid. 2020;27(4):217–22. https://doi.org/10.1080/13506129.2020.1835263.
148. Papa R, Lachmann HJ. Secondary, AA, amyloidosis. Rheum Dis Clin North Am. 2018;44(4):585–603. https://doi.org/10.1016/j.rdc.2018.06.004.
149. Taimur S, Nader C, Lloyd-Travaglini C, Seldin DC, Sanchorawala V. Microbiologically documented infections in patients undergoing high-dose melphalan and autologous stem cell transplantation for the treatment of light chain amyloidosis. Transpl Infect Dis. 2013;15(2):187–94.
150. Kyle RA, Gertz MA, Greipp PR, et al. A trial of three regimens for primary amyloidosis: colchicine alone, melphalan and prednisone, and melphalan, prednisone, and colchicine. N Engl J Med. 1997;336(17):1202–7. https://doi.org/10.1056/NEJM199704243361702.
151. Kastritis E, Palladini G, Minnema MC, et al. Daratumumab-based treatment for immunoglobulin light-chain amyloidosis. N Engl J Med. 2021;385(1):46–58. https://doi.org/10.1056/NEJMoa2028631.
152. Palladini G, Kastritis E, Maurer MS, et al. Daratumumab plus CyBorD for patients with newly diagnosed AL amyloidosis: safety run-in results of ANDROMEDA. Blood. 2020;136(1):71–80. https://doi.org/10.1182/blood.2019004460.
153. Van de Wyngaert Z, Carpentier B, Pascal L, et al. Daratumumab is effective in the relapsed or refractory systemic light-chain amyloidosis but associated with high infection burden in a frail real-life population. Br J Haematol. 2020;188(3):e24–7. https://doi.org/10.1111/bjh.16282.

Chapter 19
Paraproteinemia in Autoinflammatory Diseases

Antonio Vitale and Luca Cantarini

Abbreviations

AA	Amyloid A
AD	Autosomal dominant
AR	Autosomal recessive
CT	Computed tomography
ASCT	Autologous stem cells transplantation
IgM	Immunoglobulins M
IgG	Immunoglobulins G
IL-1	Interleukin-1
JAK	Janus Kinase
MVK	Mevalonate kinase gene
MyD88	Myeloid differentiation primary response 88
MRI	Magnetic resonance imaging
NF-kB	Nuclear factor kappa-light-chain-enhancer of activated B cells
NLRP3	NOD-like receptor-related protein 3
PET	Positron emission tomography
MKD	Mevalonate kinase deficiency
PFAPA	Periodic fever, aphthous stomatitis, pharyngitis and cervical adenitis
POEMS	Polyneuropathy, Organomegaly, Endocrinopathy, Monoclonal gammopathy, and Skin changes

A. Vitale · L. Cantarini (✉)
Research Center of Systemic Autoinflammatory Diseases, Behçet's Disease and Rheumatology-Ophthalmology Collaborative Uveitis Center, Department of Medical Sciences Surgery and Neurosciences, University of Siena, Siena, Italy

© The Author(s), under exclusive license to Springer Nature Switzerland AG 2022

G. Ragab et al. (eds.), *Paraproteinemia and Related Disorders*,
https://doi.org/10.1007/978-3-031-10131-1_19

TNFRSF1A	Tumor Necrosis Factor Receptor Superfamily Member 1A
TRAPS	Tumor necrosis factor receptor-associated periodic fever syndrome
UBA1	Ubiquitin-like modifier activating enzyme 1 gene
VEGF	Vascular endothelial growth factor
VEXAS	Vacuoles, E1 enzyme, X-linked, Autoinflammatory, Somatic

Introduction

Autoinflammatory diseases represent a group of clinical entities characterized by recurrent inflammatory attacks in the absence of infections, neoplasms, or deregulation of the adaptive immune system [1]. The autoinflammatory diseases were originally recognized as monogenic diseases caused by mutations in specific genes involved in the regulation of innate immunity. In this sense, the monogenic autoinflammatory diseases originally recognized were: familial Mediterranean fever, an autosomal recessive (AR) condition caused by mutations in the *MEFV* gene that encodes for pyrin, a protein associated with the inflammasome, an intracellular multiprotein complex involved in the maturation of interleukin (IL)-1β and IL-18; tumor necrosis factor (TNF) receptor-associated periodic fever syndrome (TRAPS), an autosomal dominant (AD) disorder related to mutations involving type 1 TNF receptor (*TNFRSF1A*); cryopyrin-associated periodic syndrome (CAPS), a group of AD disorders associated with mutations in the *NLRP3* gene that encodes for cryopyrin, a component of the NOD-like receptor-related protein 3 (NLRP3) inflammasome; mevalonate kinase deficiency (MKD), the second AR disease caused by *MVK* mutations and loss of function of the mevalonate kinase enzyme, the first in the cholesterol biosynthesis enzymatic pathway. Subsequently, on the basis of common clinical and pathogenetic features shared with monogenic autoinflammatory diseases, but also by virtue of a common excellent response to interleukin-1 (IL-1) inhibitors, several multifactorial diseases were classified as multifactorial autoinflammatory diseases even though not determined by specific gene mutations [2, 3].

Among the multifactorial autoinflammatory diseases, a leading role is played by Behçet's syndrome, adult-onset Still's disease, and systemic onset juvenile idiopathic arthritis, which correspond respectively to the adult and pediatric versions of the same immune affection, periodic fever, aphthous stomatitis, pharyngitis and cervical adenitis (PFAPA) syndrome, Schnitzler's syndrome, the gouty arthritis, and other types of microcrystal arthritis [1, 4].

Thanks to continuous research efforts, the list of monogenic and multifactorial autoinflammatory diseases is quickly widening year by year. In this regard, a specific chapter referring to autoinflammatory disorders associated with paraproteinemia is also emerging, thus arousing considerable clinical and scientific interest. Actually, suspecting or identifying a paraproteinemia in patients presenting with inflammatory symptoms is quite frequent since the routine tests for a patient presenting with fever and inflammatory features have to necessarily include plasma protein electrophoresis. Indeed, this simple laboratory exam is useful to identify an increase in gamma globulins, which would impose a differential diagnosis with infectious diseases or autoimmune diseases. Conversely, a reduction in gamma globulins would suggest a congenital or acquired immunodeficiency with consequent opportunistic infections. On the other hand, the identification of a monoclonal peak opens up different scenarios and makes it necessary to evaluate the patient in a hematological context in order to understand the significance of the finding and the possibility of multiple myeloma.

In this chapter, we will not focus on the correct diagnostic investigations and staging of patients with suspected myeloma or other hematological neoplasms, but instead address the issue of autoinflammatory diseases associated with paraproteinemia, which should be suspected in case the clinical picture acquires particular inflammatory features.

Paraproteinemia and Autoinflammatory Diseases

In the context of autoinflammatory diseases, the role of paraproteinemia is primarily expressed in Schnitzler's syndrome, which is a striking example of an acquired multifactorial autoinflammatory disease, as mentioned above. However, more recently other systemic inflammatory conditions have been included in the field of autoinflammatory conditions associated with paraproteinemia and other bone marrow disorders. In particular, VEXAS syndrome, POEMS syndrome, monoclonal gammopathy, arthralgias, and recurrent fever syndrome, and Mullins' syndrome deserve to be precisely explored.

Schnitzler's Syndrome

Firstly described in 1972, Schnitzler's syndrome is clinically characterized by fever, urticarial rash, bone and/or joint pain sustained by osteosclerosis or bone remodeling, enlarged lymph nodes, and hepatomegaly/splenomegaly. During laboratory assessment, in addition to the highly increased inflammatory markers, it is associated with a monoclonal gammopathy, which is typically of IgM type, but the IgG type is not a rare exception (to date reported in less than 10% of cases). Schnitzler's syndrome main complication is the development of a lymphoproliferative disorder, especially Waldenström's macroglobulinemia, that occurs in about 15–20% of cases after 10 to 20 years of evolution; AA amyloidosis is another rare complication in untreated patients [5]. Figure 19.1 illustrates the typical urticarial rash in a female patient with Schnitzler's syndrome.

The pathophysiology has not yet been clearly elucidated. In particular, it is not yet known if monoclonal gammopathy is the cause of clinical manifestations or represents a feature of the disease like any other. Noteworthy, delayed development of an IgM paraprotein has been described to occur approximately 4 years after the

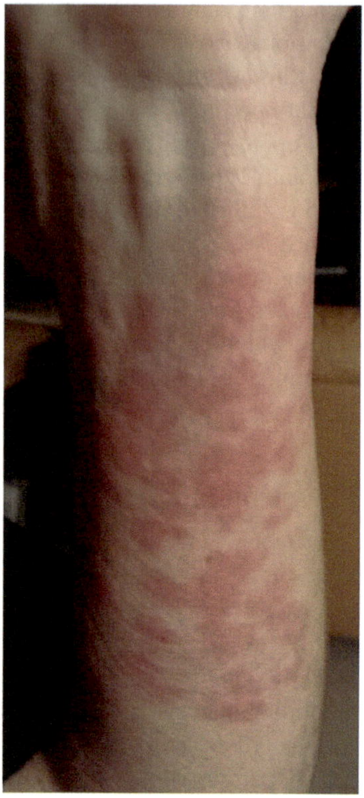

Fig. 19.1 Typical urticarial rash observed in the volar region of the left forearm in a 61-year-old female patient diagnosed with Schnitzler's syndrome

onset of symptoms in one patient [6]. Also, the association between Waldenström's macroglobulinemia and mutations in MyD88 [7], which is an adaptor in IL-1 signaling by interacting with IL-1 receptor complex and IL-1 receptor-associated kinase, could suggest that clonal IgM production may be stimulated by an increased IL-1 stimulation. Schnitzler's syndrome might be also the result of the increased NF-κβ activation, as observed in patients with monoclonal gammopathy of uncertain significance or Waldenström's macroglobulinemia. As, both MyD88 and NF-κβ have a role in controlling the NLRP3 inflammasome, that is the major source of IL-1 cellular production, the presence of a certain single nucleotide polymorphism or mosaic mutation in *NLRP3* gene has been hypothesized to induce the disease when the paraproteinemia affects MyD88 and/or NF-κβ functions [8]. In any case, it has to be noted that the level of the monoclonal component at diagnosis is highly variable, as it can only be present at a very low level or else be very high.

Patients with Schnitzler's syndrome responsive to IL-1 blocking agents, but with no evidence of monoclonal gammopathy could definitely suggest the lack of a pathogenic role for paraproteinemia in such syndrome [9, 10]. Nevertheless, great caution should be applied when diagnosing Schnitzler's syndrome without monoclonal component. Indeed, skin and musculoskeletal manifestations may closely resemble other clinical conditions possibly arising during adulthood and responsive to IL-1 inhibition, especially acquired CAPS and Still's disease. Therefore, a thorough differential diagnosis including the definite exclusion of mosaic *NLRP3* gene mutations should have been performed for diagnostic confirmation in such cases. In addition, other as yet unknown autoinflammatory conditions cannot be ruled out with sufficient certainty [11].

If the role of paraproteinemia is still a mystery, the autoinflammatory nature of Schnitzler's syndrome is now well established not only on the basis of the striking clinical similarity with monogenic autoinflammatory diseases, in particular CAPS, but also in view of the results obtained from basic research and the extraordinary response to anti-IL-1 biologic agents. Indeed, increased IL-1β secretion by lipopolysaccharide-stimulated peripheral blood mononuclear cells has been observed and is perhaps due to dermal mast cells secretion. Also IL-6 serum levels are increased and seem to be correlated with disease activity [12–14]. The adaptive immunity itself is involved, as a consequence of IL-1 overproduction: in particular a profound loss of anti-inflammatory Th17 cell functionalities has been observed, with suppression of IL-10 [15, 16].

Diagnosis of Schnitzler's syndrome requires the exclusion of many other mimicking clinical entities, especially adult-onset Still's disease, CAPS (including acquired forms associated with genetic mosaicism), cryoglobulinemia, urticarial vasculitis, autoimmune diseases with urticarial rash, infectious diseases, mastocytosis, lymphoma, and Waldenström's disease. After having ruled out these conditions, specific sets of diagnostic criteria may be applied. The first set of criteria was proposed in 2001 by Lipsker et al. and are depicted in Table 19.1. These criteria require the presence of urticarial rash and monoclonal IgM component in addition to two other clinical or laboratory features [17]. In 2013, the Strasbourg criteria were proposed by Simon et al. [18]. This set of criteria, reported in Table 19.2, introduced the distinction between IgM and IgG gammopathy and included the possibility of a "probable" diagnosis in addition to the "definite" diagnosis. Also the Strasbourg

Table 19.1 Diagnostic criteria for Schnitzler's syndrome proposed by Lipsker et al. [17]

Mandatory items	Urticarial rash
	Monoclonal IgM component
Additional items	Fever
	Arthralgia or arthritis
	Bone pain
	Palpable lymph nodes
	Liver or spleen enlargement
	Increased erythrocyte sedimentation rate
	Leukocytosis
	Abnormal findings on bone morphologic investigations

In this case, the diagnosis may be performed in case the patient fulfils both mandatory items and at least two of the additional items

Table 19.2 Strasbourg diagnostic criteria for the diagnosis of Schnitzler's syndrome [18]

Obligate criteria
Chronic urticarial skin rash
IgM or IgG monoclonal gammopathy
Minor criteria
Unexplained recurrent fever (body temperature >38 °C)
Abnormal bone remodeling assessed by bone scintigraphy, MRI, or bone alkaline phosphatase
Neutrophilic dermal infiltrate at skin biopsy with no fibrinoid necrosis or significant dermal edema
Leukocytosis (neutrophils >10.000/mm^3) and/or elevated C-reactive protein (>30 mg/L)

In this case, a "definite" diagnosis is justified by the fulfillment of the two obligate criteria and at least two minor criteria in patients with IgM monoclonal gammopathy or three minor criteria in patients with IgG monoclonal gammopathy. Diagnosis is "probable" when the two obligate criteria are fulfilled in addition to at least one minor criteria in patients with IgM monoclonal gammopathy or two minor criteria in patients with IgG monoclonal gammopathy
IgM immunoglobulins M, *IgG* immunoglobulins G, *MRI* magnetic resonance imaging

criteria include obligate items (chronic urticarial rash and IgM or IgG monoclonal gammopathy) and additional items. Particularly, in patients with IgM monoclonal gammopathy a definite diagnosis of Schnitzler's syndrome is justified by the fulfillment of the two obligate items and at least two minor criteria; diagnosis is probable when the two obligate criteria are fulfilled in addition to at least one minor criteria. In patients with IgG monoclonal gammopathy, a definite diagnosis of Schnitzler's syndrome is justified by the fulfillment of the two obligate items and at least three minor criteria; diagnosis is probable when the two obligate criteria are fulfilled in addition to at least two minor criteria.

Skin biopsy is often useful for diagnosis, as it accounts for a minor item in the diagnostic criteria. Histology is characterized by a neutrophilic urticarial dermatosis with perivascular and interstitial infiltrate of neutrophils and leukocytoclasia [19]. Vasculitis may be observed, but with no fibrinoid necrosis and no dermal edema [20].

With regard to treatment, non-steroidal anti-inflammatory drugs, antihistamines, and colchicine are useful in less severe cases. Also systemic corticosteroids are useful in controlling clinical and laboratory manifestations, but they cannot be used at high dosage for a long time because of the well-known side effects; in addition, corticosteroids seem to not avoid complications [21]. Conversely, the inhibition of IL-1 with anakinra, canakinumab, and rilonacept has proved to induce a quick and sustained control of all clinical and laboratory manifestations. The IL-1 receptor antagonist anakinra is the most currently used biologic agent to treat Schnitzler's syndrome and permit the disease control within a few hours from the first injection; the posology is generally 100 mg/day. Also the anti-IL-1β monoclonal agent canakinumab has proved to be highly effective in inducing disease remission. In this case, the posology required to control Schnitzler's disease may vary from 150 mg every 8 weeks to 300 mg every 4 weeks. The anti-IL-1 fusion protein rilonacept is also effective at the dosage of 320 mg followed by 160 mg/week. However, this agent is not available on the European market [22–24].

Anti-IL-1 agents do not seem to have a role on the monoclonal component and probably do not prevent lymphoproliferation [23, 25]; however, current data are quite poor on this matter.

As a whole, complete remission with IL-1 blocking therapies is obtained in about 83% of patients [23]. The remaining patients achieve partial remission, mainly with persistence of joint pain. This subgroup of patients could benefit from IL-6 inhibition. However, a recent open-label study involving 8 patients showed the efficacy of the anti-IL-6 agent tocilizumab in controlling clinical and laboratory disease manifestations, but also a high frequency of loss of efficacy in the short-time. The authors themselves suggested to primarily consider tocilizumab after the failure of other cytokine-targeted therapies [26].

VEXAS Syndrome

At the end of 2020, myeloid-restricted somatic X-linked inactivating mutations of *UBA1* gene have been identified to lead to an acquired autoinflammatory condition clinically characterized by late-onset, treatment-refractory inflammatory manifestations with associated hematologic abnormalities. The disease onset occurs in the fifth to seventh decade of life; clinical features of the disease include recurrent fever, alveolitis, skin lesions (neutrophilic dermatosis and cutaneous vasculitis), auricular and nasal chondritis, myalgia, arthralgia, erythema nodosum, and thromboembolic disease. In any case, the clinical picture may vary from a relatively easy-to-treat condition to a life-threatening macrophage activation syndrome [27, 28].

Hematologic abnormalities progressively involve all patients and correspond to macrocytic anemia, thrombocytopenia, and myeloid dyspoiesis; to date, overt hematologic malignant condition has not been reported. Of note, many patients fulfill diagnostic criteria for other systemic inflammatory diseases, such as relapsing polychondritis, polyarteritis nodosa, giant-cell arteritis, and Sweet's syndrome. Other patients fulfill criteria for myelodysplastic syndrome and multiple myeloma or monoclonal gammopathy of undetermined significance. Actually, myeloid-restricted somatic mutations in *UBA1* may underlie myelodysplastic disease accompanied by systemic inflammation capable of resembling many other systemic disorders [27].

UBA1 is a gene encoding the ubiquitin-activating enzyme 1 (E1 enzyme), which is necessary for the initiation of ubiquitylation, a post-translational modification of proteins involved in the regulation of various aspects of cellular biology, such as intracellular signaling and protein degradation by proteasome or autophagy–lysosome system.

Data currently available seem to suggest that this disorder involves males exclusively and that the additional allele in females protects against the effects of the mutant allele; however, it is necessary to understand whether the effect of the skewed X-inactivation could induce a milder disease in women.

From a laboratory point of view, patients present with highly increased levels of acute-phase reactants. Bone marrow analysis allows us to observe hypercellularity, ring sideroblasts, and vacuolization restricted to myeloid and erythroid precursors; electron microscopy highlights myeloid cells undergoing cell death and showing vacuoles of lipid droplets along with disordered cellular organelles, including degenerating mitochondria.

On the basis of all the prominent features this disorder has been named VEXAS (vacuoles, E1 enzyme, X-linked, autoinflammatory, somatic) syndrome.

Disease-modifying anti-rheumatic drugs are often ineffective, while high-dose glucocorticoids are effective in improving inflammatory symptoms. However, cyclosporine was proven to induce some benefit. Also anti-IL-6 agents and JAK inhibitors (ruxolitinib or tofacitinib) seem to have a good therapeutic role. On the contrary, the use of anakinra is associated with more pronounced than expected severe skin reactions [28, 29]. Further research is needed to explore bone marrow transplantation or gene-editing therapies as potential treatment modalities.

POEMS Syndrome

Polyneuropathy, organomegaly, endocrinopathy, monoclonal gammopathy, and skin changes (POEMS) syndrome is a rare multisystem autoinflammatory disease. In addition to the features corresponding to the acronym, papilledema, extravascular volume overload, sclerotic bone lesions, and thrombocytosis are often observed. Endocrinopathy includes more often hypogonadism and hypopituitarism manifesting with erectile dysfunction and gynecomastia in men, and early menopausal symptoms in women. Diabetes mellitus, parathyroid, and thyroid involvements are also frequent. Regarding skin lesions, patients present dome shaped red-brown papular (sometimes pedunculated) nodules on the trunk or proximal extremities. POEMS syndrome is caused by an underlying plasma cell proliferative disorder that can induce a severe cytokine-driven inflammatory response, in particular vascular endothelial growth factor (VEGF) [30]. VEGF induces capillary leakage and, in turn, papilledema, poor gas transfer in the lungs, ascites, and pericardial effusions in most severe cases.

Diagnosis is based on the fulfillment of clinical criteria proposed by Dispenzieri et al. and reported in Table 19.3 [31]. In particular, the diagnosis is made with the two mandatory criteria, at least one out of the three other major criteria, and at least one of the minor criteria are fulfilled. Diabetes mellitus and thyroid abnormalities should not be used as diagnostic items if accounting for the only endocrine manifestation because of their high prevalence in the general population.

Despite diagnostic criteria, the heterogeneity of clinical presentations and the frequent identification of patients with only a limited number of the classical features contribute to diagnostic delay. In addition, bone marrow biopsy may be minimally or not at all compromised by monoclonal plasma cells. In this context, VEGF represents a useful biomarker for disease detection and monitoring; other examinations include serum protein electrophoresis, immunofixation, and serum free light chain analysis to detect a subtle plasma cell disorder. Bone marrow aspirate or

Table 19.3 Diagnostic criteria for polyneuropathy, organomegaly, endocrinopathy, monoclonal gammopathy, and skin changes (POEMS) syndrome [31]

Mandatory major criteria	Polyneuropathy
	Monoclonal plasma cell proliferative disorder
Other major criteria	Castleman disease
	Sclerotic bone lesions
	Raised vascular endothelial growth factor
Minor criteria	Organomegaly (spleen/liver/lymph nodes)
	Extravascular volume overload
	Endocrinopathy (adrenal, thyroid, pituitary, gonadal, parathyroid, pancreatic)
	Skin changes
	Papilledema
	Thrombocytosis/polycythemia
Other useful features	Clubbing, weight loss, hyperhidrosis, pulmonary hypertension/restrictive lung disease, thrombotic diathesis, diarrhea, low vitamin B12

Diagnosis is possible when the patient meets both the two mandatory criteria *plus* at last one out of the three other major criteria *plus* at least one of the minor criteria. Note that diabetes mellitus and thyroid abnormalities should not be used as diagnostic criteria if not associated with other endocrine disorders, as their high prevalence makes them too little specific

biopsy specimen histopathology are also necessary for a valuable diagnosis and staging. Similarly, skeletal X-ray and computed tomography (CT) of the chest, abdomen, and pelvis can be useful to identify mixed sclerotic and lytic bone lesions. Alternatively, whole body magnetic resonance imaging is often employed as a screening tool; positron emission tomography (PET)/CT is the most useful imaging modality to identify the plasmacytoma or lymph nodes for biopsy [32] (Chap. 21).

Treatment is directed at the underlying clonal plasma cell disorder and is tailored on the extension and distribution of bone marrow involvement. Radiotherapy is useful for localized disease (one or two plasmacytoma), while autologous stem cells transplantation (ASCT) combined chemotherapy is the gold standard for patients with three or more plasmacytomas at imaging or positive bone marrow histology. Chemotherapy includes the use of alkylating agents (such as melphalan or cyclophosphamide) and dexamethasone [33, 34]. Thalidomide and lenalidomide are also emerging as treatments for POEMS syndrome [35].

Monoclonal Gammopathy, Arthralgias, and Recurrent Fever Syndrome

A work dated 2019 has pointed out the possibility of a new autoinflammatory disease characterized by fever lasting 3–12 days, arthralgia involving the peripheral joints or the spine, myalgia, and occasionally pleuritis, after having ruled out Schnitzler's syndrome, infectious and neoplastic diseases. Patients show a monoclonal gammopathy of IgG or IgM without specificity for the light chain, and increased C-reactive protein during febrile episodes. Unlike what is described for Schnitzler's syndrome, urticarial rash, osteosclerosis, or bone remodeling are lacking. Noteworthy, IL-1 inhibition seems to represent a useful treatment approach [36].

Also in this case, the significance of the monoclonal gammopathy is unclear and the authors bring up the hypotheses already considered for Schnitzler's syndrome. Fascinating as it is, this proposed new clinical condition needs to be confirmed on a broader basis, and it is necessary to understand whether patients with monoclonal gammopathy and recurrent febrile episodes share a common pathogenic link or they suffer from disparate still unclassified clinical conditions.

Mullins' Syndrome

Mullins' syndrome has been described in 2015 as an acquired autoinflammatory condition associated with IgG paraproteinemia. It is clinically similar to Schnitzler's syndrome and patients may fulfill Strasbourg clinical criteria [36]. Nevertheless, some differences have been highlighted between Mullins' syndrome and Schnitzler's syndrome. In particular, the former is characterized by: (1) complement depletion following initial symptoms, while complement is normal or increased in Schnitzler's syndrome; (2) transient leukopenia and thrombocytopenia, instead of leukocytosis; (3) lack of response to anakinra. In any case, the description of this syndrome is currently limited to a case report [37] and, on the basis of the clinical features, it would be interesting to find out whether the patient was suffering from VEXAS syndrome, which was not yet identified at the time of the case presentation.

Conclusions

While Schnitzler's syndrome, described in 1972, has been relatively better understood over the last two or three decades, the chapter of paraproteinemia in relation to the autoinflammatory diseases is starting to emerge. In fact, however intriguing, little is known about these clinical conditions and how bone marrow cells may contribute to the activation of the pathogenic process associated with innate immunity affections. In this regard, the very recent identification of the VEXAS syndrome has undoubtedly opened up a new scientific chapter that will definitely achieve a quick development in the next few years. This will probably give rise to considerable new diagnostic possibilities for many adult patients currently classified as suffering from undifferentiated autoinflammatory diseases. Actually, the need to research the cause of many unexplained inflammatory conditions in bone marrow cells—many of which are a central part of innate immunity—is demonstrated by the various attempts made in recent times to identify specific clinical entities based on the selection of evocative symptoms clustering. Scientific research in this field is only just beginning, but we believe that this could be the decade in which this chapter will grow substantially.

References

1. Masters SL, Simon A, Aksentijevich I, Kastner DL. Horror autoinflammaticus: the molecular pathophysiology of autoinflammatory disease. Annu Rev Immunol. 2009;27:621–68.
2. McGonagle D, McDermott MF. A proposed classification of the immunological diseases. PLoS Med. 2006;3(8):e297.
3. Vitale A, Insalaco A, Sfriso P, Lopalco G, Emmi G, Cattalini M, et al. A snapshot on the on-label and off-label use of the interleukin-1 inhibitors in Italy among rheumatologists and pediatric rheumatologists: a nationwide multi-center retrospective observational study. Front Pharmacol. 2016;7:380.
4. Rigante D, Lopalco G, Vitale A, Lucherini OM, Caso F, De Clemente C, et al. Untangling the web of systemic autoinflammatory diseases. Mediat Inflamm. 2014;2014:948154.
5. Gusdorf L, Lipsker D. Schnitzler syndrome: a review. Curr Rheumatol Rep. 2017;19(8):46.
6. Mulla E, Neame R. Delayed development of the IgM paraprotein in Schnitzler's syndrome. Scand J Rheumatol. 2015;44(6):521–2.
7. Treon SP, Xu L, Yang G, Zhou Y, Liu X, Cao Y, et al. MYD88 L265P somatic mutation in Waldenström's macroglobulinemia. N Engl J Med. 2012;367(9):826–33.
8. van Leersum FS, Potjewijd J, van Geel M, Steijlen PM, Vreeburg M. Schnitzler's syndrome—a novel hypothesis of a shared pathophysiologic mechanism with Waldenström's disease. Orphanet J Rare Dis. 2019;14(1):151.
9. Bixio R, Rossini M, Giollo A. Efficacy of interleukin-1 blockade in Schnitzler's syndrome without detectable monoclonal gammopathy: a case-based review. Clin Rheumatol. 2021;40(7):2973–7.
10. Fujita Y, Asano T, Sakai A, Norikawa N, Yamamoto T, Matsumoto H, et al. A case of Schnitzler's syndrome without monoclonal gammopathy successfully treated with canakinumab. BMC Musculoskelet Disord. 2021;22(1):257.
11. Wang C. Can therapeutic response to IL-1 blockade confirm the diagnosis of Schnitzler syndrome? Clin Rheumatol. 2021;40(2):805.
12. Ryan JG, de Koning HD, Beck LA, Booty MG, Kastner DL, Simon A. IL-1 blockade in Schnitzler syndrome: ex vivo findings correlate with clinical remission. J Allergy Clin Immunol. 2008;121(1):260–2.
13. de Koning HD, Schalkwijk J, Stoffels M, Jongekrijg J, Jacobs JFM, Verwiel E, et al. The role of interleukin-1 beta in the pathophysiology of Schnitzler's syndrome. Arthritis Res Ther. 2015;17:187.
14. de Koning HD, van Vlijmen-Willems IMJJ, Rodijk-Olthuis D, van der Meer JWM, Zeeuwen PLJM, Simon A, et al. Mast-cell interleukin-1β, neutrophil interleukin-17 and epidermal antimicrobial proteins in the neutrophilic urticarial dermatosis in Schnitzler's syndrome. Br J Dermatol. 2015;173(2):448–56.
15. Zielinski CE, Mele F, Aschenbrenner D, Jarrossay D, Ronchi F, Gattorno M, et al. Pathogen-induced human TH17 cells produce IFN-γ or IL-10 and are regulated by IL-1β. Nature. 2012;484(7395):514–8.
16. Noster R, de Koning HD, Maier E, Prelog M, Lainka E, Zielinski CE. Dysregulation of proinflammatory versus anti-inflammatory human TH17 cell functionalities in the autoinflammatory Schnitzler syndrome. J Allergy Clin Immunol. 2016;138(4):1161–1169.e6.
17. Lipsker D, Veran Y, Grunenberger F, Cribier B, Heid E, Grosshans E. The Schnitzler syndrome. Four new cases and review of the literature. Medicine (Baltimore). 2001;80(1):37–44.
18. Simon A, Asli B, Braun-Falco M, De Koning H, Fermand J-P, Grattan C, et al. Schnitzler's syndrome: diagnosis, treatment, and follow-up. Allergy. 2013;68(5):562–8.
19. Kieffer C, Cribier B, Lipsker D. Neutrophilic urticarial dermatosis: a variant of neutrophilic urticaria strongly associated with systemic disease. Report of 9 new cases and review of the literature. Medicine (Baltimore). 2009;88(1):23–31.
20. Lipsker D. The Schnitzler syndrome. Orphanet J Rare Dis. 2010;5:38.

21. Lipsker D, Lenormand C. Management of Schnitzler's syndrome. Expert Opin Orphan Drugs. 2014;2(9):947–55.
22. Betrains A, Staels F, Vanderschueren S. Efficacy and safety of canakinumab treatment in Schnitzler syndrome: a systematic literature review. Semin Arthritis Rheum. 2020;50(4):636–42.
23. Néel A, Henry B, Barbarot S, Masseau A, Perrin F, Bernier C, et al. Long-term effectiveness and safety of interleukin-1 receptor antagonist (anakinra) in Schnitzler's syndrome: a French multicenter study. Autoimmun Rev. 2014;13(10):1035–41.
24. Krause K, Weller K, Stefaniak R, Wittkowski H, Altrichter S, Siebenhaar F, et al. Efficacy and safety of the interleukin-1 antagonist rilonacept in Schnitzler syndrome: an open-label study. Allergy. 2012;67(7):943–50.
25. Gameiro A, Gouveia M, Pereira M, Tellechea O, Gonçalo M. Clinical characterization and long-term follow-up of Schnitzler syndrome. Clin Exp Dermatol. 2016;41(5):461–7.
26. Bonnekoh H, Frischbutter S, Roll S, Maurer M, Krause K. Tocilizumab treatment in patients with Schnitzler syndrome: an open-label study. J Allergy Clin Immunol Pract. 2021;9(6):2486–2489.e4.
27. Beck DB, Ferrada MA, Sikora KA, Ombrello AK, Collins JC, Pei W, et al. Somatic mutations in UBA1 and severe adult-onset autoinflammatory disease. N Engl J Med. 2020;383(27):2628–38.
28. Staels F, Betrains A, Woei-A-Jin S, Boeckx N, Beckers M, Bervoets A, et al. Case report: VEXAS syndrome: from mild symptoms to life-threatening macrophage activation syndrome. Front Immunol. 2021;12:678927.
29. Bourbon E, Heiblig M, Gerfaud Valentin M, Barba T, Durel C-A, Lega JC, et al. Therapeutic options in VEXAS syndrome: insights from a retrospective series. Blood. 2021;137(26):3682–4.
30. Miralles GD, O'Fallon JR, Talley NJ. Plasma-cell dyscrasia with polyneuropathy. N Engl J Med. 1992;327(27):1919–23.
31. Dispenzieri A, Kyle RA, Lacy MQ, Rajkumar SV, Therneau TM, Larson DR, et al. POEMS syndrome: definitions and long-term outcome. Blood. 2003;101(7):2496–506.
32. Keddie S, D'Sa S, Foldes D, Carr AS, Reilly MM, Lunn MPT. POEMS neuropathy: optimising diagnosis and management. Pract Neurol. 2018;18(4):278–90.
33. Dispenzieri A. POEMS syndrome: 2017 update on diagnosis, risk stratification, and management. Am J Hematol. 2017;92(8):814–29.
34. Kuwabara S, Dispenzieri A, Arimura K, Misawa S, Nakaseko C. Treatment for POEMS (polyneuropathy, organomegaly, endocrinopathy, M-protein, and skin changes) syndrome. Cochrane Database Syst Rev. 2012;(6):CD006828.
35. Zagouri F, Kastritis E, Gavriatopoulou M, Sergentanis TN, Psaltopoulou T, Terpos E, et al. Lenalidomide in patients with POEMS syndrome: a systematic review and pooled analysis. Leuk Lymphoma. 2014;55(9):2018–23.
36. Terré A, Talbot A, Louvrier C, Picque JB, Mahévas M, Boutboul D, et al. Monoclonal gammopathy, arthralgias, and recurrent fever syndrome: a new autoinflammatory syndrome? J Rheumatol. 2019;46(11):1535–9.
37. Longhurst HJ, Yong PFK, Manson AL, Cavenagh JD, Grigoriadou S, Buckland MS. Mullins' syndrome: a new gammopathy-related autoinflammatory syndrome resistant to anakinra. QJM. 2015;108(6):497–501.

Chapter 20
Paraproteins Associated with Malignancy

Pietro Enrico Pioltelli

Abbreviations

CIDP Chronic inflammatory demyelinating polyneuropathy with M component
MC Mixed cryoglobulinaemia
MGUS Monoclonal gammopathy of undetermined significance

Introduction

The interaction between the neoplastic tissue and the host immune system has been extensively explored both on the side of the inhibitory/tolerogenic effects and that of defensive reaction [1–7].

A family of specific highly immunogenic antigens have been detected to be shared among many disorders [8–13], and many authors have reported the presence of an adaptive antibody-mediated response to neoplastic antigens in a wide range of epithelial neoplasms [14], mainly in the antigen-rich tumours such as melanoma [15] but also in cases with weak immunogenic neoplasms such as gastric [16] pulmonary [17–20], mammary [21], pancreatic [22], colonic [23–25], oesophageal [26], ovarian [27] or prostatic cancers [28], and glioma [29]. Similar findings have been detected directed against neoplastic molecules linked to tumour biology [20]. Moreover, the presence of antibodies recognizing functional molecules as p53 [12, 30], c-MYC [31], interferon [32], or overexpressed or mutated in the neoplastic tissue has been reported in a considerable number of papers and reviewed in meta-analysis. Those findings more often have been proposed to serve as tools for early

P. E. Pioltelli (✉)
Haematology Unit, Milano-Bicocca University, San Gerardo Hospital, Monza, Italy

© The Author(s), under exclusive license to Springer Nature Switzerland AG 2022
G. Ragab et al. (eds.), *Paraproteinemia and Related Disorders*,
https://doi.org/10.1007/978-3-031-10131-1_20

diagnosis [33–37] or as markers of aggressive behaviour [30], and also their possible influence in improving prognosis has been reported [30, 36, 37].

Whatever the role and clinical usefulness of those antibodies, their presence confirms the immune system reaction to cancer cells or to their metabolic activity and the presence of a chronic and long-lasting triggering by a restricted antigen family.

According to the antigen-driven monoclonal expansion, in those situations, the selection, growth, and differentiation of a lymphocyte clone could be conceivable, eventually with production of monoclonal immunoglobulins.

Available Data

Despite this theoretical premise, the presence of paraproteins in cancer series has been evaluated very seldom in recent papers. Seth found cryoglobulins in 95% of 48 patients with cervical cancer and reported a link between the paraproteins and the disease severity [38]; Norris reported the presence of cryoprecipitating immune complexes in seven out of 13 melanoma patients [39].

Data from Case Reports

More often, these findings were reported in single case descriptions: Hradská described a case of a 77-year-old man with hypercalcaemia, osteolytic lesions, and IgAk monoclonal paraprotein with parathyroid adenoma but without plasma cell myeloma infiltrates [40]; Chen described a patient bearing monoclonal IgGk associated with colon adenocarcinoma who had a complete serologic recovery after surgical removal of his tumour [41]; Pramanik reported a case of prostate carcinoma with monoclonal gammopathy as its presenting feature [42]; Wronski documented a case of cryoglobulinaemic vasculitis associated with a non-malignant schwannoma [43]; finally, Cobcroft reported a female patient with cryoglobulins associated with an atrial myxoma [44].

Data from Case Series

More detailed data can be found among the series of patients with cryoglobulins or monoclonal gammopathies of undetermined significance (MGUS) or in studies on paraneoplastic autoimmune manifestations (Table 20.1). In a follow-up study on 453 patients with non-HCV cryoglobulinaemia, Eble reported a 16% incidence of solid tumours [45]. La Raja, in a case series of 8197 blood donors, identified 104

Table 20.1 Studies evaluating the presence of epithelial neoplasms in gammopathy series

Author (year)	Study population	Years of median follow-up (range)	N° cases	Cancers
Eble (2016)	Non-HCV MC	na	453	75
La Raja (2012)	MGUS	7.7 (2–11)	104	6 (*)
Kuwabara (2018)	Non-IgM MGUS	6.4 (0–9.5)	1009	54 (*)
Gore (1979)	MGUS (multiband)	na	56	1 (*)
Antoine (1996)	CIDP	na	33	1 (*)
Ferri (2004)	MC	15	231	7 (*)
Invernizzi (1983)	MC	8 (7–9)	166	None
Kyle (1995)	MGUS	48	213	None
Robert-Thompson (2002)	MGUS	na	613	None
Anagnostopoulos (2002)	MGUS	6.7	75	None
Rosinol (2007)	MGUS	20	359	None
Madan (2009)	MGUS	14	214	None
Sandecka (2017)	MGUS	4	1887	None
Ma (2019)	MGUS	0.5	49	None

CIDP chronic inflammatory demyelinating polyneuropathy with M component, *MC* mixed cryoglobulinemia, *MGUS* monoclonal gammopathy of undetermined significance
(*) see text for details of diagnoses

cases of MGUS, among them over a 92-months follow-up; three developed prostate cancer, two bladder cancer, and one colon cancer accounting for near one cancer per 133 patient/year. Surprisingly only two overt myelomas and one lymphoma were observed [46]. Kuwabara, in a 20-years follow-up of 1009 cases of non-IgM MGUS, reported the death of 168 patients: 30 cases of multiple myeloma, 2 of amyloidosis, 8 of lymphomas, 6 of myelodysplastic syndromes, 73 of non-neoplastic causes, and 54 of epithelial cancers: These were diagnosed as 11 lung cancers, 7 colon cancers, 7 gastric cancers, 7 bladder cancers, 5 hepatocarcinomas, 4 hepatobiliary cancers, 3 breast cancers, and 3 cancers of head and neck, and 7 cancers not specified, accounting for an incidence of about one cancer death in 594 patient/year [47]. In a series of 56 MGUS with multiple paraproteins, Gore included 33 cases of immunoproliferative disorders as myelomas or macroglobulinaemia, 3 lymphomas, 19 non-malignant diseases, and one case of gastric cancer at presentation [48]. Antoine et al., in a series of 33 patients with peripheral neuropathies, described the presence of cancer in three patients, one pancreatic carcinoma, and one rectosigmoid adenocarcinoma without paraprotein and one 61-year-old man with cholangiocarcinoma associated with a monoclonal IgMk [49] but in a following paper, among 26 similar patients bearing cancers, the authors found anti-onconeural antibodies in 7 of them; 5 with lung cancer, one mediastinal undifferentiated carcinoma, and one prostatic cancer but none of them showed monoclonal pattern [50].

Confounding Factors

In 2004, Ferri reported 7 liver carcinoma cases in a series of 231 patients suffering from cryoglobulinaemic syndrome and followed for about 15 years, accounting for one case over 561 patient/years. Still, the link between cancer and the paraproteins implied by this finding is rather questionable because of the presence of chronic Hepatitis C virus infection which can cause both the cryoglobulin production and the development of liver cancer [51].

Counter Arguments

Over 30 years, a large body of papers each referring to a series of paraproteins, mainly MGUS, that were performed in a wide range of countries, reported some incidence of immunoproliferative or lymphoid neoplasm and autoimmune diseases but no cases of epithelial cancer.

Invernizzi followed for 7–9 years the evolution of the disease in 166 cryoglobulinaemic patients, 87 had already been diagnosed for lymphoproliferative or hepatic diseases, within the 79 considered idiopathic, 35 of them could be followed for a period ranging from 8 to 17 years, 14 without unfavourable evolution, 13 developed membranous proliferative nephropathy, 4 hepatic disorder, and 4 lymphoproliferative neoplasm but none developed cancer [52]. Kyle followed, for as long as 48 years, 213 MGUS patients [53], and Roberts-Thomson retrospectively evaluated 613 cases of paraproteins and both found many lymphomas, but not a single case of cancer [54]. Anagnostopoulos in a population-based study including 1564 elderly patients found 197 epithelial neoplasms, none of whom had a monoclonal gammopathy. Moreover, among 75 patients bearing monoclonal gammopathy, none developed cancer over a follow-up period of 71 months [55]. Rosinol, following for 20 years 359 MGUS cases, reported a single incidence of myeloma [56]. Madan reported similar data on a series of 214 MGUS cases followed for about 14 years [57]. Bida in his search for pathogenetic causes in 17,398 MGUS reported only a single case of colon cancer, stating that its incidence is the same in MGUS as it is in the general population [58]. Sandecká analyzed 1887 MGUS cases over 4 years without detecting any cancer [59]. Similar findings were reported by Ma in a smaller series of 49 MGUS patients [60].

Summarizing Remarks

Summarizing these data, it is clear that paraproteins and cryoprecipitating complexes could be found frequently in sera of patients with epithelial neoplasms, and their presence could be a marker of worse prognosis, but the evidence supporting this statement is very weak, and studies that are more accurate are needed. In any case, this suggestion lends support to the hypothesis that a long-lasting exposure to a restricted family of neoantigens can induce a clonal lymphocyte growth and a monoclonal antibody synthesis.

Conclusion

The evidence for further evolution of this clonal growth is lacking and may be impossible to obtain because of the features of the underlying disease and the cytotoxic treatments applied. Overall, the conclusion is that a tight link of paraproteins, both monoclonal globulins and cryoprecipitating complexes having a monoclonal component, with epithelial cancer is very unreliable. Although quite abundant, the reports are scanty and uneven, and the absence of sound population studies prevents any attempt not only for a meta-analysis but also for stating a hypothesis about this issue. Though it has been very roughly evaluated, the incidence of cancer among the cryoglobulins or MGUS bearing people seems to be the same as in the general population. However, the distribution of cancer type in the general population is not mirrored in MGUS series, as the most frequently diagnosed cancers, i.e. breast or colon cancer, are less frequently encountered in the MGUS population whereas prostate and bladder cancers showed a relatively higher frequency. So, as a rule of thumb, a urological evaluation and the search for neoplastic cells in urine should be considered in the screening of a patient with MGUS or cryoglobulins.

References

1. Shimizu J, Yamazaki S, Sakaguchi S. Induction of tumor immunity by removing CD25+CD4+ T cells: a common basis between tumor immunity and autoimmunity. J Immunol. 1999;163(10):5211–8.
2. Itoh M, Takahashi T, Sakaguchi N, Kuniyasu Y, Shimizu J, Otsuka F, Sakaguchi S. Thymus and autoimmunity: production of CD25+CD4+ naturally anergic and suppressive T cells as a key function of the thymus in maintaining immunologic self-tolerance. J Immunol. 1999;162:5317–26.
3. Zou W, Chen L. Inhibitory B7-family molecules in the tumour microenvironment. Nat Rev Immunol. 2008;8(6):467–77.
4. Gjerstorff M, Burns JS, Nielsen O, Kassem M, Ditzel H. Epigenetic modulation of cancer-germline antigen gene Antigenion in tumorigenic human mesenchymal stem cells: implications for cancer therapy. Am J Pathol. 2009;175(1):314–23.
5. Akers SN, Odunsi K, Karpf AR. Regulation of cancer germline antigen gene expression: implications for cancer immunotherapy. Future Oncol. 2010;6(5):717–32.
6. Campoli M, Ferrone S. HLA antigen and NK cell activating ligand expression in malignant cells: a story of loss or acquisition. Semin Immunopathol. 2011;33(4):321–34.
7. Florke Gee RR, Chen H, Lee AK, Daly CA, Wilander BA, Fon Tacer K, Potts PR. Emerging roles of the MAGE protein family in stress response pathways. J Biol Chem. 2020;295(47):16121–55.

8. Scanlan MJ, Gure AO, Jungbluth AA, Old LJ, Chen YT. Cancer/testis antigens: an expanding family of targets for cancer immunotherapy. Immunol Rev. 2002;188:22–32.
9. Stockert E, Jager E, Chen YT, et al. A survey of the humoral immune response of cancer patients to a panel of human tumor antigens. J Exp Med. 1998;187(8):1349–54.
10. Omenn GS. Plasma proteomics, the human proteome project, and cancer-associated alternative splice variant proteins. Biochim Biophys Acta. 2014;1844(5):866–73.
11. Alsarkhi LK, Weber GF. Anti-osteopontin autoantibodies in various types of cancer. Oncol Rep. 2018;40(6):3879–89.
12. Angelopoulou K, Diamandis EP, Sutherland DJ, Kellen JA, Bunting PS. Prevalence of serum antibodies against the p53 tumor suppressor gene protein in various cancers. Int J Cancer. 1994;58(4):480–7.
13. Yang Y, Huang J, Rabii B, Rabii R, Hu S. Quantitative proteomic analysis of serum proteins from oral cancer patients: comparison of two analytical methods. Int J Mol Sci. 2014;15: 14386–95.
14. Zaenker P, Ziman MR. Serologic autoantibodies as diagnostic cancer biomarkers—a review. Cancer Epidemiol Biomark Prev. 2013;22(12):2161–81.
15. Fässler M, Diem M, Mangana J, Hasan Ali O, Berner F, Bomze D, Ring S, Niederer R, Del Carmen Gil Cruz C, Pérez Shibayama CI, Krolik M, Siano M, Joerger M, Recher M, Risch L, Güsewell S, Risch M, Speiser DE, Ludewig B, Levesque MP, Dummer R, Flatz L. Antibodies as biomarker candidates for response and survival to checkpoint inhibitors in melanoma patients. J Immunother Cancer. 2019;7:50.
16. Meistere I, Werner S, Zayakin P, Silin K, Rulle U, Pismennaja A, Santare D, Kikuste I, Isajevs S, Leja M, Kupcinskas L, Kupcinskas J, Jonaitis L, Wu CY, Brenner H, Line A, Kalnin Z. The prevalence of cancer-associated autoantibodies in patients with gastric cancer and progressive grades of premalignant lesions. Cancer Epidemiol Biomark Prev. 2017;26(10):1564–74.
17. Gao WM, Kuick R, Orchekowski RP, Misek DE, Qiu J, Greenberg AK, Rom WN, Brenner DE, Omenn GS, Haab BB, Hanash SM. Distinctive serum protein profiles involving abundant proteins in lung cancer patients based upon antibody microarray analysis. BMC Cancer. 2005;5:110.
18. Winter SF, Sekido Y, Minna JD, McIntire D, Johnson BE, Gazdar AF, Carbone DP. Antibodies against autologous tumor cell proteins in patients with small-cell lung cancer: association with improved survival. J Natl Cancer Inst. 1993;85(24):2012–8.
19. Wang T, Liu H, Pei L, Wang K, Song C, Wang P, Ye H, Zhang J, Ji Z, Ouyang S, Dai L. Screening of tumor-associated antigens based on Oncomine database and evaluation of diagnostic value of autoantibodies in lung cancer. Clin Immunol. 2020;210:108262.
20. Huang H, Luo W, Ni Y, Sun S, Wang C, Zhang L. The diagnostic efficiency of seven autoantibodies in lung cancer. Eur J Cancer Prev. 2020;29(4):315–20.
21. Chung L, Moore K, Phillips L, Boyle FM, Marsh DJ, Baxter RC. Novel serum protein biomarker panel revealed by mass spectrometry and its prognostic value in breast cancer. Breast Cancer Res. 2014;16(3):R63.
22. Dumstrei K, Chen H, Brenner H. A systematic review of serum autoantibodies as biomarkers for pancreatic cancer detection. Oncotarget. 2016;7(10):11151–64.
23. Wang H, Li X, Zhou D, Huan J. Autoantibodies as biomarkers for colorectal cancer: a systematic review, meta-analysis, and bioinformatics analysis. IJBM. 2019;34(4):334–47.
24. Chibo L, Chunqin P, Jianmin S, Haibao W, Liang Y. MALDI-TOF MS combined with magnetic beads for detecting serum protein biomarkers and establishment of boosting decision tree model for diagnosis of colorectal cancer. Int J Mol Sci. 2011;8:39–47.
25. Benvenuto M, Sileri P, Rossi P, Masuelli L, Fantini M, Nanni M, Franceschilli L, Sconocchia G, Lanzilli G, Arriga R, Faggioni G, Lista F, Orlandi A, Manzari V, Gaspari AL, Modesti A, Bei R. Natural humoral immune response to ribosomal P0 protein in colorectal cancer patients. J Transl Med. 2015;13:101.
26. Zhang H, Xia J, Wang K, Zhang J. Serum autoantibodies in the early detection of esophageal cancer: a systematic review. J Tumour Biol. 2015;36(1):95–109.
27. Fortner RT, Damms-Machado A, Kaaks R. Systematic review: tumor-associated antigen autoantibodies and ovarian cancer early detection. Gynecol Oncol. 2017;147(2):465–80.

28. Ummanni R, Duscharla D, Barett C, Venz S, Schlomm T, Heinzer H, Walther R, Bokemeyer C, Brümmendorf TH, Murthy PV, Balabanov SJ. Prostate cancer-associated autoantibodies in serum against tumor-associated antigens as potential new biomarkers. Proteomics. 2015;119:218–29.
29. He SJ, Gu YY, Yu L, Luo B, Fan R, Lin WZ, Lan XW, Lin YD, Zhang QM, Xiao SW, Xie XX. High expression and frequently humoral immune response of melanoma-associated antigen D4 in glioma. Int J Clin Exp Pathol. 2014;7(5):2350–60.
30. Lai CL, Tsai CM, Tsai TT, Kuo BIT, Chang KT, Fu HT, Perng RP, Chen JY. Presence of serum anti-p53 antibodies is associated with pleural effusion and poor prognosis in lung cancer patients. Clin Cancer Res. 1998;4:2025–30.
31. Ben-Mahrez K, Thierry D, Sorokine I, Danna-Mullerl A, Kohiyamal M. Detection of circulating antibodies against c-myc protein in cancer patient sera. Br J Cancer. 1988;57:529–34.
32. Trown PW, Kramer MJ, Dennin RA Jr, Connell EV, Palleroni AV, Quesada J, Gutterman JU. Antibodies to human leucocyte interferons in cancer patients. Lancet. 1983;1(8316):81–4.
33. Nolen BM, Lokshin AE. Autoantibodies for cancer detection: still cause for excitement? Cancer Biomark. 2010;6(5–6):229–45.
34. Wu J, Li X, Song W, Fang Y, Yu L, Liu S, Churilov LP, Zhang F. The roles and applications of autoantibodies in progression, diagnosis, treatment and prognosis of human malignant tumours. Autoimmun Rev. 2017;16(12):1270–81.
35. Yadav S, Kashaninejad N, Masud MK, Yamauchi Y, Nguyen NT, Shiddiky MJA. Autoantibodies as diagnostic and prognostic cancer biomarker: detection techniques and approaches. Biosens Bioelectron. 2019;139:111315.
36. Ebrahimnezhad S, Jazayeri M, Hassanian SM, Avan A. Current status and prospective regarding the therapeutic potential of natural autoantibodies in cancer therapy. J Cell Physiol. 2017;232(10):2649–52.
37. Triozzi PL, Fernandez AP. The role of the immune response in Merkel cell carcinoma. Cancers. 2013;5:234–54.
38. Seth P, Balachandran N, Malaviya AN, Kumar R. Circulating immune complexes in carcinoma of uterine cervix. Clin Exp Immunol. 1979;38(1):77–82.
39. Norris DA, Huff JC, Swinehart JM, Carr RI, Thorne EG, Weston WL, McIntosh RM. Cryoglobulinemia and decreased monocyte chemotaxis is malignant melanoma. J Invest Dermatol. 1980;75(3):219–23.
40. Hradská K, Jelínek T, Ďuraš J, Mihályová J, Popková T, Cvek J, Bukovanský K, Havel M, Spáčilová V, Hájek R. Osteolytic bone lesions, hypercalcemia and paraprotein, but not a myeloma: case report and review of literature. Vnitr Lek. 2020;66(5):90–5.
41. Chen HP, Carroll JA. Monoclonal gammopathy in carcinoma of the colon. Am J Clin Pathol. 1980;73(4):607–10.
42. Pramanik S, Gazi J, Das AK, Debnath NB, Pal SK. Monoclonal gammopathy in prostate carcinoma: a case report and review of literature. J Med Case Rep. 2018;12:325.
43. Wroński J, Zielińska A, Głuszko P, Szołkowska M. Systemic vasculitis induced by schwannoma—paraneoplastic syndrome caused by the benign tumor. Am J Med. 2020;133(11):e676–7.
44. Cobcroft RG, Shearer A, Gill DS, Forgan-Smith J. Fluctuating symptomatic cryofibrinogenaemia in a patient with left atrial myxoma. Br J Haematol. 1994;88(1):213–4.
45. Eble V, Legallicier B, Joly P, Vittecoq O, Caron F, Tamion F, Ducrotte P, Levesque H, Menard JF, Jouen F, Guerrot D, Marie I. Long term outcome of patients with low level of cryoglobulin (<0.05g/L). Autoimmun Rev. 2016;15(5):440–6.
46. La Raja M, Barcobello M, Bet N, Dolfini P, Florean M, Tomasella F, De Angelis V, Mascaretti L. Incidental finding of monoclonal gammopathy in blood donors: a follow-up study. Blood Transfus. 2012;10:338–43.
47. Kuwabara C, Sakuma Y, Kume A, Tamura Y, Shimizu R, Iwai R, Ishii A, Tanaka H. Characteristics and prognosis of patients with non-immunoglobulin-M monoclonal gammopathy of undetermined significance: a retrospective study. Int J Hematol. 2019;109:154–61.
48. Gore ME, Riches PG, Kohn J. Identification of the paraproteins and clinical significance of more than one paraprotein in serum of 56 patients. J Clin Pathol. 1979;32:313–7.

49. Antoine JC, Mosnier JF, Lapras J, Convers P, Absi L, Laurent B, Michel D. Chronic inflammatory demyelinating polyneuropathy associated with carcinoma. J Neurol Neurosurg Psychiatry. 1996;60:188–90.
50. Antoine JC, Mosnier JF, Absi L, Convers P, Honnorat J, Michel D. Carcinoma associated paraneoplastic peripheral neuropathies in patients with and without anti-onconeural antibodies. Neurol Neurosurg Psychiatry. 1999;67:7–14.
51. Ferri C, Sebastiani M, Giuggioli D, Cazzato M, Longombardo G, Antonelli A, Puccini R, Michelassi C, Zignego AL. Mixed cryoglobulinemia: demographic, clinical, and serologic features and survival in 231 patients. Semin Arthritis Rheum. 2004;33(6):355–74.
52. Invernizzi F, Galli M, Serino G, Monti G, Meroni PL, Granatieri C, Zanussi C. Secondary and essential cryoglobulinemias. Frequency, nosological classification, and long-term follow-up. Acta Haematol. 1983;70(2):73–82.
53. Kyle RA. Monoclonal gammopathy of undetermined significance (MGUS). Baillieres Clin Haematol. 1995;8(4):761–81.
54. Roberts-Thomson PJ, Nikoloutsopoulos T, Smith AJ. Paraproteins: a regional south Australian experience. Asian Pac J Allergy Immunol. 2002;20(3):187–95.
55. Anagnostopoulos A, Evangelopoulou A, Sotou D, Gika D, Mitsibounas D, Dimopoulos MA. Incidence and evolution of monoclonal gammopathy of undetermined significance (MGUS) in Greece. Ann Hematol. 2002;81:357–61.
56. Rosinol L, Cibeira MT, Montoto S, Rozman M, Esteve J. Monoclonal gammopathy of undetermined significance: predictors of malignant transformation and recognition of an evolving type characterized by a progressive increase in M protein size. Mayo Clin Proc. 2007;82(4):428–34.
57. Madan S, Greipp PR. The incidental monoclonal protein: current approach to management of monoclonal gammopathy of undetermined significance (MGUS). Blood Rev. 2009;23(6):257–65.
58. Bida JP, Kyle RA, Therneau TM, Melton LJ III, Plevak MF, Larson DR, Dispenzieri A, Katzmann JA, Rajkumar SV. Disease associations with monoclonal gammopathy of undetermined significance: a population-based study of 17,398 patients. Mayo Clin Proc. 2009;84(8):685–93.
59. Sandecká V, Hájek R, Pour L, Špička I, Ščudla V, Gregora E, Radocha J, Walterová L, Kessler P, Zahradová L, Adamová D, Valentova K, Vonke I, Obernauerová J, Starostka D, Wróbel M, Brožová L, Jarkovský J, Mikulášová A, Říhová L, Ševčíková S, Straub J, Minařík J, Adam Z, Krejčí M, Král Z, Maisnar V, on behalf of the Czech Myeloma Group. A first Czech analysis of 1887 cases with monoclonal gammopathy of undetermined significance. Eur J Haematol. 2017;99:80–90.
60. Ma L, Xu S, Qu J, Hou J, Wang Y, Wen L, Liu Y, Kang Y, Jiang M, Fu W, Du J, Zhou L, Huang X, Zhang Z, Lu J. Monoclonal gammopathy of undetermined significance in Chinese population: a prospective epidemiological study. Hematol Oncol. 2019;37:75–9.

Chapter 21
Monoclonal Gammopathies with Miscellaneous Associations

Pietro Enrico Pioltelli, T. Prescott Atkinson, Mervat Mattar, Amr Edrees, Hamdy M. A. Ahmed, Ahmed Laymouna, Mona R. E. Abdel-Halim, and Gaafar Ragab

Abbreviations

AIHA	Autoimmune hemolytic anemia
BM	Bone marrow
BMA	Bone marrow aspirate
CA	Cold agglutinin

P. E. Pioltelli
Haematology Unit, Milano-Bicocca University, San Gerardo Hospital, Monza, Italy

T. P. Atkinson
Department of Pediatrics, University of Alabama at Birmingham, Birmingham, AL, USA
e-mail: PAtkinson@peds.uab.edu

M. Mattar
Clinical Hematology Unit, Kasr Alainy Faculty of Medicine, Cairo University, Cairo, Egypt

A. Edrees
Department of Internal Medicine, University of Missouri-Kansas City, Kansas, MO, USA
e-mail: edreesa@umkc.edu

H. M. A. Ahmed
Division of Rheumatology, Department of Medicine, University of South Alabama, Mobile, AL, USA

A. Laymouna
Department of Medicine, Rheumatology and Clinical Immunology Unit, Faculty of Medicine, Cairo University, Cairo, Egypt

M. R. E. Abdel-Halim
Dermatology Department, Faculty of Medicine, Cairo University, Cairo, Egypt

G. Ragab (✉)
Rheumatology and Clinical Immunology Unit, Internal Medicine Department, Faculty of Medicine, Cairo University, Cairo, Egypt

School of Medicine, Newgiza University (NGU), Giza, Egypt

© The Author(s), under exclusive license to Springer Nature Switzerland AG 2022
G. Ragab et al. (eds.), *Paraproteinemia and Related Disorders*,
https://doi.org/10.1007/978-3-031-10131-1_21

CAD	Cold agglutinin disease
CD	Castleman disease
CMV	Cytomegalovirus
CVID	Common variable immunodeficiency
DAT	Direct antiglobulin test
EBV	Epstein–Barr virus
EED	Erythema elevatum diutinum
Gcase	Glucocerebrosidase
HHV8	Human Herpesvirus-8
IL	Interleukin
iMCD	Idiopathic multicentric castleman disease
iMCD-TAFRO	iMCD-thrombocytopenia, ascites, reticulin fibrosis, renal dysfunction and organomegaly
MCD	Multicentric Castleman disease
MG	Monoclonal gammopathy
MGUS	Monoclonal gammopathy of undetermined significance
MM	Multiple myeloma
PC	Plasma cell
PID	Primary inherited immunodeficienc6y
POEMS	Polyneuropathy, Organomegaly, Endocrinopathy, Monoclonal Protein, Skin Changes
POEMS-MCD	POEMS-associated MCD
PV	Polycythemia vera
SMM	Smoldering multiple myeloma
TEMPI	Telangiectasias, elevated erythropoietin (EPO) and erythrocytosis, monoclonal gammopathy, perinephric fluid collections, and intrapulmonary shunting
TNF	Tumor necrosis factor
UCD	Unicentric Castleman disease
VEGF	Vascular endothelial growth factor
WM	Waldenström macroglobulinemia

Introduction

The list of diseases and syndromes eventually proving to be associated with monoclonal gammopathies, or paraproteinemias is progressively expanding. In preceding chapters, the conditions that could be grouped under a specific entity or a causative agent are discussed. In this chapter, we will discuss the following miscellaneous topics that are associated with paraproteins.

- Monoclonal gammopathies (MG) after tissue transplantation
- Primary immunodeficiency
- Cold agglutinin disease (CAD)

- Castleman disease (CD)
- POEMS syndrome
- Gaucher disease (GD)
- TEMPI syndrome
- Erythema elevatum diutinum (EED)

They will be discussed with regard to our current knowledge on their pathogenesis, clinical presentations, and available therapeutic modalities.

Monoclonal Gammopathies After Tissue Transplantation

The presence of a monoclonal paraprotein in the sera of transplanted patients could have a dual significance. Aside from the obvious prognostic relevance of the paraproteins expressed by the disease justifying the transplantation itself, its presence before the transplant could influence the treatment outcome while its onset after the transplant could represent a harbinger of a new disease or the provocation of the host immune system by the donor antigens or the graft immune system when matched with the patient tissues. Moreover, in this bursting environment some viruses are often chronically present fueling a prolonged synthesis of antibodies against a restricted range of epitopes.

Available Data

Monoclonal paraproteins are reported in all transplant settings, with a wide range of incidence, depending on the type of transplant or the aim of the report.

Sound epidemiological surveys are lacking but studies on large series are available. In kidney transplants, Alfano studied 548 patients, over a 7-years median follow-up, and reported 39 cases of monoclonal gammopathy of undetermined significance (MGUS) accounting for 8.1% [1], Cuéllar-Garcia who worked on 1016 cases observed only 11 MGUS [2], Naina studying 3518 transplant cases reported 19 MGUS after transplantation [3], whereas Gagnon reported 13 MGUS in his 750 cases [4] . Caforio in a series of 308 cardiac transplants observed a risk for developing MGUS of 30% at 5 years and 50% at 10 years [5]. Similar events were observed in a large number of smaller series [6–8] and the presence of cryoprecipitating immune complexes has also been reported [9–12]. Those findings very seldom can be attributed to an autoimmune mechanism as proposed by Mitus on allogeneic bone marrow transplant where a transient mono/oligoclonal gammopathy and monoclonal B cells in peripheral blood are present [13]. Some hints suggesting a derangement in T cells subsets, favoring a B-cell uncontrolled growth from the links observed between a monoclonal gammopathy and an intensive anti-T immunosuppression [5, 7, 14], but in the great majority of series the monoclonal response is elicited by viral triggers, mainly by a lymphotropic virus such as Epstein–Barr virus (EBV), [3, 7, 15, 16] when expressed as reactivation of latent form [17–19], or hepatitis C virus RNA which has been reported both in typical MGUS [9, 11, 20] and in type II cryoglobulinemia [12, 21]. Some other viruses, in singular or concomitant infections are observed, such as Cytomegalovirus (CMV) [7, 14, 22, 23], or human herpesvirus 8 (HHV 8) [24]. Anyway, the role of an MG detected after transplantation is not clearly defined; some authors reported transient disorder without worsening activity [1, 4, 8, 14, 18, 25], but in many cases a lymphoproliferative disease after MGUS is documented, mainly in the presence of EBV [2, 3, 5, 7, 16, 26], or the more frequent onset of vasculitis [12, 25, 27] and septic episodes with enhanced risk of graft rejection [6, 8, 10, 11, 28, 29]. On the contrary, the presence of MGUS before transplant is always a poor prognostic marker for the evolution for multiple myeloma (MM) or lymphoproliferative disease [2, 4, 18, 30–33]. Some conflicting data are also reported about the role of an MGUS in donors, both harmful [34] and harmless [35]

Summarizing Remarks

In general, the MGs identified after allogeneic transplant are not directly linked to the immune derangement induced by the presence of unrelated tissues, but are triggered by a viral infection that is able to modify lymphocyte metabolism, or from a lymphoproliferative disease preceding the transplantation itself which is independent from the disease that justified this treatment. The fate of an MGUS which appeared after the transplant seems to be uncertain but rarely results in worsening of the prognosis, contrary to the presence of a MGUS before the transplantation as it worsens the outcome and must be considered as an index of poor prognosis.

Primary Immunodeficiency

Having been described to occur in 30% of MGUS cases and up to 70% of smoldering multiple myeloma (SMM), the association of hypogammaglobulinemia with these disorders is certainly very common [36, 37]. In addition, one study of 380 patients with hypogammaglobulinemia and no evidence of an M spike on serum or urine electrophoresis, nearly 10% proved to have a detectable band on immunofixation electrophoresis [38]. Moreover, cellular abnormalities in both T- and B-cell populations are also frequent and may contribute to the failure in some patients to suppress evolving plasma cell (PC) and other lymphoid malignancies [39, 40]. These findings to some extent create a "chicken or the egg" conundrum in which it is often unclear to what extent the immunologic abnormalities are the cause or the result of a developing MG.

Among patients with MGUS, evolving MM, and other gammopathies, are mixed in a small proportion of patients with underlying primary (inherited) immunodeficiencies (PID), who are many times at increased risk for the development of lymphoid malignancies. It is to the clinician's (and the patient's) advantage for this to be kept in mind as an uncommon, but real possibility. Scattered case reports through the literature document the development of MG in a variety of PID patients including Wiskott-Aldrich syndrome [41], IKBKG (NEMO, or Nuclear factor-kappa B Essential Modulator) deficiency [42], ataxia telangiectasia (AT) [43], and Good's syndrome [44]. Although malignant PC disorders are quite rare in children, MGs are not. In a large retrospective review of 695 tests from children with serum immunofixation electrophoresis results available, 83 patients proved to have an MG, and PID diagnoses in those patients included ataxia telangiectasia (18), severe combined immunodeficiency (2), and common variable immunodeficiency (CVID) (2) [45].

CVID is a heterogeneous severe antibody deficiency syndrome characterized by levels less than 2 SD below age-adjusted norms of IgG and either IgA or IgM or both IgA and IgM along with poor or absent specific antibody production and the absence of other causes of immunodeficiency [46]. Despite its name, CVID is relatively uncommon with a prevalence ranging up to 3.374/100,000 in northern European countries [47]. There is a known predisposition of CVID patients to develop lymphoproliferative disorders and lymphoid malignancies. In a study of 1091 CVID patients in the USIDNET registry, the authors found about 4% had been diagnosed with lymphoid malignancies, and three patients had been diagnosed with gammopathies: two with MM and one with MGUS [48].

Another much more common and more benign disorder, also most prevalent in northern European countries, is selective IgA deficiency, which has an estimated prevalence as high as 1 in 600 individuals of European ancestry [49]. IgA deficiency is a risk factor for the development of celiac disease (about 1 in 50 cases are IgA deficient) and so is frequently discovered during the course of evaluation of patients being evaluated for that disorder. In a recent study by Wallage and colleagues, the authors examined 60 patients with IgA deficiency identified through celiac disease testing and found that four patients had MGs: two new myeloma patients (one symptomatic and one asymptomatic), one patient with MGUS, and one known chronic lymphocytic leukemia (CLL) patient [50]. Thus, this common mild immunoglobulin deficiency may also be among the most common immunologic disorders associated with gammopathies.

In summary, the possibility that a patient found to have a gammopathy might also have an underlying primary immunodeficiency should always be kept in the back of the clinician's mind. While relatively uncommon, such disorders may require special treatment. PID patients with DNA repair disorders like AT are very sensitive to ionizing radiation and alkylating agents, and others may be particularly prone to developing overwhelming infection with such pathogens as CMV and EBV if treatment results in impairment of an already compromised host immune defense system. As our ability to obtain and analyze whole genome sequences of patients improves, it is likely that we will be able to better understand the roles of these abnormalities and develop improved strategies of treatment.

Cold Agglutinin Disease

Cold agglutinin disease (CAD) constitutes 5–30% of autoimmune hemolytic anemias (AIHA) and is characterized by a direct antiglobulin test (DAT) with a cold agglutinin (CA) measured at 4 °C. Titers of 64 or higher are considered significant. An associated positivity for complement fragment C3d is characteristic [51]. Affected cases are commonly elderly or middle-aged, with slight female predisposition. CAD is a rare disorder with a reported incidence of 1 per million per year in Norway and 1.2 per million per year in Denmark [52, 53].

The IGHV4-34 (Immunoglobulin Heavy Variable 4-34) Protein Coding gene, located on the long arm of chromosome 14 is responsible for CA IgM heavy chain production in about 81% of cases with absence of MYD88L265P mutation in bone marrow samples [54] in contra- distinction to lymphoplasmacytic lymphoma. The term CAD-associated B-cell lymphoproliferative disease has been suggested [55].

CA is commonly a monoclonal IgM κ subtype [56]. It tends to agglutinate erythrocytes by binding to the erythrocyte surface carbohydrate antigen I [54]. The process includes classic complement activation, more effectively so at a temperature of 3–4 °C [57]. The maximum temperature at which CA will bind to erythrocyte antigen is called the thermal amplitude. Cold agglutinins with a low thermal amplitude below 25–28 °C will not be clinically active causing no hemolysis [58].

Symptoms appear on cooling of fingers, toes, ears, or nose tip causing erythrocyte agglutination in peripheral capillaries with acrocyanosis, Raynaud's phenomenon, or gangrene [59].

Diagnosis entails an AIHA with an IgM DAT with strong positivity to C3d. A titer of 64 or more at 4 °C is required. Plasma protein electrophoresis, immunofixation, and thermal amplitude detection are required. The majority of CAs in CAD are of monoclonal IgMκ subtype with about 7% of the cases being λ subtype. CA of the IgG (Immunoglobulin G) class occurs in only about 5% [52].

An associated B-cell clonal lymphoproliferative disorder may be detected by flow cytometry and bone marrow trephine biopsy, but with no additional detectable clinical symptoms or signs [60].

Cold Agglutinin Syndrome (CAS) is found if the condition is associated with an overt infection (e.g., Mycoplasma pneumoniae, EBV), or if associated with an overt immune or malignant condition [59]. Polyclonal CAs are detected if CAS is secondary to infections [61]. Mycoplasma pneumonia infection is associated with anti-I-specific IgM CAs [62]. EBV and CMV infections are associated with the formation of anti-i IgG or IgM CAs [63, 64]. Both were found In CAS secondary to lymphomas, κ light chain CAs were more common in cases of Waldenström macroglobulinemia, while λ light chain CAs were more common with other B-cell lymphomas [65].

Non-drug treatment of CAD includes warming and low plasma-containing blood transfusion [66]. Plasmapheresis may be resorted to as an emergency treatment [67]. Chemo-/immunotherapy includes the use of Rituximab [68] with or without Bendamustine [69]. Bruton kinase inhibitor use [70] may be effective. Complement-directed therapy includes the complement inhibitor eculizumab [71] and C1-esterase inhibitor concentrate [72].

Castleman Disease

CD, angiofollicular lymph node hyperplasia describes a heterogeneous group of disorders sharing together a wide range of histopathological characteristics. However, they can be attributed to various causes. They also have different manifestations, therapeutic approaches, and outcomes. Benjamin Castleman was the first to describe the disease in the 1950s. He reported mediastinal lymph node swelling with increased lymphoid follicles with germinal centers involution as well as marked capillary proliferation. This included follicular and interfollicular endothelial hyperplasia [73]. Afterwards, Flendrig reported, in 1969, the PC variants, the hyalinized, and the "intermediate" histopathological ones. The second variant is also referred to as the mixed variant [74]. By the mid-1980s of the twentieth century, CD was classified into unicentric CD (UCD), when involving a single lymph node or region of lymph nodes, and multicentric CD (MCD), when involving multiple stations [75].

MCD is further subdivided into idiopathic MCD (iMCD), HHV8-associated MCD (HHV8-MCD) and polyneuropathy, organomegaly, endocrinopathy, monoclonal plasma cell disorder, and skin changes (POEMS)-associated MCD (POEMS-MCD). The iMCD is again subdivided into iMCD—thrombocytopenia, ascites, reticulin fibrosis, renal dysfunction, and organomegaly (TAFRO) and iMCD-not otherwise specified (iMCD-NOS) [76]. In 1996, the relation of CD with HHV8 was recognized. All cases of human immunodeficiency virus (HIV)-positive and some HIV-negative MCD cases were related to HHV 8 [77]. In 2010, Takai and his group identified a severe form of iMCD with characteristic findings. It is named TAFRO syndrome, the acronym for Thrombocytopenia, Ascites, reticulin Fibrosis, Renal dysfunction, and Organomegaly [78] (Fig. 21.1).

PCs are usually polyclonal, but monoclonality has been reported, mainly lambda light chain restricted (IgG or IgA), particularly if the PC-CD is associated with osteosclerotic myeloma or POEMS syndrome. However, MG is rare and its detection may be a harbinger of progression to lymphoma [79]. Yang et al. reported a case of MCD that transformed into IgG MM [80], thus adding to the list of complications.

Monoclonal PCs may be the causative drivers of POEMS-MCD [81]. We do not know the exact difference in the cellular or cytokine characteristics when comparing POEMS-MCD and classic POEMS syndrome. In classic POEMS syndrome, an abundance of vascular endothelial growth factor (VEGF) and IL-12 production caused by PCs somatic mutation is well recognized [82]. All POEMS syndrome cases will have a proof of monoclonal PCs proliferation, either on serum and/or urine immunofixation studies, on immunostaining or flow cytometric studies done on the BM or lymph node in the case of coexisting CD.

Therapy

- Surgical removal is the main treatment for UCD, regardless of pathology. Complete surgical excision is always curative with resolution of all clinical and laboratory abnormalities [83].
- Rituximab-based therapy has significantly improved the 5-year survival for HHV8-MCD from 33 to 90% [84].

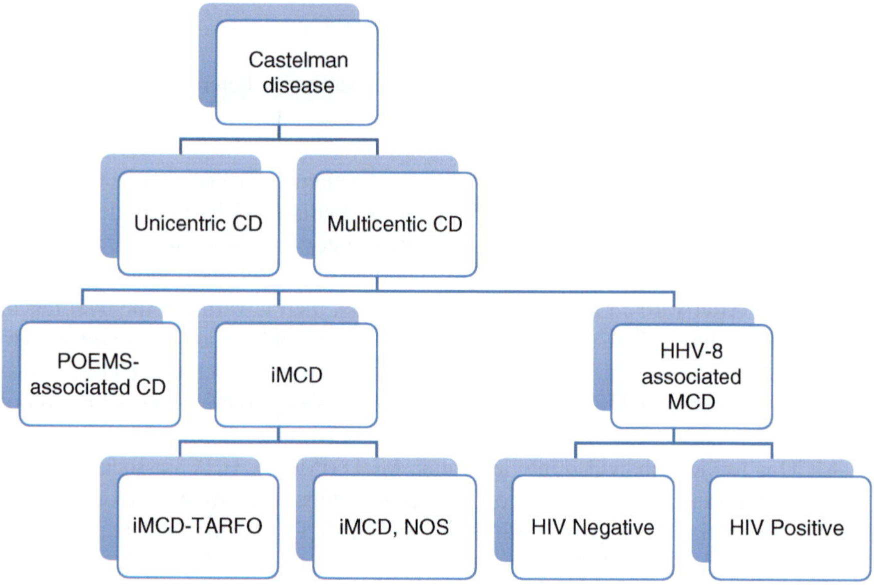

Fig. 21.1 Castleman disease classification. *CD* Castleman disease, *iMCD* idiopathic MCD, *TAFRO* thrombocytopenia, ascites, reticulin fibrosis, renal dysfunction, and organomegaly

- Patients with POEMS syndrome and MCD with osteosclerotic lesions and predominant peripheral neuropathy symptoms are managed with standard MM therapy, usually by ASCT preceded by high-dose chemotherapy. When ASCT is not to be considered, other drugs borrowed from the MM armamentarium may be considered. The list includes melphalan, cyclophosphamide, lenalidomide, thalidomide, bortezomib, carfilzomib, and daratumumab. When bone lesions are not present in POEMS-MCD, we don't have sufficient data. If there is high IL-6, Sarilumab can be considered [85].
- iMCD patients should be classified based on disease severity. For patients with mild symptomatology, a limited course of rituximab can be considered. Other biological drugs targeting IL-6 may also be considered, including siltuximab (recently licensed for iMCD) or tocilizumab. If organ dysfunction worsens at any time, initiation of combination chemotherapy should be considered with oral thalidomide, cyclophosphamide, and prednisone [86].

POEMS Syndrome

Definition

The syndrome was first described in 1968 by Crow and Fukase; however, the acronym POEMS was first reported in 1980 [87]. It stands for Polyneuropathy, Organomegaly, Endocrinopathy, Monoclonal protein, Skin changes. It has other less common names as osteosclerotic myeloma, Crow–Fukase syndrome and Takatsuki syndrome [88, 89].

Epidemiology

The incidence of POEMS syndrome is exceedingly rare. According to a 2003 Japanese national survey, the prevalence of POEM is 0.3 per 100,000 [90]. This could be related to failure to recognize the syndrome by clinicians as it often requires more than one specialty to make the diagnosis [91]. Overall, its prevalence is higher in men than women with variable ratios depending on the origin of the cohort. The median age at incidence varies between cohorts with a range of 46–53 years [81, 90, 91].

Clinical Picture

Clinical characteristics of POEMS are not limited to the acronym. In fact, not all characteristics mentioned in the acronym are required to make the diagnosis. Besides, there are other features that were not recognized in the initial reports and later became essential for the diagnosis. Other clinical characteristics include thrombocytosis, papilledema, volume overload manifesting with peripheral edema, pleural effusion and ascites, pulmonary hypertension, meningeal thickening, clubbing, sclerotic bone

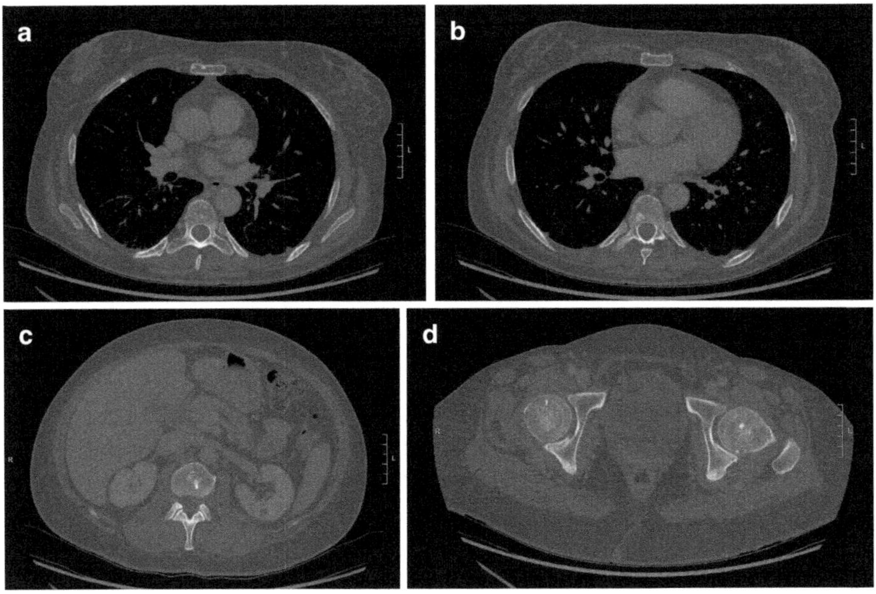

Fig. 21.2 CT scans with bone window showing osteosclerotic lesions at different sites in the course of POEMS syndrome (vertebral bodies) (**a**–**c**); sternum, ribs (**a**, **b**); femoral heads and pelvis (**d**). (Courtesy of Dr. Luca Quartuccio, Department of Medicine, University of Udine, School of Rheumatology, Italy)

lesions, and CD. Cytopenia is usually absent unless CD is present [85, 92, 93]. CD may coexist with POEMS and there is an association with anti-HHV-8 antibodies. The prevalence of CD in POEMS ranges between 15 and 25% [81, 89, 94, 95].

Bone lesions are usually multiple small osteosclerotic lesions (Fig. 21.2); however, sometimes they may present with mixed sclerotic and lytic parts (hence the name osteosclerotic myeloma). Lesions are usually found in the pelvis, thoracolumbar spine, and ribs [96–98].

Pathology

Bone marrow biopsy in POEMS typically includes a rim of PCs, mostly lambda restricted, around hypercellular reactive or normal appearing lymphoid aggregates of mixed B- and T-cells [99, 100]. Monoclonal PCs are usually <5%. However, plasmacytosis (>20%) may be present in 5% of the patients). Hyperplastic and atypical megakaryocytes may be seen. In patients with localized disease, biopsy from the iliac crest may be normal [81, 89, 94].

Pathogenesis

The exact etiology of POEMS remains unknown. Several proinflammatory cytokines were found to not only increase in patients with POEMS but also increase in patients with active disease compared with those in remission. This includes interleukins, IL-1B, IL-6, IL-12, and tumor necrosis factor alpha (TNF-alpha) along with VEGF [101, 102]. VEGF appears to be responsible for multiple clinical features such as polyneuropathy, organomegaly, volume overload, increased vascular permeability, angiogenesis, vascular wall thickening, pulmonary hypertension, and papilledema [93, 103–105]. VEGF levels can be used to monitor response to therapy and as a prognostic marker [106]. Despite the importance of VEGF in POEMS syndrome, anti-VEGF (Bevacizumab) failed to show promising results in its treatment [107–112].

Diagnosis

The International Myeloma Group Criteria for diagnosing POEMS requires the presence of both mandatory, one of the major and one of the minor criteria as follows [113]:

Mandatory
1. Polyneuropathy
2. Monoclonal plasma cell proliferation (almost always lambda)

Major

1. Sclerotic bone lesions
2. CD
3. Elevated levels of VEGF (Criteria did not specify a cut off level)

Minor

1. Organomegaly (splenomegaly, hepatomegaly, or lymphadenopathy)
2. Extravascular volume overload (edema, pleural effusion, or ascites)
3. Endocrinopathy (adrenal, thyroid, pituitary, gonadal, parathyroid, pancreas) (Not including diabetes and hypothyroidism)
4. Skin changes (hyperpigmentation, hypertrichosis, glomeruloid hemangioma, plethora, acrocyanosis, flushing, white nails)
5. Papilledema
6. Thrombocytosis and or polycythemia

POEMS Syndrome Versus Other Paraproteinemias

POEMS syndrome differs from other paraproteinemic syndromes in a few aspects. Its predominant symptoms are related to neuropathy, endocrinopathy, and volume overload and not to paraproteinemia, plasma cell infiltration, hypercalcemia, or renal involvement. It is also distinguished by the high VEGF levels and the presence of sclerotic bone lesions [85]. The distinction is important given the difference in treatment and prognosis.

Even when plasma cell proliferation is present, paraproteinemia may not be present in all patients [93, 99, 100]. Serum M protein is usually less than 2 g/dL, and it is usually IgG or IgA with almost always a lambda chain [81, 89]. In less than half of the patients, M protein may be found in urine [89, 114]. However, there are case reports with exceptions such as a case of POEMS with IgM lambda paraprotein, another with bi-clonal IgG lambda and IgA kappa gammopathy and a case with IgG kappa paraprotein [114–117].

Treatment

Given the rarity of the disease, there are no controlled trials and there is no standard treatment. Depending on the extent of PC infiltration and the extent of bony lesions, radiation therapy, chemotherapy, and stem cell transplantation are the main options that can be used for treatment along with supportive measures for various manifestations and organ involvement.

Prognosis is better compared to MM. With treatment, the median survival rate can reach up to 13 years. However, this depends on the clinical presentation as well as the complications and timing of therapy initiation [81, 88, 89, 94].

Gaucher Disease

It is a rare lysosomal storage disease due to glucocerebrosidase (GCase) enzyme deficiency; however, it is more rarely caused by deficiency of saposin C, its activator. This causes glucocerebrosidase, its substrate, to be accumulated in the macrophages. It can be detected in hepatic, splenic, myeloid, cerebral, or pulmonary macrophages [118]. It is inherited in a Mendelian fashion as an autosomally recessive trait [118]. GBA is the gene which encodes GCase enzymes. It comprises 11 exons and is present on the long arm of chromosome 1 (1q21) [119], GD is the most common among sphingolipidoses disorders [120], and it has a broad phenotypic expression, starting from subclinical to fatal forms [121].

GD is classified according to its neurological involvement into three distinct phenotypes:Type 1, the most prevalent type, accounts for 90–95% in western countries and is characterized by inflicting no neurological damage. Type 3 typically causes neurological damage in the form of ophthalmoplegia, epilepsy, myoclonus, ataxia, and/or dementia. Type 2, however, typically manifests early in life by severe nervous system involvement causing damage. It can lead to death in the first three years of life [122].

Generally, patients may express fatigue [123]. They may have splenomegaly, which is sometimes huge [124] and hepatomegaly [125]. Hematological manifestations include bleeding tendency that can rarely be severe and is usually due to thrombocytopenia [126] or rarely due to platelet dysfunction [127] and anemia which is observed in 50% of cases. The majority of cases will show mild to moderate thrombocytopenia and splenomegaly [128]

Bone disorders include avascular necrosis and bone marrow failure [129, 130]. Osteopenia, osteoporosis, and pathological fractures occur more frequently in this group and may be correlated with other complications whether osseous or visceral [131]. There are very rare reports of osteosarcomas, osteoblastomas, or other secondary osseous neoplasms [132].

To confirm the diagnosis, it is mandatory to measure glucosylcerebrosidase activity in total leucocytes, mononuclear cells, or fibroblasts in culture. In GD samples, activity drops to as low as 10–15% of normal [133].

Bone marrow aspirate (BMA) is not a routine procedure. BMA, sometimes, detects the so-called pseudo-Gaucher cells which can't be easily differentiated from true Gaucher cells [134]. They can be found in other hematological conditions or some infections [134]. The list of these associations is summarized in Table 21.1.

Genetic analysis is recommended prenatally [139]. Polyclonal gammaglobulinemia was reported in 25–91% of patients while paraproteins were detected less frequently (1–35% of patients) [140, 141]. These figures, however, reflect different

Table 21.1 Pseudo-Gaucher cells reported associations

Disease	References
MM with histiocytic accumulation of IG crystals	[134]
WM and other lymphomas with paraproteins	[135]
CML	[136]
Myelodysplasia	[137]
Infections like atypical mycobacteria	[138]

MM multiple myeloma, *CML* Chronic myeloid leukemia, *WM* Waldenström's macroglobulinemia, *IG* Immunoglobulin crystals

findings which impact the outcome of therapy on the IG and results in a reduction of the hypergammaglobulins but does not influence the paraproteins [142].

There are two lines of therapy available for GD patients, the first one aims to replenish the cellular GCase enzyme, enzyme replacement therapy (ERT), (imiglucerase, velaglucerase, or taliglucerase) while the second is directed towards the substrate to impede enzymatic biosynthesis. This approach is referred to as substrate reduction therapy (SRT). This includes miglustat and eliglustat [118]. Therapy aims to avoid GD complications like huge organomegaly, cytopenias, or osseous lesions. This, however, is not indicated for all cases.

Several studies provided data in support of an elevated incidence of hematological disorders complicating GD. The list includes gammopathies and hematological malignancies [142–144], amyloidosis, B-cell non-Hodgkin lymphoma (NHL) [143, 145–147], polyclonal gammopathy (PG) [148], and MGUS with a prevalence ranging from 2.2 to 25% [143]. However, in Nguyen et al. series, PG prevalence was 48%, while MG was 32% among their 278 GD cases [121]. In a systematic review by Arends et al., the prevalence of PG and MGUS in GD patients ranged from 25% to 91% and from 0% to 35%, respectively [149]. The incidence of MM is also increased and it ranges from 5.9 to 51.1 times when compared to healthy populations [150].

Currently, we don't have a clear understanding of the pathophysiological mechanisms leading to such IGs aberrations. Investigators proposed many hypotheses to account for the origin of these aberrations [121].

It has been reported that the B lymphocytes in this disease are provoked by certain type II natural killer T cells, which have a T follicular helper profile where the populations in GD as well as in its murine experimental models are targeting glucosyl sphingosine, the deacylated form of glucosylceramide [151, 152], whereas in GD-associated MGUS and MM the clonal IG are directed against the glucocerebrosidase activator, Saposin C [153].

The genesis of MGUS in GD may be attributed to the lingering exposure to undergraded glucocerebroside leading to chronic antigenic provocation. In MM, cells are reported to express a wide range of toll-like receptors (TLRs) which can lend assistance to B lymphocytes in microbial antigen pattern recognition. TLR-specific ligands cause proliferation and survival of MM PCs [154]. Similarly, overexpression of the IL-6 alpha chain has been reported in MGUS PC [155]. As a consequence, dysregulation of TLR expansion and/or an overexpressed IL-6 receptor on PCs may produce an exaggerated response to microbial antigens presenting on IL-6-dependent autocrine trigger for PC to proliferate [156].

Lo et al. also studied the genetic background of GD in two siblings who developed acute lymphoblastic lymphoma. They detected a homozygous mutation in MSH6 leading to DNA repair deficiency syndrome and a homozygous mutation GBA [157].

Paraproteins in GD were studied in small-patient groups, hence, our understanding of their risk factors, clinical importance and development is defective, and its pathophysiology is still controversial [121].

TEMPI Syndrome

In 2010, Bizari et al. [158] described a 49-year-old male patient who presented with erythrocytosis, perinephric fluid collections, and kidney disease failure who had no definite diagnosis. One year later, Sykes and his colleagues described five cases who shared similar features, and they gave it its syndromic entity "TEMPI" standing for Telangiectasias, elevated Erythropoietin (EPO) and erythrocytosis, Monoclonal gammopathy, Perinephric fluid collections, and Intrapulmonary shunting [159].

TEMPI is a rare, acquired disease which in general presents during the fourth or fifth decades of age [160]. It inflicts both genders and has no discernible ethnic or geographic predisposing factors [160]. It has an insidious onset and a slow progressive course [161]. Deep vein thrombosis, MGUS, and MM have been reported in a subset of TEMPI syndrome cases [162]. The syndrome is presumed to be due to PCs proliferation as patients respond dramatically to PC-targeted medications [163].

Table 21.2 Immunoglobulin of 15 case reports of TEMPI syndrome

Investigator	Patient number	Age (years)	Monoclonal band
Sykes et al. (2011) [159]	1	42	IgGκ (0.7 g/dL)
	2	36	IgGκ (0.7 g/dL)
	3	39	IgGκ (0.7 g/dL
	4	35	Not reported
	5	56	IgG
	6	36	Not reported
Schroyens et al. (8) (2012) [164]	7	49	IgGκ
Mohammadi et al. (9) (2012) [165]	8	58	IgAλ (1.4 g/dL)
Kwok et al. (10) (2012) [166]	9	56	IgGλ (3.6 g/dL)
Viglietti et al. (11) (2012) [167]	10	49	IgAλ (0.2 g/dL)
Ryden et al. (12) (2013) [168]	11	50	IgGκ
Jasim et al. (13) (2014) [169]	12	61	IgAλ (1.4 g/dL)
Kenderian et al. (14) (2015) [170]	13	49	IgGκ (1.8 g/dL)
Belizaire et al. (15) (2015) [171]	14	54	IgGκ (0.8 g/dL)
Pascart et al. (16) (2015) [172]	15	65	IgGκ (2.3 g/dL)

IgA immunoglobulin A, *IgG* immunoglobulin G, *κ* kappa light chain, *λ* lambda light chain

There is scant data on its genomic background unlike many PC neoplasms; hence, its pathophysiology evades our understanding. The characteristic feature of the syndrome is the MG [163]. We present 15 patients who were reported in the literature and their IGs characteristics in Table 21.2. In spite of their MG, they lack the CRAB criteria of MM and they have less than 10% PC in their BM at the time of diagnosis [173].

Free light chain levels and free light chain ratios in serum are either normal or only show marginal changes [160]. BM biopsy is similar to that of MGUS or smoldering myeloma, and PCs percentages are mildly elevated (5–10% by immunohistochemistry) [173].

A subset of patients with TEMPI syndrome have developed venous thrombosis as has also been described in patients with MGUS and MM [162].

Flow cytometry is oftentimes the preferred laboratory techniques to confirm PC clonality, which is performed using a broad panel of antibodies [174].

Polycythemia vera (PV) should be differentiated from TEMPI syndrome when erythrocytosis can be the initial manifestation. This is important to avoid wrong diagnosis, mismanagement, and its complications including venesection [170]. More than 95% of PV possess Janus kinase 2 (JAK2) V617F acquired genetic mutation, whereas it is absent in TEMPI syndrome [175]. Also, serum EPO readings in PV cases, along with other types of primary erythrocytosis are low (mean < 3.3 mU/mL), which further helps in the differentiation [173].

Successful management of TEMPI syndrome can lead to dramatic improvement in patients' quality of life [166]. Thalidomide, bevacizumab, and sirolimus were all tried but proved unsuccessful when experimented by Sykes and his group [159]. Bortezomib significantly improved the clinical manifestations and successfully eliminated the MG. This remarkable success was featured in many cases [165, 166, 169]. ASCT can be tried, for eligible cases, when bortezomib-based protocols prove unsuccessful [170]. The benefits of ASCT have to be weighed judiciously against its potential risks mainly infection and autoimmune hemolysis [176].

The successful response to bortezomib therapy, whether partial or complete, in a subgroup of cases lends support to the early presumption that MG is involved in pathophysiology of TEMPI syndrome [164, 166]. Another subgroup responded to ASCT following melphalan [170].

As daratumumab proved successful in clinical trials on MM patients in 2015, it was given approval by the FDA promptly [177]. Sykes and his group reported two cases that showed complete response to daratumumab as a single agent [178]. One of their patients showed incomplete response to three therapeutic regimens in line, IV bortezomib, a combination of bortezomib and lenalidomide ending with ASCT. The second one had received IV bortezomib with recurrence of illness 6 years after complete remission [178]. Treatment with single-agent daratumumab in their two cases proved remarkably successful with elimination of their gammopathies and restoring their hematocrit and EPO readings back to normal while having acceptable safety profile [178].

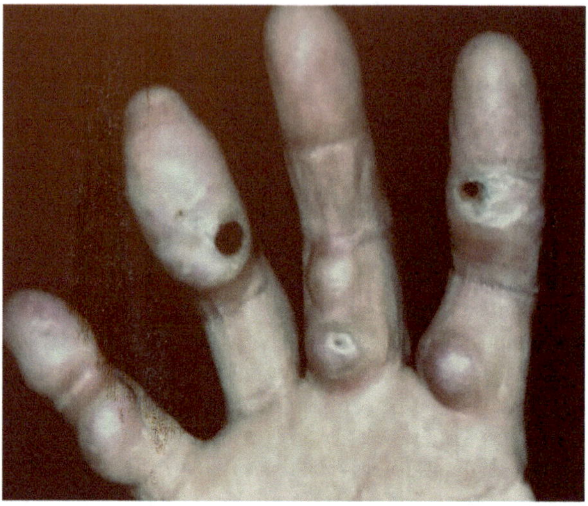

Fig. 21.3 Erythema elevatum diutinum lesions on the palmer aspect of the right hand of a patient. (Courtesy of Dr. Luca Quartuccio, Department of Medicine, University of Udine, School of Rheumatology, Italy)

Erythema Elevatum Diutinum

EED is a peculiar skin condition frequently associated with an underlying medical condition. It was first described by Hutchinson in 1888 [179]. It has no racial predilection and affects mainly adults with only 5.2% of cases affecting patients aged less than 19 years. Men are affected slightly more than women [180].

Clinically, EED is characterized by reddish brown or violaceous nodules and plaques that mainly involve the extensor surfaces of the extremities with dorsal hands being the most frequently involved sites followed by elbows, legs, knees, and feet [180] (Fig. 21.3). Atypical presentations include verrucous lesions [181], vesiculobullous lesions [179, 182], involvement of flexor surfaces, genital, and oral ulcerations [180]. The lesions run a chronic relapsing course, hence the term "diutinum." They are usually asymptomatic, but sometimes patients may experience pain, itching, or associated joint pain [183].

Despite being a chronic disorder, early lesions of EED show histopathological features of acute leukocytoclastic vasculitis with perivascular neutrophilic infiltrates, , endothelial swelling, and fibrin deposition in the wall of small dermal blood vessels, also known as "toxic hyaline". The infiltrate also contains lymphocytes, histiocytes, few eosinophils, and rare extravasated erythrocytes [184]. As lesions progress, neutrophils fill the dermis and basophilic nuclear dust may get encrusted on collagen fibers. Late lesions show variable fibrosis with fascicles of spindle cells, yet small foci of neutrophilic vasculitis can still be seen [184, 185]. Secondary deposition of cholesterol within the lesions have also been reported [179].

The main etiopathogenic mechanism in its development which is the deposition of immune complexes in the wall of small dermal blood vessels. These complexes may develop secondary to infectious agents such as streptococci, TB, and viruses including HIV [180, 186]. EED is also associated with many autoimmune diseases such as systemic lupus erythematosus, rheumatoid arthritis, relapsing polychondritis, Crohn's disease, and celiac disease [179, 186–189] reflecting an effect of immune dysregulation in eliciting the inflammatory reaction that causes the skin lesions. It is also reported in association with internal malignancies especially lymphoma and MM including IgA myeloma [190–192].

The association between EED and paraproteinemia is well established, being most frequently associated with IgA paraproteinemia followed by IgG, IgM, and IgD paraproteinemias [180]. The exact mechanism by which paraproteins contribute to the development of EED is unknown. They can damage the vessels via complement-mediated inflammation. Dermal deposits of IgA have been found in some cases [193]. Patients may develop EED lesions long before the immunoglobulins are elevated and later on, frank myeloma may develop [192]. Accordingly, patients with EED must be routinely monitored by serum immunofixation electrophoresis since it is more sensitive than immunoelectrophoresis in detecting small amounts of immunoglobulins both in serum and urine (16). IgA ANCA was frequently present in patients with EED more than IgG ANCA. It plays a role in neutrophil activation in these cases [194]. Associated diabetes mellitus has been reported [179] and patients with EED may complain of ocular and pulmonary manifestations [195, 196].

Dapsone is the most frequently used therapeutic modality due to its anti-neutrophilic properties. Treatment with dapsone and the resultant clinical response was reported in 75 cases. Of those, 36 patients (48%) achieved full resolution of lesions without relapse, while 24 patients (32%) had a partial response or temporary resolution of disease manifestations. No response to dapsone was reported in only seven cases (9.3%). Furthermore, eight reports described an adverse reaction to dapsone that required discontinuation [180].

Other lines of treatment included topical or systemic corticosteroids [197], topical dapsone 5% [198], colchicine [199], cyclosporine [200], plasma exchange [201], and surgery [202]. Moemen and colleagues [202] proposed an algorithm for the treatment of EED composed of six steps. The first step is targeted treatment of the underlying systemic disorder followed by dapsone monotherapy as the second step, dapsone combined with another agent as the third step, antibiotics as the fourth step, colchicine as the fifth step, and oral steroids as the final step.

Other Associations

The list of paraproteinemias' associations is broad and is incessantly expanding. Beside the entities described in this chapter and the preceding ones, the list includes the following:

- Crystal-storing histiocytosis [203]
- Crystalline keratopathy [204]
- C1 inhibition deficiency [205]

- Bullous skin diseases [206]
- Von Willebrand diseases [207]
- Xanthomatosis [208]
- Systemic capillary leak syndrome [209]
- Scleromyxedema [210]
- Acquired cutis laxa [211]
- Neutrophilic dermatosis [212]
  - Pyoderma gangrenosum
  - Sweet syndrome
  - Subcorneal pustular dermatosis
- Sporadic late onset nemaline myopathy [213]

Conclusion

The discipline of MG, or paraproteinemias, is steadily growing with expanding horizons. With reported entanglements or associations with many other fields, clinicians should be alert to the possibility of its existence in many situations. A deep understanding of the nature and significance of this phenomenon will be extremely rewarding as it will shed light on the pathogenesis, course, and fate of many illnesses. Furthermore, it will offer more therapeutic options with potential benefits.

References

1. Alfano G, Fontana F, Colaci E, et al. Monoclonal gammopathy of undetermined significance after kidney transplantation: single-center experience. Transplantation. 2017;101(11):e337–42.
2. Cuellar-Garcia C, Sevillano Ruiz-Mateos C, Mazuecos Blanca MA, et al. Follow-up monoclonal gammopathy of undetermined significance in kidney transplant. Transplant Proc. 2015;47(1):78–80.
3. Naina HV, Harris S, Dispenzieri A, et al. Long-term follow-up of patients with monoclonal gammopathy of undetermined significance after kidney transplantation. Am J Nephrol. 2012;35(4):365–71.
4. Gagnon MF, Cardinal H, Emond JP, et al. The evolution of monoclonal gammopathy of undetermined significance in kidney transplant recipients. Transplant Direct. 2019;5(10):e489.
5. Caforio AL, Gambino A, Belloni Fortina A, et al. Monoclonal gammopathy in heart transplantation: risk factor analysis and relevance of immunosuppressive load. Transplant Proc. 2001;33(1–2):1583–4.
6. Bhasin B, Szabo A, Wu R, et al. Monoclonal gammopathies after renal transplantation: a single-center study. Clin Lymphoma Myeloma Leuk. 2020;20(8):e468–73.
7. Chakalarovski C, Lang P, Buisson C, et al. Monoclonal immunoglobulins in patients with renal transplants: characterization, evolution and risk factors. Transpl Int. 1992;5(Suppl 1):S23–5.
8. Galioto A, Morando F, Rosi S, et al. Monoclonal gammopathy after liver transplantation: a risk factor for long-term medical complications other than malignancies. Transpl Int. 2012;25(1):25–33.

9. Abrahamian GA, Cosimi AB, Farrell ML, et al. Prevalence of hepatitis C virus-associated mixed cryoglobulinemia after liver transplantation. Liver Transpl. 2000;6(2):185–90.
10. Basse G, Ribes D, Kamar N, et al. Rituximab therapy for mixed cryoglobulinemia in seven renal transplant patients. Transplant Proc. 2006;38(7):2308–10.
11. Hammoud H, Haem J, Laurent B, et al. Glomerular disease during HCV infection in renal transplantation. Nephrol Dial Transplant. 1996;11(Suppl 4):54–5.
12. Sens YA, Malafronte P, Souza JF, et al. Cryoglobulinemia in kidney transplant recipients. Transplant Proc. 2005;37(10):4273–5.
13. Mitus AJ, Stein R, Rappeport JM, et al. Monoclonal and oligoclonal gammopathy after bone marrow transplantation. Blood. 1989;74(8):2764–8.
14. Passweg J, Thiel G, Bock HA. Monoclonal gammopathy after intense induction immunosuppression in renal transplant patients. Nephrol Dial Transplant. 1996;11(12):2461–5.
15. Giordano M, Santangelo L, Scarasciulli ML, et al. Monoclonal gammopathy of undetermined significance in pediatric kidney transplant: a possible role of Epstein-Barr virus. Pediatr Transplant. 2014;18(1):42–6.
16. Mehra V, Rhone E, Widya S, et al. Epstein-Barr virus and monoclonal gammopathy of clinical significance in autologous stem cell transplantation for multiple sclerosis. Clin Infect Dis. 2019;69(10):1757–63.
17. Babel N, Schwarzmann F, Pruss A, et al. Monoclonal gammopathy of undetermined significance (MGUS) is associated with an increased frequency of Epstein-Barr virus (EBV) latently infected B lymphocytes in long-term renal transplant patients. Transplant Proc. 2004;36(9):2679–82.
18. Badley AD, Portela DF, Patel R, et al. Development of monoclonal gammopathy precedes the development of Epstein-Barr virus-induced posttransplant lymphoproliferative disorder. Liver Transpl Surg. 1996;2(5):375–82.
19. Chiusolo P, Metafuni E, Cattani P, et al. Prospective evaluation of Epstein-Barr virus reactivation after stem cell transplantation: association with monoclonal gammopathy. J Clin Immunol. 2010;30(6):894–902.
20. Hestin D, Hussenet F, Frimat L, et al. Hepatitis C after renal transplantation: histopathological correlations. Nephrol Dial Transplant. 1996;11(Suppl 4):52–3.
21. Duvoux C, Tran Ngoc A, Intrator L, et al. Hepatitis C virus (HCV)-related cryoglobulinemia after liver transplantation for HCV cirrhosis. Transpl Int. 2002;15(1):3–9.
22. Fernández EJ, Auyanet I, Guerra R, et al. [Primary cytomegalovirus infection causing a kidney transplant patient to develop cryoagglutinins and cryoglobulins]. Nefrologia. 2010;30(2):267–268.
23. Drouet E, Chapuis-Cellier C, Bosshard S, et al. Oligo-monoclonal immunoglobulins frequently develop during concurrent cytomegalovirus (CMV) and Epstein-Barr virus (EBV) infections in patients after renal transplantation. Clin Exp Immunol. 1999;118(3):465–72.
24. Regamey N, Hess V, Passweg J, et al. Infection with human herpesvirus 8 and transplant-associated gammopathy. Transplantation. 2004;77(10):1551–4.
25. Jimenez-Zepeda VH, Heilman RL, Engel RA, et al. Monoclonal gammopathy of undetermined significance does not affect outcomes in patients undergoing solid organ transplants. Transplantation. 2011;92(5):570–4.
26. Sečník P Jr, Jabor A, Lavríková P, et al. Immunoglobulin abnormalities in 1677 solid organ transplant recipients. Implications for posttransplantation follow-up. Transpl Immunol. 2019;57:101229.
27. Shimoni A, Körbling M, Champlin R, et al. Cryofibrinogenemia and skin necrosis in a patient with diffuse large cell lymphoma after high-dose chemotherapy and autologous stem cell transplantation. Bone Marrow Transplant. 2000;26(12):1343–5.
28. Rayhill SC, Kirby PA, Voigt MD, et al. Positive serum cryoglobulin is associated with worse outcome after liver transplantation for chronic hepatitis C. Transplantation. 2005;80(4):448–56.
29. Rasouli-Arsala J, Huebner TA, Drachenberg CB, et al. Accelerated renal allograft failure due to monoclonal gammopathy of undetermined significance. Transplantation. 2012;93(e27):e26–7.

30. Cadnapaphornchai P, Sillix D. Recurrence of monoclonal gammopathy-related glomerulonephritis in renal allograft. Clin Nephrol. 1989;31(3):156–9.
31. Dysseleer A, Michaux L, Cosyns JP, et al. Benign monoclonal gammopathy turning to AL amyloidosis after kidney transplantation. Am J Kidney Dis. 1999;34(1):166–9.
32. Goebel TE, Schiltz NK, Woodside KJ, et al. Neoplastic and non-neoplastic complications of solid organ transplantation in patients with preexisting monoclonal gammopathy of undetermined significance. Clin Transplant. 2015;29(9):851–7.
33. Nobacht S, Kusters B, Breukink MB, et al. Recurrence of paraproteinemic crystalline keratopathy after corneal transplantation: a case of monoclonal gammopathy of ocular significance. Am J Ophthalmol Case Rep. 2020;19:100803.
34. Felldin M, Ekberg J, Polanska-Tamborek D, et al. Donor monoclonal gammopathy may cause lymphoproliferative disorders in solid organ transplant recipients. Am J Transplant. 2016;16(9):2676–83.
35. Serra N, Revuelta I, Bladé J, et al. Monoclonal gammopathy of undetermined significance: a contraindication for living kidney donation? NDT Plus. 2011;4(4):256–7.
36. Lomas OC, Mouhieddine TH, Tahri S, et al. Monoclonal gammopathy of undetermined significance (MGUS)—not so asymptomatic after all. Cancers (Basel). 2020;12(6):1554.
37. Zemble RM, Takach PA, Levinson AI. The relationship between hypogammaglobulinemia, monoclonal gammopathy of undetermined significance and humoral immunodeficiency: a case series. J Clin Immunol. 2011;31(5):737–43.
38. Lakshminarayanan R, Li Y, Janatpour K, et al. Detection by immunofixation of M proteins in hypogammaglobulinemic patients with normal serum protein electrophoresis results. Am J Clin Pathol. 2007;127(5):746–51.
39. Joshua D, Suen H, Brown R, et al. The T cell in myeloma. Clin Lymphoma Myeloma Leuk. 2016;16(10):537–42.
40. Dosani T, Mailankody S, Korde N, et al. Host-related immunodeficiency in the development of multiple myeloma. Leuk Lymphoma. 2018;59(5):1127–32.
41. Rikhi R, Bhattad S, Jindal A, et al. Monoclonal gammopathy of unclear significance in a child with Wiskott-Aldrich syndrome: a rare occurrence. J Clin Immunol. 2019;39(1):7–10.
42. Pachlopnik Schmid JM, Junge SA, Hossle JP, et al. Transient hemophagocytosis with deficient cellular cytotoxicity, monoclonal immunoglobulin M gammopathy, increased T-cell numbers, and hypomorphic NEMO mutation. Pediatrics. 2006;117(5):e1049–56.
43. McDonald PS, Cora-Bramble D, De Palma L. Monoclonal gammopathy of the immunoglobulin A class in a two-year-old girl with ataxia telangiectasia. Pediatr Dev Pathol. 1998;1(4):319–21.
44. Oehler E, Heuberger L, Ghawche F, et al. Good's syndrome and IgA monoclonal gammopathy of undetermined significance. BMJ Case Rep. 2012;2012:bcr2012007601.
45. Karafin MS, Humphrey RL, Detrick B. Evaluation of monoclonal and oligoclonal gammopathies in a pediatric population in a major urban center. Am J Clin Pathol. 2014;141(4):482–7.
46. Bonilla FA, Barlan I, Chapel H, et al. International Consensus Document (ICON): common variable immunodeficiency disorders. J Allergy Clin Immunol Pract. 2016;4(1):38–59.
47. Weifenbach N, Schneckenburger AAC, Lötters S. Global distribution of common variable immunodeficiency (CVID) in the light of the UNDP human development index (HDI): a preliminary perspective of a rare disease. J Immunol Res. 2020;2020:8416124.
48. Yakaboski E, Fuleihan RL, Sullivan KE, et al. Lymphoproliferative disease in CVID: a report of types and frequencies from a US patient registry. J Clin Immunol. 2020;40(3):524–30.
49. Schroeder HW Jr, Zhu ZB, March RE, et al. Susceptibility locus for IgA deficiency and common variable immunodeficiency in the HLA-DR3, -B8, -A1 haplotypes. Mol Med. 1998;4(2):72–86.
50. Wallage M, Dutton D, Lock RJ. Low immunoglobulin A levels detected via the tissue transglutaminase assay can reveal previously undetected monoclonal proteins. Ann Clin Biochem. 2016;53(Pt 3):409–11.
51. Jäger U, Barcellini W, Broome CM, et al. Diagnosis and treatment of autoimmune hemolytic anemia in adults: recommendations from the First International Consensus Meeting. Blood Rev. 2020;41:100648.

52. Berentsen S, Ulvestad E, Langholm R, et al. Primary chronic cold agglutinin disease: a population based clinical study of 86 patients. Haematologica. 2006;91(4):460–6.
53. Bylsma LC, Gulbech Ording A, Rosenthal A, et al. Occurrence, thromboembolic risk, and mortality in Danish patients with cold agglutinin disease. Blood Adv. 2019;3(20):2980–5.
54. Małecka A, Trøen G, Tierens A, et al. Immunoglobulin heavy and light chain gene features are correlated with primary cold agglutinin disease onset and activity. Haematologica. 2016;101(9):e361–4.
55. Małecka A, Trøen G, Tierens A, et al. Frequent somatic mutations of KMT2D (MLL2) and CARD11 genes in primary cold agglutinin disease. Br J Haematol. 2018;183(5):838–42.
56. Swiecicki PL, Hegerova LT, Gertz MA. Cold agglutinin disease. Blood. 2013;122(7):1114–21.
57. Ulvestad E, Berentsen S, Bø K, et al. Clinical immunology of chronic cold agglutinin disease. Eur J Haematol. 1999;63(4):259–66.
58. Berentsen S. How I manage patients with cold agglutinin disease. Br J Haematol. 2018;181(3):320–30.
59. Berentsen S. New insights in the pathogenesis and therapy of cold agglutinin-mediated autoimmune hemolytic anemia. Front Immunol. 2020;11:590.
60. Randen U, Trøen G, Tierens A, et al. Primary cold agglutinin-associated lymphoproliferative disease: a B-cell lymphoma of the bone marrow distinct from lymphoplasmacytic lymphoma. Haematologica. 2014;99(3):497–504.
61. Berentsen S, Tjønnfjord GE. Diagnosis and treatment of cold agglutinin mediated autoimmune hemolytic anemia. Blood Rev. 2012;26(3):107–15.
62. Linz DH, Tolle SW, Elliot DL. Mycoplasma pneumoniae pneumonia. Experience at a referral center. West J Med. 1984;140(6):895–900.
63. Berlin BS, Chandler R, Green D. Anti-"i" antibody and hemolytic anemia associated with spontaneous cytomegalovirus mononucleosis. Am J Clin Pathol. 1977;67(5):459–61.
64. Luzuriaga K, Sullivan JL. Infectious mononucleosis. N Engl J Med. 2010;362(21):1993–2000.
65. Crisp D, Pruzanski W. B-cell neoplasms with homogeneous cold-reacting antibodies (cold agglutinins). Am J Med. 1982;72(6):915–22.
66. Hoyer KK, Kuswanto WF, Gallo E, et al. Distinct roles of helper T-cell subsets in a systemic autoimmune disease. Blood. 2009;113(2):389–95.
67. Schwartz J, Padmanabhan A, Aqui N, et al. Guidelines on the use of therapeutic apheresis in clinical practice-evidence-based approach from the writing committee of the American Society for Apheresis: the seventh special issue. J Clin Apher. 2016;31(3):149–62.
68. Berentsen S. Rituximab for the treatment of autoimmune cytopenias. Haematologica. 2007;92(12):1589–96.
69. Berentsen S, Randen U, Oksman M, et al. Bendamustine plus rituximab for chronic cold agglutinin disease: results of a Nordic prospective multicenter trial. Blood. 2017;130(4):537–41.
70. Jalink M, Berentsen S, Castillo JJ, et al. Effect of ibrutinib treatment on hemolytic anemia and acrocyanosis in cold agglutinin disease/cold agglutinin syndrome. Blood. 2021;138(20):2002–5.
71. Makishima K, Obara N, Ishitsuka K, et al. High efficacy of eculizumab treatment for fulminant hemolytic anemia in primary cold agglutinin disease. Ann Hematol. 2019;98(4):1031–2.
72. Wouters D, Stephan F, Strengers P, et al. C1-esterase inhibitor concentrate rescues erythrocytes from complement-mediated destruction in autoimmune hemolytic anemia. Blood. 2013;121(7):1242–4.
73. Castleman B, Iverson L, Menendez VP. Localized mediastinal lymphnode hyperplasia resembling thymoma. Cancer. 1956;9(4):822–30.
74. Festen C, Flendrig JA, Schillings PH. [Giant lymphomas]. Ned Tijdschr Geneeskd. 1969;113(43):1918–1919.
75. Frizzera G, Banks PM, Massarelli G, et al. A systemic lymphoproliferative disorder with morphologic features of Castleman's disease. Pathological findings in 15 patients. Am J Surg Pathol. 1983;7(3):211–31.

76. Fajgenbaum DC, Uldrick TS, Bagg A, et al. International, evidence-based consensus diagnostic criteria for HHV-8-negative/idiopathic multicentric Castleman disease. Blood. 2017;129(12):1646–57.
77. Gessain A, Sudaka A, Brière J, et al. Kaposi sarcoma-associated herpes-like virus (human herpesvirus type 8) DNA sequences in multicentric Castleman's disease: is there any relevant association in non-human immunodeficiency virus-infected patients? Blood. 1996;87(1):414–6.
78. Takai K, Nikkuni K, Shibuya H, et al. [Thrombocytopenia with mild bone marrow fibrosis accompanied by fever, pleural effusion, ascites and hepatosplenomegaly]. Rinsho Ketsueki. 2010;51(5):320–5.
79. van Rhee F, Stone K, Szmania S, et al. Castleman disease in the 21st century: an update on diagnosis, assessment, and therapy. Clin Adv Hematol Oncol. 2010;8(7):486–98.
80. Yang D, Zhou X, Zhao Y, et al. A rare case of multicentric Castleman's disease transforms into multiple myeloma and its successful treatment. Cancer Biol Ther. 2018;19(11):949–52.
81. Dispenzieri A, Kyle RA, Lacy MQ, et al. POEMS syndrome: definitions and long-term outcome. Blood. 2003;101(7):2496–506.
82. Kanai K, Sawai S, Sogawa K, et al. Markedly upregulated serum interleukin-12 as a novel biomarker in POEMS syndrome. Neurology. 2012;79(6):575–82.
83. Mandreoli M, Casanova S, Vianelli N, et al. Remission of nephrotic syndrome due to AA amyloidosis and initiation of glomerular repair after surgical resection of localized Castleman's disease. Nephron. 2002;90(3):336–40.
84. Bower M, Newsom-Davis T, Naresh K, et al. Clinical features and outcome in HIV-associated multicentric Castleman's disease. J Clin Oncol. 2011;29(18):2481–6.
85. Dispenzieri A. POEMS syndrome: 2019 update on diagnosis, risk-stratification, and management. Am J Hematol. 2019;94(7):812–27.
86. Dispenzieri A, Fajgenbaum DC. Overview of Castleman disease. Blood. 2020;135(16):1353–64.
87. Bardwick PA, Zvaifler NJ, Gill GN, et al. Plasma cell dyscrasia with polyneuropathy, organomegaly, endocrinopathy, M protein, and skin changes: the POEMS syndrome. Report on two cases and a review of the literature. Medicine (Baltimore). 1980;59(4):311–22.
88. Takatsuki K, Sanada I. Plasma cell dyscrasia with polyneuropathy and endocrine disorder: clinical and laboratory features of 109 reported cases. Jpn J Clin Oncol. 1983;13(3):543–55.
89. Nakanishi T, Sobue I, Toyokura Y, et al. The Crow-Fukase syndrome: a study of 102 cases in Japan. Neurology. 1984;34(6):712–20.
90. Nasu S, Misawa S, Sekiguchi Y, et al. Different neurological and physiological profiles in POEMS syndrome and chronic inflammatory demyelinating polyneuropathy. J Neurol Neurosurg Psychiatry. 2012;83(5):476–9.
91. Wang Y, Huang LB, Shi YH, et al. Characteristics of 1946 cases of POEMS syndrome in Chinese subjects: a literature-based study. Front Immunol. 2019;10:1428.
92. Dispenzieri A. POEMS syndrome. Blood Rev. 2007;21(6):285–99.
93. Brown R, Ginsberg L. POEMS syndrome: clinical update. J Neurol. 2019;266(1):268–77.
94. Soubrier MJ, Dubost JJ, Sauvezie BJ. POEMS syndrome: a study of 25 cases and a review of the literature. French Study Group on POEMS syndrome. Am J Med. 1994;97(6):543–53.
95. Bélec L, Mohamed AS, Authier FJ, et al. Human herpesvirus 8 infection in patients with POEMS syndrome-associated multicentric Castleman's disease. Blood. 1999;93(11):3643–53.
96. Albertí MA, Martinez-Yélamos S, Fernandez A, et al. 18F-FDG PET/CT in the evaluation of POEMS syndrome. Eur J Radiol. 2010;76(2):180–2.
97. Shibuya K, Misawa S, Horikoshi T, et al. Detection of bone lesions by CT in POEMS syndrome. Intern Med. 2011;50(13):1393–6.
98. Pan Q, Li J, Li F, et al. Characterizing POEMS syndrome with 18F-FDG PET/CT. J Nucl Med. 2015;56(9):1334–7.

99. Dao LN, Hanson CA, Dispenzieri A, et al. Bone marrow histopathology in POEMS syndrome: a distinctive combination of plasma cell, lymphoid, and myeloid findings in 87 patients. Blood. 2011;117(24):6438–44.
100. Kulkarni GB, Mahadevan A, Taly AB, et al. Clinicopathological profile of polyneuropathy, organomegaly, endocrinopathy, M protein and skin changes (POEMS) syndrome. J Clin Neurosci. 2011;18(3):356–60.
101. Gherardi RK, Bélec L, Soubrier M, et al. Overproduction of proinflammatory cytokines imbalanced by their antagonists in POEMS syndrome. Blood. 1996;87(4):1458–65.
102. Soubrier M, Dubost JJ, Serre AF, et al. Growth factors in POEMS syndrome: evidence for a marked increase in circulating vascular endothelial growth factor. Arthritis Rheum. 1997;40(4):786–7.
103. Lesprit P, Godeau B, Authier FJ, et al. Pulmonary hypertension in POEMS syndrome: a new feature mediated by cytokines. Am J Respir Crit Care Med. 1998;157(3 Pt 1):907–11.
104. Scarlato M, Previtali SC, Carpo M, et al. Polyneuropathy in POEMS syndrome: role of angiogenic factors in the pathogenesis. Brain. 2005;128(Pt 8):1911–20.
105. Briani C, Fedrigo M, Manara R, et al. Pachymeningeal involvement in POEMS syndrome: MRI and histopathological study. J Neurol Neurosurg Psychiatry. 2012;83(1):33–7.
106. Misawa S, Sato Y, Katayama K, et al. Vascular endothelial growth factor as a predictive marker for POEMS syndrome treatment response: retrospective cohort study. BMJ Open. 2015;5(11):e009157.
107. Badros A, Porter N, Zimrin A. Bevacizumab therapy for POEMS syndrome. Blood. 2005;106(3):1135.
108. Straume O, Bergheim J, Ernst P. Bevacizumab therapy for POEMS syndrome. Blood. 2006;107(12):4972–3; author reply 4973–4.
109. Samaras P, Bauer S, Stenner-Liewen F, et al. Treatment of POEMS syndrome with bevacizumab. Haematologica. 2007;92(10):1438–9.
110. Dietrich PY, Duchosal MA. Bevacizumab therapy before autologous stem-cell transplantation for POEMS syndrome. Ann Oncol. 2008;19(3):595.
111. Ohwada C, Nakaseko C, Sakai S, et al. Successful combination treatment with bevacizumab, thalidomide and autologous PBSC for severe POEMS syndrome. Bone Marrow Transplant. 2009;43(9):739–40.
112. Sekiguchi Y, Misawa S, Shibuya K, et al. Ambiguous effects of anti-VEGF monoclonal antibody (bevacizumab) for POEMS syndrome. J Neurol Neurosurg Psychiatry. 2013;84(12):1346–8.
113. Rajkumar SV, Dimopoulos MA, Palumbo A, et al. International myeloma working group updated criteria for the diagnosis of multiple myeloma. Lancet Oncol. 2014;15(12):e538–48.
114. Abe D, Nakaseko C, Takeuchi M, et al. Restrictive usage of monoclonal immunoglobulin lambda light chain germline in POEMS syndrome. Blood. 2008;112(3):836–9.
115. Romas E, Storey E, Ayers M, et al. Polyneuropathy, organomegaly, endocrinopathy, M-protein and skin change (POEMS) syndrome with IgG kappa paraproteinemia. Pathology. 1992;24(3):217–20.
116. Colaco SM, Miller T, Ruben BS, et al. IgM-lambda paraproteinemia with associated cutaneous lymphoplasmacytic infiltrate in a patient who meets diagnostic criteria for POEMS syndrome. J Am Acad Dermatol. 2008;58(4):671–5.
117. Ham JY, Suh JS, Lee WK, et al. POEMS syndrome with IgG-λ/IgA-κ biclonal gammopathy and abnormal serum free light chain ratio: a case report. Ann Clin Lab Sci. 2015;45(6):702–6.
118. Stirnemann J, Belmatoug N, Camou F, et al. A review of Gaucher disease pathophysiology, clinical presentation and treatments. Int J Mol Sci. 2017;18(2):441.
119. Koprivica V, Stone DL, Park JK, et al. Analysis and classification of 304 mutant alleles in patients with type 1 and type 3 Gaucher disease. Am J Hum Genet. 2000;66(6):1777–86.
120. Scriver CR. The metabolic & molecular bases of inherited disease. New York: McGraw-Hill; 2001.

121. Nguyen Y, Stirnemann J, Lautredoux F, et al. Immunoglobulin abnormalities in Gaucher disease: an analysis of 278 patients included in the French Gaucher Disease Registry. Int J Mol Sci. 2020;21(4):1247.
122. Sidransky E. Gaucher disease: complexity in a "simple" disorder. Mol Genet Metab. 2004;83(1–2):6–15.
123. Kaplan P, Andersson HC, Kacena KA, et al. The clinical and demographic characteristics of nonneuronopathic Gaucher disease in 887 children at diagnosis. Arch Pediatr Adolesc Med. 2006;160(6):603–8.
124. Neudorfer O, Hadas-Halpern I, Elstein D, et al. Abdominal ultrasound findings mimicking hematological malignancies in a study of 218 Gaucher patients. Am J Hematol. 1997;55(1):28–34.
125. Stirnemann J, Vigan M, Hamroun D, et al. The French Gaucher's disease registry: clinical characteristics, complications and treatment of 562 patients. Orphanet J Rare Dis. 2012;7:77.
126. Rosenbaum H. Hemorrhagic aspects of Gaucher disease. Rambam Maimonides Med J. 2014;5(4):e0039.
127. Gillis S, Hyam E, Abrahamov A, et al. Platelet function abnormalities in Gaucher disease patients. Am J Hematol. 1999;61(2):103–6.
128. Thomas AS, Mehta A, Hughes DA. Gaucher disease: haematological presentations and complications. Br J Haematol. 2014;165(4):427–40.
129. Clarke LA, Hollak CE. The clinical spectrum and pathophysiology of skeletal complications in lysosomal storage disorders. Best Pract Res Clin Endocrinol Metab. 2015;29(2):219–35.
130. Marcucci G, Zimran A, Bembi B, et al. Gaucher disease and bone manifestations. Calcif Tissue Int. 2014;95(6):477–94.
131. Pastores GM, Wallenstein S, Desnick RJ, et al. Bone density in Type 1 Gaucher disease. J Bone Miner Res. 1996;11(11):1801–7.
132. Zver S, Bracko M, Andoljsek D. Primary bone angiosarcoma in a patient with Gaucher disease. Int J Hematol. 2010;92(2):374–7.
133. Neufeld EF. Lysosomal storage diseases. Annu Rev Biochem. 1991;60:257–80.
134. Costello R, O'Callaghan T, Sébahoun G. Gaucher disease and multiple myeloma. Leuk Lymphoma. 2006;47(7):1365–8.
135. Robak T, Urbańska-Ryś H, Jerzmanowski P, et al. Lymphoplasmacytic lymphoma with monoclonal gammopathy-related pseudo-Gaucher cell infiltration in bone marrow and spleen—diagnostic and therapeutic dilemmas. Leuk Lymphoma. 2002;43(12):2343–50.
136. Yang HS, Cho KS, Park TS. Chronic myeloid leukemia with marked splenomegaly and pseudo-Gaucher cells. Blood Res. 2013;48(4):241.
137. Stewart AJ, Jones RD. Pseudo-Gaucher cells in myelodysplasia. J Clin Pathol. 1999;52(12):917–8.
138. Busarla SV, Sadruddin FA, Sohani AR. Pseudo-Gaucher cells in disseminated mycobacterial infection. Am J Hematol. 2013;88(2):155.
139. Yoshida S, Kido J, Matsumoto S, et al. Prenatal diagnosis of Gaucher disease using next-generation sequencing. Pediatr Int. 2016;58(9):946–9.
140. Grosbois B, Rose C, Noël E, et al. Gaucher disease and monoclonal gammopathy: a report of 17 cases and impact of therapy. Blood Cells Mol Dis. 2009;43(1):138–9.
141. de Fost M, Out TA, de Wilde FA, et al. Immunoglobulin and free light chain abnormalities in Gaucher disease type I: data from an adult cohort of 63 patients and review of the literature. Ann Hematol. 2008;87(6):439–49.
142. Brautbar A, Elstein D, Pines G, et al. Effect of enzyme replacement therapy on gammopathies in Gaucher disease. Blood Cells Mol Dis. 2004;32(1):214–7.
143. de Fost M, Vom Dahl S, Weverling GJ, et al. Increased incidence of cancer in adult Gaucher disease in Western Europe. Blood Cells Mol Dis. 2006;36(1):53–8.
144. Jurecka A, Gregorek H, Kleinotiene G, et al. Gaucher disease and dysgammaglobulinemia: a report of 61 patients, including 18 with GD type III. Blood Cells Mol Dis. 2011;46(1):85–7.
145. Paulson JA, Marti GE, Fink JK, et al. Richter's transformation of lymphoma complicating Gaucher's disease. Hematol Pathol. 1989;3(2):91–6.

146. Haran MZ, Feldberg E, Berrebi A. Incidental diagnosis of Gaucher's disease in an elderly patient with lymphoma. Leuk Lymphoma. 2001;40(3–4):445–6.
147. Bertram HC, Eldibany M, Padgett J, et al. Splenic lymphoma arising in a patient with Gaucher disease. A case report and review of the literature. Arch Pathol Lab Med. 2003;127(e245):e242–5.
148. Ayto R, Hughes DA. Gaucher disease and myeloma. Crit Rev Oncog. 2013;18(3):247–68.
149. Arends M, van Dussen L, Biegstraaten M, et al. Malignancies and monoclonal gammopathy in Gaucher disease; a systematic review of the literature. Br J Haematol. 2013;161(6):832–42.
150. Rosenbloom BE, Weinreb NJ, Zimran A, et al. Gaucher disease and cancer incidence: a study from the Gaucher Registry. Blood. 2005;105(12):4569–72.
151. Nair S, Boddupalli CS, Verma R, et al. Type II NKT-TFH cells against Gaucher lipids regulate B-cell immunity and inflammation. Blood. 2015;125(8):1256–71.
152. Nair S, Branagan AR, Liu J, et al. Clonal immunoglobulin against lysolipids in the origin of myeloma. N Engl J Med. 2016;374(6):555–61.
153. Preuss KD, Hollak CEM, Fadle N, et al. Saposin C is a frequent target of paraproteins in Gaucher disease-associated MGUS/multiple myeloma. Br J Haematol. 2019;184(3):384–91.
154. Jego G, Bataille R, Geffroy-Luseau A, et al. Pathogen-associated molecular patterns are growth and survival factors for human myeloma cells through Toll-like receptors. Leukemia. 2006;20(6):1130–7.
155. Pérez-Andrés M, Almeida J, Martín-Ayuso M, et al. Clonal plasma cells from monoclonal gammopathy of undetermined significance, multiple myeloma and plasma cell leukemia show different expression profiles of molecules involved in the interaction with the immunological bone marrow microenvironment. Leukemia. 2005;19(3):449–55.
156. Rajkumar SV. Multiple myeloma. Curr Probl Cancer. 2009;33(1):7–64.
157. Lo SM, Choi M, Liu J, et al. Phenotype diversity in type 1 Gaucher disease: discovering the genetic basis of Gaucher disease/hematologic malignancy phenotype by individual genome analysis. Blood. 2012;119(20):4731–40.
158. Bazari H, Attar EC, Dahl DM, et al. Case records of the Massachusetts General Hospital. Case 23-2010. A 49-year-old man with erythrocytosis, perinephric fluid collections, and renal failure. N Engl J Med. 2010;363(5):463–75.
159. Sykes DB, Schroyens W, O'Connell C. The TEMPI syndrome—a novel multisystem disease. N Engl J Med. 2011;365(5):475–7.
160. Sykes DB, O'Connell C, Schroyens W. The TEMPI syndrome. Blood. 2020;135(15):1199–203.
161. Swerdlow SH, Campo E, Harris NL, Jaffe ES, Pileri SA, Stein H, Thiele J. WHO classification of tumours of haematopoietic and lymphoid tissues. Lyon: International Agency for Research on Cancer; 2008.
162. Kristinsson SY, Pfeiffer RM, Björkholm M, et al. Arterial and venous thrombosis in monoclonal gammopathy of undetermined significance and multiple myeloma: a population-based study. Blood. 2010;115(24):4991–8.
163. Zhang X, Fang M. TEMPI syndrome: erythrocytosis in plasma cell dyscrasia. Clin Lymphoma Myeloma Leuk. 2018;18(11):724–30.
164. Schroyens W, O'Connell C, Sykes DB. Complete and partial responses of the TEMPI syndrome to bortezomib. N Engl J Med. 2012;367(8):778–80.
165. Mohammadi F, Wolverson MK, Bastani B. A new case of TEMPI syndrome. Clin Kidney J. 2012;5(6):556–8.
166. Kwok M, Korde N, Landgren O. Bortezomib to treat the TEMPI syndrome. N Engl J Med. 2012;366(19):1843–5.
167. Viglietti D, Sverzut JM, Peraldi MN. Perirenal fluid collections and monoclonal gammopathy. Nephrol Dial Transplant. 2012;27(1):448–9.
168. Ryden A, Wei K, Rodriguez R, et al. Too much blood: a case of the newly described TEMPI syndrome. Chest. 2013;144(4):927A.
169. Jasim S, Mahmud G, Bastani B, et al. Subcutaneous bortezomib for treatment of TEMPI syndrome. Clin Lymphoma Myeloma Leuk. 2014;14(6):e221–3.

170. Kenderian SS, Rosado FG, Sykes DB, et al. Long-term complete clinical and hematological responses of the TEMPI syndrome after autologous stem cell transplantation. Leukemia. 2015;29(12):2414–6.
171. Belizaire R, Sykes DB, Chen YB, et al. Difficulties in hematopoietic progenitor cell collection from a patient with TEMPI syndrome and severe iatrogenic iron deficiency. Transfusion. 2015;55(9):2142–8.
172. Pascart T, Herbaux C, Lemaire A, et al. Coexistence of rheumatoid arthritis and TEMPI syndrome: new insight in microangiogenic-related diseases. Joint Bone Spine. 2016;83(5):587–8.
173. Rosado FG, Oliveira JL, Sohani AR, et al. Bone marrow findings of the newly described TEMPI syndrome: when erythrocytosis and plasma cell dyscrasia coexist. Mod Pathol. 2015;28(3):367–72.
174. Stetler-Stevenson M, Paiva B, Stoolman L, et al. Consensus guidelines for myeloma minimal residual disease sample staining and data acquisition. Cytometry B Clin Cytom. 2016;90(1):26–30.
175. Malhotra J, Kremyanskaya M, Schorr E, et al. Coexistence of myeloproliferative neoplasm and plasma-cell dyscrasia. Clin Lymphoma Myeloma Leuk. 2014;14(1):31–6.
176. Zeher M, Papp G, Szodoray P. Autologous haemopoietic stem cell transplantation for autoimmune diseases. Expert Opin Biol Ther. 2011;11(9):1193–201.
177. Lokhorst HM, Plesner T, Laubach JP, et al. Targeting CD38 with daratumumab monotherapy in multiple myeloma. N Engl J Med. 2015;373(13):1207–19.
178. Sykes DB, Schroyens W. Complete responses in the TEMPI syndrome after treatment with daratumumab. N Engl J Med. 2018;378(23):2240–2.
179. Haber H. Erythema elevatum diutinum. Br J Dermatol. 1955;67(4):121–45.
180. Doktor V, Hadi A, Hadi A, et al. Erythema elevatum diutinum: a case report and review of literature. Int J Dermatol. 2019;58(4):408–15.
181. Barzegar M, Davatchi CC, Akhyani M, et al. An atypical presentation of erythema elevatum diutinum involving palms and soles. Int J Dermatol. 2009;48(1):73–5.
182. Agusti-Mejias A, Messeguer-Badia F, Rodriguez M, et al. Erythema elevatum diutinum mimicking a vesiculobullous disease. Int J Dermatol. 2011;50(9):1126–8.
183. Wilkinson SM, English JS, Smith NP, et al. Erythema elevatum diutinum: a clinicopathological study. Clin Exp Dermatol. 1992;17(2):87–93.
184. Caputo R, Alessi E. Unique aspects of a lesion of erythema elevatum diutinum. Am J Dermatopathol. 1984;6(5):465–9.
185. LeBoit PE, Yen TS, Wintroub B. The evolution of lesions in erythema elevatum diutinum. Am J Dermatopathol. 1986;8(5):392–402.
186. Wahl CE, Bouldin MB, Gibson LE. Erythema elevatum diutinum: clinical, histopathologic, and immunohistochemical characteristics of six patients. Am J Dermatopathol. 2005;27(5):397–400.
187. Chan Y, Mok CC, Tang WY. Erythema elevatum diutinum in systemic lupus erythematosus. Rheumatol Int. 2011;31(2):259–62.
188. Orteu CH, McGregor JM, Whittaker SJ, et al. Erythema elevatum diutinum and Crohn disease: a common pathogenic role for measles virus? Arch Dermatol. 1996;132(12):1523–5.
189. Rodriguez-Serna M, Fortea JM, Perez A, et al. Erythema elevatum diutinum associated with celiac disease: response to a gluten-free diet. Pediatr Dermatol. 1993;10(2):125–8.
190. Futei Y, Konohana I. A case of erythema elevatum diutinum associated with B-cell lymphoma: a rare distribution involving palms, soles and nails. Br J Dermatol. 2000;142(1): 116–9.
191. Albitar S, Bourgeon B, Genin R, et al. POEMS syndrome, steroid-dependent diabetes mellitus, erythema elevatum diutinum, and rheumatoid arthritis as extramedullary manifestations of plasma cell dyscrasia. Am J Kidney Dis. 1998;31(4):E3.
192. Archimandritis AJ, Fertakis A, Alegakis G, et al. Erythema elevatum diutinum and IgA myeloma: an interesting association. Br Med J. 1977;2(6087):613–4.
193. Chowdhury MM, Inaloz HS, Motley RJ, et al. Erythema elevatum diutinum and IgA paraproteinaemia: 'a preclinical iceberg'. Int J Dermatol. 2002;41(6):368–70.

194. Crichlow SM, Alexandroff AB, Simpson RC, et al. Is IgA antineutrophil cytoplasmic antibody a marker for patients with erythema elevatum diutinum? A further three cases demonstrating this association. Br J Dermatol. 2011;164(3):675–7.
195. Takiwaki H, Kubo Y, Tsuda H, et al. Peripheral ulcerative keratitis associated with erythema elevatum diutinum and a positive rheumatoid factor: a report of three cases. Br J Dermatol. 1998;138(5):893–7.
196. Creus L, Salleras M, Sola MA, et al. Erythema elevatum diutinum associated with pulmonary infiltrates. Br J Dermatol. 1997;137(4):652–3.
197. Cordier JF, Faure M, Hermier C, et al. Pleural effusions in an overlap syndrome of idiopathic hypereosinophilic syndrome and erythema elevatum diutinum. Eur Respir J. 1990;3(1):115–8.
198. Frieling GW, Williams NL, Lim SJ, et al. Novel use of topical dapsone 5% gel for erythema elevatum diutinum: safer and effective. J Drugs Dermatol. 2013;12(4):481–4.
199. Maruthappu T, Tharakaram S, Calonje E, et al. Erythema elevatum diutinum with oral ulceration. Br J Dermatol. 2012;167(1):222–4.
200. Takahashi H, Fukami Y, Honma M, et al. Successful combination therapy with dapsone and cyclosporine for erythema elevatum diutinum with unusual appearance. J Dermatol. 2012;39(5):486–7.
201. Chow RK, Benny WB, Coupe RL, et al. Erythema elevatum diutinum associated with IgA paraproteinemia successfully controlled with intermittent plasma exchange. Arch Dermatol. 1996;132(11):1360–4.
202. Zacaron LH, Gonçalves JC, Curty VM, et al. Clinical and surgical therapeutic approach in erythema elevatum diutinum—case report. An Bras Dermatol. 2013;88(6 Suppl 1):15–8.
203. Kanagal-Shamanna R, Xu-Monette ZY, Miranda RN, et al. Crystal-storing histiocytosis: a clinicopathological study of 13 cases. Histopathology. 2016;68(4):482–91.
204. Milman T, Kao AA, Chu D, et al. Paraproteinemic keratopathy: the expanding diversity of clinical and pathologic manifestations. Ophthalmology. 2015;122(9):1748–56.
205. Gobert D, Paule R, Ponard D, et al. A nationwide study of acquired C1-inhibitor deficiency in France: characteristics and treatment responses in 92 patients. Medicine (Baltimore). 2016;95(33):e4363.
206. Aractingi S, Bachmeyer C, Prost C, et al. Subepidermal autoimmune bullous skin diseases associated with B-cell lymphoproliferative disorders. Medicine (Baltimore). 1999;78(4):228–35.
207. Dicke C, Schneppenheim S, Holstein K, et al. Distinct mechanisms account for acquired von Willebrand syndrome in plasma cell dyscrasias. Ann Hematol. 2016;95(6):945–57.
208. Szalat R, Arnulf B, Karlin L, et al. Pathogenesis and treatment of xanthomatosis associated with monoclonal gammopathy. Blood. 2011;118(14):3777–84.
209. Druey KM, Parikh SM. Idiopathic systemic capillary leak syndrome (Clarkson disease). J Allergy Clin Immunol. 2017;140(3):663–70.
210. James K, Fudenberg H, Epstein WL, et al. Studies on a unique diagnostic serum globulin in papular mucinosis (lichen myxedematosus). Clin Exp Immunol. 1967;2(2):153–66.
211. Jachiet M, Harel S, Saussine A, et al. Cutis laxa associated with monoclonal gammopathy: 14 new cases and review of the literature. J Am Acad Dermatol. 2018;79(5):945–7.
212. Szalat R, Monsel G, Le Goff W, et al. The spectrum of neutrophilic dermatoses associated with monoclonal gammopathy: association with IgA isotype and inflammatory profile. J Am Acad Dermatol. 2015;73(5):809–20.
213. Uruha A, Benveniste O. Sporadic late-onset nemaline myopathy with monoclonal gammopathy of undetermined significance. Curr Opin Neurol. 2017;30(5):457–63.

Part III
Experimental Therapies

Chapter 22
Novel and Experimental Clone-Directed Therapies

Mohamed Elemary and Ibraheem Othman

Abbreviations

Abs	Antibodies
ACT	Adoptive cell transfer
ADC	Antibody-drug conjugate
ADCC	Antibody-dependent cellular cytotoxicity
ADCP	Antibody-dependent cellular phagocytosis
APRIL	A proliferation-inducing ligand
ASCT	Autologous stem cell transplantation
ATRA	All-trans retinoic acid
BAFF	B-cell activation factor
BCMA	B-cell mutation antigen
BiTE	Bispecific-T-cell engagers
BM	Bone marrow
BTK	Bruton's tyrosine kinase
CAR-T	Chimeric antigen receptor-T cells
CDC	Complement-dependent cytotoxicity
Cilta-Cel	Ciltacabtagene Autoleucel
CR	Complete remission
CRS	Cytokine release syndrome

M. Elemary (✉)
Saskatoon Cancer Centre and College of Medicine, University of Saskatchewan, Saskatoon, SK, Canada
e-mail: mohamed.elemary@saskcancer.ca

I. Othman
Alain Blair Cancer Centre and College of Medicine, University of Saskatchewan, Saskatoon, SK, Canada
e-mail: Ibraheem.othman@saskcancer.ca

© The Author(s), under exclusive license to Springer Nature Switzerland AG 2022

G. Ragab et al. (eds.), *Paraproteinemia and Related Disorders*,
https://doi.org/10.1007/978-3-031-10131-1_22

CTLA-4	Cytotoxic T lymphocyte antigen-4
CXCR4	C-X-C Motif Chemokine Receptor 4
DoR	Duration of response
DXM	Dexamethasone
eEF1A2	Elongation factor 1-α 2
ICD	Immunogenic cell death
Ide-Cel	Idecabtagene Vicleucel
IDR	Ixazomib, dexamethasone, and rituximab
IMiDs	Immunomodulatory drugs
KarMMa	Clinical study of Ide-Cel
mABs	Monoclonal antibodies
MC	Myeloma cell
MIg	Monoclonal immunoglobulin
MM	Multiple myeloma
MRD	Minimal residual disease
MYD88	Toll-like receptor MYD88 protein
NF- κB	Nuclear factor κB
NK	Natural killer
ORR	Overall response rate
Orva-Cel	Orvacabtagene Autoleucel
OS	Overall survival
PC	Plasma cells
PFS	Progression-free survival
PI3K	Phosphatidylinositol 3-kinase
PIs	Proteasome inhibitors
R/R	Relapsed refractory
Rd	Revlimid and dexamethasone
RRMM	Relapsed refractory multiple myeloma
TLR	Toll-like receptor
VGPR	Very good partial response
WHIM	Warts, hypogammaglobulinemia, infections, and myelokathexis syndrome
WM	Waldenström macroglobulinemia
WT	Wild type
XPO-1	Exportin-1

Introduction

Most of the clonal disorders are either malignant or premalignant and often result in incurable diseases. By virtue of their by-products, they result in organ damage. Therefore, treatment should aim to preserve or improve organ function by targeting the monoclonal immunoglobulin (MIg)-producing plasma or B-cell clone. Although many disorders are not associated with an evidently malignant clone per se, and as in cases of overt malignancy, current evidence strongly supports a clone-directed therapy strategy. The best results are possibly achieved when targeting the underlying clone induces the most profound hematologic response [1]. The isotype of the underlying clone in the bone marrow (BM) (IgG, IgA, or LCs only versus IgM clone), the renal metabolism, and potential renal and neurological toxicity of the therapeutic protocol will guide the treatment strategy [2].

A-Plasma Cell Clone and Multiple Myeloma

Multiple myeloma (MM) is the second most frequent hematological malignancy. It often represents an evolution from the premalignant, monoclonal gammopathy of undetermined significance (MGUS). The development of end-organ damage signals this progression. The proliferation of aberrant plasma cells (PC) in the complex BM microenvironment leads to a genetically complex and heterogeneous disease [3]. Many secondary genetic events have been reported leading to increased cell cycling, the loss of cell cycle arrest or aberrant signaling that provides many prosurvival and growth signals to MM cells [4, 5]. Over the last decade, the knowledge about the different cellular expressions and bone marrow microenvironmental changes in MM patients and the characteristics of PCs lead to the development of many new therapeutic agents (Chap. 4). Proteasome inhibitors (PIs), immunomodulatory drugs (IMiDs), conventional chemotherapeutic agents, and monoclonal antibodies (mAbs) are now routinely administered to patients in different combinations alone or in conjunction with high-dose therapy followed by autologous stem cell transplantation (ASCT). Nowadays, treatment is almost tailored to individual patients with significant improvement in outcomes. Despite this, MM is still considered an incurable disease. Patients will go into remissions, alternating with relapse/progression episodes and eventually culminating into a resistant disease. Patients who become refractory to PIs, IMiDs, and mAbs are particularly at risk of inferior outcomes [6, 7].

With a better understanding of the cellular mechanisms involved in MM, many new agents are being developed to address this incurable disease. These could be classified into medications targeting the aberrant PCs and others affecting the bone marrow milieu.

Agents Targeting Aberrant Plasma Cells

Plasma cells have characteristic clusters of differentiations studded on their membrane. Both normal and aberrant plasma cells express CD38 (bright) and CD138, which are more specific but less sensitive. Normal peripheral blood plasma cells are CD45+. Two subsets of plasma cells coexist in the bone marrow: one major CD45 positive and a smaller negative one. Coexpression of bright CD38 with CD56 identifies abnormal populations of PCs by flow cytometry.

In contrast to normal plasma cells, abnormal plasma cells are also CD19, whereas normal and abnormal plasma cells do not express CD20. Combined assessment of CD38 and CD138 identifies BM plasma cells (PC) [8].

In contrast, more heterogeneous lists of markers are used to further distinguish between normal/reactive PCs and myeloma PCs. Among the later markers, CD19, CD45, CD27, and CD81, together with CD56, CD117, CD200, and CD307, have emerged as particularly informative with no single marker providing enough specificity for clear discrimination. Combined assessment of CD138 and CD38, together with CD45, CD19, CD56, CD27, CD81, and CD117, would ideally suit minimal residual disease (MRD) monitoring in most MM patients [9]. Furthermore, MM cells express SLAMF7, which is targeted by elotuzumab currently used for MM treatment.

Daratumumab is a targeted therapy (IgG1k human monoclonal antibody) that targets CD38. It is currently widely used in standard treatment protocols of MM [10, 11]. Furthermore, MM cells express SLAMF7, which is targeted by elotuzumab. It yielded superior response rates and PFS when combined with lenalidomide/dexamethasone as part of many standard protocols. Many new experimental monoclonal antibodies are being developed targeting cell surface antigens. Interestingly, many other approaches are being experimented, focusing on other surface or intracellular targets directly or an intermediate target to deliver cytotoxic agents avoiding toxicity to non-target tissues.

In their detailed, comprehensive review, Leow and Low (2021) reviewed the biology of plasma cell neoplasm and the potential targets of the new therapeutic agents [12].

Experimental Monoclonal Antibodies Against Cell Surface Antigens

Targeting CD 38

Since CD38 is highly expressed on malignant plasma cells with a minimal expression on normal lymphoid and myeloid cells, its role in cell signaling has made it an attractive antibody target [13]. Interestingly, all-trans retinoic acid (ATRA) increased CD38 expression levels and reduced expression of the complement-inhibitory proteins CD55 and CD59 in both cell lines and primary MM cells in vitro.

Isatuximab is a chimeric monoclonal antibody that binds to CD38, leading to cell death via different mechanisms. It leads to direct apoptosis, triggers antibody-dependent cellular cytotoxicity (ADCC), complement-dependent cytotoxicity (CDC), and antibody-dependent cellular phagocytosis (ADCP) [14]. Antimyeloma activity is enhanced when Isatuximab is combined with pomalidomide or PIs such as bortezomib or carfilzomib [15].

MOR202, on the other hand, is a bispecific antibody that binds to CD38 on myeloma cells and natural killer (NK) cells, leading to the destruction of myeloma cells. MOR202 showed safety and efficacy [16] and is currently being assessed in phase III trial in relapsed refractory MM (RRMM).

Other mAbs under development targeting CD 38 include TAK-079, TAK-169, and TAK 573, tested in Phase 1 trials [17–19].

Targeting CD 138

CD138 is expressed on malignant plasma cells. Indatuximab ravtansine binds to CD138, causing cell cycle arrest via tubulin binding followed by apoptosis [20]. It showed limited efficacy as a single agent but promising activity when combined with Lenalidomide or Pomalidomide [21]. VIS832 is another novel CD138-targeting monoclonal antibody that showed synergism with IMiDs or bortezomib in vitro and in vivo. It is currently tested in clinical trials [22].

B-Cell Maturation Antigen (BCMA)

Mature B lymphocytes preferentially express BCMA. Its overexpression and activation are associated with MM in preclinical models and humans, supporting its potential utility as a therapeutic target. Moreover, it is considered a prognostic biomarker [23]. It has no expression on naïve and memory B lymphocytes, T cells, and other nonlymphoid organs. It promotes myeloma cell growth, chemotherapy resistance, and survival of neoplastic plasma cells by

interacting with overexpressed intracellular receptors for a proliferation-inducing ligand (APRIL) and B-cell activating factor (BAFF) that protect myeloma cells from apoptosis [24, 25]. Thus, BCMA is an attractive target and can be addressed by antibody-drug conjugate (ADC), bispecific T-cell engagers (BiTE), or CAR-T.

Antibody-Drug Conjugates (ADCs)

ADCs represent a new class of target therapy in the management of MM. They deliver cytotoxic agents into MM cells, leading to targeted tumor cell lysis with reduced toxicity in non-targeted tissues. They are usually composed of three elements: an mAb, a linker connecting the drug to the antibody, and the cytotoxic drug [26].

Belantamab Mafodotin (Belamaf) is a humanized IgG1 ADC conjugated with the potent antimitotic agent maleimidocaproyl monomethyl auristatin. It binds specifically to BCMA and is the first in this class of ADCs. It can induce cell death by multiple mechanisms, including ADC and internalize into the cell after binding it, ADCC and ICD (immunogenic cell death) through the expression of antigens specific to dying tumor cells [26].

It showed efficacy as a single agent in the DREAMM-2 study with a clinically meaningful overall response rate (ORR) of 31% in patients who had received a median of seven prior lines of treatment ($n = 97$). Although the median duration of response (DoR) was not reached at the 6-month analysis, 73% of responders had a DoR equal to or greater than 6 months. However, severe ocular adverse events occurred commonly in 77% of the 218 patients. They ranged from keratopathy to changes in visual acuity, blurred vision and dry eye. Ocular adverse events lead to treatment discontinuation in 2.1% of patients [27].

Belantamab Mafodotin is currently under many phases II and III clinical trials as a single agent or combination in newly diagnosed and relapsed MM and was recently approved by the European licensing authorities [26].

Other ADCs against BCMA such as MED12228, CC-99712, AMG-224, and HDP-101 are under phase I/II clinical trials.

Bispecific Antibodies and Bispecific T-Cell Engagers (BiTE)

Bispecific monoclonal antibodies consist of an Fc domain, a Fab region (including a variable domain and a constant domain) and two binding sites, one for CD3 on T cells and the other for the specific target on cancer cells. The binding of the bispecific Abs activates cytotoxic T cells and promotes the killing of tumor cells.

On the other hand, bispecific T-cell engagers (BiTE) differ in the presence of two single-chain variable fragments connected by a linker and the lack of the Fc domain, which gives them a short half-life requiring frequent or continuous dosing [28].

Most of the agents in this class target BCMA on the myeloma cell and bind to CD3 found on the surface of T cells with multiple BCMA bispecific including Elranatamab and Teclistamab and BiTE antibodies currently under clinical development; most, however, are still in phase I dose-escalation or phase II trials [29]. Teclistamab was tested in the relapsed refractory setting [30].

Promising phase I trials as a single agent with an acceptable toxicity profile has led to combining BCMA targeting BiTE antibodies in combination with standard therapies [29, 30].

Chimeric Antigen Receptor-T Cell (CAR T) Therapy

Adoptive cell transfer (ACT) is a rapidly emerging immunotherapy approach for treating cancer and hematologic malignancies. Patients' own immune cells are collected and redirected to treat their cancer. As its name implies, the backbone of CAR T-cell therapy is T cells. It represents the new frontier in treating hematologic malignancies, and it consists of genetically modified T cells to induce cytotoxic ability by targeting specific tumor antigens [31].

An ideal target for CARs is a surface antigen that is uniformly expressed on tumor cells but not on normal cells to minimize toxicity [32]. In MM cells, this requirement is ideal in the BCMA to be the target antigen on malignant plasma cells [33].

Idecabtagene Vicleucel (Ide-Cel)

Idecabtagene vicleucel (ide-cel, bb2121) is a CAR-T product against BCMA with a lentiviral vector. In a phase I trial (CRB-401) in RRMM patients who have gone through a median of five prior lines of therapy. It showed good efficacy with an overall response rate (ORR) of 85% and a complete remission (CR) achieved in 45% of cases. The median progression-free survival (PFS) was 11.3 months [34]. Neutropenia and thrombocytopenia were the most common adverse events noted. Cytokine release syndrome (CRS) developed in more than two-thirds of cases.

Ide-cel was also evaluated in phase II pivotal KarMMa study in 128 heavily pretreated patients who failed at least three previous regimens, including a proteasome inhibitor, an immunomodulatory agent, and an anti-CD38 antibody. At a median follow-up of 13.3 months, ORR was achieved in 73, with CR in 33% of cases. With MRD negativity in 26% of cases. Patients who received higher doses of CAR-T cells had a better response and PFS. CRS and cytopenias were the most reported side effects [35].

Ide-cel is currently being investigated in Phase III KarMMa-3 trial (NCT03651128), comparing ide-cel with standard regimens in RRMM and Phase I KarMMa-4 (NCT04196491) is a study of ide-cel in patients with high-risk newly diagnosed MM.

Ciltacabtagene Autoleucel (Cilta-Cel, JNJ-4528)

LCAR-B38M (JNJ-4528), also known as Ciltacabtagene Autoleucel (Cilta-Cel), is a CAR-T cell with two BCMA-targeting single-domain antibodies. The LEGEND-2 phase I study [36] showed a remarkable response with an ORR of 88%, median PFS of 19.9 months, and median overall survival (OS) of 36.1 months. CRS grade 3 occurred in 7%.

CARTITUDE-1 study [34], a phase 1b/ 2 study, evaluated Cilta-cel in 97 patients who received three or more previous lines of therapy that had failed PIs, IMiDs, and anti-CD 38 mAbs. The ORR was 97% in the study, with 67% of patients achieving a stringent complete response. The OS rate was 89% [37].

The safety profile was consistent with LEGEND-2, with mainly grade 3–4 cytopenias resolved after 60 days. In contrast, the CRS occurred in 95% of patients (4% were grade 3 or 4), with a median time to onset of 7 days and median duration of 4.0 days. Neurotoxicity occurred in 21% of cases [36, 37].

Orvacabtagene Autoleucel (Orva-Cel, JCAR-H125)

Orva-cel is another BCMA CAR-T cell with a fully human binder and a manufacturing process enriching the central memory T-cell phenotype. The phase I/II EVOLVE study [38] showed promising results in 62 heavily pretreated RRMM who have received a median of six previous lines of therapy. ORR was 92%, with 68% achieving a very good partial response (VGPR) and 36% CR.

Orva-cell safety profile was reasonable, with the most common side effects being hematologic cytopenias. Grade 3–4 CRS and neurotoxicity occurred only in 3% and 2%, respectively.

Other CAR-T Cell Products

Several other BCMA-targeted CAR-T cell products are under investigation in phase I/II studies with promising efficacy and safety data [39–42].

Targeting Intracellular Aminopeptidases

Melphalan is a classic alkylating agent commonly used in treating MM. It inhibits DNA and RNA synthesis, causing the death of both dividing and non-dividing tumor cells and has been used to treat MM since the 1960s. It is the agent of choice for conditioning before ASCT.

Melphalan-flufenamide (Melflufen) is a first-in-class peptide-drug conjugate targeting intracellular aminopeptidases [43]. Being highly lipophilic, it passively diffuses across the cellular membrane to bind aminopeptidases and releases melphalan which remains inside the hydrophilic cells. It penetrates the nucleus and induces DNA damage leading to cellular apoptosis [44].

Phase I/II studies showed promising results with ORR in the range of 70% in heavily pretreated RRMM [45–48]. Phase III trials are undergoing.

Inhibitor of Nuclear Cytoplasmic Transport Receptors: Exportin 1

Aberrant plasma cells overexpress exportin-1 (XPO-1), the principal regulator of intracellular oncoprotein transport [49]. It induces nuclear retention of tumor suppression protein and suppresses oncoprotein expression [50]. Selinexor is a potent oral XPO-1 inhibitor that was investigated in clinical trials as monotherapy or in combinations. Phase III BOSTON trial compared bortezomib-dexamethasone with or without selinexor in 402 pretreated patients who received one to three prior lines. Triplet therapy containing selinexor showed significantly better PFS. The main toxicities were hematologic and gastrointestinal [51].

Cereblon E3 Ligase Modulators (CELMoDs)

Cereblon E3 ligase modulators (CELMoDs) represent a novel category of agents in the management of RRMM. Like IMiDs, such as lenalidomide or pomalidomide, they mediate their anti-myeloma activity via cereblon that degrades Ikaros and Aiolos.

CELMoDs belong to the next-generation IMIiDs and are functionally different and more potent. They induce myeloma cell (MC) apoptosis. As they stimulate the immune system, they could help overcome resistance to certain drugs. Iberdomide (CC-220) showed an ORR of 31% associated with dexamethasone in the first-in-human phase 1b/2a multicenter dose-escalation study [52, 53].

An ORR between 40 and 60% was obtained when Iberdomide was combined with daratumumab or bortezomib. The main adverse events were neutropenia and infections [54].

Another novel and possibly more powerful CELMoD currently investigated is CC-92480 [55].

Bruton's Tyrosine Kinase (BTK) Inhibitors

Ibrutinib is an oral drug approved for several B-cell malignancies. BTK is overexpressed in MM cells favoring proliferation and migration of plasma cells, bone destruction, and dexamethasone resistance. Moreover, ibrutinib enhances the activity of PIs and IMiDs [56]. A phase I/II trial of ibrutinib in combination with carfilzomib and dexamethasone yielded an ORR of 71% and PFS of 7.4 months. No unexpected side effects were seen with this association [57].

BCL-2 Inhibitor

Myeloma cells overexpress anti-apoptotic proteins heterogeneously, making their dependency on the BCL-2 survival signal somewhat variable. Therefore, overexpression of BCL-2 in a subset of MCs with BCL-2 survival dependency provides an attractive therapeutic target. MM cells harboring t(11;14) translocation are associated mainly with increased dependency upon BCL-2 for plasma cell survival [58]. Venetoclax (formerly known as ABT-199) is a first-in-class, orally bioavailable BH3 43 mimetic designed by reverse engineering to produce a compound highly selective for BCL-2.

Phase III BELLINI trial [59] compared bortezomib plus dexamethasone to triplet combination venetoclax, bortezomib, and dexamethasone in 291 RRMM patients. Patients receiving combinations with venetoclax had a significantly longer PFS; however, substantially worse OS due to early deaths due to infection in the venetoclax arm. Subgroup analysis showed impressive prolonged PFS in patients with t(11;14) or high BCL-2 expression without significant differences early. Phase III trial (CANOVA; NCT03539744) comparing venetoclax plus dexamethasone vs pomalidomide plus dexamethasone in patients with RRMM with t(11;14) or high BCL-2 expression is undergoing.

Immune Checkpoint Inhibitors

Anti-PD1

MM plasma cells overexpress immune checkpoints, which lead to drug resistance and immune reactions. They were appealing targets for MM therapy. Two randomized trials compared Revlimid and dexamethasone (Rd) vs Rd and pembrolizumab, an anti-PD1 (KEYNOTE 185) [60] as first-line therapy (KEYNOTE 183) [61] or in the RRMM setting. Both studies were halted and concluded in an interim unplanned analysis that triple therapy had an unfavorable risk-benefit profile due to an inferior PFS. An excess of attributable mortality in the pembrolizumab arm was reported.

Anti-CD47

Various cancers and MM cells express CD47, an immune checkpoint known as the "don't eat me" signal. It sends inhibitory signals to macrophages to impede phagocytosis and immune response. In plasma cell clonal disorders, its expression directly correlates with the stage of the disease, from normal to MGUS to MM. Blocking of CD47 using an anti-CD47 antibody induces immediate activation of macrophages with phagocytosis and killing of MM cells. AO176 may be a potential candidate for this experimental approach [62, 63].

Cytotoxic T Lymphocyte Antigen-4 (CTLA-4)

Cytotoxic T lymphocyte antigen-4 (CTLA-4) are important risk factors associated with autoimmune diseases and malignancies. Like PD-1 (CD279), CTLA-4 regulates immune responses at very different levels by very different mechanisms. It is a global regulator of T-cell activation.

CTLA-4 polymorphism reduced the progression-free survival and the overall survival of patients with MM who received bortezomib-based therapy [64]. It is also an attractive therapeutic target currently being investigated with ipilimumab.

Other Experimental Therapies

Targeting C-X-C-Motif Chemokine Receptor 4 (CXCR4), which plays an essential role in disseminating MM cells out of the BM, is another appealing approach to treat MM. Ulocuplumab represents the first-in-class fully mAb targeting CXCR4; it showed activity in RRMM in a phase Ib/II study [65].

The anticancer effects of the marine-derived antitumor agent plitidepsin primarily rely on the interaction with elongation factor 1-α 2 (eEF1A2). eEF1A2 is known to be overexpressed in breast cancer and MM cells. Targeting this protein leads to a proapoptotic response. In Australia, plitidepsin was approved in combination with the corticosteroid agent dexamethasone to treat MM patients who failed or became resistant to other therapies, covering the third- and fourth-line treatment settings [66]. The randomized phase III ADMYRE trial evaluated plitidepsin plus dexamethasone (DXM) versus DXM alone in patients with RRMM and demonstrated superiority in PFS and OS when plitidepsin was added [67].

AL extracellular proteins deposit in tissues and aggregate in ß-pleated sheets arranged in an antiparallel fashion, distorting tissue architecture and exerting significant tissue toxicity in AL amyloidosis. Adjuvant doxycycline may enhance anti-amyloid effects. The DUAL (Doxycycline to Upgrade response in AL amyloidosis) study is based on the fact that doxycycline has been reported to produce fibril disruption, reduces AL deposits, and controls light chain toxicity. Doxycycline is safe and effective when administered with concurrent chemotherapy, with encouraging results in cardiac patients [68, 69]. Furthermore, enhancer of zeste homolog 2 is a histone methyltransferase that is of great interest in human cancer and its inhibition may represent a future treatment option.

Myeloma-Developing Regimens Using Genomics (MyDRUG)

Advances in MM biology knowledge paved the way to transition from a patient- and drug characteristic-guided therapy to biomarker-driven therapy.

The MyDRUG study is a Precision Medicine trial to treat patients with drugs targeting the affected specific mutated genes. Patients with a greater than 25% mutation to any of the following genes: CDKN2C, FGFR3, KRAS, NRAS, BRAF V600E, IDH2, or t(11;14) are enrolled in one of the treatment arms. These arms have treatments directed explicitly to the mutated genes. Patients that do not have a greater than 25% mutation to the genes listed are enrolled in a non-actionable treatment arm [70].

Figure 22.1 illustrates the various target sites of newly developed agents on aberrant plasma cells.

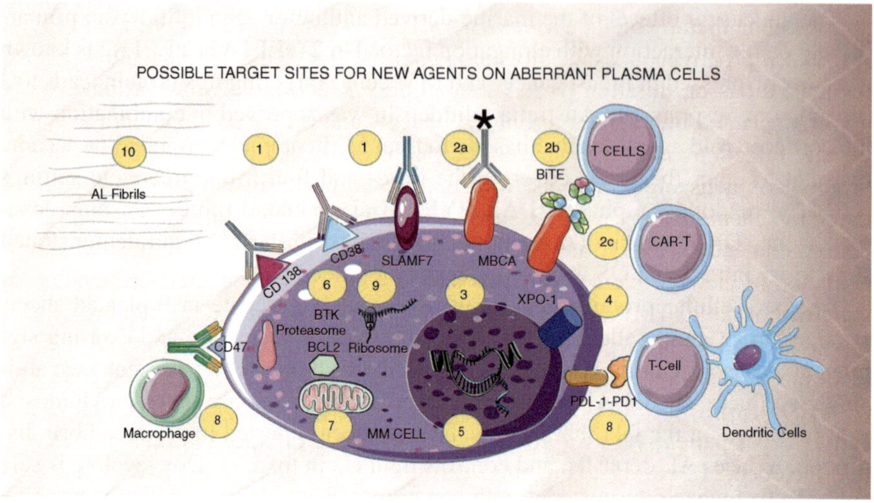

Fig. 22.1 Possible target sites for new agents on aberrant plasma cells. (1) Targeting cell surface receptors including SLAMF7, CD38, and CD138. (2) (**a**) Targeting B-cell maturation antigen (BCMA) by antibody-drug conjugate, (**b**) by BiTE or bispecific antibodies, (**c**) by CAR-T. (3) Targeting aminopeptidase. (4) Targeting exportin 1. (5) Site of action of Cereblon E3 ligase modulators. (6) Targeting BTK. (7) Targeting BCL-2. (8) Checkpoint inhibitors affecting PD1/PDL-1 axis and CD47. (9) Targeting ribosome with marine-derived antitumor agents. (10) Interfering with AL fibrils

B-B-Cell Plasmacytic Clone and Waldenström Macroglobulinemia

For B-cell plasmacytic clones and Waldenström Macroglobulinemia (WM), the anti-CD20 monoclonal antibody rituximab is the backbone of the most commonly used treatment combinations [71]. However, the treatment landscape of the disease changed with the introduction of the first-in-class BTK inhibitor, the oral ibrutinib, administered continuously until disease progression. Responses were best in patients with CXCR4 wild type (^{WT})/Toll-like receptor MYD88 protein with L265P mutation (MYD88^{L265P}) and lowest in patients with CXCR4^{WT}/MYD88^{WT} highlighting the unmet need and treatment gaps for those patients [72].

Patients with germline mutation with warts, hypogammaglobulinemia, infections, and myelokathexis syndrome (WHIM syndrome) (CXCR4^{WHIM}) have a distinct clinical presentation with more inadequate responses to BTK inhibition.

Furthermore, the development of resistance to ibrutinib attributed to a decreased intrinsic binding affinity to this binding site is an emerging problem [73].

Therefore, the challenges and research goals are to develop a fixed duration treatment with sustained disease control. It will probably include BTK inhibition along with agents that target alternative pathways to address resistance mechanisms. Interestingly, a better understanding of the molecular pathway of cellular proliferation with BTK paves the way for developing these new agents. BTK works upstream and leads to downstream activation of phosphoinositide-3-kinase (PI3K)-AKT pathway, PLC, PKC, and nuclear factor κB (NF-κB) with B-cell proliferation, differentiation, and enhanced survival [74].

Agents Targeting B-Cell IgM Producing Clones

Newer Anti-CD20 mABs

In the current practice, anti-CD 20 rituximab is the backbone treatment for B-cell clones secreting IgM and expressing CD20. It is often administered as a part of the initial chemotherapy combined with alkylating agents followed by maintenance monotherapy. Other anti-CD20 mAB includes ublituximab that has been advocated by some authors [75], whereas ofatumumab, the first human anti-CD20 mAb, has also shown potential in treating Waldenström's macroglobulinemia [76].

Newer BTK Inhibitors

In some centers, BTK inhibitors have replaced classic chemoimmunotherapy based on MYD88 and CXCR4 genotypes. Despite their convenient oral administration, intolerable side effects and reduced efficacy in the $MYD88^{WT}$ cohort may limit their use [77].

Acalabrutinib (ACP-196) was developed to be more potent and selective than ibrutinib [77]. In phase 2 multicenter study of 106 WM patients, oral acalabrutinib administered until disease progression or toxic effects developed achieved an ORR of 93% [78]. Zanubrutinib is another potent irreversible next-generation BTK inhibitor. It demonstrated superiority when compared to ibrutinib with fewer reported adverse cardiac events [79]. No randomized controlled trials have compared BTK to chemoimmunotherapy and therapy, therefore, should be individualized to the patient and mutational profile.

BCL2 Inhibitors

Venetoclax, the small oral molecule that selectively inhibits BCL2, has significantly improved patient outcomes with relapsed/refractory (R/R) WM with an ORR of 87% [80]. A combination trial of venetoclax and ibrutinib in treatment-naive patients is underway [73]. Novel covalent and noncovalent BTK inhibitors (tirabrutinib, vecabrutinib, LOXO-305, ARQ-531) are undergoing clinical trials in WM [81].

Proteosome Inhibitors

The potential role of proteasome inhibitors in the treatment of WM patients has been established based on previous data on bortezomib activity, but more clinical trials are ongoing.

Ixazomib is an oral proteasome inhibitor that blocks the chymotrypsin-like activity of the β5 subunit of the 20S proteasome [82].

When ixazomib, dexamethasone, and rituximab (IDR) were administered to 26 treatment-naive patients with WM as 6-monthly induction cycles followed by six maintenance cycles every 2 months, the overall, major, and VGPR rates were 96%, 77%, and 19%, respectively [83].

PI3K Inhibitors

The phosphatidylinositol 3-kinase (PI3K) pathway plays a significant role in the initiation and progression of malignancies as it enhances cell survival and stimulates cell proliferation [84] PI3Kδ inhibitors have been shown to induce cell death in WM cell lines [85]. Idelalisib is a potent, highly selective, oral PI3Kδ/AKT inhibitor that promotes apoptosis. A phase 1b, in patients with relapsed B-cell malignancies, demonstrated an ORR of 55% in 9 patients with WM [73]. Less hepatotoxic PI3K inhibitors, such as duvelisib and umbralisib, are currently being evaluated in WM [86, 87].

CXCR4 Inhibitors

Targeting CXCR4 leads to a significant downstream reduction of proliferative signals and hence tumor reduction [88]. New agents targeting CXCR4 were developed to improve WM patients' outcomes with the $CXCR4^{WHIM}$ mutation [73, 89]. The results of a Phase I trial of the CXCR4-antagonist ulocuplumab with ibrutinib to target CXCR4Mut in WM were recently published [90].

The major and VGPR response rates were 100% and 33%, respectively, with VGPRs observed at lower ulocuplumab dose cohorts. Median times to minor and major responses were 0.9 and 1.2 months, respectively. With a median follow-up of 22.4 months, the estimated 2-year PFS was 90% [90].

Mavorixafor (AMD-070) is another small oral, potent, noncompetitive antagonist of CXCR4 which demonstrated a favorable safety profile and resulted in meaningful hematological improvement in patients with WHIM syndrome is currently investigated in WM [73].

Furthermore, plerixafor (AMD3100) is a CXCR4 antagonist that disrupts the CXCR4/SDF-1α bond. It is used in combination with granulocyte colony-stimulating factor for hematopoietic stem and progenitor cell mobilization in patients with lymphoma and multiple myeloma [91].

Other Emerging Therapies

MYD88 and CXCR4 trigger mTOR, part of the P13 K/AKT resulting in prosurvival signaling.

Everolimus, an mTOR inhibitor, has been evaluated as monotherapy in 33 treatment-naive WM patients with some success [92].

Other therapeutic agents such as PD-1 inhibitors or ImiDs were also experimented with WM in many trials.

Focusing on the plasma cell component of the lymphoplasmacytic clone is another exploratory approach. Plasma cells in WM express CD38 which could be targeted by daratumumab, which being assessed in a single-arm phase II study in patients with RR WM. Another study involves the combination of daratumumab and ibrutinib. CAR-T will also likely be a new therapeutic option [73].

Selinexor, a potent oral XPO-1 inhibitor previously investigated in MM, has also been tried on a small cohort of WM in its dose-escalation phase [93].

Castillo et al. reviewed the novel approach to manage WM and lymphoplasmacytic clones [81, 89, 94].

Figure 22.2 illustrates the potential target sites of novel agents on the B-cell lymphoplasmacytic clone.

Therefore, numerous new therapeutic agents are being developed as the molecular and genetic basis of disease development and progression are being better understood. These agents range from monoclonal antibodies targeting surface markers to

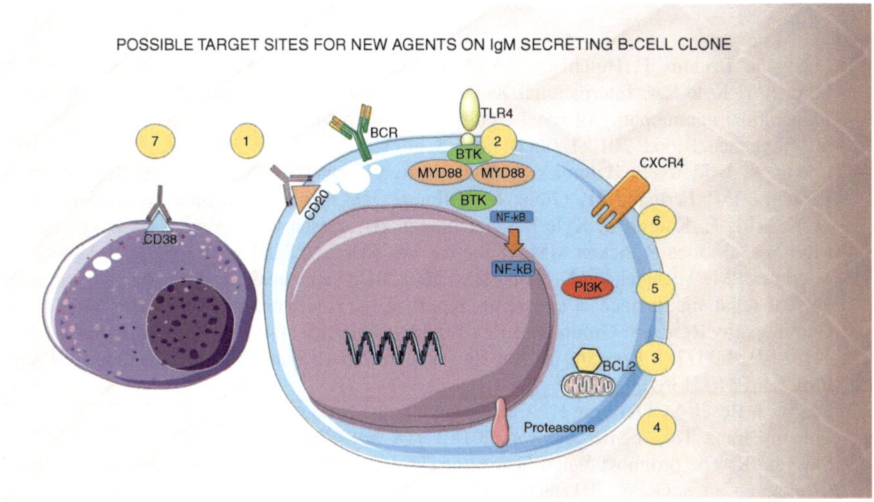

Fig. 22.2 Potential target sites of novel agents on the B-cell lymphoplasmacytic clone. (1) Novel anti-CD20, (2) BTK inhibitors, (3) BCL-2 inhibitors, (4) Proteasome inhibitors, (5) PI3K Phosphatidylinositol 3-kinase inhibitors, (6) CXCR4 inhibitors and blockers, (7) Novel mechanisms including anti-CD38

more complex antibody-drug conjugates, bispecific antibodies or CAR-T. This arsenal of new agents will likely represent a significant addition to the armamentarium used for other disciplines in the non-neoplastic arena.

Conclusions

Understanding the microenvironmental characteristics and the different signal pathways that lead to cellular proliferation in plasma cell and B-cell clones can translate into a precision approach to therapy.

MM is a heterogeneous and complex disease with many driving mechanisms and mutations. Understanding the biology of the disease and the structural characteristics of the aberrant plasma cells and its surrounding bone marrow microenvironment allows us to experiment with numerous targeted therapies. The future of MM therapy is a fascinating challenge to achieve a cure and a good quality of life for all MM patients.

For WM and the lymphoplasmacytic clones, once more, understanding the intracellular proliferative signals and their molecular interactions are paving the way for a patient-tailored therapy that will change the way we manage such cases.

We will likely soon meet the challenge to develop a fixed duration treatment with sustained disease control with the novel agents.

References

1. Leung N, Bridoux F, Hutchison CA, Nasr SH, Cockwell P, Fermand JP, Dispenzieri A, Song KW, Kyle RA, International Kidney and Monoclonal Gammopathy Research Group. Monoclonal gammopathy of renal significance: when MGUS is no longer undetermined or insignificance. Blood. 2012;120(22):4292–5. https://doi.org/10.1182/blood-2012-07-445304.
2. Leung N, Bridoux F, Batuman V, Chaidos A, Cockwell P, D'Agati VD, Dispenzieri A, Fervenza FC, Fermand JP, Gibbs S, Gillmore JD, Herrera GA, Jaccard A, Jevremovic D, Kastritis E, Kukreti V, Kyle RA, Lachmann HJ, Larsen CP, Ludwig H, Markowitz GS, Merlini G, Mollee P, Picken MM, Rajkumar VS, Royal V, Sanders PW, Sethi S, Venner CP, Voorhees PM, Wechalekar AD, Weiss BM, Nasr SH. The evaluation of monoclonal gammopathy of renal significance: a consensus report of the International Kidney and Monoclonal Gammopathy Research Group. Nat Rev Nephrol. 2019;15(1):45–59. https://doi.org/10.1038/s41581-018-0077-4. Erratum in: Nat Rev Nephrol. 2019 Feb;15(2):121. PMID: 30510265; PMCID: PMC7136169.
3. Stakiw J, Bosch M, Goubran H. A closer look at the bone marrow microenvironment in multiple myeloma. Tumor Microenviron. 2018;1:1–8. https://doi.org/10.4103/2395-7182.203049.
4. Sawyer JR. The prognostic significance of cytogenetics and molecular profiling in multiple myeloma. Cancer Genet. 2011;204:3–12.
5. Keats JJ, Fonseca R, Chesi M, Schop R, Baker A, Chng WJ, Van Wier S, Tiedemann R, Shi CX, Sebag M, et al. Promiscuous mutations activate the noncanonical NF-kappaB pathway in multiple myeloma. Cancer Cell. 2007;12:131–44.

6. Offidani M, Corvatta L, Morè S, Olivieri A. Novel experimental drugs for treatment of multiple myeloma. J Exp Pharmacol. 2021;13:245–64. Published online 2021 Mar 9. PMCID: PMC7955760. https://doi.org/10.2147/JEP.S265288.
7. Kumar SK, Dimopoulos MA, Kastritis E, et al. Natural history of relapsed myeloma, refractory to immunomodulatory drugs and proteasome inhibitors: a multicenter IMWG study. Leukemia. 2017;31:2443–8.
8. Flores-Montero J, de Tute R, Paiva B, Perez JJ, Böttcher S, Wind H, Sanoja L, Puig N, Lecrevisse Q, Vidriales MB, van Dongen JJ, Orfao A. Immunophenotype of normal vs. myeloma plasma cells: toward antibody panel specifications for MRD detection in multiple myeloma. Cytometry B Clin Cytom. 2016;90(1):61–72. https://doi.org/10.1002/cyto.b.21265. Epub 2015 Jul 31. PMID: 26100534.
9. Dimopoulos MA, Oriol A, Nahi H, San-Miguel J, Bahlis NJ, Usmani SZ, Rabin N, Orlowski RZ, Komarnicki M, Suzuki K, Plesner T, Yoon SS, Ben Yehuda D, Richardson PG, Goldschmidt H, Reece D, Lisby S, Khokhar NZ, O'Rourke L, Chiu C, Qin X, Guckert M, Ahmadi T, Moreau P, POLLUX Investigators. Daratumumab, lenalidomide, and dexamethasone for multiple myeloma. N Engl J Med. 2016;375(14):1319–31. https://doi.org/10.1056/NEJMoa1607751. PMID: 27705267.
10. Facon T, Kumar S, Plesner T, Orlowski RZ, Moreau P, Bahlis N, Basu S, Nahi H, Hulin C, Quach H, Goldschmidt H, O'Dwyer M, Perrot A, Venner CP, Weisel K, Mace JR, Raje N, Attal M, Tiab M, Macro M, Frenzel L, Leleu X, Ahmadi T, Chiu C, Wang J, Van Rampelbergh R, Uhlar CM, Kobos R, Qi M, Usmani SZ, MAIA Trial Investigators. Daratumumab plus Lenalidomide and dexamethasone for untreated myeloma. N Engl J Med. 2019;380(22):2104–15. https://doi.org/10.1056/NEJMoa1817249. PMID: 31141632.
11. Lin P, Owens R, Tricot G, Wilson CS. Flow cytometric immunophenotypic analysis of 306 cases of multiple myeloma. Am J Clin Pathol. 2004;121:482–8.
12. Leow CC-Y, Low MSY. Targeted therapies for multiple myeloma. J Pers Med. 2021;11:334. https://doi.org/10.3390/jpm11050334.
13. Van de Domnk NW, Usmani SZ. CD38 antibodies in multiple myeloma: mechanisms of action and modes of resistance. Front Immunol. 2018;9:2134.
14. Martin TG, Corzo K, Chiron M, et al. Therapeutic opportunities with pharmacological inhibition of CD38 with isatuximab. Cell. 2019;8:1522.
15. Raab MS, Engelhardt M, Blank A, et al. MOR202, a novel anti-CD38 monoclonal antibody, in patients with relapsed or refractory multiple myeloma: a first-in-human, multicenter, phase 1-2a trial. Lancet Hematol. 2020;7:e381–94.
16. Krishnan AY, Patel KK, Hari P, et al. A phase Ib study of TAK-079, an investigational anti-CD38 monoclonal antibody (mAb) in patients with relapsed/refractory multiple myeloma (RRMM): preliminary results. J Clin Oncol. 2020;38(15_suppl):8539.
17. Bruins WSC, Zheng W, Higgins JP, et al. TAK-169, a novel recombinant immunotoxin specific for CD38, induces powerful preclinical activity against patient-derived multiple myeloma cells. Blood. 2020;136(Supplement 1):11–2.
18. Vogl DT, Kaufman JL, Holstein SA, et al. TAK-573, an anti-CD38/attenuated Ifnα fusion protein, has clinical activity and modulates the Ifnα receptor (IFNAR) pathway in patients with relapsed/refractory multiple myeloma. Blood. 2020;136(Supplement 1):37–8.
19. Ikeda H, Hideshima T, Fulciniti M, et al. The monoclonal antibody nBT062 conjugated to cytotoxic maytansinoids has selective cytotoxicity against CD138-positive multiple myeloma cells in vitro and in vivo. Clin Cancer Res. 2009;15:4028–37.
20. Kelly KR, Siegel DS, Chanan-Khan AA, et al. Indatuximab Ravtansine (BT062) in combination with low-dose dexamethasone and lenalidomide or pomalidomide: clinical activity in patients with relapsed/refractory multiple myeloma. Blood. 2016;128:4486.
21. Yu T, Chaganty B, Lin L, et al. VIS832, a novel CD138-targeting monoclonal antibody, potently induces killing of human multiple myeloma and further synergizes with IMiDs or bortezomib in vitro and in vivo. Blood Cancer J. 2020;10:110.

22. Shah N, Chari A, Scott E, Mezzi K, Usmani SZ. B-cell maturation antigen (BCMA) in multiple myeloma: rationale for targeting and current therapeutic approaches. Leukemia. 2020;34(4):985–1005. https://doi.org/10.1038/s41375-020-0734-z. Epub 2020 Feb 13. PMID: 32055000.
23. Moreaux J, Legou E, Jourdan E, et al. BAFF and APRIL protect myeloma cells from apoptosis induced by interleukin 6 deprivation and dexamethasone. Blood. 2004;103:3148–57.
24. Dalla Palma B, Marchica V, Catarozzo MT, Giuliani N, Accardi F. Monoclonal and bispecific anti-BCMA antibodies in multiple myeloma. J Clin Med. 2020;9(9):3022. https://doi.org/10.3390/jcm9093022. PMID: 32961764.
25. McMillan A, Warcel D, Popat R. Antibody-drug conjugates for multiple myeloma. Expert Opin Biol Ther. 2021;21(7):889–901.
26. Lassiter G, Bergeron C, Guedry R, Cucarola J, Kaye AM, Cornett EM, Kaye AD, Varrassi G, Viswanath O, Urits I. Belantamab mafodotin to treat multiple myeloma: a comprehensive review of disease, drug efficacy and side effects. Curr Oncol. 2021;28(1):640–60. https://doi.org/10.3390/curroncol28010063. PMID: 33494319.
27. Lonial S, Lee HC, Badros A, Trudel S, Nooka AK, Chari A, Abdallah AO, Callander N, Lendvai N, Sborov D, Suvannasankha A, Weisel K, Karlin L, Libby E, Arnulf B, Facon T, Hulin C, Kortüm KM, Rodríguez-Otero P, Usmani SZ, Hari P, Baz R, Quach H, Moreau P, Voorhees PM, Gupta I, Hoos A, Zhi E, Baron J, Piontek T, Lewis E, Jewell RC, Dettman EJ, Popat R, Esposti SD, Opalinska J, Richardson P, Cohen AD. Belantamab mafodotin for relapsed or refractory multiple myeloma (DREAMM-2): a two-arm, randomised, open-label, phase 2 study. Lancet Oncol. 2020;21(2):207–21. https://doi.org/10.1016/S1470-2045(19)30788-0. Epub 2019 Dec 16. PMID: 31859245.
28. Lancman G, Richter J, Chari A. Bispecific, trispecific, and other novel immune treatments in myeloma. Hematology. 2020;2020:264–71.
29. Caraccio C, Krishna S, Phillips DJ, Schürch CM. Bispecific antibodies for multiple myeloma: a review of targets, drugs, clinical trials, and future directions. Front Immunol. 2020;11:501.
30. Garfall AL, Usmani SZ, Mateos M-V, et al. Updated phase 1 results of Teclistamab, a B-cell maturation antigen (BCMA) × CD3 Bispecificc antibody, in relapsed and/or refractory multiple myeloma (RRMM). Blood. 2020;136:27.
31. Sadelain M, Brentjens R, Riviere I. The basic principles of chimeric antigen receptor design. Cancer Discov. 2013;3:338–98.
32. Mikkilinemi L, Kochenderfer JN. Chimeric antigen receptor T-cell therapies for multiple myeloma. Blood. 2017;130:2594–602.
33. Raje N, Berdeja J, Lin Y, et al. Anti-BCMA CAR T-cell therapy bb2121 in relapsed or refractory multiple myeloma. N Engl J Med. 2019;380:1726–37.
34. Lin Y, Raje NS, Berdeja JG, et al. Idecabtagene vicleucel (ide-cel, bb2121), a BCMA-directed CAR T cell therapy, in patients with relapsed and refractory multiple myeloma: updated results from phase 1 CRB-401 study. Blood. 2020;136(Suppl. 1):26–7.
35. Munshi NC, Anderson LD Jr, Shah N, et al. Idecabtagene vicleucel in relapsed and refractory multiple myeloma. N Engl J Med. 2021;384(8):705–16.
36. Wang B-Y, Zhao W-H, Liu J, et al. Long-term follow-up of a phase 1, first-in-human open-label study of LCAR-B38M, a structurally differentiated chimeric antigen receptor T (CAR-T) cell therapy targeting B-cell maturation antigen (BCMA) in patients with relapsed/refractory multiple myeloma. Blood. 2019;134(Suppl. 1):579.
37. Berdeja JG, Madduri D, Usmani SZ, et al. Ciltacabtagene autoleucel, a B-cell maturation antigen-directed chimeric antigen receptor T-cell therapy in patients with relapsed or refractory multiple myeloma (CARTITUDE-1): a phase 1b/2 open-label study. Lancet. 2021;398(10297):314–24.
38. Mailankody S, Jakuboviak A, Htut M, et al. Orvacabtagene autoleucel (orva-cel), a B-cell maturation antigen (BCMA)-directed CAR T cell therapy for patients with relapsed/refractory multiple myeloma: update of the phase 1/2 EVOLVE study (NCT03430011). J Clin Oncol. 2020;38(Suppl):8504.

39. Alsina M, Shah N, Raje NS, et al. Updated results from the phase I CRB-402 study of anti-BCMA CAR-T cell therapy bb21217 in patients with relapsed and refractory multiple myeloma: correlation of expansion and duration of response with T cell phenotypes. Blood. 2020;136(Suppl. 1):130.
40. Hao S, Jin J, Jiang S, et al. Two-years follow-up of investigator-initiated phase 1 trials of the safety and efficacy of fully human anti-bcma CAR T cells (CT053) in relapsed/refractory multiple myeloma. Blood. 2020;136(Suppl. 1):132.
41. Costello VCL, Cohen AD, Patel KK, et al. Phase 1/2 study of the safety and response of P-BCMA-101 CAR-T cells in patients with relapsed/refractory multiple myeloma (PRIME) with novel therapeutic strategies. Blood. 2020;136(Suppl. 1):29–30.
42. Jiang H, Dong B, Gao L, et al. Clinical results of a multicenter study of the first-in-human dual BCMA and CD19 targeted novel platform fast CAR-T cell therapy for patients with relapsed/refractory multiple myeloma. Blood. 2020;136(Suppl. 1):25–6.
43. Chauhan D, Ray A, Viktorsson K, et al. In vitro and in vivo antitumor activity of a novel alkylating agent, melphalan-flufenamide, against multiple myeloma cells. Clin Cancer Res. 2013;19:3019–31.
44. Oriol A, Larocca A, Leleu X, et al. Melflufen for relapsed and refractory multiple myeloma. Expert Opin Investig Drugs. 2020;29:1069–78.
45. Larocca A, Richardson PG, Oriol A, et al. HORIZON (OP-106): melflufen plus dexamethasone in patients with relapsed/refractory multiple myeloma-age subgroup analysis of elderly patients. Blood. 2020;136(Suppl 1):44–6.
46. Mateos M-V, Oriol A, Larocca A, et al. HORIZON (OP-106): melflufen plus dexamethasone in patients with relapsed/refractory multiple myeloma with high-risk cytogenetics-subgroup analysis. Blood. 2020;136(Suppl 1):41–3.
47. Rodriguez-Otero P, Mateos M-V, Oriol A, et al. HORIZON (OP-106): melflufen plus dexamethasone in patients with relapsed/refractory multiple myeloma exposed to prior alkylator therapy-subgroup analysis. Blood. 2020;136(Suppl 1):22–3.
48. Ocio EM, Efebera YA, Hajek R, et al. ANCHOR (OP-104): melflufen plus dexamethasone and daratumumab or bortezomib in relapsed/refractory multiple myeloma refractory to an IMiD and/or a proteasome inhibitor-updated efficacy and safety. Blood. 2020;136(Suppl 1):3124.
49. Hill R, Cautain B, De Pedro N, et al. Targeting nucleocytoplasmic transport in cancer therapy. Oncotarget. 2014;5:11–28.
50. Gravina GL, Senapedis W, McCauley D, et al. Nucleo-cytoplasmic transport as a therapeutic target of cancer. J Hematol Oncol. 2014;7:85.
51. Grosicki S, Simonova M, Spicka I, et al. Once-per-week selinexor, bortezomib, and dexamethasone versus twice-per-week bortezomib and dexamethasone in patients with multiple myeloma (BOSTON): a randomized, open-label, phase 3 trial. Lancet. 2020;396:1563–73.
52. Bjorklund CC, Kang J, Amatangelo M, et al. Iberdomide (CC-220) is a potent cereblon E3 ligase modulator with antitumor and immunostimulatory activities in lenalidomide- and pomalidomide-resistant multiple myeloma cells with dysregulated CRBN. Leukemia. 2020;34:1197–20.
53. Bobin A, Liuu E, Moya N, Gruchet C, Sabirou F, Lévy A, Gardeney H, Nsiala L, Cailly L, Guidez S, Tomowiak C, Systchenko T, Javaugue V, Durand G, Leleu X, Puyade M. Multiple myeloma: an overview of the current and novel therapeutic approaches in 2020. Cancers (Basel). 2020;12(10):2885. https://doi.org/10.3390/cancers12102885. PMID: 33050025.
54. Van de Donk N, Popat R, Larsen J, et al. First results of iberdomide (IBER; CC-220) in combination with dexamethasone and daratumumab or bortezomib in patients with relapsed/refractory multiple myeloma. Blood. 2020;136(Suppl 1):16–7.
55. Hansen JD, Correa M, Nagy MA, et al. Discovery of CRBN E3 ligase modulator CC-92480 for the treatment of relapsed and refractory multiple myeloma. J Med Chem. 2020;63:6648–76.
56. Tai YT, Chang BY, Kong SY, et al. Bruton tyrosine kinase inhibition is a novel therapeutic strategy targeting tumor in the bone marrow microenvironment in multiple myeloma. Blood. 2012;120:1877–87.

57. Chari A, Corbnell RF, Gasparetto C, et al. Final analysis of a phase 1/2b study of ibrutinib combined with carfilzomib/dexamethasone in patients with relapsed/refractory multiple myeloma. Hematol Oncol. 2020;38:353–62.
58. Touzeau C, Dousset C, Le Gouill S, et al. The bcl-2 specific BH3 mimetic ABT-199: a promising targeted therapy for t(11;14) multiple myeloma. Leukemia. 2014;28:210–2.
59. Kumar SK, Harrison SJ, Cavo M, et al. Venetoclax or placebo in combination with bortezomib and dexamethasone in patients with relapsed or refractory multiple myeloma (BELLINI): a randomized, double-blind, multicenter, phase 3 trial. Lancet Oncol. 2020;21:1630–42.
60. Usmani SZ, Schjesvold F, Oriol A, et al. Pembrolizumab plus lenalidomide and dexamethasone for patients with treatment-naïve multiple myeloma (KEYNOTE-185): a randomized, open-label, phase 3 trial. Lancet Hematol. 2019;6:e448–58.
61. Mateos M-V, Blacklock H, Schjesvold F, et al. Pembrolizumab plus pomalidomide and dexamethasone for patients with relapsed or refractory multiple myeloma (KEYNOTE-183): a randomized, open-label, phase 3 trial. Lancet Hematol. 2019;6:e459–69.
62. Sun J, Muz B, Alhallak K, Markovic M, Gurley S, Wang Z, Guenthner N, Wasden K, Fiala M, King J, Kohnen D, Salama NN, Vij R, Azab AK. Targeting CD47 as a novel immunotherapy for multiple myeloma. Cancers (Basel). 2020;12(2):305. https://doi.org/10.3390/cancers12020305. PMID: 32012878.
63. Puro RJ, Bouchlaka MN, Hiebsch RR, Capoccia BJ, Donio MJ, Manning PT, Frazier WA, Karr RW, Pereira DS. Development of AO-176, a next-generation humanized anti-CD47 antibody with novel anticancer properties and negligible red blood cell binding. Mol Cancer Ther. 2020;19(3):835–46. https://doi.org/10.1158/1535-7163.MCT-19-1079. Epub2019 Dec 26. PMID: 31879362.
64. Qin XY, Lu J, Li GX, Wen L, Liu Y, Xu LP, Chang YJ, Liu KY, Jiang ZF, Huang XJ. CTLA-4 polymorphisms are associated with treatment outcomes of patients with multiple myeloma receiving bortezomib-based regimens. Ann Hematol. 2018;97(3):485–95. https://doi.org/10.1007/s00277-017-3203-7. Epub 2017 Dec 21. PMID: 29264740.
65. Ghobrial IM, Liu C-J, Redd R, et al. A phase Ib/II trial of the first-in-class anti-CXCR4 antibody ulocuplumab in combination with lenalidomide or bortezomib plus dexamethasone in relapsed multiple myeloma. Clin Cancer Res. 2020;26:344–53.
66. Gomes NGM, Valentão P, Andrade PB, Pereira RB. Plitidepsin to treat multiple myeloma. Drugs Today (Barc). 2020;56(5):337–47. https://doi.org/10.1358/dot.2020.56.5.3135886. PMID: 32406881.
67. Spicka I, Ocio EM, Oakervee HE, Greil R, Banh RH, Huang SY, D'Rozario JM, Dimopoulos MA, Martínez S, Extremera S, Kahatt C, Alfaro V, Carella AM, Meuleman N, Hájek R, Symeonidis A, Min CK, Cannell P, Ludwig H, Sonneveld P, Mateos MV. Randomized phase III study (ADMYRE) of plitidepsin in combination with dexamethasone vs. dexamethasone alone in patients with relapsed/refractory multiple myeloma. Ann Hematol. 2019;98(9):2139–50. https://doi.org/10.1007/s00277-019-03739-2. Epub 2019 Jun 25. PMID: 31240472.
68. D'Souza A, Szabo A, Flynn KE, Dhakal B, Chhabra S, Pasquini MC, Weihrauch D, Hari PN. Adjuvant doxycycline to enhance anti-amyloid effects: results from the dual phase 2 trial. EClinicalMedicine. 2020;23:100361. https://doi.org/10.1016/j.eclinm.2020.100361. eCollection 2020 Jun. PMID: 32529175.
69. Wechalekar AD, Whelan C. Encouraging impact of doxycycline on early mortality in cardiac light chain (AL) amyloidosis. Blood Cancer J. 2017;7(3):e546. https://doi.org/10.1038/bcj.2017.26. PMID: 28338670 PMCID: PMC5380910.
70. Auclair D, Anderson KC, Avigan D, et al. The myeloma-developing regimens using genomics (MyDRUG) master protocol. Journal of Clinical Oncology 2019;37:15_suppl, TPS8057-TPS8057.
71. Buske C, Sadullah S, Kastritis E, et al. Treatment and outcome patterns in European patients with Waldenstrom's macroglobulinaemia: a large, observational, retrospective chart review. Lancet Haematol. 2018;5(7):e299–309.

72. Treon S, Meid K, Gustine J, et al. Long-term follow-up of previously treated patients who received ibrutinib for symptomatic Waldenstrom's macroglobulinemia: update of pivotal clinical trial. Blood. 2017;130:2776.
73. Despina F, Meletios Athanasios D, Efstathios K. Emerging drugs for the treatment of Waldenstrom macroglobulinemia. Expert Opin Emerg Drugs. 2020;25(4):433–44. https://doi.org/10.1080/14728214.2020.1822816. Epub 2020 Sep 21. PMID: 32955949.
74. Stevenson FK, Krysov S, Davies AJ, et al. B-cell receptor signaling in chronic lymphocytic leukemia. Blood. 2011;118(16):4313–20.
75. Le Garff-Tavernier M, Herbi L, de Romeuf C, Azar N, Roos-Weil D, Bonnemye P, Urbain R, Leblond V, Merle-Beral H, Vieillard V. The optimized anti-CD20 monoclonal antibody ublituximab bypasses natural killer phenotypic features in Waldenstrom macroglobulinemia. Haematologica. 2015;100(4):e147–51. https://doi.org/10.3324/haematol.2014.118083. Epub 2014 Dec 31. PMID: 25552707.
76. Gupta IV, Jewell RC. Ofatumumab, the first human anti-CD20 monoclonal antibody for the treatment of B cell hematologic malignancies. Ann N Y Acad Sci. 2012;1263:43–56. https://doi.org/10.1111/j.1749-6632.2012.06661.x. Epub 2012 Jul 25. PMID: 22830942.
77. Grimont CN, Castillo Almeida NE, Gertz MA. Current and emerging treatments for Waldenstrom macroglobulinemia. Acta Haematol. 2021;144(2):146–57. https://doi.org/10.1159/000509286. Epub 2020 Aug 18. PMID: 32810857.
78. Owen RG, McCarthy H, Rule S, D'Sa S, Thomas SK, Tournilhac O, et al. Acalabrutinib monotherapy in patients with Waldenström macroglobulinemia: a single-arm, multicentre, phase 2 study. Lancet Haematol. 2020;7(2):e112–21.
79. West C. BeiGene announces results of phase 3 ASPEN trial of zanubrutinib compared to ibrutinib for the treatment of patients with Waldenström's macroglobulinemia BeiGene. 2019. http://ir.beigene.com/news-releases/news-release-details/beigeneannounces-results-phase-3-aspen-trial-zanubrutinib.
80. Castillo JJ, Gustine J, Meid K, Dubeau T, Keezer A, Allan JN, et al. Multicenter prospective phase II study of venetoclax in patients with previously treated Waldenstrom macroglobulinemia. Blood. 2018;132(Suppl 1):132.
81. Castillo JJ, Treon SP. Management of Waldenstrom macroglobulinemia in 2020. Hematology Am Soc Hematol Educ Program. 2020;2020(1):372–9. https://doi.org/10.1182/hematology.2020000121. PMID: 33275726.
82. Xie J, Wan N, Liang Z, Zhang T, Jiang J. Ixazomib—the first oral proteasome inhibitor. Leuk Lymphoma. 2019;60(3):610–8.
83. Castillo JJ, Meid K, Flynn CA, Chen J, Demos MG, Guerrera ML, Kofides A, Liu X, Munshi M, Tsakmaklis N, Patterson CJ, Yang G, Hunter Z, Treon SP. Ixazomib, dexamethasone, and rituximab in treatment-naive patients with Waldenstrom macroglobulinemia: long-term follow-up. Blood Adv. 2020;4(16):3952–9. https://doi.org/10.1182/bloodadvances.2020001963. PMID: 32822482.
84. Pene F, Claessens YE, Muller O, Viguié F, Mayeux P, Dreyfus F, et al. Role of the phosphatidylinositol 3-kinase/Akt and mTOR/ P70S6-kinase pathways in the proliferation and apoptosis in multiple myeloma. Oncogene. 2002;21(43):6587–97.
85. Yang G, Zhou Y, Liu X, Xu L, Cao Y, Manning RJ, et al. A mutation in MYD88 (L265P) supports the survival of lymphoplasmacytic cells by activation of Bruton tyrosine kinase in Waldenström macroglobulinemia. Blood. 2013;122(7):1222–32.
86. NIH. Study to assess the efficacy and safety of umbralisib in patients with non-follicular indolent non-Hodgkin's lymphoma. https://clinicaltrials.gov/ct2/show/study/NCT03364231.
87. Flinn IW, O'Brien S, Kahl B, Patel M, Oki Y, Foss FF, et al. Duvelisib, a novel oral dual inhibitor of PI3K-δ,γ, is clinically active in advanced hematologic malignancies. Blood. 2018;131(8):877–87.
88. Roccaro AM, Sacco A, Jimenez C, et al. C1013G/CXCR4 acts as a driver mutation of tumor progression and modulator of drug resistance in lymphoplasmacytic lymphoma. Blood. 2014;123(26):4120–31.

89. Castillo JJ, Treon SP. What is new in the treatment of Waldenstrom macroglobulinemia? Leukemia. 2019;33(11):2555–62. https://doi.org/10.1038/s41375-019-0592-8. Epub 2019 Oct 7. PMID: 31591468.
90. Treon SP, Meid K, Hunter ZR, Flynn CA, Sarosiek SR, Leventoff CR, White TP, Cao Y, Roccaro AM, Sacco A, Demos MG, Guerrera ML, Kofides A, Liu X, Xu L, Patterson CJ, Munshi M, Tsakmaklis N, Yang G, Ghobrial IM, Branagan AR, Castillo JJ. Phase I study of ibrutinib and the CXCR4 antagonist ulocuplumab in CXCR4 mutated Waldenstrom macroglobulinemia. Blood. 2021;138(17):1535–9. https://doi.org/10.1182/blood.2021012953. Online ahead of print. PMID: 34289017.
91. DiPersio JF, Stadtmauer EA, Nademanee A, Micallef IN, Stiff PJ, Kaufman JL, et al.; 3102 Investigators. Plerixafor and G-CSF versus placebo and G-CSF to mobilize hematopoietic stem cells for autologous stem cell transplantation in patients with multiple myeloma. Blood. 2009;113(23):5720–5726.
92. Treon SP, Meid K, Tripsas C, et al. Prospective, multicenter clinical trial of everolimus as primary therapy in Waldenstrom macroglobulinemia (WMCTG 09-214). Clin Cancer Res. 2017;23(10):2400–4.
93. Chen C, Siegel D, Gutierrez M, Jacoby M, Hofmeister CC, Gabrail N, Baz R, Mau-Sorensen M, Berdeja JG, Savona M, Savoie L, Trudel S, Areethamsirikul N, Unger TJ, Rashal T, Hanke T, Kauffman M, Shacham S, Reece D. Safety and efficacy of selinexor in relapsed or refractory multiple myeloma and Waldenstrom macroglobulinemia. Blood. 2018;131(8):855–63. https://doi.org/10.1182/blood-2017-08-797886. Epub 2017 Dec 4. PMID: 29203585.
94. Castillo JJ, Advani RH, Branagan AR, Buske C, Dimopoulos MA, D'Sa S, Kersten MJ, Leblond V, Minnema MC, Owen RG, Palomba ML, Talaulikar D, Tedeschi A, Trotman J, Varettoni M, Vos JM, Treon SP, Kastritis E. Consensus treatment recommendations from the tenth international workshop for Waldenstrom macroglobulinaemia. Lancet Haematol. 2020;7(11):e827–37. https://doi.org/10.1016/S2352-3026(20)30224-6. PMID: 33091356.

Chapter 23
Non-pharmacological Management of Paraproteinemia

Hadi Goubran, Mark Bosch, and Thierry Burnouf

Abbreviations

AIDP	Acute inflammatory demyelinating polyneuropathy
AKI	Acute kidney injury
CDPN	Chronic immune peripheral neuropathies
CIDP	Chronic inflammatory demyelinating polyneuropathy
DAAs	Direct antiviral agents
DFPP	Double filtration plasmapheresis
FLC	Free light chain
GBS	Guillain Barré syndrome
HCV	Hepatitis C virus
HEV	Hepatitis E virus
HVS	Hyperviscosity syndrome
MC	Mixed cryoglobulinemia
MGRS	Monoclonal gammopathy of renal significance
MGUS	Monoclonal gammopathy of undetermined significance
MM	Multiple myeloma
MV	Measles virus
OCT-A	Optical coherence tomography angiography

H. Goubran (✉) · M. Bosch
Saskatoon Cancer Centre and College of Medicine, University of Saskatchewan, Saskatoon, SK, Canada
e-mail: hadi.goubranmessiha@saskcancer.ca; Mark.bosch@saskcancer.ca

T. Burnouf
Graduate Institute of Biomedical Materials and Tissue Engineering, College of Biomedical Engineering, Taipei Medical University, Taipei, Taiwan

International Ph.D. Program in Biomedical Engineering, College of Biomedical Engineering, Taipei Medical University, Taipei, Taiwan

© The Author(s), under exclusive license to Springer Nature Switzerland AG 2022

G. Ragab et al. (eds.), *Paraproteinemia and Related Disorders*,
https://doi.org/10.1007/978-3-031-10131-1_23

OS	Overall survival
POEMS	Polyneuropathy, organomegaly, endocrinopathy, M protein, and skin changes syndrome
PPN	Paraprotein neuropathies
sFLC	Serum free light chain
SLAM	Signaling lymphocytic activation molecule
SP	Solitary plasmacytoma
TPE	Therapeutic plasma exchange
WM	Waldenström's macroglobulinemia

Introduction

Paraproteinemia results from an immunoproliferative hematological disorder characterized by producing excessive amounts of a single monoclonal gamma globulin in the blood.

The main therapeutic goal in paraproteinemia is to target the cell clones responsible for producing these abnormal pathological proteins, known as paraproteins. Until a reduced production is achieved, paraproteins can cause irreversible damage to various body tissues and organs. Non-pharmacological means to eliminate paraproteins are routinely employed in the initial treatment phases or combined with clone-specific therapies to induce or maintain the therapeutic response.

Whenever paraproteinemia presents with severe or life-threatening complications, plasmapheresis has been used successfully as an emergency tool to reduce the paraproteins' level temporarily until clone-specific therapies achieve a reduction of synthesis. It has also been used as long-term adjuvant therapy in cases of slowly proliferating conditions.

Paraprotein-related complications that plasmapheresis can address include hyperviscosity syndrome (HVS), hypervolemia, hemorrhagic diathesis, cryoglobulinemic manifestations, and end-organ affections with rapidly deteriorating kidney functions, neurological symptoms, or visual loss [1].

The Hyperviscosity Syndrome and Plasmapheresis

HVS, reported in paraproteinemia, develops most commonly in Waldenström's macroglobulinemia (WM) followed by multiple myeloma (MM). The incidence of symptomatic hyperviscosity in WM is 10–30%, while in IgG MM it is 2–6% [2–5]. HVS leads to significant morbidity and mortality. The variables that affect the development of HVS include the plasma concentration and the molecular size of the specific paraprotein. The threshold for the onset of HVS for IgG is >150 g/L, for polymerized IgG3 >40–50 g/L, for IgA >100–110 g/L; for polymerized IgA >60–70 g/L and is only >30–40 g/L for pentameric IgM. Table 23.1 illustrates the various concentrations of paraproteins capable of causing HVS.

Table 23.1 Paraproteins levels associated with hyperviscosity syndrome (derived from [2])

Paraproteins	Levels inducing HVS
IgG	150 g/L
Polymerized IgG3	>40–50 g/L
IgA	100–110 g/L
Polymerized IgA	60–70 g/L
IgM	30–40 g/L

The pathological complications of HVS are due to increased plasma viscosity and increased erythrocyte aggregation leading to increased whole blood viscosity. Hyperviscosity impairs the microcirculation in various organs; It can also lead to a broad spectrum of neurological disorders and may affect the heart, the kidney, and the skin. The retina is often targeted with HVS leading to sluggish circulation and hemorrhages around the small retinal blood vessels. Early diagnosis and urgent institution of plasmapheresis may abort blindness caused by retinal hemorrhages and/or possible detachment.

Clinically, the syndrome has a neurologic constellation of symptoms: headaches, tinnitus, dizziness, visual changes, renal functional deterioration mounting to failure, and cardiac decompensation from increased plasma volume and viscosity. The impact on hemostasis is variable. Thrombotic complications are frequent, but paradoxically, bleeding complications due to impairment of platelet function can be life-threatening [6].

Since the 1960s, therapeutic plasmapheresis has been widely used as primary or adjunctive therapy in the United States. Several plasmapheresis procedures are tailored to treat various diseases. Therapeutic plasma exchange (TPE) with a centrifugal plasma separator, using replacement fluid, is the most widely used method. Other forms of plasmapheresis rely on the concept of membrane filtration or adsorption and include membrane plasma separation, membrane fractionation, microfiltration apheresis, cryofiltration, immunoadsorption, and chemical affinity column pheresis [5]. Unlike in the cases of thrombotic thrombocytopenic purpura where the replacement is usually by fresh frozen plasma (FFP) or cryosupernatant, the most commonly used replacement fluid is either 4–5% human albumin in physiologic saline or rarely FFP, which is used in patients with coagulation abnormalities.

Since most TPEs performed for paraprotein-related disorders use albumin, the risk of blood-borne virus transmission is minimal. Albumin is pasteurized (heat-treated at 60 °C for 10 h) and has never been associated with the transmission of blood-borne viruses. On the other hand, when FFP is used, there exists a small potential for virus transmission. Despite the use of pathogen-reduced plasma, some studies have identified TPE as a risk factor for post-transplantation infection by hepatitis E viral (HEV), a non-enveloped resistant virus, and transaminase elevation [7]. Therefore, screening for HEV RNA should preferably be carried out on plasma used to treat immunocompromised patients [8]. Fortunately, paraprotein-specific complications of therapeutic plasmapheresis are rare outside of central line complications. As an ancillary treatment, therapeutic plasmapheresis has expanded the therapeutic tools in managing paraproteinemia and has not been shown to influence the underlying malignant process [1].

Plasmapheresis is an effective tool for inducing immediate symptomatic relief, and it is often continued until acute symptoms abate. In hepatitis C virus (HCV)-related mixed cryoglobulinemia (MC), plasmapheresis is indicated in rapidly evolving life-threatening disease in combination with steroids, rituximab or cyclophosphamide [9]. In non-infectious MC, on the other hand, plasmapheresis represents the second-line option for severe disease manifestations, in particular for acute motor neuropathy, acute renal failure, or alveolar hemorrhage [10]. In WM patients with HVS and IgM > 40 g/L, preemptive plasmapheresis may be required to prevent an IgM flare from potentially occurring with the initial use of rituximab [6, 11]. Certain IgG/A monoclonal gammopathy of undetermined significance (MGUS)-associated neuropathy patients may benefit from plasmapheresis. When cast nephropathy is suspected or confirmed by biopsy, plasmapheresis is recommended as early as possible when the serum free light chain (sFLC) is ≥500 mg/L. Theoretically, without efficient tumor killing, extracorporeal removal alone could not reduce sFLC due to high production tumor mass and rapid rebound and redistribution between compartments [6].

Cryoglobulinemia

Cryoglobulinemia is defined by the presence of immunoglobulins that precipitate in the serum when the temperature is <37 °C, and redissolve after rewarming. The presence of both polyclonal IgG and monoclonal IgM (type II) or polyclonal IgG and polyclonal IgM (type III) identifies the MC. The identification of an HCV infection in most cases represents a cornerstone in understanding the pathogenesis of this condition.

The clinical spectrum presentations of MC are heterogeneous, ranging from arthralgias, mild palpable purpura, and fatigue to severe vasculitic features with necrotic skin patterns. Peripheral neuropathy and, less commonly, lungs, central nervous system, gastrointestinal tract, and heart involvement are also frequently reported [12]. On the other hand, kidney involvement represents the most common target-organ affection, and glomerulonephritis is crucial when considering prognosis [13].

HCV infection affects about 170 million people worldwide. For years, TPE combined with steroids and/or rituximab was the cornerstone therapy in advanced MC with multiorgan involvement. At the same time, the triggering HCV used to be controlled with the classic combination of interferon and ribavirin. After the introduction of the new direct antiviral agents (DAAs), the medical community abandoned the combination of pegylated interferon and ribavirin. DAAs therapy is now used as a first-line approach. In patients with severe vasculitis, DAAs therapy and second-line treatment with rituximab with or without apheresis represent the standard of care [14, 15].

Four MC cases showing severe and progressive clinical manifestations, including skin purpura, nephrotic syndrome, acute kidney injury, and peripheral neuropathy, have been subjected to cryofiltration, a dedicated apheresis procedure for removal of cryoprecipitates, in conjunction with conventional pharmacological therapies resulting in a significant reduction in cryoglobulins [16]. In addition to the symptomatic improvement, monitoring the cryocrit throughout TPE sessions can guide the response to treatment and determine the ideal length of therapy [17].

Cryocrystalglobulinemia, on the other hand, is a rare variant of cryoglobulinemia in which monoclonal immunoglobulins self-assemble into crystalline arrays. DeLyria et al. (2016) [18] described a case of a 53-year-old man who presented with systemic thrombotic microangiopathy causing multiorgan failure with missing features of the typical leukocytoclastic vasculitis, affecting most of his organs; the kidneys, lungs, and gastrointestinal tract as well as causing skin necrosis and mental status changes. Tissue biopsy specimens showed intravascular thrombi, along with renal spindled crystalline deposits. Crystals precipitated in the cryoglobulin assay, and immunofixation showed them to be composed of monoclonal immunoglobulin G κ light chains. The ultrastructural analysis demonstrated the deposits to have an array-like substructure. The patient was successfully treated with a combination of plasmapheresis, steroids, and bortezomib but experienced a relapse and died 12 months after his initial diagnosis. This entity is now classified as monoclonal gammopathy of renal significance (MGRS) (covered in Chap. 13) [18].

Multiple Myeloma

Since the late 1960s, plasmapheresis has been used to address complications of MM [19].

In MM patients, TPE in combination with chemotherapy, or novel agents like bortezomib, could significantly remove both the paraproteins and the free light chains (FLC) that lead to acute kidney injury (AKI). Urgent application of TPE has improved both renal recovery and patient survival. In a trial of 29 patients, a higher number of plasma exchange sessions significantly reduced FLCs compared to bortezomib. Still, the non-pharmacological procedure must be combined with other clonal-directed chemotherapeutic agents to prolong renal recovery and patient survival [20].

In 2021, Merz et al. reported an excellent clinical response to plasmapheresis in a young, undiagnosed MM patient presenting with bilateral HVS-related retinopathy. As fundoscopy leads to the diagnosis of HVS, the authors considered it advisable to screen all patients with MM and perform plasmapheresis as soon as possible to save their sight [21].

The immunoglobulin (Ig) D type is a rare variant of MM as it accounts for only 1–2% of all cases. The diagnosis is difficult to carry as IgD assay is not part of the routine initial workup for myeloma patients. Patients presenting with IgD MM have more severe symptoms at presentation with a poorer prognosis when compared to the other types. Ueda et al. demonstrated in 2020 the benefits of a bortezomib-based regimen in combination with TPE for IgD MM with acute kidney disease [22].

Kanda et al. reported renal Improvement with Molecular-Selective Plasma Exchange in a patient with Bence-Jones Type MM [23]. Others have advocated for double-filtration plasmapheresis to treat acute renal failure in MM patients [24].

Patients may present with a solitary plasmacytoma (SP) on rare occasions. SP may be a solitary bone lesion or may represent an extramedullary SP. Patients with SP should be primarily treated with radiotherapy with or without surgery. The choice of therapy and its dose is often dependent on the location of the lesion and its accessibility. Although local control rates are high after radiotherapy, progression to MM frequently occurs [25]. (MM is discussed in detail in Chap. 11).

Oncolytic virotherapy uses the natural ability of viruses to infect and kill cells to eliminate cancer cells. Adenovirus serotype 5 (Ad5) has been approved for use in humans as a therapy for solid cancers. Ad5 and low-seroprevalence adenoviruses were evaluated as oncolytics for MM as they infect and replicate in myeloma cell lines and mediate oncolytic cell killing [26].

The growth-inhibitory activity of recombinant CD40 ligand (CD40L) is also well documented in MM. It acts in concert with viral oncolysis to produce MM growth inhibition through activation of cellular apoptosis [27].

These findings drew the attention of researchers to consider vaccine strains of measles virus (MV) as agents with an impressive range of oncolytic activity in preclinical and early clinical trials with safety and efficacy evidence. Overexpression of the MV receptor CD46 in many tumor cells may direct the virus to preferentially enter transformed cells. There is increasing awareness of their importance in mediating nectin-4 and signaling lymphocytic activation molecule (SLAM) oncolysis. Attenuated Edmonston lineage measles virus (MV-Edm) vaccine strains can preferentially infect and lyse many cancer cells, including myeloma [28]. Furthermore, successful attempts to retarget MV by inserting tumor-specific antigen genes and engineering the virus to express synthetic microRNA targeting sequences may represent an exciting means of increasing viral specificity and enhancing the oncolytic effect [29].

Therefore, oncolytic virotherapy can function as an antigen agnostic vaccine, increasing cytotoxic T-lymphocyte responses against tumor-associated antigens in patients with MM [30].

Several different myeloma gene therapy approaches, including cell-based ones, are also currently being explored and will likely influence MM therapy in various ways [31, 32].

Another non-pharmacological approach involves the gut microbiome. It is being investigated by a clinical trial at the Mayo Clinic in patients with lymphoma or MM as it may alter the outcome of patients undergoing stem cell transplantation [33]. Other trials investigate the impact of implicating patients in clinical trials on their quality of life and performance [34].

Waldenström's Macroglobulinemia

The most common cause of HVS is WM [35], as 10–30% of patients exhibit an HVS. As the large pentameric IgM accumulates in the circulation, viscosity builds up until a full-blown picture of symptomatic hyperviscosity, a well-established phenomenon of WM, develops. The predictors of symptomatic HVS and outcomes related to this complication remain slightly unclear. Still, a study in 2018 proposed that IgM >60 g/L be considered a new criterion for initiating therapy in otherwise asymptomatic (smouldering) WM to pre-empt hyperviscosity-related injury [36]. In their study on 997 WM patients evaluated for 11 years, Abeykoon et al. reported that symptomatic HVS was observed in 13% of them. Overall survival (OS) of these patients was similar to patients without symptomatic hyperviscosity. On multivariate analysis, only viscosity >1.8 cp assessed at the initial diagnosis was an independent predictor for the development of subsequent symptomatic HVS [36]. In another study, a serum IgM level >60 g/L at diagnosis was associated with a median time to symptomatic hyperviscosity of 3 months. In contrast, the median time for patients with serum IgM levels of 50–60 g/L was approximately 3 years. Adjusting for other clinical factors, the odds of developing symptomatic HVS were 370-fold higher with serum IgM levels >60 g/L. Once more, symptomatic hyperviscosity did not influence OS [11]. The previous findings support the use of serum IgM level >60 g/L as a criterion for initiation of therapy in otherwise asymptomatic patients with smouldering WM. Therefore, it seems reasonable that in the absence of other symptoms or signs, high serum IgM can be safely observed without the initiation of WM-directed therapy as per the consensus recommendations.

Retinal affection, on the other hand, represents a challenge. IgM's long-term toxicity to the retinal pigment epithelium may impede the resolution of the persistent serous macular detachment, resulting in an inability to recover the vision. This may represent an urgent indication for intervention to reduce paraproteins [37]. After plasmapheresis, TPE improved optical coherence tomography angiography (OCT-A) with an objective decrease in retinal capillary and large vessel density. This technique has the potential to guide treatment and surveillance for patients with hyperviscosity-related retinopathy [38]. Prophylactic plasmapheresis should be considered in patients at risk for HVS after rituximab therapy to avoid an IgM flare [6, 39]. Due to the concern of IgM flare, some centers prefer to have the IgM <40 g/L before proceeding with anti-CD20 therapies like rituximab.

In their very comprehensive 2019 review, Dimopoulos and Kastritis highlighted that plasmapheresis can reduce the IgM levels significantly after 2–3 sessions, thereby bridging the time required for systemic clone-directed therapy to be effective whenever immediate IgM reduction is needed (such as for HVS, symptomatic cryoglobulinemia, severe hemolysis from cold agglutinin disease.) [40]. It was also pointed out that blood warmers should be considered during apheresis if cryoglobulins are present [41].

However, the question remains on the optimal modality of application of apheresis. TPE and double filtration plasmapheresis (DFPP) are effective treatment options for HVS caused by WM. Nonetheless, few data are available for the relationship between the prescribed regimen of apheresis and the reduction rate of target IgM, especially in the modalities using membrane separation. Studies have demonstrated that DFPP is superior to TPE [42]. (The treatment of WM is covered in Chap. 14.)

Paraproteinemia Associated with Neurological Disorders

Chronic inflammatory demyelinating polyneuropathy (CIDP) is a rare neurological disorder of nerve roots and peripheral nerves that destroys the myelin sheath of the nerve fibers. It represents a chronic form of acute inflammatory demyelinating polyneuropathy (AIDP), the most common form of Guillain Barré syndrome (GBS). TPE has been proposed as a treatment option for chronic immune peripheral neuropathies (CDPN). However, guidelines and protocols are limited, and only few studies have been published. A subset of CIDP, anti-MAG peripheral neuropathy, accounting for 5% of CIDP-like disorders, can be treated successfully with TPE [35]. Anti-MAG occurs when the body's immune system develops antibodies against a critical glycoprotein (myelin-associated glycoprotein, or MAG). MAG is required to maintain a healthy peripheral nervous system. In the absence of evident paraproteinemia, however, the use of intravenous gamma globulins seems to be more appropriate as patients who underwent TPE experienced prolonged hospitalization with a poorer outcome and a more significant hospitalization [43].

A 10-year retrospective study assessed the effectiveness and tolerance of TPE in CDPN. Among the 206 patients who received TPE during the study period, 30 (14.6%) met the diagnostic criteria of CDPN. Four of the five paraprotein neuropathies (PPN) patients (80%) and 8 of the 11 chronic inflammatory demyelinating polyneuropathies (CIDP) patients (72.7%) responded to TPE. Six of the nine anti-MAG neuropathy patients (66.7%) responded to treatment [44]. TPE appears to be effective in CIDP and PPN and ineffective in Lewis-Sumner and the polyneuropathy, organomegaly, endocrinopathy, M protein, skin changes syndrome; and (Crow-Fukase) (POEMS) syndromes [44] (Chap. 21).

Conclusions

Clone-directed therapies are the most logical therapeutic options for the long-term management of paraproteinemia. Paraproteins, however, can have very detrimental effects on various body tissues and organs, inflicting rapid irreversible damage. In this setting, plasmapheresis is a cornerstone life-saving tool in symptomatic patients with hyperviscosity syndrome by eliminating paraproteins quickly.

Other promising modalities including oncolytic virotherapy and gene therapy are currently under investigation. If they prove to be successful, they will add to the medical armamentarium in this battlefield.

References

1. Euler HH, Schmitz N, Löffler H. Plasmapheresis in paraproteinemia. Blut. 1985;50(6):321–30. https://doi.org/10.1007/BF00320925. PMID: 3890984.
2. Garcia-Sanz R, Montoto S, Torrequebrada A, de Coca AG, Petit J, Sureda A, et al. Waldenstrom macroglobulinemia: presenting features and outcome in a series with 217 cases. Br J Haematol. 2001;115:575–82. https://doi.org/10.1046/j.1365-2141.2001.03144.x.
3. Kyrtsonis MC, Vassilakopoulos TP, Angelopoulou MK, Siakantaris P, Kontopidou FN, Dimopoulou MN, et al. Waldenstrom's macroglobulinemia: clinical course and prognostic factors in 60 patients. Experience from a single hematology unit. Ann Hematol. 2001;80:722–7. https://doi.org/10.1007/s00277-001-0385-8.
4. Riccardi A, Gobbi PG, Ucci G, Bertoloni D, Luoni R, Rutigliano L, et al. Changing clinical presentation of multiple myeloma. Eur J Cancer. 1991;27:1401–5. https://doi.org/10.1016/0277-5379(91)90020-E.
5. Siami GA, Siami FS. Plasmapheresis and paraproteinemia: cryoprotein-induced diseases, monoclonal gammopathy, Waldenström's macroglobulinemia, hyperviscosity syndrome, multiple myeloma, light chain disease, and amyloidosis. Ther Apher. 1999;3(1):8–19. https://doi.org/10.1046/j.1526-0968.1999.00146.x.
6. Kalayoglu-Besisik S. The use of emergency apheresis in managing plasma cell disorders. Transfus Apher Sci. 2018;57(1):35–9. https://doi.org/10.1016/j.transci.2018.02.014. Epub 2018 Feb 20. PMID: 29477943.
7. https://www.who.int/news-room/fact-sheets/detail/hepatitis-e
8. Mallet V, Sberro-Soussan R, Roque-Afonso AM, Vallet-Pichard A, Deau B, Portal A, Chaix ML, Hauser L, Beylouné A, Mercadier A, Izopet J, Legendre C, Pol S. Transmission of hepatitis E virus with plasma exchange in kidney transplant recipients: a retrospective cohort study. Transplantation. 2018;102(8):1351–7. https://doi.org/10.1097/TP.0000000000002185. PMID: 29561324.
9. Marson P, Monti G, Montani F, Riva A, Mascia MT, Castelnovo L, Filippini D, Capuzzo E, Moretto M, D'Alessandri G, Marenchino D, Zani R, Fraticelli P, Ferri C, Quartuccio L, De Silvestro G, Oreni L, Accorsi P, Galli M. Apheresis treatment of cryoglobulinemic vasculitis: a multicentre cohort study of 159 patients. Transfus Apher Sci. 2018;57(5):639–45. https://doi.org/10.1016/j.transci.2018.06.005. Epub 2018 Jun 26. PMID: 30228046.
10. Quartuccio L, Bond M, Isola M, Monti S, Felicetti M, Furini F, Murgia S, Berti A, Silvestri E, Pazzola G, Bozzolo E, Leccese P, Raffeiner B, Parisi S, Leccese I, Cianci F, Bettio S, Sainaghi P, Ianniello A, Ravagnani V, Bellando Randone S, Faggioli P, Lomater C, Stobbione P, Ferro F, Colaci M, Alfieri G, Carubbi F, Erre GL, Giollo A, Franzolini N, Ditto MC, Balduzzi S, Padoan R, Bortolotti R, Bortoluzzi A, Cariddi A, Padula A, Di Scala G, Gremese E, Conti F, D'Angelo S, Matucci Cerinic M, Dagna L, Emmi G, Salvarani C, Paolazzi G, Roccatello D, Govoni M, Schiavon F, Caporali R, De Vita S. Italian Study Group on Lung Involvement in Rheumatic Diseases and the Italian Vasculitis Study Group. Alveolar haemorrhage in ANCA-associated vasculitis: long-term outcome and mortality predictors. J Autoimmun. 2020;108:102397. https://doi.org/10.1016/j.jaut.2019.102397. Epub 2020 Jan 9. PMID: 31926833.
11. Gustine JN, Meid K, Dubeau T, Hunter ZR, Xu L, Yang G, Ghobrial IM, Treon SP, Castillo JJ. Serum IgM level as predictor of symptomatic hyperviscosity in patients with Waldenström macroglobulinaemia. Br J Haematol. 2017;177(5):717–25. https://doi.org/10.1111/bjh.14743. Epub 2017 May 9. PMID: 28485115.
12. Treppo E, Quartuccio L, Ragab G, Vita DE, S. Rheumatologic manifestations of hepatitis C virus. Minerva Med. 2021;112(2):201–14. https://doi.org/10.23736/S0026-4806.20.07158-X. Epub 2020 Dec 2. PMID: 33263372.
13. Rossi D, Sciascia S, Fenoglio R, Ferro M, Baldovino S, Kamgaing J, Ventrella F, Kalikatzaros I, Viziello L, Soffietti L, Barreca A, Roccatello D. Cryoglobulinemic glomerulonephritis: clinical presentation and histological features, diagnostic pitfalls and controversies in the management. State of the art and the experience on a large monocentric cohort treated with B cell depletion therapy. Minerva Med. 2021;112(2):162–74. https://doi.org/10.23736/S0026-4806.20.07076-7.

14. Muro K, Toda N, Yamamoto S, Yanagita M. The successful treatment of a case of HCV-associated cryoglobulinemic glomerulonephritis with rituximab, direct-acting antiviral agents, plasmapheresis and long-term steroid despite serologically persistent cryoglobulinemia. Intern Med. 2021;60(4):583–9. https://doi.org/10.2169/internalmedicine.5461-20. PMID: 32999232.
15. Galli M, Monti G, Marson P, Scaini P, Pietrogrande M, Candela M, Castelnovo L, Faggioli P, Novati P, Zani R, Mascia MT, Saccardo F, Mazzaro C, Sarzi-Puttini P, Sebastiani M, Quartuccio L, De Vita S. Recommendations for managing the manifestations of severe and life-threatening mixed cryoglobulinemia syndrome. Autoimmun Rev. 2019;18(8):778–85. https://doi.org/10.1016/j.autrev.2019.06.008. Epub 2019 Jun 8. PMID: 31181326.
16. Taniyama Y, Nakatani Y, Matsuoka T, Takahashi M, Shimizu K, Yamamoto S, Inoue Y, Ohnishi S, Kobayashi N, Nakano Y, Takami M, Arima S. Efficacy of cryofiltration for treatment of mixed cryoglobulinemia: a report of four cases. Ther Apher Dial. 2017;21(3):238–42. https://doi.org/10.1111/1744-9987.12556. PMID: 28661098.
17. Olson N, Yarrabothula S, Dunbar N. Successful use of cryocrit for monitoring response to therapeutic plasma exchange in type 1 cryoglobulinemia. J Clin Apher. 2016;31(4):403–4. https://doi.org/10.1002/jca.21414. Epub 2015 Jul 21. PMID: 26194475.
18. DeLyria PA, Avedschmidt SE, Yamada C, Farkash EA. Fatal cryocrystalglobulinemia with intravascular and renal tubular crystalline deposits. Am J Kidney Dis. 2016;67(5):787–91. https://doi.org/10.1053/j.ajkd.2015.11.014. Epub 2016 Jan 14. PMID: 26775022.
19. Tan BL, Cleton FJ, van Beusekom GT, Veltkamp JJ, van Rood JJ. Plasmapheresis treatment of haemorrhagic complications in a patient with multiple myeloma. Folia Med Neerl. 1967;10(6):174–9. PMID: 5590976.
20. Premuzic V, Batinic J, Roncevic P, Basic-Jukic N, Nemet D, Jelakovic B. Role of plasmapheresis in the management of acute kidney injury in patients with multiple myeloma: should we abandon it? Ther Apher Dial. 2018;22(1):79–86. https://doi.org/10.1111/1744-9987.12606. Epub 2017 Dec 14. PMID: 29239143.
21. Merz T, Marchesoni I, Caminiti G, Romanelli F. Efficacy of plasmapheresis as treatment for bilateral hyperviscosity syndrome related retinopathy in multiple myeloma. Eur J Ophthalmol. 2022;32(4):NP48–51. https://doi.org/10.1177/1120672121997069. PMID: 33601903.
22. Ueda H, Kuno H, Takahashi D, Katsuma A, Kimura A, Nakashima A, Kato J, Momoki M, Ohba R, Dobashi N, Yamamoto I, Kawamura T, Miyazaki Y, Yokoo T. Plasma exchange combined with bortezomib-based chemotherapy is effective for early renal recovery in a patient with IgD-λ type multiple myeloma. CEN Case Rep. 2020;9(2):165–72. https://doi.org/10.1007/s13730-020-00448-y.
23. Kanda M, Sanada S, Kowata H, Mizuno S, Yamakage S, Sato M, Sato T, Taguma Y. Renal improvement with molecular-selective plasma exchange in a patient with Bence-Jones type multiple myeloma. Ther Apher Dial. 2016;20(4):420–2. https://doi.org/10.1111/1744-9987.12472.
24. Jiang X, Feng J, Ye Y. Double-filtration plasmapheresis for treatment of acute renal failure in a multiple myeloma patient. Ther Apher Dial. 2014;18(3):318–9. https://doi.org/10.1111/1744-9987.12187. Epub 2014 May 12. PMID: 24820823.
25. König L, Herfarth K. [Benefits of radiotherapy for patients with solitary plasmacytoma or multiple myeloma]. Radiologe. 2022;62(1):30–34. https://doi.org/10.1007/s00117-021-00935-y. Epub 2021 Nov 11. PMID: 34762165.
26. Senac JS, Doronin K, Russell SJ, Jelinek DF, Greipp PR, Barry MA. Infection and killing of multiple myeloma by adenoviruses. Hum Gene Ther. 2010;21(2):179–90. https://doi.org/10.1089/hum.2009.082. PMID: 19788385.
27. Fernandes MS, Gomes EM, Butcher LD, Hernandez-Alcoceba R, Chang D, Kansopon J, Newman J, Stone MJ, Tong AW. Growth inhibition of human multiple myeloma cells by an oncolytic adenovirus carrying the CD40 ligand transgene. Clin Cancer Res. 2009;15(15):4847–56. https://doi.org/10.1158/1078-0432.CCR-09-0451. Epub 2009 Jul 21. PMID: 19622582.
28. Msaouel P, Opyrchal M, Dispenzieri A, Peng KW, Federspiel MJ, Russell SJ, Galanis E. Clinical trials with oncolytic measles virus: current status and future prospects. Curr Cancer Drug Targets. 2018;18(2):177–87. https://doi.org/10.2174/1568009617666170222125035. PMID: 28228086.

29. Aref S, Bailey K, Fielding A. Measles to the rescue: a review of oncolytic measles virus. Viruses. 2016;8(10):294. https://doi.org/10.3390/v8100294. PMID: 27782084.
30. Packiriswamy N, Upreti D, Zhou Y, Khan R, Miller A, Diaz RM, Rooney CM, Dispenzieri A, Peng KW, Russell SJ. Oncolytic measles virus therapy enhances tumor antigen-specific T-cell responses in patients with multiple myeloma. Leukemia. 2020;34(12):3310–22. https://doi.org/10.1038/s41375-020-0828-7. Epub 2020 Apr 23. PMID: 32327728.
31. Adachi Y, Yoshio-Hoshino N, Nishimoto N. Gene therapy for multiple myeloma. Curr Gene Ther. 2008;8(4):247–55. https://doi.org/10.2174/156652308785160683. PMID: 18691020.
32. Voelker R. Cell-based gene therapy is new option for multiple myeloma. JAMA. 2021;325(17):1713. https://doi.org/10.1001/jama.2021.6401. PMID: 33944887.
33. https://www.mayo.edu/research/clinical-trials/cls-20347031
34. https://www.mayo.edu/research/clinical-trials/cls-20341681
35. Perez Rogers A, Estes M. Hyperviscosity syndrome. In: StatPearls [Internet]. Treasure Island: StatPearls Publishing; 2022. PMID: 30085505.
36. Abeykoon JP, Zanwar S, Ansell SM, Winters J, Gertz MA, King RL, Murray D, Habermann T, Dingli D, Muchtar E, Go RS, Leung N, Inwards DJ, Buadi FK, Dispenzieri A, Lacy MQ, Lin Y, Gonsalves WI, Kourelis T, Witzig TE, Thompson C, Vincent Rajkumar S, Kyle RA, Kumar S, Kapoor P. Predictors of symptomatic hyperviscosity in Waldenstrom macroglobulinemia. Am J Hematol. 2018;93(11):1384–93. https://doi.org/10.1002/ajh.25254. Epub 2018 Oct 2. PMID: 30121949.
37. Lai CC, Chang CH. Hyperviscosity-related retinopathy and serous macular detachment in Waldenstrom's macroglobulinemia: a mortal case in 5 years. Eur J Ophthalmol. 2022;32(4):NP109–14. https://doi.org/10.1177/1120672121 1002066. Online ahead of print. PMID: 33719618.
38. Schatz MJ, Wilkins CS, Otero-Marquez O, Chui TYP, Rosen RB, Gupta M. Multimodal imaging of Waldenstrom macroglobulinemia-associated hyperviscosity-related retinopathy treated with plasmapheresis. Case Rep Ophthalmol Med. 2021;2021:6816195. https://doi.org/10.1155/2021/6816195. eCollection 2021. PMID: 34956683.
39. Stone MJ, Bogen SA. Role of plasmapheresis in Waldenstrom's macroglobulinemia. Clin Lymphoma Myeloma Leuk. 2013;13(2):238–40. https://doi.org/10.1016/j.clml.2013.02.013. Epub 2013 Mar 20. PMID: 23522642.
40. Dimopoulos MA, Kastritis E. How I treat Waldenström macroglobulinemia. Blood. 2019;134(23):2022–35.
41. Stone MJ. Waldenström's macroglobulinemia: hyperviscosity syndrome and cryoglobulinemia. Clin Lymphoma Myeloma. 2009;9(1):97–9.
42. Miyamoto Y, Hamasaki Y, Matsumoto A, Doi K, Noiri E, Nangaku M. Prediction of immunoglobulin M reduction via therapeutic dose of simple plasma exchange and double filtration plasmapheresis using membrane separation in patients with hyperviscosity syndrome caused by Waldenstrom macroglobulinemia. J Clin Apher. 2018;33(5):611–5. https://doi.org/10.1002/jca.21655. Epub 2018 Sep 6. PMID: 30188580.
43. Beydoun HA, Beydoun MA, Hossain S, Zonderman AB, Eid SM. Nationwide study of therapeutic plasma exchange vs intravenous immunoglobulin in Guillain-Barre syndrome. Muscle Nerve. 2020;61(5):608–15. https://doi.org/10.1002/mus.26831. Epub 2020 Feb 22. PMID: 32052454.
44. Codron P, Cousin M, Subra JF, Pautot V, Letournel F, Verny C, Cassereau J. Therapeutic plasma exchange in chronic dysimmune peripheral neuropathies: a 10-year retrospective study. J Clin Apher. 2017;32(6):413–22. https://doi.org/10.1002/jca.21530. Epub 2017 Mar 1. PMID: 28247959.

Correction to: Amyloidosis: Pathogenesis, Types, and Diagnosis

Shereef Elmoamly and Laura Obici

Correction to

Chapter 7 in: G. Ragab et al. (eds.), *Paraproteinemia and Related Disorders*, https://doi.org/10.1007/978-3-031-10131-1_7

The figures and captions in the chapter were published incorrectly. The corrections are provided below:

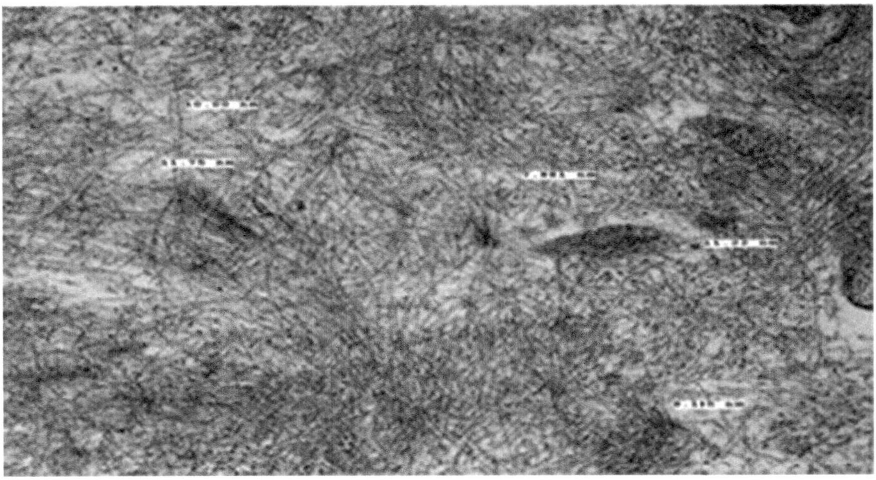

Fig. 7.1 Electron microscopy appearance of amyloid (in renal amyloidosis). Photo courtesy of Dr. B Vydianath, University Hospitals Birmingham NHS Foundation Trust.

The updated original version of the chapter can be found at
https://doi.org/10.1007/978-3-031-10131-1_7

© The Author(s), under exclusive license to Springer Nature Switzerland AG 2022
G. Ragab et al. (eds.), *Paraproteinemia and Related Disorders*,
https://doi.org/10.1007/978-3-031-10131-1_24

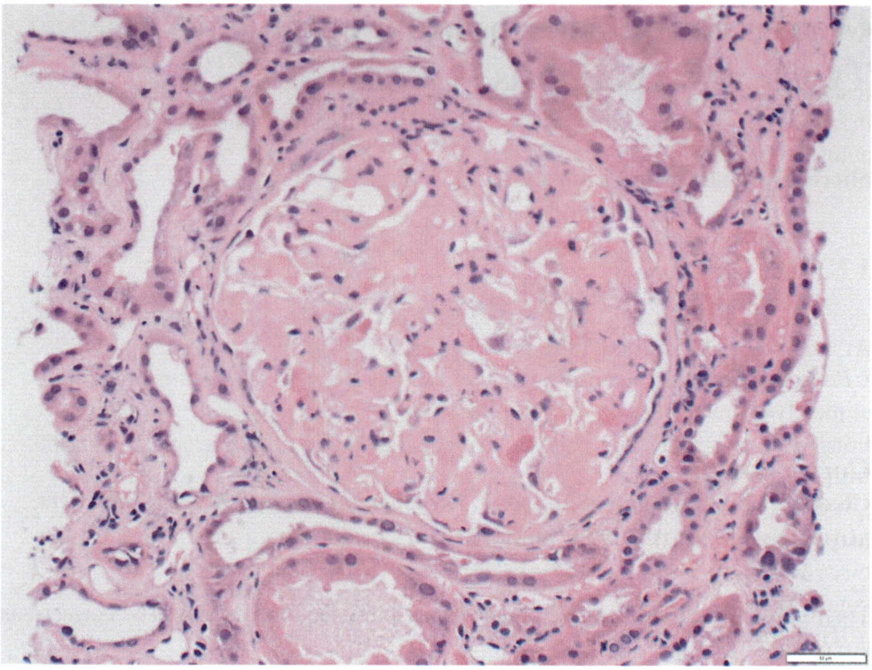

Fig. 7.2 Amyloid deposition in a renal glomerulus as seen on Haematoxylin and Eosin stain. Original magnification x 200, Photo courtesy of Dr. Y Hock, University Hospitals Birmingham NHS Foundation Trust.

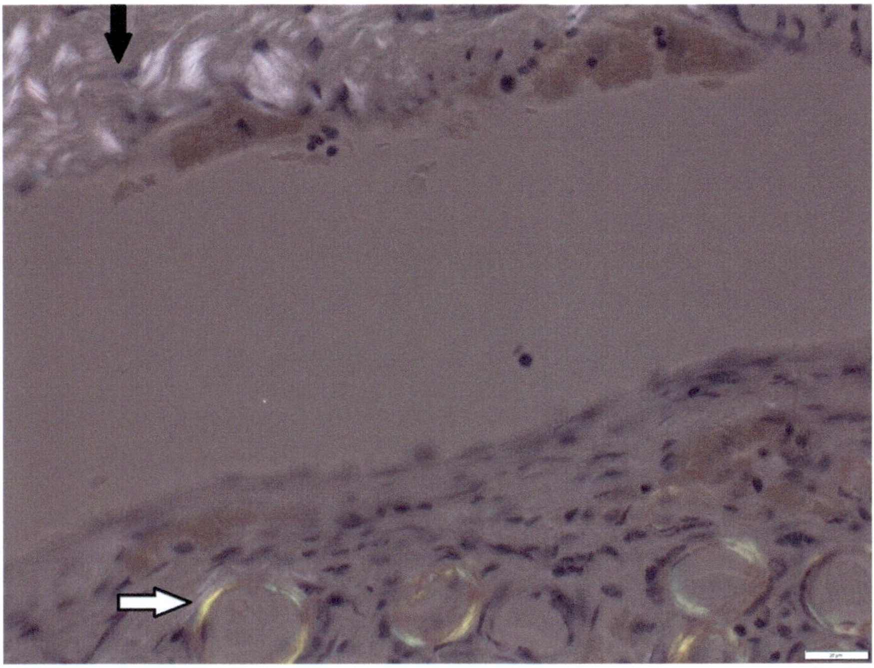

Fig. 7.3 Abundant amyloid deposition in renal blood vessels as seen by Congo red staining (with polarization). Apple green birefringence of amyloid in blood vessels can be seen in the lower part (white arrow) with non-birefringent collagen fibres in the upper part for comparison (black arrow). Original magnification x 200, Photo courtesy of Dr. Y Hock, University Hospitals Birmingham NHS Foundation Trust.

Fig. 7.4 Abundant amyloid deposition in liver as seen on Congo red stain (with polarization demonstrating apple green birefringence). Original magnification x 200, Photo courtesy of Dr. Y Hock, University Hospitals Birmingham NHS Foundation Trust.

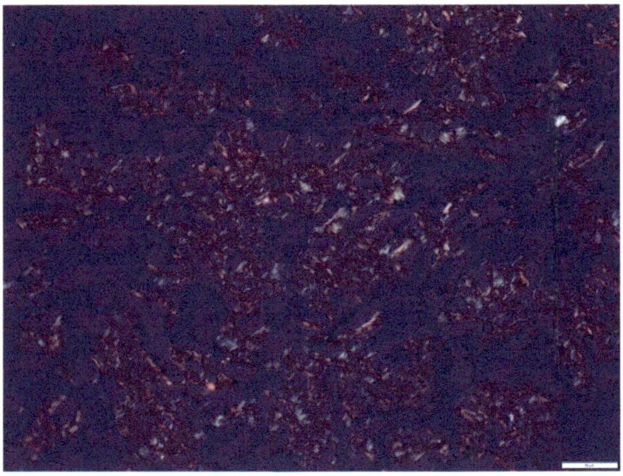

Index

© The Editor(s) (if applicable) and The Author(s), under exclusive license to Springer Nature Switzerland AG 2022
G. Ragab et al. (eds.), *Paraproteinemia and Related Disorders*,
https://doi.org/10.1007/978-3-031-10131-1

GPSR Compliance

The European Union's (EU) General Product Safety Regulation (GPSR) is a set of rules that requires consumer products to be safe and our obligations to ensure this.

If you have any concerns about our products, you can contact us on ProductSafety@springernature.com

In case Publisher is established outside the EU, the EU authorized representative is:

Springer Nature Customer Service Center GmbH
Europaplatz 3
69115 Heidelberg, Germany

Batch number: 10732076

Printed by Printforce, the Netherlands